Immunoregulation in Health and Disease

Experimental and Clinical Aspects

Immunoregulation in Health and Disease

Experimental and Clinical Aspects

edited by

Miodrag L. Lukić
Immunology Unit, Department of Microbiology
Faculty of Medicine and Health Sciences
UAE University, Al Ain
United Arab Emirates

Miodrag Čolić
Institute for Medical Research
Military Medical Academy, Belgrade
Yugoslavia

Marija Mostarica-Stojković
Institute of Microbiology and Immunology
School of Medicine, University of Belgrade
Yugoslavia

Kosta Čuperlović
Institute for the Application of Nuclear Energy
Zemun, Yugoslavia

ACADEMIC PRESS
San Diego London Boston
New York Sydney Tokyo Toronto

This book is printed on acid-free paper.

Academic Press, Inc.
525 B Street, Suite 1900, San Diego, California 92101-4495, USA
http://www.apnet.com

Academic Press Limited
24–28 Oval Road, London NW1 7DX, UK
http://www.hbuk.co.uk/ap/

ISBN 0-12-459460-3

A catalogue record for this book is available from the British Library

Typeset by Keyset Composition, Colchester, Essex, UK
Printed in Great Britain by Hartnolls Limited, Bodmin, Cornwall

97 98 99 00 01 02 EB 9 8 7 6 5 4 3 2 1

Contents

Contributors

Pavle R. Andjus Institute of Physiology and Biochemistry, School of Biology, University of Belgrade, Belgrade, Yugoslavia

Slobodan Apostolski Institute of Neurology, School of Medicine, University of Belgrade, Belgrade, Yugoslavia

Helen Arrol Department of Rheumatology, The Medical School, University of Birmingham, Edgbaston, Birmingham, UK

Valentina Arsić Institute of Microbiology and Immunology, School of Medicine, University of Belgrade, Yugoslavia

Vladimir Badovinac Institute for Biological Research, University of Belgrade, Belgrade, Yugoslavia

Alexandru Constantin Bancu Department of Immunochemistry, Institute 'Victor Babes', Bucharest, Romania

Tatjana Banović Institute for Medical Research, MMA, Belgrade, Yugoslavia

Nadežda Basara Institute of Haematology, Clinical Centre of Serbia, Belgrade, Yugoslavia

Milovan Bojić Department of Cardiology, 'Dedinje' Cardiovascular Clinic, Belgrade, Yugoslavia

Darinka Bošković Institute of Hematology, Clinical Centre of Serbia, Belgrade, Yugoslavia

Marinela Bostan Department of Immunochemistry, Institute 'Victor Babes', Bucharest, Romania

Srđjan Brkić Department of Cardiology, 'Dedinje' Cardiovascular Clinic, Belgrade, Yugoslavia

Vladimir Bumbaširević Institute of Histology, School of Medicine, University of Belgrade, Belgrade, Yugoslavia

Enrico Cherubini Biophysics Sector, International School for Advanced Studies (SISSA), Trieste, Italy

Maria Chirilă 'Christiana' Medical Association, Bucharest, Romania

Bogoljub Ćirić Immunology Research Centre, 'Branislav Janković', Belgrade, Yugoslavia

Jerry Clarke 16 Belitha Villas, London N1 1PD, UK

Miodrag Čolić Institute for Medical Research, MMA, Belgrade, Yugoslavia

Kosta Čuperlović Institute for the Application of Nuclear Energy (INEP), University of Belgrade, Zemun, Yugoslavia

Margita Čuperlović Institute for the Application of Nuclear Energy (INEP), University of Belgrade, Zemun, Yugoslavia

Angelika Daser Department of Clinical Biochemistry, Rudolph Virchow University Hospital, Berlin, Germany

Ljilijana Dimitrijević Immunology Research Centre, 'Branislav Janković', Belgrade, Yugoslavia

Charles A. Dinarello University of Colorado, Health Sciences Center, Denver, Colorado, USA

Bogdan Djuričić Institute of Biochemistry, School of Medicine, University of Belgrade, Belgrade, Yugoslavia

Predrag Đorđević Diabetes Centre, Institute for Endocrinology, Diabetes and Metabolic Diseases, Clinical Centre of Serbia, Belgrade, Yugoslavia

Nebojša Dovezenski Institute of Medical Research, Belgrade, Yugoslavia

Biljana Drašković-Pavlović Institute for Medical Research, MMA, Belgrade, Yugoslavia
Jelena Drulović Institute of Neurology, Clinical Centre of Serbia, Belgrade, Yugoslavia
Aleksandar Dujić Institute for Medical Research, MMA, Belgrade, Yugoslavia
Aleksandar Džamić Institute of Microbiology and Immunology, School of Medicine, University of Belgrade, Yugoslavia
Lota Ejdus Institute for Biological Research 'Siniša Stanković', University of Belgrade, Yugoslavia
Edita Grego Zvezdara University Medical Centre, Belgrade, Yugoslavia
Assen Gudev Department of Internal Medicine, Faculty of Medicine, Sofia Medical University, Sofia, Bulgaria
Ljiljana Hajduković-Dragojlović Institute for the Application of Nuclear Energy (INEP), University of Belgrade, Zemun, Yugoslavia
Ronald B. Herberman Departments of Medicine and Pathology, University of Pittsburgh School of Medicine and Pittsburgh Cancer Institute, Pittsburgh, USA
Vesna Ilić Institute for Medical Research, MMA, Belgrade, Yugoslavia
Zoran Ivanović Institute of Medical Research, Belgrade, Yugoslavia
Ratko Jankov Faculty of Chemistry, University of Belgrade, Belgrade, Yugoslavia
Roy Jefferis Department of Immunology, The Medical School, University of Birmingham, Edgbaston, Birmingham, UK
Kanchan G. Jhaver Michael Heidelberger Division of Immunology, Department of Pathology and Kaplan Comprehensive Cancer Center, NYU Medical Center, New York, USA
Aleksandra Jotić Diabetes Centre, Institute for Endocrinology, Diabetes and Metabolic Diseases, Clinical Centre of Serbia, Belgrade, Yugoslavia
Lidija Jovanović Institute for Medical Research, Belgrade, Yugoslavia
Vilma Jovičić Institute for Microbiology, Belgrade, Yugoslavia
Aleksandar Jurišić Obstetrics and Gynaecology Clinic 'Narodni front', Belgrade, Yugoslavia
Djordjije Karadaglić Clinic for Dermatovenerology, MMA, Belgrade, Yugoslavia
Branka Karapetrović Immunology Research Centre, 'Branislav Janković', Belgrade, Yugoslavia
Milena Kataranovski Institute for Medical Research, MMA, Belgrade, Yugoslavia
Ivan Kehayov Department of Molecular Immunology, Institute of Biology and Immunology of Reproduction, Bulgarian Academy of Sciences, Sofia, Bulgaria
Leonard Khiroug Biophysics Sector, International School for Advanced Studies (SISSA), Trieste, Italy
Dimitris Kioussis National Institute for Medical Research, Mill Hill, London, UK
Sanja Kolarević Institute for Biological Research, University of Belgrade, Yugoslavia
Gordana Konjević Institute of Oncology and Radiology of Serbia, Belgrade, Yugoslavia
Duško Kosec Immunology Research Centre, 'Branislav Janković', Belgrade, Yugoslavia
Vesna Kovačević-Jovanović Immunology Research Centre, 'Branislav Janković', Belgrade, Yugoslavia

Ivana Kranjčić-Zec Institute of Microbiology and Immunology, School of Medicine, University of Belgrade, Yugoslavia

Zorka Kukić Institute for Medical Research, MMA, Belgrade, Yugoslavia

Stanimir Kyurkchiev Department of Molecular Immunology, Institute of Biology and Immunology of Reproduction, Bulgarian Academy of Sciences, Sofia, Bulgaria

Branislav Lako Institute for Microbiology, MMA, Belgrade, Yugoslavia

Katarina Lalić Diabetes Centre, Institute for Endocrinology, Diabetes and Metabolic Diseases, Clinical Centre of Serbia, Belgrade, Yugoslavia

Nebojša M. Lalić Diabetes Centre, Institute for Endocrinology, Diabetes and Metabolic Diseases, Clinical Center of Serbia, Belgrade, Yugoslavia

Norman Latov Department of Neurology, College of Physicians and Surgeons of Columbia University, New York, USA

Roland Lauster Deutsches Rheumaforschung Zentrum Berlin, Germany

Gordana Leposavić Immunology Research Centre, 'Branislav Janković', Belgrade, Yugoslavia

Zvonimir Lević Institute of Neurology, Clinical Centre of Serbia, Belgrade, Yugoslavia

Eddy Liew Department of Immunology, University of Glasgow, Glasgow, UK

Alexandra Livescu Department of Immunochemistry, Institute 'Victor Babes', Bucharest, Romania

Miodrag L. Lukić Immunology Unit, Department of Medical Microbiology, Faculty of Medicine and Health Sciences, UAE University, Al Ain, United Arab Emirates

Tatjana Lukić Institute for Medical Research, MMA, Belgrade, Yugoslavia

Enrico Maggi Department of Clinical Immunology, University of Florence, Italy

Zvonko Magić Institute for Medical Research, MMA, Belgrade, Yugoslavia

Clio Mamalaki Institute of Molecular Biology and Biotechnology, Crete, Greece

Gina Manda Department of Immunochemistry, Institute 'Victor Babes', Bucharest, Romania

Vanya Manolova Department of Molecular Immunology, Institute of Biology and Immunology of Reproduction, Bulgarian Academy of Sciences, Sofia, Bulgaria

Elena Mazîlu 'Christiana' Medical Association, Bucharest, Romania

Terence McAlarney Department of Neurology, College of Physicians and Surgeons of Columbia University, New York, USA

Andreas Mertz Universität Klinikum 'Benjamin Franklin', Berlin, Germany

Šarlota Mesaroš Institute of Neurology, Clinical Centre of Serbia, Belgrade, Yugoslavia

Sanja Mijatović Institute for Biological Research 'Siniša Stanković', University of Belgrade, Belgrade, Yugoslavia

Pavle Milenković Institute of Medical Research, Belgrade, Yugoslavia

Vojislav D. Miletić Department of Pediatrics, Duke University Medical Center, Durham, North Carolina, USA

Novica M. Milićević Institute of Histology and Embryology, School of Medicine, University of Belgrade, Belgrade, Yugoslavia

Živana Milićević Institute of Histology and Embryology, School of Medicine, University of Belgrade, Belgrade, Yugoslavia

Mirjana Milinković Institute for Medical Research, MMA, Belgrade, Yugoslavia

Danica Milobratović Institute of Microbiology and Immunology, School of Medicine, University of Belgrade, Yugoslavia

Nada Milošević-Jovčić Institute of Medical Research, Belgrade, Yugoslavia

Aleksandar Mirčić Institute of Histology, School of Medicine, University of Belgrade, Belgrade, Yugoslavia
Milutin Mirić Department of Cardiology, 'Dedinje' Cardiovascular Clinic, Belgrade, Yugoslavia
Avrion Mitchison Deutsches Rheuma-Forschungszentrum Berlin, Monbijoustrasse 2, D-10117, Berlin, Germany
Hannah Mitchison Department of Pediatrics, University College London Medical School, London, UK
Sanja Mitrović Institute of Microbiology and Immunology, School of Medicine, University of Belgrade, Yugoslavia
Masayuki Miyasaka Department of Bioregulation, Medical School, Osaka University, Osaka, Japan
Marija Mostarica Stojković Institute of Microbiology and Immunology, School of Medicine, University of Belgrade, Belgrade, Yugoslavia
Miodrag Movsesijan Institute for the Application of Nuclear Energy (INEP), University of Belgrade, Zemun, Yugoslavia
Brigitte Müller Deutsches Rheuma-Forschungszentrum Berlin, Germany
Marianna Murdjeva Higher Medical Institute, Department of Microbiology and Immunology, Plovdiv, Bulgaria
Chudomir Nachev Department of Internal Medicine, Faculty of Medicine, Sofia Medical University, Sofia, Bulgaria
Shigeki Nagashima Department of Pathology, University of Pittsburgh School of Medicine and Pittsburgh Cancer Institute, Pittsburgh, USA
Monica Neagu Department of Immunochemistry, Institute 'Victor Babes', Bucharest, Romania
Dragana Nešić Michael Heidelberger Division of Immunology, Department of Pathology and Kaplan Comprehensive Cancer Center, NYU Medical Centre, New York, USA
Milena Nešić Institute for the Application of Nuclear Energy (INEP), University of Belgrade, Zemun, Yugoslavia
Goran A. Nikolić Blood Transfusion Institute, Belgrade, Yugoslavia
Andrea Nistri Biophysics Sector, International School for Advanced Studies (SISSA), Trieste, Italy
Trisha Norton National Institute for Medical Research, Mill Hill, London, UK
Sandra Obradović Immunology Research Centre, 'Branislav Janković', Belgrade, Yugoslavia
William Ollier ARC Epidemiology Research Unit, University of Manchester, UK
Chryssa Papasteriades Department of Immunology and Histocompatibility, Evangelismos Hospital, Athens, Greece
Helen Pappas Department of Immunology and Histocompatibility, Evangelismos Hospital, Athens, Greece
Miloš D. Pavlović Department of Dermatology, MMA, Belgrade, Yugoslavia
Nada Pejnović Institute for Medical Research, MMA, Belgrade, Yugoslavia
Bogdan Petrunov National Centre of Infectious and Parasitic Diseases, Sofia, Bulgaria
Laurentiu Mircea Popescu Department of Immunochemistry, Institute 'Victor Babes', Bucharest, Romania
Ljiljana Popović Institute for Medical Research, MMA, Belgrade, Yugoslavia
Petar Popović Institute for Medical Research, MMA, Belgrade, Yugoslavia
Zoran Popović Department of Cardiology, 'Dedinje' Cardiovascular Clinic, Belgrade, Yugoslavia

Vera Pravica Institute of Microbiology and Immunology, School of Medicine, University of Belgrade, Belgrade, Yugoslavia

Čedomir Radojičić Institute for Medical Research, MMA, Belgrade, Yugoslavia

Nina Radošević Institute of Hematology, Clinical Centre of Serbia, Belgrade, Yugoslavia

Jelena Radulović Immunology Research Centre, 'Branislav Janković', Belgrade, Yugoslavia

Marko Radulović Immunology Research Centre, 'Branislav Janković', Belgrade, Yugoslavia

Zorica Ramić Institute of Microbiology and Immunology, School of Medicine, University of Belgrade, Yugoslavia

Bojana Rodić Blood Transfusion Institute, Centre for Tissue Typing and Immunochemistry, Belgrade, Yugoslavia

Sergio Romagnani Department of Clinical Immunology, University of Florence, Italy

Kjersti S. Rønningen Institute of Transplantation Immunology, The National Hospital, Oslo, Norway

Dijana Šefer Institute of Hematology, Clinical Centre of Serbia, Belgrade, Yugoslavia

Allen Shahin Immunology Unit, Faculty of Medicine, UAE University, Al Ain, United Arab Emirates

Yehuda Shoenfeld Department of Medicine 'B', Sheba Medical Centre, Tel-Hashomer, Israel

Joachim Sieper Deutsches Rheumaforschung Zentrum and Universität Klinikum 'Benjamin Franklin', Berlin, Germany

Andjelija Škaro-Milić Institute for Pathology and Forensic Medicine, MMA, Belgrade, Yugoslavia

Ljiljana Sofronić-Milosavljević Institute for the Application of Nuclear Energy (INEP), University of Belgrade, Zemun, Yugoslavia

Dragoslav Sokić Institute of Neurology, Clinical Centre of Serbia, Belgrade, Yugoslavia

Ivan Spužić Institute of Oncology and Radiology of Serbia, Belgrade, Yugoslavia

Maria Stamenova Department of Molecular Immunology, Institute of Biology and Immunology of Reproduction, Bulgarian Academy of Sciences, Sofia, Bulgaria

Stanislava Stanojević Immunology Research Centre, 'Branislav Janković', Belgrade, Yugoslavia

Nebojša Stojsavljević Institute of Neurology, Clinical Centre of Serbia, Belgrade, Yugoslavia

Stanislava Stošić-Grujičić Institute for Biological Research 'Siniša Stanković', University of Belgrade, Belgrade, Yugoslavia

Vesna Tadić Institute for Medical Research, MMA, Belgrade, Yugoslavia

Yujiro Tanaka National Institute for Medical Research, Mill Hill, London, UK

Katerina Tarassi Department of Immunology and Histocompatibility, Evangelismos Hospital, Athens, Greece

Mauro Tolaini National Institute for Medical Research, Mill Hill, London, UK

Ljiljana Tomašević Department of Clinical Immunology, University of Florence, Italy

Vladimir Trajković Institute of Microbiology and Immunology, University of Belgrade, Belgrade, Yugoslavia

Sanja Ugrinović Universität Klinikum 'Benjamin Franklin', Berlin, Germany

Marighoula Varla-Leftherioti Department of Immunology, General District–Maternity Hospital 'Helena Venizelou', Athens, Greece
Jovan D. Vasiljević Department of Cardiology, 'Dedinje' Cardiovascular Clinic, Belgrade, Yugoslavia
Tatjana Vasiljević Immunology Research Centre, 'Branislav Janković', Belgrade, Yugoslavia
Biljana Vidić Danković Immunology Research Centre, 'Branislav Janković', Belgrade, Yugoslavia
Danilo Vojvodić Institute for Medical Research, MMA, Belgrade, Yugoslavia
Dragana Vučević Institute for Medical Research, MMA, Belgrade, Yugoslavia
Nikola L. Vujanović Department of Pathology, University of Pittsburgh School of Medicine and Pittsburgh Cancer Institute, Pittsburgh, USA
Vesna Vujić Institute of Chemistry, School of Medicine, University of Belgrade, Belgrade, Yugoslavia
Mirjana Vukičević Department of Cardiology, 'Dedinje' Cardiovascular Clinic, Belgrade, Yugoslavia
Stanislav Vukmanović Michael Heidelberger Division of Immunology, Department of Pathology and Kaplan Comprehensive Cancer Center, NYU Medical Center, New York, USA
Theresa L. Whiteside Department of Otolaryngology and Pathology, University of Pittsburgh School of Medicine and Pittsburgh Cancer Institute, Pittsburgh, USA
Miroslava Zamaklar Diabetes Centre, Institute for Endocrinology, Diabetes and Metabolic Diseases, Clinical Centre of Serbia, Belgrade, Yugoslavia
Snežana Živančević-Simonović Faculty of Medicine, Kragujevac, Yugoslavia
Vladimir Živanović Institute of Histology and Embryology, School of Medicine, University of Belgrade, Belgrade, Yugoslavia

Preface

In the past decade we have made monumental advances in our understanding of the molecular and cellular basis of immune functions. These data shed new light on the mechanisms of disordered immune regulation underlying many immune mediated diseases. *Immunoregulation in Health and Disease* contains papers related to the immunoregulatory mechanisms and their alterations as reflected in acquisition of T-cell repertoire and T-cells maturation, Th-1 - Th-2 cell dichotomy and cross-regulation, development of autoimmune diseases and hypersensitivity state, cytokine imbalance in inflammatory response and host reactivity to graft, tumor and infection. The volume contains contributions from the major research groups involved in the studies of immunoregulation led by N. A. Mitchison, S. Romagnani, R. Herberman, Y. Shoenfeld, D. Kioussis and others. The papers represent the viewpoints, mini-reviews and original works related to the different immunoregulatory mechanisms and their dysfunction which shape our protection against pathogens or result in harmful immune responses to innocuous antigens. They reflect the lively discussions and data presented at the Balkan Immunology Conference, the first of its kind held recently (December 1995) in Belgrade. The editors were asked to select, within the available space, the presentations for publication in this volume. Under the general title of '*Immunoregulation in health and disease*', they attempted to collect the contributions which will best represent the quality of the meeting. The editors wish to thank the contributors for timely providing their manuscripts and to Academic Press for competent editorial assistance and hope that this volume will contribute to the knowledge in the science and practice of immunology.

M. L. Lukić
Al Ain, 1997

Acknowledgement

This publication is supported by ICN Pharmaceuticals, Inc., Costa Mesa, California, USA.

Section 1

Regulatory, effectory and accessory cells of the immune response

1

Overcoming the TCR Signalling Defect of β_2-microglobulin Deficient CD8$^+$ T Cells in Response to Wildtype Syngeneic MHC Class I

Kanchan G. Jhaver, Dragana Nešić and Stanislav Vukmanović

CD8$^+$ T lymphocytes are stimulated by T-cell receptor (TCR) mediated recognition of antigens presented as short peptides complexed to MHC class I molecules (1). Upon antigen recognition CD8$^+$ cells initiate the expression of perforin and granzymes – molecules with cytolytic potential that are stored in cytoplasmic granules in inactive form. The expression of these molecules allows CD8$^+$ cells to differentiate into effector cytotoxic cells (2,3). Subsequent encounter with the antigen results in the release of perforin and granzymes from the granules into the intercellular space between the effector and target cells, which results in the death of the target cell. In addition to the perforin/granzyme-mediated lysis, interaction of the Fas ligand with the Fas molecule (if expressed by target cells) induces Fas to initiate signals in target cells that lead to apoptosis (4–6). In addition to the cytolytic attack, CD8$^+$ effector cells respond to recall antigen recognition by production of lymphokines, such as interferon-γ (IFNγ) IL-3, TNFα, and GM-CSF, amongst others. In some cases secretion of these lymphokines may be an indirect effector mechanism of destruction of target cells (7), whereas in others direct killing mechanisms seem to be exclusively involved (8). Finally, with the help of IL-2 (secreted sometimes by CD8$^+$ cells themselves, but more often by CD4$^+$ cells) effector CD8$^+$ cells will respond to antigen by proliferation as well. The proliferation will result in the generation of sufficient numbers of effector cells for the ongoing immune response, some of which will be the carriers of the immunological memory.

Immunoregulation in Health and Disease
ISBN 0–12–459460–3

Early signalling events after TCR ligation include activation of tyrosine kinases (such as CD3-associated ZAP70 and $p59^{fyn}$, as well as CD4- and CD8-associated $p56^{lck}$), which phosphorylate a number of substrates including CD3ζ chain (9). These early tyrosine phosphorylation events are believed to result in activation of two major signalling pathways. The first pathway is the activation of phospholipase C that catalyzes hydrolysis of phosphoinositolbisphosphate into diacylglycerol (DAG) and inositoltriphosphate (IP_3). IP_3 stimulates calcium uptake, while DAG acts as an activator of protein kinase C (PKC). Because calcium ionophores and phorbol esters (PKC activators), can mimic almost all aspects of T-cell activation (10), it was believed that this calcium flux and PKC activation are the only signalling pathways induced in the T-cell activation. However, a second major activation pathway has been discovered. This is the activation of $p21^{ras}$, a guanine nucleotide-binding protein whose activity is regulated by a GTP-binding cycle (11). Stimulation of the TCR results in rapid accumulation of biologically active, GTP-bound form (10). The activation of $p21^{ras}$ through the TCR seems to be independent of the calcium flux or the PKC, while PMA mediated $p21^{ras}$ activation is achieved indirectly through PKC (12).

Calcium flux and $p21^{ras}$, through activating calcineurin, induce translocation of the nuclear factor of activated T cells (NFATc) from the cytoplasm to the nucleus (13), while activation of PKC induces translocation of the NF-kB as well as induction of many nuclear factors, including AP1 (consisting of c-jun and c-fos) (14). NFATc and AP1 bind to and activate transcription of many lymphokine genes, including genes for IL-3, GM-SCF, and IFNγ (15). In addition, the IL-2 gene can infrequently be expressed in $CD8^+$ cells. The interaction of IL-2 (secreted by $CD8^+$ cells themselves or more frequently by $CD4^+$ cells) with its receptor leads to the initiation of the cell cycle and proliferation. The recent discovery that single amino acid substituted antigenic peptides may antagonize T-cell responses (16) or may induce split cellular responses (production of IL-4, but not proliferation by Th2 clones) (17, 18) raises the possibility that selective signals may be responsible for the induction of individual cellular responses and that a single TCR can transmit qualitatively different signals. We do not know, however, whether some of the above-mentioned signalling pathways may be exclusively required for the induction of particular responses.

Due to the low MHC class I expression in β2M−/− mice, positive selection of $CD8^+$ cells in the thymus is impaired. However, although $CD8^+$ T cells are virtually absent from peripheral lymphoid tissues of β2M−/− mice as determined by flow cytometric analysis (19, 20), immunization of β2M−/− mice with allogeneic, as well as syngeneic, tumour cells results in the appearance of small numbers of $TCR\alpha\beta^+CD8^+$, MHC class I specific, CTLs at the site of injection (21–23). It was suggested that due to the low ligand density of MHC class I, negative selection does not remove T cells capable of recognizing cells with normal MHC class I density, thus permitting the generation of an autoreactive T-cell repertoire in these knock-out mice (23). In vitro experiments seem to support this hypothesis, since syngeneic β2M+/+ target cells are lysed by β2M−/− CD8$^+$ cells, irrespective of the tumour haplotype used for in vivo immunization. In vivo experiments, however, do not provide a clear-cut support for this notion. If β2M−/− mice are challenged with MHC class I expressing tumours they will reject allogeneic but not syngeneic tumours, by a CD8$^+$ dependent mechanism (22,24). This is true for several different tumour lines. Thus, despite the ability of β2M−/− mice to raise a cytotoxic response directed at syngeneic cells, the growth of syngeneic tumours is not inhibited. These findings suggested that β2M−/− CD8$^+$ cells might be partially tolerant to syngeneic MHC class I expressed at wildtype levels. We have recently demonstrated that this tolerance in vivo correlated with the failure of β2M−/− CD8$^+$ cells to proliferate and secrete cytokines upon in vitro stimulation with syngeneic tumour cells (25). A cytotoxic response to syngeneic cells, on the other hand, was readily detectable. At the same time allogeneic cells could elicit all of the above responses. This lack of full responsiveness to the syngeneic MHC class I may be a result of the immunological tolerance to syngeneic MHC class I induced by the low levels of properly conformed MHC class I found in β2M−/− mice (20,26). We here demonstrate that the reactivity in vivo of β2M−/− CD8$^+$ cells fits the criteria of immunological tolerance, and that they originate from thymus. We further demonstrate that full reactivity in vitro to syngeneic MHC class I can be restored by synergistic action of phorbol esters, and we explore the nature of this synergy.

MATERIALS AND METHODS

Experimental procedures used to perform the experiments presented here have been described in detail elsewhere (25).

RESULTS AND DISCUSSION

Tumour growth of EL4 cells in β2M−/− mice is dependent on the recipient background

If partial non-responsiveness is indeed a result of tolerance to self, a prediction could be made that full responsiveness of CD8$^+$ cells to the H-2^b class I and rejection of H-2^b tumours would be expected in β2M−/− mice lacking the H-2^b heavy chains. To test this prediction, we have challenged BALB/c (H-2^d) β2M−/− mice with EL4 as well as P815 tumour cells (Table 1.1). P815 tumour was effectively rejected in both BALB/c and C57Bl/6 backgrounds. This is not unexpected, since P815 tumour was isolated from

Table 1.1 H-2^d or H-2^k but not H-2^b β2M-/- mice reject EL4 tumours. Mice were injected subcutaneously into the left inguinum with 1×10^6 indicated tumour cells, and were scored for palpable tumour growth twice a week. Only continuous growth of tumours was scored positive–mice that showed initial tumour growth followed by complete regression were scored negative. In the case of C3H mice, mice were injected intraperitoneally with anti-CD8 monoclonal antibody YTS 169 (500 μg/injection), or with PBS, on days −7, 0, 7, and 14 relative to the tumour injection on day 0.

Recipient β2M−/− mouse background	mAb treatment	Tumour injected	Tumour incidence
C57Bl/6 (H-2^b)	–	P815 (H-2^d)	0/4
C57Bl/6 (H-2^b)	–	EL4 (H-2^b)	4/4
BALB/c (H-2^d)	–	P815 (H-2^d)	0/3
BALB/c (H-2^d)	–	EL4 (H-2^b)	1/4
C3H/HeJ (H-2^k)	–	EL4 (H-2^b)	0/3
C3H/HeJ (H-2^k)	Anti-CD8	EL4 (H-2^b)	3/3

DBA/2 background, which shares only the MHC locus with BALB/c mice. There are a number of minor histocompatibility differences between DBA/2 and BALB/c mice. It has been demonstrated that BALB/c β2M−/− mice can raise CD8$^+$ responses specific for at least one of the minor antigens, tum− (27). Thus, cells with specificities for this and other minor antigens might be responsible for the rejection of P815 cells in BALB/c β2M−/− mice. In the case of EL4 tumour, however, unlike in C57BI/6 background where all mice injected with EL4 cells exhibited tumour growth, only one out of four mice in BALB/c background developed the tumour. There is thus a clear difference in the ability of the two mouse strains to react in vivo to the EL4 tumour. Further, β2M−/− mice bred on the C3H/HeJ background (H-2^k) also completely reject EL4 tumours, and this rejection is mediated by CD8$^+$ cells as all mice treated in vivo with anti-CD8 monoclonal antibody developed tumours. We therefore conclude that CD8$^+$ cells are tolerant in vivo to EL4 cells (H-2^b) only if they are themselves of H-2^b origin.

Thymic origin of the β2M−/− CD8$^+$ T cells

The CD8$^+$ T cell compartment in the wildtype mouse is comprised of cells that have differentiated in the thymus or in the intestine. Although gut-derived CD8$^+$ cells usually reside locally, it is possible that some migrate to the spleen, lymph node, and peritoneal cavity, and that CD8$^+$ cells we isolate from the β2M−/− mice in fact originate from the intestines. There are several features that distinguish intestinal CD8$^+$ cells from those of thymic origin, the make-up of the CD8 molecule being the most prominent.

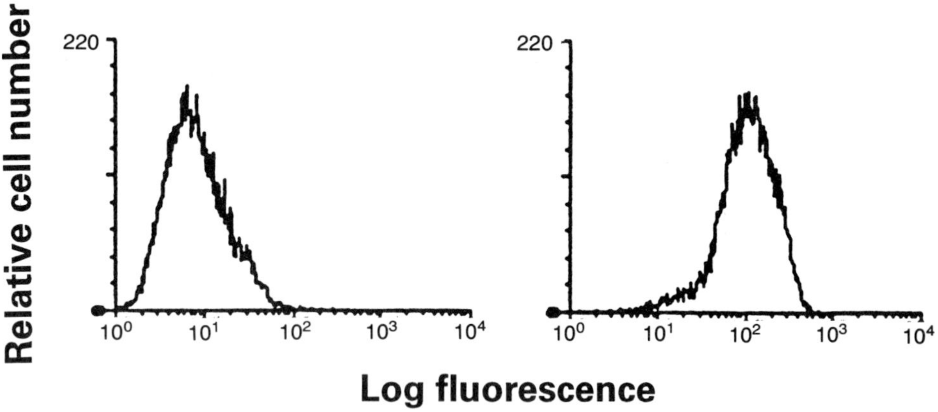

Fig. 1.1 CD8β is expressed by β2M−/− CD8$^+$ cells. Immunofluorescence profile of line 5 cells stained with anti-CD8β-FITC monoclonal antibody (right panel), or left unstained (left panel), and analyzed by flow cytometry.

CD8 molecules on thymic CD8$^+$ cells are $\alpha\beta$ heterodimers, while intestinal cells express $\alpha\alpha$ homodimers (28). In addition to T cells, some NK cells may express the CD8 molecule as well, but again in the form of $\alpha\alpha$ homodimers (29). It appears that the expression of the CD8β chain reflects the thymic origin of lymphocytes. β2M−/− CD8$^+$ cells express high levels of CD8β (Fig. 1.1), but not NK 1.1 antigens (data not shown), suggesting that the β2M−/− CD8$^+$ lines originate from thymic T cells and not from NK cells.

Syngeneic MHC class I molecules synergise with PMA, but not with ionomycin, to activate β2M−/− CD8$^+$ cells to proliferate

The split responsiveness of β2M−/− CD8$^+$ cells observed upon stimulation with syngeneic MHC class I provides an ideal model to study the differential TCR signalling events leading to the isolated cytotoxic T-cell response. To explore the nature of the signals delivered to the β2M−/− CD8$^+$ cells by syngeneic MHC class I, we asked whether stimulation with phorbol esters or calcium ionophores could restore full responsiveness upon stimulation with syngeneic cells. We stimulated β2M−/− CD8$^+$ cells with syngeneic EL4 cells in the absence or presence of either ionomycin or PMA, and measured proliferation (Table 1.2). In the absence of EL4 cells neither stimulus induced proliferation, and the combination of EL4 cells and ionomycin was also ineffective. However, EL4 cells in the presence of PMA induced proliferation. Similar findings were observed when IL-3/GM-CSF secretion by β2M−/− CD8$^+$ cells was assayed (data not shown). Although stimulation with ionomycin and PMA do not activate calcium ion flux and PKC, respectively, in precisely the same way as the engagement of the TCR does,

Table 1.2 Proliferation of β2M−/− CD8$^+$ cells upon stimulation with EL4 cells and either PMA or ionomycin. 5×10^4 β2M−/− CD8$^+$ cells were cultured for 72 h in the absence or presence of 3×10^4 irradiated EL4 cells, with or without PMA or ionomycin at indicated concentrations. Cultures were pulsed for 16 h with 0.5 μCi [^{3}H]-thymidine, and incorporation of [^{3}H]-thymidine into newly synthesized DNA determined by scintillation counting. Shown are means of triplicate cultures and standard deviations. Mean obtained in the cultures with irradiated EL4 cells alone was 1297 ($\pm$ 120) cpm, and has been subtracted where appropriate.

	^{3}H-thymidine incorporation (cpm^{-1})				
EL4	–	PMA (10^{-8} M)	PMA (5×10^{-8} M)	Ionomycin (0.1 μM)	Ionomycin (0.5 μM)
–	227 ± 41	260 ± 51	268 ± 16	272 ± 3	417 ± 5
+	−804	11205 ± 2250	63006 ± 11041	3206 ± 952	3211 ± 1087

these results nevertheless suggest that recognition of syngeneic MHC class I stimulates calcium ion flux.

The presence of a PKC inhibitor differentially affects cytolysis and IL-3/GM-CSF secretion by β2M−/− CD8$^+$ effector cells

The simplest explanation for the synergy between EL4 cells and PMA in stimulating β2M−/− CD8$^+$ cells would be that EL4 cells completely failed to activate the PKC, but did induce calcium ion flux. This may seem to be difficult to explain from the biochemical point of view as second messengers for both PKC activation and calcium ion flux arise from the same molecule, PIP_2. However, a second wave of DAG production that is required for the sustained PKC activation may be a result of phosphatidylcholine degradation that follows after calcium ion flux has occurred (30). If EL4 cells failed to activate PKC, it would follow that the PKC activation was not required for the cytolytic activity of CD8$^+$ T cells since EL4 cells were lysed by β2m−/− CD8$^+$ cells owing to perforin/granzyme release. If that is the case then PKC inhibitors should not affect the cytolytic activity of CD8$^+$ cells. To test this hypothesis we asked whether bisindolylmaleimide (BIM), a selective inhibitor of all PKC isoforms that acts as a competitor for ATP-binding sites (31), can inhibit the EL4- or P815-directed cytotoxic activity of β2M−/− CD8$^+$ cells. However, BIM blocked cytolysis of both EL4 and P815 cells in a dose-dependent manner, 10μM concentration being sufficient for complete inhibition of cytolysis (Fig. 1.2). 10μM BIM completely inhibited the activation of at least three PKC isoforms (βI, βII, and ζ) in anti-CD3 stimulated β2M−/− CD8$^+$ cells, as demonstrated by their inability to translocate to the membrane fraction of cells (data not shown). These results

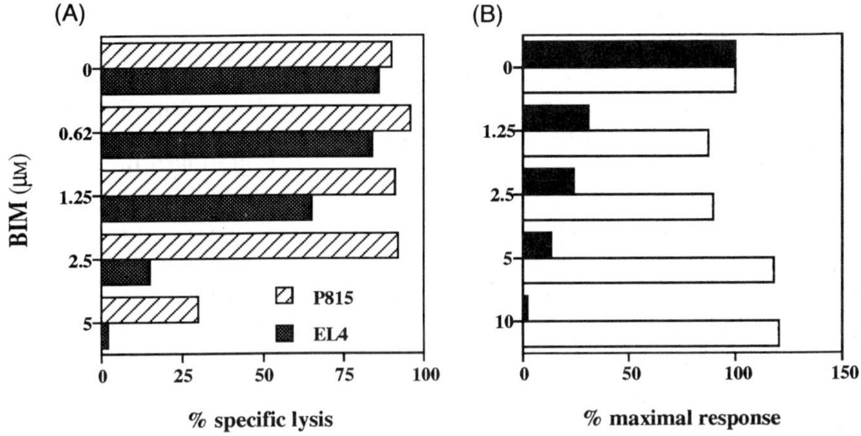

Fig 1.2 The effects of a selective PKC inhibitor, BIM, on cytotoxic response or IL-3/GM-CSF release of β2M−/− CD8^{+} cells. A: β2M−/− CD8^{+} cells were used in cytotoxic assay with P815 or EL4 target cells at an effector-to-target ratio of 20:1. Bisindolylmaleimide was preincubated with effector cells for 60 min before the addition of target cells. B: β2M−/− cells were stimulated with P815 cells in the presence of the indicated concentration of BIM and their ability to secrete IL-3/GM-CSF (white bars) or to lyse P815 cells (black bars) determined. The results are expressed as a percentage maximal stimulation obtained in the absence of inhibitor.

suggest that PKC activation is in fact induced by both target cells, and is required for the lysis by β2M−/− CD8^{+} cells.

The next possibility is that EL4 cells only weakly activate the PKC, the level of activation being sufficient to induce the CTL activity but not reaching the threshold required for lymphokine secretion. This possibility seems plausible since two-to-fourfold higher concentrations of BIM were required for the inhibition of lysis of P815 cells than for the lysis of EL4 cells. If indeed lower threshold of PKC activation is required for the activation of the lytic machinery than for the lymphokine secretion, then one might predict that an incomplete block of the PKC activation by suboptimal concentrations of BIM might result in no lymphokine release with at least partially preserved cytotoxicity. To our surprise, however, we could not observe inhibition of IL-3/GM-CSF secretion by any dose of BIM (Fig. 1.2). These results were also confirmed for the IFNγ at the mRNA expression level (data not shown).

Thus, the induction of the isolated cellular response in β2M−/− CD8^{+} cells by syngeneic MHC class I cannot be explained by lower requirement for the PKC activation of the granule exocytosis compared to the cytokine secretion. In fact, antigen (P815 cells)-induced activation of the lymphokine secretion programme by β2M−/− CD8^{+} cells is completely independent, whereas cytolysis may be entirely dependent on the PKC activation. These findings can be explained by the possibility that PMA synergizes for the full responsiveness by activating directly or indirectly another signalling molecule, in another signalling cascade. Vav might be the candidate molecule as it has been demonstrated that phorbol esters activate Vav directly (32). However, PKC inhibitor prevented the IFNγ mRNA accumulation induced by synergistic action of EL4 cells and PMA (data not shown), suggesting a PKC dependent role for PMA. The key finding that can explain our results, we believe, comes from the studies of Izquierdo *et al.*, which demonstrates that the activation of $p2l^{ras}$ through the TCR seems to be independent of the calcium ion flux or the PKC, while PMA-mediated $p21^{ras}$ activation is achieved indirectly through PKC (12). We therefore believe that EL4 cells are in our model inducing both calcium ion flux and PKC activation, but fail to activate $p21^{ras}$, and that addition of PMA activates $p21^{ras}$ indirectly through the PKC. We are currently testing this hypothesis. If true, it would imply that PKC is selectively required for the cytolytic function, whereas $p21^{ras}$ is selectively required for the cytokine secretion by effector $CD8^+$ cells.

CONCLUSION

Few $CD8^+$ T cells that are allowed to mature in the thymus of β2M−/− mice are tolerant to the syngeneic MHC class I, as demonstrated by the failure of β2M−/− mice to reject syngeneic β2M+/+ tumours in vivo, and a partial response of β2M−/− $CD8^+$ T cells to β2M+/+ stimulators in vitro. The partial response, consisting of cytotoxic attack in the absence of proliferation or cytokine secretion, can be converted to the full response by synergistic action of syngeneic MHC class I and phorbol esters. Phorbol ester-induced activation of the ras pathway seems to be responsible for reverting to the phenotype, suggesting that ras activation is required for cytokine secretion and proliferation of $CD8^+$ cells. PKC activation, on the other hand, seems to be selectively required for perforin/granzyme release. This conclusion is based on findings that PKC inhibitor affects cytolytic activity of β2M−/− $CD8^+$ cells, with no effect on cytokine secretion. The induction of cytolysis and of cytokine secretion by effector $CD8^+$ cells seems to be regulated by different TCR signalling pathways.

ACKNOWLEDGEMENTS

The authors gratefully acknowledge Derry Roopenian for providing β2M−/− mice on various backgrounds, and John Hirst for the FACS analysis. This work was supported by the Markey Charitable Trust Award, ACS Institutional Grant No. IRG-14-38, and the NCI Core Support Grant 5P30 CA 16087-18.

REFERENCES

1. Townsend, A. R. M., J. Rothbard, F. M. Gotch, G. Bahadur, D. Wraith and A. J. McMichael. 1986. The epitopes of Influenza nucleoprotein recognized by cytotoxic T lymphocytes can be defined with short synthetic peptides. *Cell* **44**:959–68.
2. Liu, C.-C., S. Rafii, A. Granelli-Piperno, J. A. Trapani and J. D.-E. Young. 1989. Perforin and serine esterase gene expression in stimulated human T cells. Kinetics, mitogen requirements, and effects of cyclosporin A. *J. Exp. Med.* **170**:2105– 8.
3. Liu, C.-C., J. S. V., B. S. Kwon and J. D.-E. Young. 1990. Induction of perforin and serine esterases in a murine cytotoxic T lymphocyte clone. *J. Immunol.* **144**:1196–201.
4. Rouvier, E., M.-F. Luciani and P. Goldstein. 1993. Fas involvement in Ca^{2+}-independent T cell-mediated cytotoxicity. *J. Exp. Med.* **177**:195–200.
5. Kagi, D., F. Vignaux, B. Ledermann, K. Burki, V. Depraetere, S. Nagata, H. Hengartner and P. Goldstein. 1994. Fas and perforin pathways as major mechanisms of T cell-mediated cytotoxicity. *Science* **265**:528–30.
6. Lowin, B., M. Hahne, C. Mattmann and J. Tschopp. 1994. Cytolytic T-cell cytotoxicity is mediated through perforin and Fas lytic pathways. *Nature* **370**:650–2.
7. Suzuki, Y. and J. S. Remington. 1990. The effect of anti-IFN-γ antibody on the protective effect of Lyt-2^+ immune T cells against toxoplasmosis in mice. *J. Immunol.* **144**:1954–6.
8. Harty, J. T. and M. J. Bevan. 1995. Specific immunity to *Listeria monocytogenes* in the absence of IFNγ. *Immunity* **3**:109–17.
9. Perlmutter, R. M., S. D. Levin, M. W. Appleby, S. J. Anderson and J. Alberolalla. 1993. Regulation of lymphocyte function by protein phosphorylation. *Ann. Rev. Immunol.* **11**:451–99.
10. Downward, J., J. D. Graves, P. H. Warne, S. Rayter and D. A. Cantrell. 1990. Stimulation of $p21^{ras}$ upon T cell activation. *Nature* **346**:719–23.
11. Bourne, H. R., D. A. Sanders and F. McCormick. 1991. The GTPase superfamily: Conserved structure and molecular mechanism. *Nature* **349**:117–27.
12. Izquierdo, M., J. Downward, J. D. Graves and D. A. Cantrell. 1992. Role of protein kinase C in T-cell antigen receptor regulation of $p21^{ras}$. Evidence that two $p2l^{ras}$ regulatory pathways coexist in T cells. *Mol. Cell. Biol.* **12**:3305–12.
13. Woodrow, M., N. A. Clipstone and D. Cantrell. 1993. $p21^{ras}$ and calcineurin synergize to regulate the nuclear factor of activated T cells. *J. Exp. Med.* **178**:1517–22.
14. Goodbourn, S. 1994. Transcriptional regulation in activated T cells. *Curr. Biol.* **4**:930–2.
15. Rao, A. 1994. NF-ATp: a transcription factor required for the co-ordinate induction of several cytokine genes. *Immunol. Today* **15**:274–81.
16. De Magistris, M. T., J. Alexander, M. Coggeshall, A. Altman, F. C. A. Gaeta, H. N. Grey and A. Sette. 1992. Antigen analog-major histocompatibility complexes act as antagonists of the T cell receptor. *Cell* **68**:625–34.

17. Evavold, B. D. and P. M. Allen. 1991. Separation of IL-4 production from Th cell proliferation by an altered T cell receptor ligand. *Science* **252**:1308–10.
18. Sloan-Lancaster, J., B. D. Evavold and P. M. Allen. 1994. Th2 cell clonal anergy as a consequence of partial activation. *J. Exp. Med.* **180**:1195–205.
19. Koller, B. H., P. Marrack, J. W. Kappler and O. Smithies. 1990. Normal development of mice deficient in β2M, MHC class I proteins, and CD8$^+$ T cells. *Science* **248**:1227–30.
20. Zijlstra, M., M. Bix, N. E. Simister, J. M. Loring, D. H. Raulet and R. Jaenisch. 1990. β2-microglobulin deficient mice lack CD4-CD8$^+$ cytolytic T cells. *Nature* **344**:742–6.
21. Apasov, S. and M. Sitkovski. 1993. Highly lytic CD8$^+$, $\alpha\beta$ T cell receptor cytotoxic T cells with major histocompatibility complex (MHC) class I antigen-directed cytotoxicity in β2-microglobulin, MHC class I-deficient mice. *Proc. Natl. Acad. Sci. USA* **90**:2837–41.
22. Lamouse-Smith, E., V. K. Clements and S. Ostrand-Rosenberg. 1993. β2M-*l*-knockout mice contain low levels of CD8$^+$ cytotoxic T lymphocyte that mediate specific tumor rejection. *Immunol.* **151**:6283–90.
23. Glas, R., C. Ohlen, P. Hoglund and K. Karre. 1994. The CD8$^+$ T cell repertoire in β2-microglobulin deficient mice is biased towards reactivity against self-major histocompatibility class I. *J. Exp. Med.* **179**:661–72.
24. Apasov, S. G. and M. V. Sitkovsky. 1994. Development of antigen specificity of CD8$^+$ cytotoxic T lymphocytes in β2-microglobulin-negative, MHC class I-deficient mice in response to immunization with tumor cells. *J. Immunol.* **152**:2087–97.
25. Jhaver, K. G., T. D. Rao, A. B. Frey and S. Vukmanovic. 1995. Apparent split tolerance of CD8$^+$ T cells from β2-microglobulin-deficient (β2m−/−) mice to syngeneic β2m+/+ cells. *J. Immunol.* **154**:6252–61.
26. Bix, M. and D. Raulet. 1992. Functionally conformed free class I heavy chains exist on the surface of β2 microglobulinnegative cells. *J. Exp. Med.* **176**:829–34.
27. Cook, J. R., J. C. Solheim, J. M. Connolly and T. H. Hansen. 1995. Induction of peptide-specific CD8$^+$ CTL clones in β2-microglobulin-deficient mice. *J. Immunol.* **154**:47–57.
28. Guy-Grand, D., B. Rocha, P. Mintz, M. Malassis-Seris, F. Selz, B. Malissen and P. Vassalli. 1994. Different use of T cell receptor transducing modules in two populations of gut intraepithelial lymphocytes are related to distinct pathways of T cell differentiation. *J. Exp. Med.* **180**:673–9.
29. Torres-Nagel, N., E. Kraus, M. H. Brown, G. Tiefenthaler, R. Mitnacht, A. F. Williams and T. Hunig. 1992. Differential thymus dependence of rat CD8 isoform expression. *Eur. J. Immunol.* **22**:2841–8.
30. Nishizuka, Y. 1992. Intracellular signaling by hydrolysis of phospholipids and activation of protein kinase C. *Science* **258**:607–14.
31. Toullec, D., P. Pianetti, H. Coste, P. Bellevergue, T. Grand-Perret, M. Ajakane, V. Baudet, P. Boissin, E. Boursier, F. Loriolle, L. Duhamel, D. Charon and J. Kirilovsky. 1991. The bisindolylmaleimide GF 109203X is a potent and selective inhibitor of protein kinase C. *J. Biol. Chem.* **266**:15771–81.
32. Gulbins, E., K. M. Coggeshall, G. Baier, D. Telford, C. Langlet, G. Baier-Bitterlich, N. Bonnefoy-Berard, P. Burn, A. Wittinghofer and A. Altman. 1994. Direct stimulation of Vav guanine nucleotide exchange activity for Ras by phorbol esters and diglycerides. *Mol. Cell. Biol.* **14**:4749–58.

2

Adhesion Molecules in the Thymic Microenvironment: Interactions Between Thymocytes and Cloned Thymic Epithelial Cell Lines

Miodrag Čolić, Dragana Vučević, Miloš D. Pavlović, Tatjana Lukić, Mirjana Milinković, Ljiljana Popović, Petar Popović and Aleksandar Dujić

The thymus plays a crucial role in the generation of T cells. It provides an appropriate milieu within which thymocytes can proliferate, differentiate, mature, develop their antigen receptor repertoire restricted by the self major histocompatibility complex (MHC), and become tolerant to self antigens (reviewed in 1,2). Thymocyte differentiation starts from the earliest multipotential $CD3^-CD4^{-/low}CD8^-$ precursors (predominantly located in the subcapsular area), continues through the stage of immature (cortical) thymocytes which at first are $CD3^-CD4^+CD8^{-/low}$ or $CD3^-CD4^{-/low}CD8^+$ and then $CD3^{low/intermediate}CD4^+CD8^+$ and terminates by forming mature (medullary) $CD3^{hi}CD4^+CD8^-$ or $CD3^{hi}CD4^-CD8^+$ thymocytes (3). This pathway of T-cell development involves a series of sequential, symbiotic interactions between thymocytes and different components of the thymic microenvironment such as epithelial cells, dendritic cells, macrophages, fibrous stroma, and extracellular matrix (4,5). Numerous factors may contribute to this complicated multistep process including soluble mediators (cytokines and thymic hormones) and direct cell–cell contacts (4,5).

Close cellular interactions seem to be an essential event in T-cell development since isolated progenitor cells have only a limited capacity to

Immunoregulation in Health and Disease
ISBN 0-12-459460-3

proliferate and differentiate in vitro (6). However, the role of individual components of the thymic microenvironment in these processes has not been fully elucidated.

MORPHOLOGICAL HETEROGENEITY OF THE THYMIC EPITHELIUM

Thymic epithelial cells (TEC) form a supporting network of the thymus and represent the major component of the thymic microenvironment (7,8,9). They are located both in the cortex and in the medulla and are in close contact with developing thymocytes and other non-lymphoid cells. TEC in the cortex have very long cytoplasmic processes forming a fine reticular network. Medullary TEC are oval cells with shorter, spatulate processes, sometimes loosely connected with each other. Some of the medullary TEC form concentric whorls of epithelial, highly keratinized cells, named Hassall's corpuscles, which considerably vary in size. They are large in humans, but very small and atypical in mouse and rat (7–9).

Electron microscopy has revealed considerable heterogeneity within the thymic epithelium. In human at least six different TEC types have been described (9). Similar types can be observed in mouse and rat (10, Čolić, personal observation). Type 1 cells are the subcapsular/subtrabecular sheet-like TEC which also line the perivascular spaces. These cells are involved in formation of the blood–thymus barrier and secrete thymic hormones, cytokines and haemotactic peptides for thymocyte progenitors.

The cortex is populated with type 2 (pale), type 3 (intermediate), and type 4 (dark) cells which may represent different stages of a single population of TEC. These cells are characterized by long cytoplasmic processes that extend between thymocytes. Numerous vacuoles containing osmiophilic granules, different particles, or membranous structures are visible in their cytoplasm. Some of these cells (especially type 2 and 3) completely enclose a number of thymocytes and represent thymic nurse cells (TNC). Scanning electron microscopy has demonstrated that thymocytes can freely enter and exit from TNC. Type 4 are electron dense, probably dying TEC localized predominantly in the deep cortex.

In the medulla type 5 and 6 cells are present. Type 5 TEC are localized in small groups at the corticomedullary border. They are undifferentiated cells, have short processes and do not appear to be active secretors. The type 6 cells form a loose network in the medulla and frequently contain secretory granules and cluster-like vacuoles with microvilli filled with a floccular content (9). These cells are believed to produce different cytokines and thymic hormones (11). Some of them correspond to the hypertrophic epithelial cells which can develop large cytoplasmic cysts (12).

Reticular epithelial cells (12) similar to cortical types 3 and 4 are also located in the medulla. However, these cells in mouse and rat do not contain vacuoles characteristic for cortical TEC (13). Type 6 and reticular medullary TEC form Hassall's corpuscles (13).

PHENOTYPIC HETEROGENEITY OF THE THYMIC EPITHELIUM

Hybridoma technology has enabled the generation of a large panel of monoclonal antibodies (mAbs) reactive with different components of the thymic microenvironment (14,15). Such reagents have revealed considerable phenotypic heterogeneity within the thymic epithelium. They have been characterized in several laboratories, including ours, and compared in a series of workshops. Based on immunohistochemical staining patterns on the thymus and other organs anti-TEC antibodies are grouped in five major 'clusters of thymic epithelial staining' (CTES) (14,15).

CTES I are panepithelial mAbs. CTES II mAbs bind to subcapsular/perivascular and most medullary TEC. CTES III reagents detect different molecules on cortical TEC. CTES IV mAbs stain medullary TEC and Hassall's corpuscles, whereas CTES V reagents are restricted to Hassall's corpuscles only and sometimes to a surrounding halo of the medullary epithelium. Among each cluster further heterogeneity of the mAb was observed (14,15).

In our laboratory, we have raised a panel of mAbs to rat thymic epithelium (16–19). Some of them have been submitted to these CTES workshops. Immunohistochemistry confirmed similar phenotypic heterogeneity of rat TEC, too. It was demonstrated that cortical TEC which express R-MC 13–R-MC 17, PT10B7 and R-TNC 2G9 are phenotypically different from subcapsular/perivascular TEC. Subcapsular/perivascular TEC which are positive with R-MC 18–R-MC 20 and PT13D11 mAb share common antigens with most medullary TEC. In contrast, some medullary TEC, including Hassall's corpuscles, possess their own antigenic profiles (R-MC 22, TE-R 4F10).

We also found that distinct regions of the thymic epithelium also differ in the expression of cytokeratin (CK) polypeptides (20), as reported for other species (21,22). It is known that cytokeratins form cytoskeletal intermediate filaments of epithelial cells. They are heterogeneous proteins which belong to a family of at least 20 different polypeptides. Small molecular mass CK (40–56 kDa) are acidic (type I) while larger molecular mass CK (53–68 kDa) are basic (type II). Type I and II cytokeratins are frequently expressed as specific pairs depending on the type of epithelium, period of epithelial differentiation or embryonic development (23). Using a panel of mAbs to different CK polypeptides or CK pairs we found that in adult rat thymus CK 8 is a panepithelial marker. Subcapsular/perivascular and most medullary TEC express CK 7, CK 16 and CK 19. Cortical TEC and a subset of medullary TEC possess CK 18, whereas the expression of CK 10 is restricted

Table 2.1 Phenotypic characteristics of different TEC subsets (TEC-PH) in adult rat thymus

	TEC subsets					
Markers	TEC-PH 1	TEC-PH 2	TEC-PH 3	TEC-PH 4	TEC-PH 5	TEC-PH 6
R-MC 14	−	+	−	−	−	−
R-MC 16	−	+	−	−	−	−
R-MC 18	+	±	+	+	+	±
R-MC 20	+	−	+	±	+	−
PT13D11	+	−	+	+	+	−
CK 7	+	−	±	−	−	−
CK 8	+	+	+	+	+	+
CK 10	−	−	−	+	+	−
CK 18	−	+	±	+	−	−
CK 19	+	−	+	+	−	−
TE-R 4F10	−	−	−	+	±	−

TEC subsets were determined using double or triple immunofluorescence labelling as previously described (20).
+ = strong positivity; ± = weak positivity; − = negative

to a subset of medullary TEC including Hassall's corpuscles (20). In addition, we demonstrated that CK are differently expressed in fetal, neonatal, and adult thymus (24).

Multimarker phenotypic analysis using double and triple staining with anti-CK and/or anti-TEC antibodies showed that at least six phenotypic different TEC subsets (TEC PH 1-6) could be identified in adult rat thymus (Table 2.1). Cortical TEC (TEC-PH 2) possess their own antigenic characteristics. Subcapsular/perivascular TEC (TEC PH-1) share common phenotypic profiles with a subset of medullary TEC. Another four different TEC subsets (TEC PH 3–6) are localized in the medulla. TEC PH 3, 5, and 6 are three phenotypically different TEC subsets. Among them TEC PH 5 might be terminally differentiated medullary epithelium whereas TEC PH 4 is probably a discrete stage of medullary TEC differentiation towards the type 5 cells (20).

At the moment it is not clear whether the differences observed reflect different origin of TEC subsets (endodermal cortex versus ectodermal medulla) or different stages of TEC development (especially in the medulla), or whether they represent TEC subsets with different functions.

THYMIC EPITHELIUM IN VITRO

One approach in studying functional characteristics of the thymic epithelium involves in vitro cell culture assays. However, many difficulties in maintaining pure populations of TEC have been reported (reviewed in 25). TEC growth has been promoted with low calcium, serum-free medium, medium supplemented with D-valine, using extracellular matrix or irradiated fibroblasts as filler cells (26,27). Sometimes the results were not satisfactory. Successfully cultivated TEC usually grow heterogeneous cell populations of both cortical and medullary origin or morphologically and phenotypically undifferentiated TEC (28,29).

Although this culture system is a good tool to unravel in vitro functions of TEC in T-cell development, it does not provide insight into the specific role of individual TEC subsets in these processes. To this purpose, TEC have to be cloned and grown as a cell line. Up to now, several different TEC lines have been established using various cloning techniques or immortalization procedures by treating the cells with Simian virus 40 (reviewed in 2). However, cloned TEC lines often change their phenotype in culture and it is not easy to define whether a particular line reflects a TEC subset in situ. Sometimes certain TEC in culture simultaneously express antigens typical of epithelial cells from multiple sites in the in vivo thymus (5). Moreover, some morphologically similar cells observed in in vitro cultures of the thymic epithelium have the potential to generate several different subtypes of TEC when transplanted in vivo (5).

PHENOTYPIC AND ULTRASTRUCTURAL CHARACTERISTICS OF CLONED TEC LINES

We have succeeded in cloning two different TEC lines from long-term cultures of the rat thymic epithelium which could reflect their normal counterparts in vivo (18,19,30). Both clones were characterized as epithelial lines by staining with anti-CK antibodies.

The first line, named TE-R 2.5, was positive with panepithelial anti-CK antibodies (CK 8 and K 8.13) and with R-MC 18 and R-MC 19 but not with R-MC 14, R-MC 16 and R-MC 17 mAbs (18,30). As previously mentioned, these reagents recognize subcapsular/perivascular and most medullary TEC, and cortical TEC, respectively (16,20) (Table 2.2). Based on these results we concluded that this line might represent a cell type originating either from the subcapsule or from the medulla. The positivity of TE-R 2.5 cells with *Ulex europaeus* agglutinin which binds to medullary TEC including Hassall's corpuscles and Mar3 mAb recognizing antigens expressed on thymic macrophages and a subset of medullary TEC and Hassall's corpuscles (16) further confirmed that this line is of medullary origin.

Ultrastructural analysis has also revealed that TE-R 2.5 represents a type of medullary but not subcapsular TEC (Fig. 2.1a). This was documented by the presence of cluster-like vacuoles containing microvilli which are characteristics for hypertrophic epithelial cells (12) (probably type 6 in the study

Table 2.2 Phenotypic characteristics of cloned TEC lines

		R-TNC.1		TE-R 2.5	
MAbs	Specificity	IFNγ(−)	IFNγ(+)	IFNγ(−)	IFNγ(+)
K 8.13	CK 1,5–8, 10,11,18	98 (++)	87 (++)	99 (+++)	96 (+++)
CK 8	CK 8	6 (+)	12 (+)	96 (+++)	98 (+++)
K 8.12	CK 13/16	0	0	79 (++)	76 (++)
CK 18	CK 18	76 (+)	59 (+)	0	0
CK 19	CK 19	0	0	6 (+)	2 (+)
KL 1	CK 3/10	0	0	0	0
R-MC 14	–	66 (+)	64 (+)	0	0
R-MC 16	–	58 (+)	59 (+)	0	0
R-MC 17	–	49 (++)	51 (+)	0	0
R-MC 18	–	0	0	76 (++)	49 (++)
R-MC 19	–	0	0	78 (++)	59 (++)
R-MC 20	–	0	0	4 (+)	2 (+)
UEA	–	13 (+)	5 (+)	86 (++)	79 (++)
Mar 3	–	0	0	99 (+++)	95 (+++)
OX-6	IA	0	43 (++)	2 (+)	96 (++)
OX-18	Class I MHC	94 (++)	98 (+++)	98 (++)	97 (+++)
1A29	ICAM-1	0	53 (++)	16 (+)	84 (++)
TE-R 4F10	–	0	0	75 (++)	94 (+++)
4D1	–	36 (+)	24 (+)	69 (++)	73 (++)
1D6	–	12 (+)	20 (+)	92 (++)	89 (++)
G7E6	–	96 (+++)	99 (+++)	95 (+++)	94 (+++)
3F10	–	99 (+++)	99 (+++)	98 (+++)	99 (+++)

Cytospins of TEC lines were stained by mAbs using a streptavidin–biotin immunoperoxidase method and analysed as described (18,19). TEC were cultivated without or with recombinant rat IFNγ for 2 days (100 u/ml). Values are the percentages of positive cells from one representative experiment.
Intensity of labelling: + = weak; ++ = moderate; +++ = strong.

of van Wijgnaert) (9), localized in situ in the medulla including the corticomedullary border. Final experiments using TE-4F10 mAb raised against the TE-R 2.5 cell antigen confirmed again the medullary origin of this line (18). Namely, this mAb stains only a subset of medullary TEC including HC but not any other TEC subpopulations. Cumulatively, the TE-R 2.5 cell line might represent an in vitro equivalent of hypertrophic epithelial cells, type 6 as defined by electron microscopic examinations and types TEC-PH 4 and 5 by our phenotypic analysis. It is obvious that TE-R 2.5 did not possess all the markers expressed by these TEC subsets in situ such as CK 10 or CK 19 (20). Up to now, lines with similar phenotypic and ultrastructural characteristics have not been described. It is therefore a useful tool for studying the function of medullary TEC subsets in T cell development.

The second line, named R-TNC.1, was characterized as a type of cortical

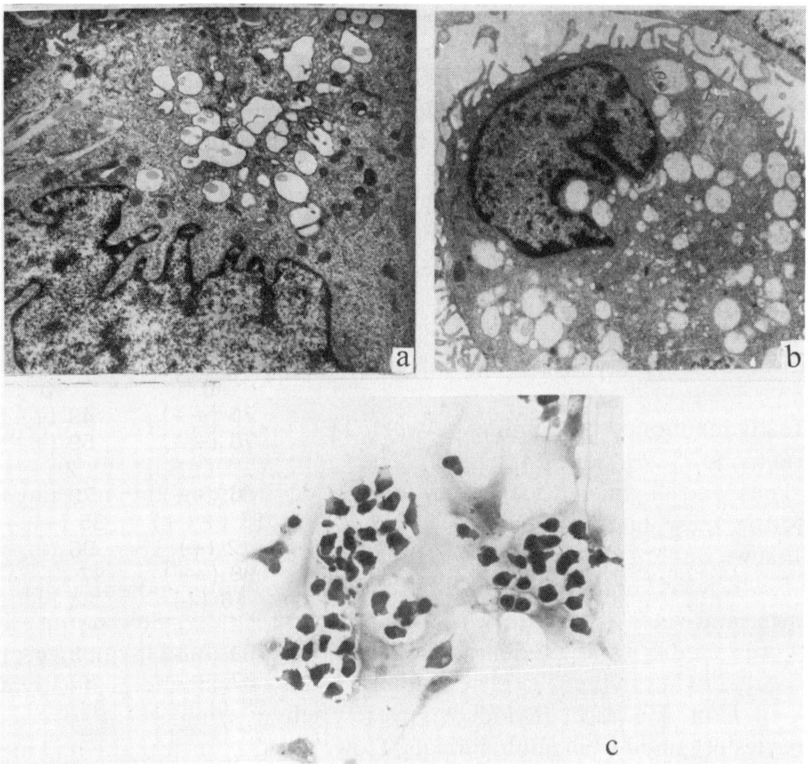

Fig. 2.1 Typical ultrastructural characteristics of epithelial cells of TE-R 2.5 (a) and R-TNC.1 lines (b). (c) engulfment of the BWRT3 thymocyte hybridoma by R-TNC.1 cells in the monolayer culture.

TEC on the basis of its reactivity with R-MC 14, R-MC 16, R-MC 17, CK 18 and R-TNC 2G9 but not with reagents defining subcapsular and medullary TEC (R-MC 19, R-MC 20, TE-R 4F10 and KL 1) (Table 2.2). It is interesting that initially this line did not express CK 8, which appeared in the majority of cells after prolonged cultivation (19).

Electron microscopic examinations showed numerous microvilli at the cell surface. Small or large vacuoles containing vesicles or osmiophilic granules characteristic of cortical TEC in situ were also present (Fig. 2.1b) (19).

It was further demonstrated that the R-TNC.1 cell line possesses nursing activity manifested by the binding and subsequent engulfment of thymocytes or thymocyte hybridoma (Fig. 2.1c). Based on these criteria it was identified as a thymic nurse cell (TNC) line (31). The properties are identical, with mouse stromal cell lines forming characteristic complex structures both with thymocytes in the monolayer and a hanging drop culture system (32–34). To our knowledge this is the first line with nursing characteristics established from the rat thymus.

It is known that TNC express MHC class I and class II molecules as well as several neuropeptides that may reflect a neuroendocrine origin but to date there are no mAbs specific for TNC despite their unique structure and apparent function (4). They share antigens with the rest of cortical epithelium, being the same for R-TNC.1 cells (19). Thus, the R-TNC.1 cell line corresponds to the type 2 or 3 by electron microscopic analysis (9) and TEC-PH 2 as established by our phenotypic analysis.

DIFFERENCES IN THYMOCYTE BINDING TO TEC LINES

As already mentioned the binding between TEC and thymocytes is of crucial importance for T-cell development (2). Therefore, in vitro experiments using TEC lines and thymocytes are very helpful in defining the mechanisms involved in these interactions.

At first we wanted to investigate whether our TEC lines bind thymocytes and other T cells, whether there are any differences in the binding potential of these two lines, and what are the factors which influence these interactions. The results presented in Table 2.3 demonstrate that both lines bind thymocytes, but only poorly bind peripheral T cells. Binding was higher when fetal or activated (PMA or Con A + IL-2) thymocytes were used in comparison to resting thymocytes obtained from adult animals. However, the cortical line had much higher adhesion capability. In addition, R-TNC.1 bound significantly less neonatal and hydrocortisone-resistant thymocytes. In contrast, the TE-R 2.5 line bound these cells as equally as strongly as adult thymocytes.

Phenotypic analysis (Fig. 2.2) demonstrates that R-TNC.1 cells bound exclusively double positive ($CD4^+CD8^+$) cells with low expression of $\alpha\beta$TCR. The finding might be relevant for the in vivo situation because $CD4^+CD8^+$ $\alpha\beta TCR^{+/-}$ thymocytes are the predominant population of immature, cortical thymocytes. This is also in agreement with the strong attachment of BWRT-2 and BWRT-3 thymocyte hybridomas of cortical phenotype (31) (Table 2.3) to the line. Similar results were published on the phenotype of intra-TNC thymocytes in freshly isolated murine TNC (32) or thymocytes engulfed by mouse TNC lines (33,34). An exception was published by Nishimura *et al.* (35) who demonstrated that both $CD4^+CD8^+$ and $CD4^-CD8^-$ immature mouse thymocytes preferentially interacted with the TNC-R 3.1 cell line.

The medullary line also predominantly bound $CD4^+CD8^+$ thymocytes but minor subsets of other thymocytes ($CD4^+CD8^-$ and $CD4^-CD8^+$) were also identified. Based on the profile of $\alpha\beta$TCR expression it can be concluded that among adherent thymocytes a higher percentage of more mature ($\alpha\beta TCR^{hi}$) thymocytes was seen in comparison to those adhering to the cortical line (Fig. 2.2).

Table 2.3 Binding of different T-cell populations to TEC lines

T-cell subpopulations	Percentages of binding	
	R-TNC.1	TE-R 2.5
Adult thymocytes	40.3 ± 6.2	18.3 ± 5.3
Fetal thymocytes	53.4 ± 5.0	24.1 ± 3.7
Neonatal thymocytes	26.4 ± 3.9	16.2 ± 5.0
Cortisone-resistant thymocytes	20.2 ± 4.6	21.3 ± 7.2
Activated thymocytes (Con A + IL-2)	61.3 ± 5.9	39.2 ± 4.3
Activated thymocytes (PMA)	53.3 ± 5.4	30.2 ± 6.4
Peripheral T cells	13.2 ± 4.3	8.0 ± 3.4
BWRT-2 hybridoma	69.2 ± 4.6	29.2 ± 3.7
BWRT-3 hybridoma	79.3 ± 8.0	36.2 ± 7.3
Adult thymocytes (IFNγ stim. TEC)[a]	58.2 ± 2.7	35.1 ± 5.0

Confluent monolayers of TEC lines grown in 96-well plates were incubated with 5×10^5 thymocytes or 1×10^5 thymocyte hybridomas or Con A + IL-2 activated thymocytes for 1 h at 37°C. Fetal thymocytes were taken from thymuses of 17-day-old fetuses. Cortisone-resistant thymocytes were obtained after treatment of adult (10 weeks old) AO rats with 150 mg/kg b.w. 2 days before their sacrifice. Thymocytes were activated after stimulation with PMA (20 ng/ml) for 30 min or with Con A (1 μg/ml) + 3 U/ml of human recombinant IL-2 for 3 days. BWRT-2 ($CD4^{+/-}CD8^{+/-}\alpha\beta TCR^{+/-}$) and BWRT-3 ($CD4^{+}CD8^{+}\alpha\beta TCR^{+/-}$) thymocyte hybridomas were produced by fusing resting rat thymocytes with the BW5147 thymoma line as described (31).
[a]TEC lines were stimulated for 2 days with 100 U/ml of recombinant rat IFNγ.
Non-adherent cells were removed by washing and adherent cells were calculated. The percentages of bound thymocytes were determined and expressed as mean of quadriplicates ±SD of a representative of three similar experiments.

The binding of cortical phenotype thymocytes to the medullary TEC line is not an unexpected phenomenon, since similar results have already been published for a mouse medullary TEC line, E5 (36). We think that such a process might be relevant for in vivo interactions since hypertrophic epithelial cells are located in both the medulla and the corticomedullary zone, where immature thymocytes can be in close contact with them. In addition, our immunohistological observations in AO rats demonstrated that approximately 10–20% of thymocytes located in the medulla are $CD4^+CD8^+$ (data not shown).

The data presented in Table 2.3 also show that stimulation of thymocytes with PMA or TEC lines with IFNγ increased the adhesion process. It is known that PMA, a potent stimulator of PKC, transiently increases the affinity of LFA-1 for its ligands by inducing conformational changes in the integrin (37). This is also confirmed in our experiments (Vučević *et al.*, manuscript in preparation) that PMA stimulated thymocyte binding to TEC lines via LFA-1. IFNγ has been known to modulate the expression of different adhesion molecules on various cell lines (38). In our experiments

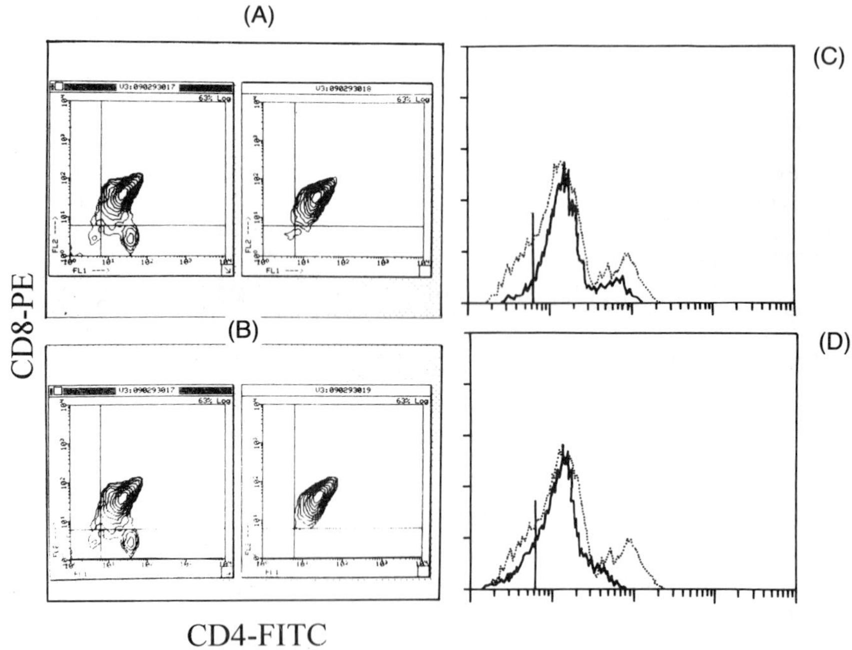

Fig. 2.2 Double immunofluorescence staining of thymocytes which bind to the TE-R 2.5 line (A) (right) and the R-TNC.1 line (B) (right) by anti-CD4 and anti-CD8 mAbs. The control (left) represents total thymocytes. Single immunofluorescence staining of thymocytes by an anti-$\alpha\beta$ TCR mAb (R-73). Solid lines represent histograms of adherent thymocytes to TE-R 2.5 cells (C) and R-TNC. 1 cells (D). Dotted lines represent histograms of total thymocytes. Thymocytes were stained by mAbs in suspension and analysed on a FACScan flow cytometer (Becton-Dickinson).

this cytokine upregulated the expression of class I on both lines and induced the expression of class II MHC molecules and ICAM-1 (Table 2.2). As seen later in antibody blocking studies, some of these findings could be relevant for increased thymocyte binding to these TEC lines.

ADHESION MOLECULES INVOLVED IN THE BINDING OF THYMOCYTES TO TEC LINES

It is known that binding between TEC and thymocytes is mediated by different cell surface molecules. Although the contact between TCR, CD4 and CD8 antigens expressed on thymocytes and MHC molecules expressed on TEC ensures the signals required for these events, its affinity is not sufficient to sustain the strong cell–cell binding (2,39).

Experiments performed in several laboratories have demonstrated that TEC–thymocyte binding is predominantly mediated via other receptor–ligand pairs. However, little is known about the differences in expression of particular adhesion molecules on TEC subsets and their involvement in adhesion to different thymocyte subsets. To study these processes we used an indirect approach by comparing the involvement of particular adhesion molecules on R-TNC.1 and TE-R 2.5 cell lines. Both lines were stimulated with IFNγ which corresponded better to their phenotypic counterparts in vivo, at least judged by the expression of MHC molecules and ICAM-1.

CD2/LFA-3 and LFA-1/ICAM-1 interactions

We found that CD2 is partly involved in the binding between thymocytes and TEC lines (Fig. 2.3). The inhibitory effect of OX-34 (anti-CD2) mAb was stronger when the TE-R 2.5 cell line was used (approximately 40% inhibition) in comparison to the R-TNC.1 cell line (25–30% inhibition). Results directly comparable with ours are those of Kinebuchi *et al.* who showed a similar inhibitory effect of OX-34 mAb on the adhesion between rat thymocytes and the Tu-D3 rat TEC line (40). Some authors reported stronger inhibition mediated by anti-CD2 mAbs in a similar assay at 4°C using non-cloned human TEC (41). The differences could also result from the expression of ligands for CD2 on TEC. It is known that LFA-3, a ligand for human CD2, is expressed on both cortical and medullary TEC in situ and in culture (41). However, little is known about the expression of CD48, a ligand for CD2 in mouse and rat (42) on TEC both in vivo and in vitro.

We demonstrated that LFA-1 and its ligand ICAM-1 are also partly involved in the binding of thymocytes to both cortical and medullary TEC lines. After prolonged incubation (3 h), inhibitory effects of these mAbs were not observed (19). The results are in agreement with those of Lepesant *et al.* (43) who showed that LFA-1 is involved in stabilization of the early, rapid phase of thymocyte adhesion to a murine TEC line which constitutively expressed ICAM-1 in culture. Other authors reported different results, showing that the binding of resting thymocytes to TEC was not dependent on LFA-1. In contrast, the adhesion of Con A + IL-2 activated human thymocytes to IFNγ-stimulated TEC was predominantly mediated by the LFA-1/ICAM-1 interaction (44,45). In our opinion, the differences among these experiments might result from the nature and origin of TEC, differences in the binding assays used, and incubation time.

Thy-1, CD4, and CD8 molecules

We also identified some other cell-surface molecules which participate in thymocyte/TEC binding. One of them is Thy 1. Anti-Thy 1 mAb partly inhibited thymocyte adhesion to both lines but its inhibitory effect was

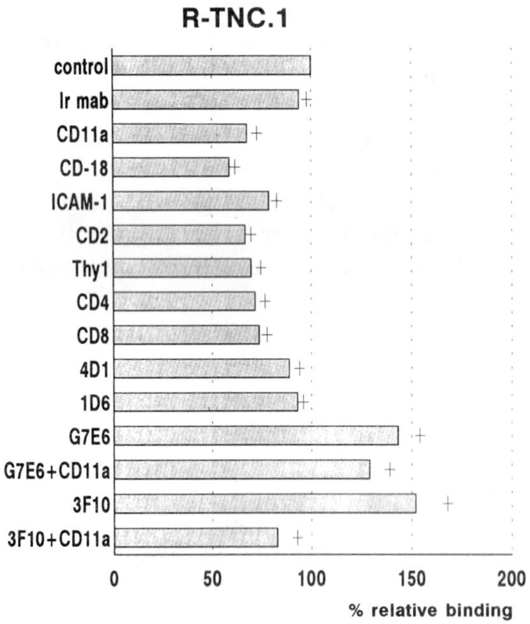

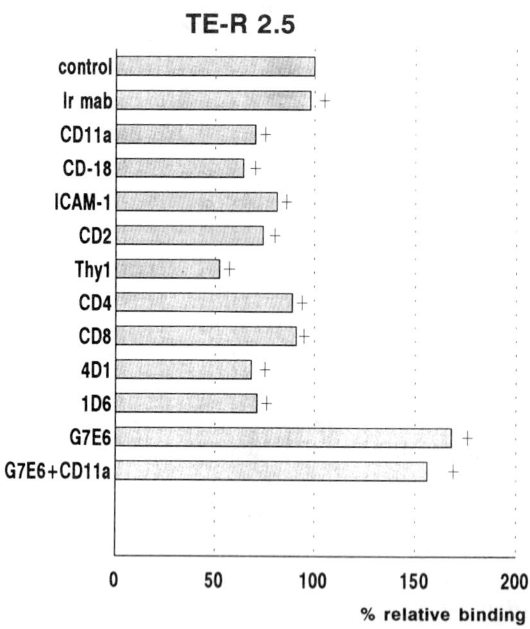

Fig. 2.3 Effect of mAbs on thymocyte binding to IFNγ stimulated TEC-lines. Thymocyte binding was determined after 45 min of cell cultures at 37°C as previously described (19). Values (mean ± SD from 4–6 different experiments) are given as percentage binding to control (without mAb).

stronger when the medullary TE-R 2.5 cell line was used (Fig. 2.3). It is known that Thy 1 is involved in both cell adhesion and signal transduction. Previous results showed that this molecule mediates cell adhesion via surface molecules on bone marrow stromal cells (46). Its importance in thymocyte/TEC interactions has already been reported by He *et al.* (47). They found that Thy 1 supported the adhesion of mouse thymocytes as well as the AKR 1 thymoma line to mouse cloned TEC lines through a calcium-independent mechanism, especially at the level of initial cell contact at 4°C. The possible ligand on TEC lines was not identified. It seems unlikely that it would be Thy 1 itself because most TEC in culture are Thy 1 negative. The same authors demonstrated later that one of ligands for Thy 1 could be sulfated glycans present on TEC surface (48).

Anti-CD4 and anti-CD8 mAbs partly inhibited thymocyte binding only to cortical, but not to medullary TEC (Fig. 2.3). Lepesant *et al.* (43) also showed that coreceptor molecules CD4 and CD8 were partly involved in adhesion of mouse thymocytes to mouse TEC lines. In contrast to our results these TEC lines were predominantly of medullary origin. Li *et al.* (49) did not find a significant role of CD4 and CD8 in the nursing activity of mouse cortical TEC line (TNC). The inhibitory effect of these mAbs in our experiments could be a consequence of the blocking of CD4 and CD8 binding to class II and class I MHC antigens, respectively, expressed on cortical TEC. This is in agreement with the upregulation (class I) or induction (class II) of expression of these molecules on IFNγ stimulated TEC lines (Table 2.2). However, OX-3 (anti-class II MHC) or OX-18 (anti-class I MHC) mAbs did not exert any significant inhibitory effect.

It is possible that the mAbs directed to MHC were not blocking or mAbs to coreceptor molecules could influence the thymocyte adhesion in some other way. Lepesant *et al.* (43) found that an anti-mouse CD4 mAb inhibited thymocyte binding to TEC lines which are MHC class II negative. The authors suggest that the CD4 molecule could interact with a transducing molecule TCR-CD3 and that anti-CD4 mAb could block thymocyte activation mediated through CD4 which is important in the enhancement of cell adhesion. A role of the TCR-CD3 molecule in these processes has been demonstrated since an anti-CD3 mAb induced thymocyte adhesion to mouse TEC which was probably a consequence of an increased affinity of LFA-1 for its ligands (50).

The reason why anti-CD4 and anti-CD8 mAbs were not efficient in blocking thymocyte adhesion to the medullary TEC line, which expressed comparable levels of class I and class II MHC as did the R-TNC.1 line is not clear. A possible explanation could be that binding of thymocytes through other adhesion molecules to the medullary line is stronger than to the cortical line, so that potential involvement of these coreceptor molecules is difficult to assess.

β_1 integrins/extracellular matrix components and lectins

All the results presented here show that different, well-defined adhesion molecules participate in thymocyte binding to TEC lines. However, the significant binding (35–50%) observed in the presence of a cocktail of these inhibitory mAbs (data not shown) suggest the involvement of other antigens as well. Among them the role of β_1 integrins and their ligands has been examined. Watt *et al.* (51) studied the expression of β_1 integrins in human thymus. They found that the majority of thymocytes expressed the integrin VLA-β_1 as well as VLA-4 and VLA-6. In addition, some transformed human TEC lines expressed VLA-β_1 and different α chains VLA-2, VLA-3 and VLA-6. These cells were also weakly positive with anti-β_3, -β_4 and -vitronectin receptor mAbs.

The thymus also contains a number of extracellular matrix (ECM) components which are ligands for β_1 integrins, including types I, III, and IV collagen, fibronectin (FN), laminin (LN) and tenascin. FN, LN, and collagen type IV which were found in basement membranes bordering the capsule, septae, and perivascular spaces were also identified inside TEC and in the spaces between TEC, suggesting that TEC can produce these ECM glycoproteins (52).

The role of VLA-4 in thymocyte development was studied by Sawada *et al.* (53) who found that it is strongly expressed on $CD4^-CD8^-$ and immature $CD4^-CD8^{+/-}$ thymocyte populations. Its expression is significantly reduced on $CD4^+CD8^+$ and $CD4^+CD8^-$ or $CD4^-CD8^+$ cells. This contrasts with the increase in levels of LFA-1 along with thymocyte maturation. DN thymocytes predominantly adhered to a monolayer of a thymic stromal cell clone, MRL 104.8a, that induces growth-maintenance and differentiation of these thymocytes. The adhesion was almost completely inhibited by simultaneous addition of antibodies to FN (a ligand for VLA-4) and mixture of peptides capable of binding to FN receptors. These findings suggest that interaction through FN expressed on stromal cells and FN receptors on DN thymocytes has a crucial role in inducing and/or supporting differentiation of these cells. The results also indicate that these adhesive interactions might occur in vivo in the cortex. Villa-Verde *et al.* (54) showed that the physiology of cortical, freshly isolated TNC is partially under the control of ECM and receptors for ECM. They showed that in vitro spontaneous thymocyte release from TNC was accelerated by FN and LN, whereas anti-ECM mAbs exhibited a blocking effect. Similar results were obtained with anti-ECM receptor (VLA 5, β_1 integrin and CD44) mAbs. Moreover, these mAbs abrogated in vitro reconstitution of TNC complexes and thymocyte adhesion to TNC-derived epithelial cultures.

Giunta *et al.* (55) described an integrin of the VLA subfamily composed of the known β_1 chain and a novel α chain. The molecule is expressed on the surface of medullary TEC and is involved in the adhesion between TEC and thymocytes, but not peripheral blood T lymphocytes.

Different lectins are also expressed on distinct subpopulations of TEC (56). Baum *et al.* have recently demonstrated that one of them, galectin 1, is synthesized by human TEC. This lectin binds to oligosaccharide ligands (core 2 *O*-glycan) on the surface of thymocytes and T lymphoblastoid cells. Binding of thymocytes to TEC in vitro was inhibited by a polyclonal antibody to galectin 1 and by two mAbs which recognize carbohydrate epitopes on CD43 and CD45 expressed on immature, but not mature, thymocytes (57). These results suggest that galectin 1 might be relevant to TEC/thymocyte interactions in the cortex.

Novel adhesion molecules

Recent findings demonstrate that human and murine thymic epithelial cells express a putative ligand for CD6 (58). CD6 is a type I transmembrane protein expressed by thymocytes, mature T cells, a subset of B cells, and some cells in the brain. Among a panel of anti-CD6 mAbs, one was able to partially block thymocyte-TEC binding. The CD6 ligand on TEC was characterized as a new adhesion molecule. It is a 100–105 kDa antigen named ALCAM (**a**ctivated **l**eukocyte **c**ell **a**dhesion **m**olecule) because it is expressed on activated leukocytes and other non-lymphoid cells (58). The antigen of similar molecular mass (107 kDa) was identified by Kina *et al.* (59) on a mouse thymic stromal cell line by the use of polyclonal antisera. The serum inhibited complex formation between this stromal line and lymphoid tumour cells. It is not known whether this adhesion molecule is identical, similar to, or different from ALCAM.

The next two adhesion molecules seem to be relevant for binding of thymocytes to cortical and medullary TEC lines, respectively. The first one, named 4F1, is expressed on cortical TEC but not on medullary TEC in mouse thymus (60). Imami *et al.* (60) showed, using western blotting, that the molecule to which 4F1 binds is expressed in four forms, 29, 32, 40 and 43 kDa. All forms carry *N*-linked carbohydrate and may exist in both transmembrane and phosphoinositol-linked forms. The molecular and functional characteristics suggest that the 4F1 antigen is a novel adhesion molecule involved in binding of thymocytes to TEC in vitro and that may be involved in intrathymic T-lymphocyte differentiation. The second one, which is identified by Couture *et al.* (61), is present on thymic medullary TEC which selectively bind $CD4^+CD8^+$ thymocytes. This adhesion molecule is composed of two non-covalently associated glycoproteins of 23 kDa and 45 kDa, respectively, both of which are needed to bind to thymocytes. The heterodimer is associated with a 90 kDa glycoprotein. Further experiments from this laboratory demonstrated that gp 23/45-mediated contact with thymocytes induced de novo tyrosine phosphorylation of gp 90 (possibly via autophosphorylation) suggesting that the protein tyrosine kinase responsible for gp 90 neophosphorylation is itself an integral part of the adhesion complex (62).

We screened a panel of mAbs raised against the antigens of our TEC lines and identified two of them (1D6 and 4D1) which partly inhibited thymocyte binding to medullary, but not to cortical TEC lines (Table 2.2, Fig. 2.3).

1D6 stains in situ both cortical and medullary epithelium as well as a subset of thymocytes. In addition it binds to nervous tissue and to some other stromal and hemopoietic cells in different organs. TE-R 2.5 cells were strongly 1D6$^+$ but both unstimulated or IFNγ stimulated R-TNC.1 cells were only weakly positive. This is probably why the antibody did not affect thymocyte binding to the cortical TEC line. Immunoprecipitation studies of TE-R 2.5 cell lysates showed a strong band of 135 kDa (Čolić *et al.*, manuscript in preparation). Some of these characteristics indicate that 1D6 might detect a rat equivalent of mouse neuronal cell adhesion molecule (NCAM) which has been shown to have a role both in homotypic and heterotypic adhesion of thymocytes in the thymus through homophilic interactions (63). However, cloning of 1D6 antigens is necessary to confirm this hypothesis.

The other mAb, 4D1 binds to TE-R 2.5 cells. In situ, it stains the subcapsular and medullary epithelium and macrophages, whereas thymocytes are negative. In addition, some epithelial cells and components in the interstitium of other organs are also positive. Up to now the nature of the antigen recognized by 4D1 mAb has not been identified but experiments are currently in progress.

Shared molecules

Monoclonal antibody technology enabled the discovery of different novel antigenic determinants on TEC. Unexpectedly, a large number of them are molecules shared between TEC and developing thymocytes (4,5). Detailed studies have confirmed that both cell types synthesize the molecules de novo and that the antigen detected on the two cell populations is genuinely the same, rather than simply sharing a cross-reactive epitope. The significance of molecules shared between two interacting cells is not clear. They could be involved in homotypic or heterotypic binding with the same or a complementary structure on the opposing cell surface, respectively. Alternatively, the molecules might act as receptors for soluble ligand produced via an autocrine or paracrine mechanisms (4,5).

One such shared molecule has been recently characterized in rat by Kinebuchi *et al.* (40) by a murine mAb named 7D3. The antigen is expressed on thymic epithelium, and most thymocytes. The mAb recognized a single polypeptide of 80 kDa on both cell types. It seems, however, that it is differentially glycosylated on these two cell populations. 7D3 is characterized as a new adhesion molecule because of its ability to inhibit thymocyte aggregation induced by phorbol esters and adhesion of thymocytes or thymic lymphoma cells to TEC. The binding was mediated by 7D3 antigen on TEC and by undefined ligand for 7D3 on thymocytes.

We also identified two antigens by G7E6 and 3F10 mAbs which are shared between thymocytes and thymic microenvironmental cells. Unlike 7D3 mAb, they significantly stimulate TEC/thymocyte binding (Fig. 2.3). We gave them working names, **t**hymic **s**hared **a**dhesion **m**odulating **a**ntigens (TSAMA) 1 and 2, respectively.

G7E6 recognizes a 61 kDa antigen expressed on thymic epithelium, 40–50% of thymocytes, all granulocytes, and monocytes, but not on peripheral lymphocytes. The R-TNC.1 and TE-R 2.5 lines are both positive. We found that G7E6 stimulates thymocyte adhesion to both TEC lines, the effect being more pronounced after prolonged cell incubation (3 h), but is neither mediated by the LFA-1 molecule, nor a consequence of simple cross-linking of relevant antigens on different cell types by the mAb. G7E6 also partly inhibits thymocyte proliferation induced by Con A and IL-2 but does not influence apoptosis of thymocytes.

3F10 mAb recognizes an antigen broadly distributed on various leukocytes and non-lymphoid cells. Almost all thymocytes and different thymocyte hybridomas are positive. Both cortical and medullary TEC lines are positive with this mAb too, and the antigen expression was down-regulated by IL-1 or TNFα, but not by IL-6 or IFNγ. Western blot analysis showed that 3F10 mAb recognizes two antigens (60 and 55 kDa) of whole thymocyte lysates. The mAb stimulates homotypic thymocyte adhesion as well as thymocyte adhesion to TEC at 37°C. Both processes completely depend on LFA-1 (Fig. 2.3).

As reported, the list of adhesion molecules mediating thymocyte/TEC interactions is very long. It is not yet complete, since at least another two important adhesion molecules have been identified on human TEC, CD40 (64) and CD23 (65). All these results clearly indicate the complexity of adhesion molecules and their ligands expressed on TEC which are necessary for optimal TEC/thymocyte contact. Some of them show different expression on particular TEC lines, supporting the concept that TEC subsets of different regions provide different signals for distinct phases of thymocyte development. At the moment we do not know the sequence of their involvement in the adhesion process, which of them act synergistically or antagonistically with others, what signals are generated upon their engagement, or their significance for TEC/thymocyte binding in vivo. The use of well-defined TEC lines which reflect their normal counterpart in vivo and specific mAbs reactive with the adhesion molecules could help in answering most of these questions.

CONCLUSION

Different subsets of TEC provide distinct stimuli to developing thymocytes in the thymus via direct cell–cell interactions and soluble molecules. A number of various receptor–ligand pairs have been described to participate in these processes, but little is known about the differences in the expression of particular adhesion molecules on TEC subpopulations and their involvement in the binding to different thymocyte subsets. We cloned two TEC lines (R-TNC.1 and TE-R 2.5) from long-term culture of the rat thymic epithelium. Based on detailed multimarker phenotypic analysis and electron microscopy it was concluded that the R-TNC.1 line is a type of cortical TEC with nursing activity whereas the TE-R 2.5 line belongs to the medullary (hypertrophic type) TEC. Using an in vitro assay we showed that R-TNC.1 and TE-R 2.5 cell lines differently bind thymocytes and T cell hybridomas. Binding of thymocytes to both lines is mediated by LFA-1/ICAM-1, CD2, and Thy 1 but the extent of binding inhibition in the presence of specific mAbs depends on TEC lines used. CD4 and CD8 as well as two novel molecules expressed on TEC, defined by 4D1 and 1D6 mAbs, are involved in adhesion of thymocytes to the medullary line. Two mAbs, G7E6 and 3F10, which detect molecules shared between thymocytes and TEC potentiate TEC/thymocyte binding via an LFA-1-dependent and an LFA-1-independent pathway, respectively.

REFERENCES

1. Sprent, J., D. Lo, E. K. Gao and Y. Ron. 1988. T cell selection in the thymus. *Immunol. Rev.* **101**:173–90.
2. Van Ewijk, W. 1991. T cell differentiation is influenced by thymic microenvironments. *Annu. Rev. Immunol.* **9**:591–615.
3. Nikolic-Zugic, J, 1991. T cell development: Phenotypic and functional stages in the intrathymic development of alpha-beta T cells. *Immunol. Today* **12**:65–70.
4. Boyd, L. R., C. L. Tucek, D. I. Godfrey *et al.* 1993. The thymic microenvironment. Inside the thymus. *Immunol. Today* **14**:445–59.
5. Ritter, M. A and R. L. Boyd. 1993. Development in the thymus: it takes two to tango. *Immunol. Today* **14**:462–9.
6. Ceredig, R. 1986. Proliferation in vitro and interleukin production by 14 day fetal and adult Lyt- 2- L3T4-mouse thymocytes. *J. Immunol.* **137**:2260–9.
7. Van Ewijk, W. 1988. Cell surface topography of thymic microenvironments. *Lab. Invest.* **59**:579–90.
8. Ritter, M. A. and I. N. Crispe. 1992. In: *The thymus* (In Focus.) Male D. ed. Oxford University Press, Oxford, p.1.
9. VanWijngaert, F. P., M. D. Kendall, H. J. Schuurman *et al.* 1984. Heterogeneity of epithelial cells in the human thymus. An ultrastructural study. *Cell. Tiss. Res.* **237**:227–37.
10. Nabarra, B. and I. Andrianarison. 1987. Ultrastructural studies of thymic reticulum: I. The epithelial component. Thymus **9**:95–121.
11. Savino, W., P. C. Huang, A. Corrigan *et al.* 1984. Thymic hormone-containing cells. V. Immunohistological detection of metallothionein within the cells bearing thymulin (a zinc-containing hormone) in human and mouse thymuses. *J. Histochem. Cytochem.* **32**:942–6.
12. van Haelst, U. 1967. In: Light and electron microscopic study of the normal

and pathological thymus of the rat. I. The normal thymus. *Z. Zellforsch.* **77**:534–53.

13. Čolić, M. 1987. Morphological and functional characteristics of thymic cells in mice subjected to combined radiation injury. PhD thesis, MMA Belgrade.
14. Kampinga, J., S. Berges, R. Boyd *et al.* 1989. Thymic epithelial antibodies: immunohistological analysis and introduction of CTES nomenclature. *Thymus* **13**:165–74.
15. Brekelmans, P. and W. van Ewijk. 1990. Phenotypic characterization of murine thymic microenvironments. *Semin. Immunol.* **2**:13–24.
16. Čolić, M., D. Matanović, L. Hegedis and A. Dujić. 1988. Immunohistochernical characterization of rat thymic non-lymphoid cells. I. Epithelial and mesenchymal components defined by monoclon alantibodies. *Immunology* **65**:277–84.
17. Pavlović, M. D., M. Čolić, D. Vučević and A. Dujić. 1993. Two novel monoclonal antibodies reactive with different components of the rat thymic epithelium. *Thymus* **21**:235–46.
18. Čolić, M., N. Stojanović, Lj. Popović and A. Dujić. 1992. Phenotypic and ultrastructural characterization of an epithelial cell line established from rat thymic cultures. *Immunology* **77**:201–7.
19. Čolić, M., D. Vučević, M. Miyasaka *et al.* 1994. Adhesion molecules involved in the binding and subsequent engulfment of thymocytes by a rat thymic epithelial cell line. *Immunology* **83**:449–56.
20. Čolić, M., S. Jovanovic, S. Mitrovic and A. Dujić. 1989. Immunohistochemical identification of six cytokeratin-defined subsets of the rat thymic epithelial cells. *Thymus* **13**:175–85.
21. Savino, W. and M. Dardenne. 1988. Development studies on expression of monoclonal antibody-defined cytokeratins by thymic epithelial cells from normal and autoimmune mice. *J. Histochem. Cytochem.* **36**:1123–9.
22. De Souza, R. L. M. and W. Savino. 1993. Modulation of cytokeratin expression in the hamster thymus: evidence for a plasticity of the thymic epithelium. *Dev. Immunol.* **3**:137–46.
23. Moll, F., W. W. Franke and D. L. Schiller. 1982. The catalog of human cytekeratins: patterns of expression on normal epithelia, tumors and cultured cells. *Cell* **31**:11–24.
24. Čolić, M., S. Jovanovic, M. Vasiljevski and A. Dujić. 1990. Ontogeny of rat thymic epithelium defined by monoclonal anticytokeratin antibodies. *Dev. Immunol.* **1**:67–75.
25. Osculati, F., G. Balercia and G. Mathe. 1988. Human thymic epithelium in culture: an experimental model for the study of thymic microenvironment. *Biomed. Pharmacother.* **42**:395–407.
26. Piltch, A., F. Naylor and J. Hayashi. 1988. A cloned rat thymic epithelial cell line established from serum-free selective culture. *In Vitro* **24**:289–99.
27. Farr, A. G., J. Eisenhardt and S. K. Anderson. 1986. Isolation of murine thymic epithelium and improved method for its propagation in vitro. *Anat. Rec.* **216**:85–94.
28. Small, M., W. van Ewijk, A. M. Grown and R. V. Rouse. 1989. Identification of subpopulations of mouse thymic epithelial cells in culture. *Immunology* **68**:371–7.
29. Fabien, N., C. Auger, M. Bounard *et al.* 1989. Quantitative analysis of cultured thymic reticulo-epithelial cells labelled by different antibodies: a flow cytometric study. *Clin. Exp. Immunol.* **75**:292–8.
30. Čolić, M., N. Pejnović, M. Kataranovski *et al.* 1991. Rat thymic epithelial cells in culture constitutively secrete IL-1 and IL-6. *Int. lmmunol.* **3**:1165–74.

31. Popović, Lj., M. Čolić and D. Kosec, 1994. Production and characterization of the rat thymic T-cell hybridomas. *Vojnosanit. Pregl.* **51**:56–9.
32. Wekerle, H. and U. P. Ketelson. 1980. Thymic nurse cells: I-A bearing epithelium involved in T lymphocyte differentiation. *Nature* **283**:402–4.
33. Hiramine, C., K. Hojo, M. Koseto *et al.* 1990. Establishment of a murine thymic epithelial cell line capable of inducing both thymic nurse cell formation and thymocyte apoptosis. *Lab. Invest.* **62**:41–64.
34. Itoh, T., H. Doi, S. Chin *et al.* 1988. Establishment of mouse thymic nurse cell clones from a spontaneous BALB/c thymic tumor. *Eur. J. Immunol.* **18**:821–4.
35. Nishimura, T., Y. Takeuchi, Y. Ichimura *et al.* 1990. Thymic stromal cell clone with nursing activity supports the growth and differentiation of murine $CD4^+8^+$ thymocytes in vitro. *J. Immunol.* **145**:4012–17.
36. Potworowski, F. E., P. Hugo and C. Couture. 1989. Binding of cortical thymocytes to a medullary epithelial cell line: a brief review. *Thymus* **13**:237–43.
37. Arnaout, M. A. 1990. Structure and function of the leukocyte adhesion molecules CD11/CD18. *Blood* **75**:1037–50.
38. Berrih, S. F., F. Arenzana-Seisdedos, S. Cohen *et al.* 1985. Interferon-gamma modulates HLA class II antigen expression on cultured thymic epithelial cells. *J. Immunol.* **135**:1165–71.
39. Patel, D. D. and B. F. Haynes. 1993. Cell adhesion molecules involved in intrathymic T cell development. *Sem. Immunol.* **5**:282–92.
40. Kinebuchi, M., T. Ide, D. Lupin *et al.* 1991. A novel cell surface antigen involved in thymocyte and thymic epithelial cell adhesion. *J. Immunol.* **146**:3721–8.
41. Vollger, L., D. T. Tuck, T. A. Springer *et al.* 1987. Thymocyte binding to human thymic epithelial cells inhibited by monoclonal antibodies to CD2 and LFA-3 antigens. *J. Immunol.* **138**:358–63.
42. Brown, H. M. S. Preston and A. N. Barclay. 1995. A sensitive assay for detecting low-affinity interactions at the cell surface reveals no additional ligands for the adhesion pair rat CD2. *Eur. J. Immunol.* **25**:3222–8.
43. Lepesant, H., H. Reggio, M. Pierres and P. Naquet. 1990. Mouse thymic epithelial cell lines interact with and select a $CD3^{low}CD4^+CD8^+$ thymocyte subset through an LFA-1-dependent adhesion–de-adhesion mechanisms. *Int. Immunol.* **2**:1021–30.
44. Singer, K. H., S. M. Denning, L. P. Whichard and B. Haynes. 1990. Thymocyte LFA-1 and thymocyte epithelial cell ICAM-1 molecules mediate binding of activated human thymocytes to thymic epithelial cells. *J. Immunol.* **144**:2931–9.
45. Nonoyama, S., M. Nakayama, T. Shijohara and J. I. Yata. 1989. Only dull $CD3^-$ thymocytes bind to thymic epithelial cells. The binding is elicited by both CD2/LFA-3 and LFA-1/ICAM-1 interactions. *Eur. J. Immunol.* **19**:1631–5.
46. Irlin, Y. and A. Peled. 1992. Thy-1 antigen-mediated adhesion of mouse lymphoid cells to stromal cells of haemopoetic origin. *Immunol. Lett.* **33**:233–8.
47. He, H. T., P. Naquet, D. Caillol and M. Pierres. 1991. Thy-1 supports adhesion of mouse thymocytes to thymic epithelial cells through a Ca^{2+}-independent mechanism. *J. Exp. Med.* **173**:515–18.
48. Hueber, A. O., M. Pierres and H. He. 1992. Sulfated glycans directly interact with mouse Thy-1 and negatively regulate Thy-1-mediated adhesion of thymocytes to thymic epithelial cells. *J. Immunol.* **148**:3692–9.
49. Li, Y., M. Pezzano, D. Philp, V. Reid and J. Guyden. 1992. Thymic nurse cells exclusively bind and internalize $CD4^+CD8^+$ thymocytes. *Cell. Immunol.* **140**:495–506.

50. Dustin, M. L. and T. A. Springer. 1989. T-cell receptor cross-linking transiently stimulates adhesiveness through LFA-1. *Nature* **341**:619–24.
51. Watt, S. M., J. A. Thomas, A. J. Edwards *et al.* 1992. Adhesion receptors are differentially expressed on developing thymocytes and epithelium in human thymus. *Exp. Hematol.* **20**:1101–11.
52. Lannes-Vieira, J., M. Dardenne and W. Savino. 1991. Extracellular matrix components of the mouse thymus microenvironment: ontogenetic studies and modulation by glucocorticoid hormones. *J. Histochem. Cytochem.* **39**:1539–46.
53. Sawada, M., J. Nagamine, K. Takeda *et al.* 1992. Expression of VLA-4 on thymocytes. Maturation stage-associated transition and its correlation with their capacity to adhere to thymic stromal cells. *J. Immunol.* **149**:3517–24.
54. Villa-Verde, D. M. S., J. Machado, L. Candido *et al.* 1994. Extracellular matrix components of the mouse thymus microenvironrnent. IV. Modulation of thymic nurse cells by extracellular matrix ligands and receptors. *Eur. J. Immunol.* **24**:659–64.
55. Guinta, M., A. Favre, D. Ramarli *et al.* 1991. A novel integrin involved in thymocyte-thymic epithelial cell interactions. *J. Exp. Med.* **173**:1537–48.
56. Wiley, E. L., J. M. Nosal and R. G. Freeman. 1990. Immunohistochemical demonstration of H antigen, peanut agglutinin receptor, and *Saphora japonica* receptor expression in infant thymuses and thymic neoplasias. *American Journal of Clinical Pathology* **93**:44–8.
57. Baum, L. G., M. Pang, N. L. Perillo *et al.* 1995. Human thymic epithelial cells express endogenous lectin, galectin-1, which binds to core 2 O-glycans on thymocytes and T lymphoblastoid cells. *J. Exp. Med.* **181**:877–87.
58. Bowen, M. A., D. D. Patel, X. Li *et al.* 1995. Cloning, mapping, and characterization of activated leukocyte-cell adhesion molecule (ALCAM), a CD6 ligand. *J. Exp. Med.* **181**:2213–20.
59. Kina, T., A. S. Majumdar, S. Heimfeld *et al.* 1991. Identification of 107-kD glycoprotein that mediates adhesion between stromal cells and hematolymphoid cells. *J. Exp. Med.* **173**:373–81.
60. Imami, N., H. M. Ladyman, E. Spanopoulou and M. A. Ritter. 1992. A novel adhesion molecule in the murine thymic microenvironment: functional and biochemical analysis. *Develop. Immunol.* **2**:161–73.
61. Couture, C., P. C. Patel and E. F. Potworowski. 1990. A novel thymic epithelial adhesion molecule. *Eur. J. Immunol.* **20**:2769–73.
62. Couture, C., G. Amarante-Mendes and E. F. Potworowski. 1992. Tyrosine kinase activation in thymic epithelial cells: necessity of thymocyte contact through the gp23/45/90 adhesion complex. *Eur. J. Immunol.* **22**:2579–85.
63. Brunet, J. F., M. R. Hirsch, P. Naquet *et al.* 1989. Developmentally regulated expression of neural cell adhesion molecule (NCAM) by mouse thymocytes. *Eur. J. Immunol.* **19**:837–41.
64. Galy, A. H. M. and H. Spits. 1992. CD40 is functionally expressed on human thymic epithelial cells. *J. Immunol.* **149**:775–82.
65. Dalloul, A. H., C. Fourcade, P. Debre and M. D. Mossalayi. 1991. Thymic epithelial cell-derived supernatants sustain the maturation of human prothymocytes: involvement of interleukin-1 and CD23. *Eur. J. Immunol.* **22**:2633–6.

3

Non-deletional Tolerant State to a Cognate Antigen in TCR Transgenic Mice

Clio Mamalaki, Marianna Murdjeva, Mauro Tolaini, Trisha Norton and Dimitris Kioussis

It is important to understand the mechanisms of induction and maintenance of tolerant state of T cells in order to be able to intervene in cases where their untimely activation causes autoimmune disease. Maintenance of T-cell tolerance is generally accomplished by elimination of self reactive cells either during development in the thymus (1,2) or after encountering self antigen in the periphery (3–6). However, some potentially autoreactive cells are not physically deleted but are rendered unresponsive to self antigens (7–9). The unresponsiveness maintained in some non-deletional tolerant states has been attributed to the downregulation of the reactive TCR (10) and/or the coreceptor CD4 or CD8 (6). In addition, other factors such as transcription levels of certain genes or efficiency in costimulation and signal transduction may be affected in this process (11).

We have generated a TCR transgenic mouse which bears on most of its T cells a TCR (F5) which recognizes a nonamer peptide (aa 366–374; NP peptide) from influenza virus nucleoprotein in the context of class I MHC (D^b) (12,13). Most T cells in F5 TCR transgenic mice are $CD8^+$ cytotoxic and can respond to the cognate antigen (peptide or viral protein) both in vivo and in vitro (14,15). To assess the development of T cells and study the mechanisms of tolerant induction in transgenic mice in which the cognate antigen influenza nucleoprotein is a self antigen, we generated transgenic mice expressing the viral protein under the broadly active H-2K^b promoter. Double transgenic mice (F5TCR/NP) were assessed for F5 T-cell development and for their ability to respond to nucleoprotein antigen.

Immunoregulation in Health and Disease
ISBN 0–12–459460–3

MATERIALS AND METHODS

Experimental animals

Mice were generated and maintained in a conventional colony free of pathogens at the National Institute for Medical Research in London. F5 TCR and H2NP transgenic mice were generated as described previously (16,13) using inbred C57BI/10 mice. Influenza nucleoprotein peptide was dissolved in PBS and injected intraperitoneally as indicated in the figure legends.

Flow cytometry

For three-colour analysis 10^6 thymocytes or lymph node cells were stained with the following antibodies in different combinations : PE-conjugated anti-CD4 (GK1.5) (Becton Dickinson), FITC-conjugated anti-CD8 (53-6.7) (Becton Dickinson), PE-conjugated anti-CD8 (YTS 169.4) (Coulter Immunology), biotinylated anti-Vβ11 (KT11) (17) and biotinylated anti-CD44 (pgp-1) followed by a second layer of tricolour-conjugated Streptavidin (Caltag) or Streptavidin red 670 (Gibco). Three-colour FACS analysis was performed with a FACS-scan laser instrument and Lysis II program (Becton Dickinson).

Isolation of antigen in presenting cells

Thymuses and spleens from adult B10, NP40 and NP47 mice were teased gently and placed in a cocktail with collagenase (Worthington, USA, 1.6 mg/ml) and DNAse (Sigma 0.1%) in RPMI for 1 h at 37°C. Dendritic cells and macrophages were isolated using the method described (18).

Cytotoxic T-cell assays

Effector cells were spleen cells of transgenic mice and targets – EL-4 cells loaded with 100 μl of 100 μM influenza nucleoprotein peptide (NP366-374). The assay was performed as described before (14). The percent specific lysis was calculated according to the formula

$$\% \text{ specific lysis} = \frac{(E - C)}{(M - C)} \times 100$$

where E denotes cpm from wells with effectors present, C is the cpm from control wells with target cells incubated in medium alone, and M = maximum released counts from target cells incubated with 5% Triton. Twelve-point regression analysis was performed for each titration curve and the percentage lysis at an effector : target ratio of 10 : 1 was taken from this curve. Significant positive lysis was taken as levels over 10% specific lysis from curves where the r^2 value lay between 0.80 and 1.00.

Proliferation assays

Responder cells were suspensions of spleen cells in RPMI with supplements. They were dispensed at 1×10^6 cells per 0.2 ml flat bottomed microtitre well for proliferative MLR cultures. Human rIL-2 was added to a final concentration of 10 IU/ml for proliferative assays. Cells used as a source of antigen were spleen cell suspensions from which red blood cells had been removed by brief exposure to hypotonic shock. B10 spleen cells were used either alone (B10) or after 45 min incubation with 100 μM peptide (NP365-379) followed by two washes in RPMI ($B10^p$). Cells were then irradiated 2500 R from a ^{60}Co source immediately before addition to cultures: 5×10^5 cells were added to each 0.2 ml microtitre well for the proliferation assay. Microtitre wells were pulsed at 72 h with 1 μCi/well ^{3}H-thymidine and harvested 6 h later for β-scintillation counting.

RESULTS

Generation of double (F5/NP) transgenic mice

In order to generate mice expressing a transgenic influenza nucleoprotein, we placed the expression of the transgene under the control of the widely expressed class I MHC promoter H-2K^b (H2NP). The construct was injected into fertilized mouse (C57BI/10) eggs and several transgenic lines were generated: four of these were used in our study (H2NP10, H2NP22, H2NP40 and H2NP47). The messenger RNA for the nucleoprotein proved to be too unstable to allow us to perform Northern analysis studies for expression. PCR on RNA from tissues of NP transgenic mice established that the transgene was expressed in these mice (data not shown). To assess the effects of an antigenic molecule expressed as a self protein on the development of F5 T cells, the H2NP transgenic mice were crossed with the F5 TCR transgenic mice. F5/H2NP double transgenic mice were analyzed by FACS analysis and their T-cell development was compared with that seen in F5 (H-2^b) single transgenic mice. The absolute numbers of thymocytes showed a tendency to be reduced in mice expressing transgenic nucleoprotein – approximately $\frac{1}{3}$ to $\frac{1}{2}$ of the number of thymocytes in F5 control mice. In all double transgenic mice the proportions of CD4$^+$CD8$^+$ and CD4$^+$ cells were not affected, whereas the proportion of thymocytes which developed into fully mature CD8$^+$ cells was reduced (Fig. 3.1A). Three-colour FACS analysis of F5 thymocytes stained with antibodies against CD4, CD8, and Vβ11 normally shows two populations of cells with different levels of TCR (Fig. 3.1C): one that stains dull for TCR (TCR^{lo}) and represents the majority of double positive thymocytes (13); and a brightly staining population (TCR^{hi}) which represents mainly single positive mature T cells and those double positive

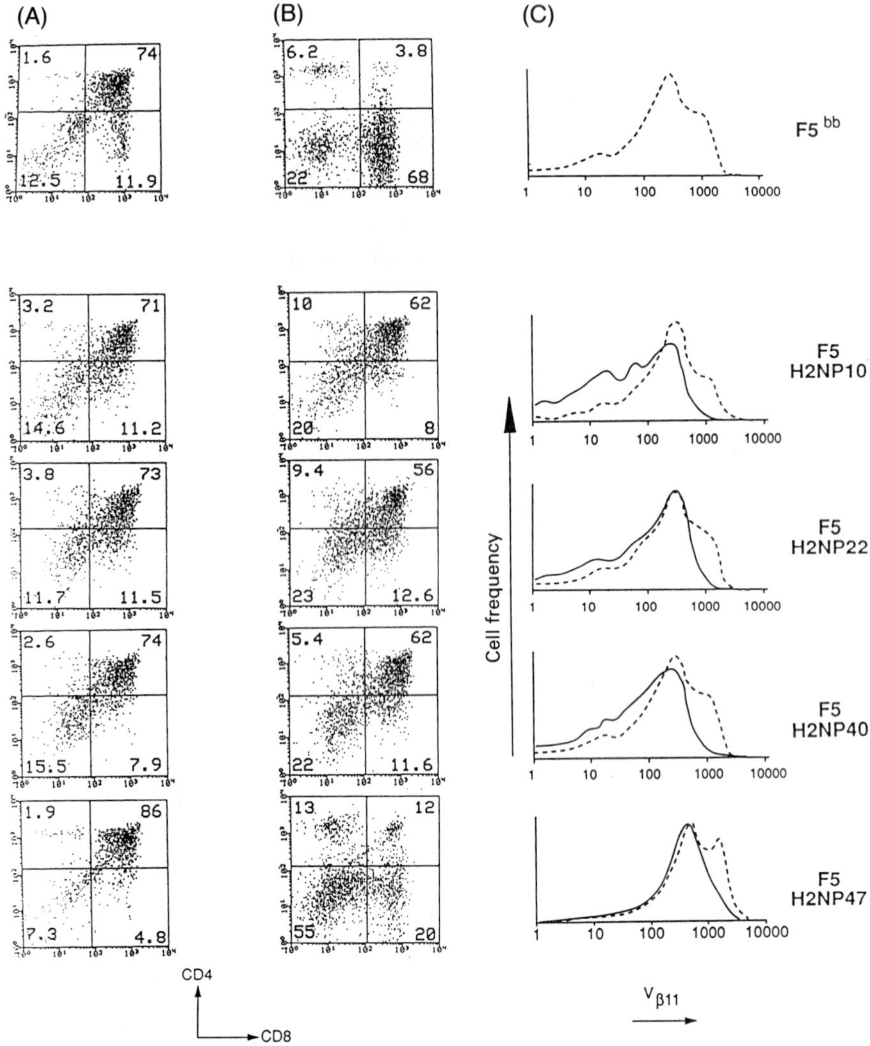

Fig. 3.1 Absence of TCR^{hi} cells in the thymus of F5/H2NP double transgenic mice. Thymocytes from TCR single transgenic or TCR/NP double transgenic mice were stained before (A) or after (B) intraperitoneal treatment for 4 days with 50 nmol antigenic peptide. Anti-CD8 FITC, anti-CD4 PE and biotinylated anti-Vβ11 antibodies were used followed by tricolour-conjugated streptavidin as described in Methods. Dot blots represent two-colour analysis of cells stained with CD4 and CD8. Numbers represent percent proportion of cells in the quadrant. (C) Three-parameter data files were software-gated to generate single-colour staining histograms of Vβ11 expression on total thymocytes. Numbers indicate the mean fluorescence of Vβ11 staining in arbitary units. Solid line: Vβ11 expression on total thymocytes from double transgenic mice. Dotted line: Vβ11 expression on total thymocytes from the F5 control.

cells which have already upregulated their TCR including the intermediate populations $CD4^{+}8^{lo}$ and $CD4^{lo}8^{+}$ (13). When the Vβ11 profile of total thymocytes from F5/NP mice was compared with that of F5 single transgenic mice it became evident that the thymus from double transgenic mice was almost devoid of TCR^{hi} population (Fig. 3.1C). Lymph nodes of the mice described above were stained for CD4, CD8, and Vβ11. Figure 3.2A shows that the proportion of $CD8^{+}$ cells was drastically reduced in the lymph nodes from various double transgenic mice. Gated $CD8^{+}$ cells had reduced levels of transgenic TCR (Fig. 3.2C). This reduction varied from line to line. Since allelic exclusion in TCR mice is not complete, particularly at the α chain gene locus, the presence of $CD4^{+}8^{+}$ thymocytes and $CD8^{+}$ $V\beta11^{+}$ peripheral cells in F5/NP mice could be explained by the fact that they may express endogenous α and β receptors which allow them to be positive selected.

To test whether physical elimination of $F5TCR^{+}$ cells is complete and whether double positive thymocytes and $CD8^{+}$ T cells seen in double transgenic mice are due to the expression of endogenous receptors, we generated F5/NP mice unable to rearrange TCR genes by breeding double transgenics with recombination activating gene-1 deficient mice ($RAG\text{-}1^{-/-}$) (19). In the absence of endogenous TCR rearrangement $CD4^{+}8^{+}$ thymocytes and peripheral $CD8^{+}$ cells are still present. $CD8^{+}$ T cells in lymphoid organs are reduced in numbers and have lower levels of TCR and its coreceptor CD8 in comparison with $CD8^{+}$ cells from $F5/RAG\text{-}1^{-/-}$ (data not shown).

Antigen-presenting cells in H2NP transgenic mice express and present influenza nucleoprotein peptide

Figure 3.3 shows the proliferation of F5 T cells after incubation with $H2^{b}$ (C57BI/10) APC, $H2^{b}$ APC loaded with NP68 peptide, or APC from H2NP40 and H2NP47 mice. The results show that peripheral (A) and thymic (B) APC from H2NP40 mice can stimulate F5 T cells with similar efficiency to $H2^{b}$ APC loaded with NP peptide. Similar results were obtained using APCs from H2NP22 mice. This confirms the expression of the NP transgene in APCs of these mice and explains the phenotype in double transgenic mice. APCs from the spleens or thymus of H2NP47 mice on the other hand stimulated F5 T cells to a lesser extent but consistently above the background. This is taken as an indication that expression of NP in H2NP47 transgenic mice is limited.

Additional evidence that the transgene NP is expressed and presented in H2NP mice comes from analysis of CD44 (pgp-1) expression on lymphocytes from F5/NP mice. The level of CD44 on $CD8^{+}$ Vβ11 spleen cells surface was upregulated in comparison with CD8 T cells from F5 mice (data not shown). Findings indicate that these T cells have encountered nucleoprotein.

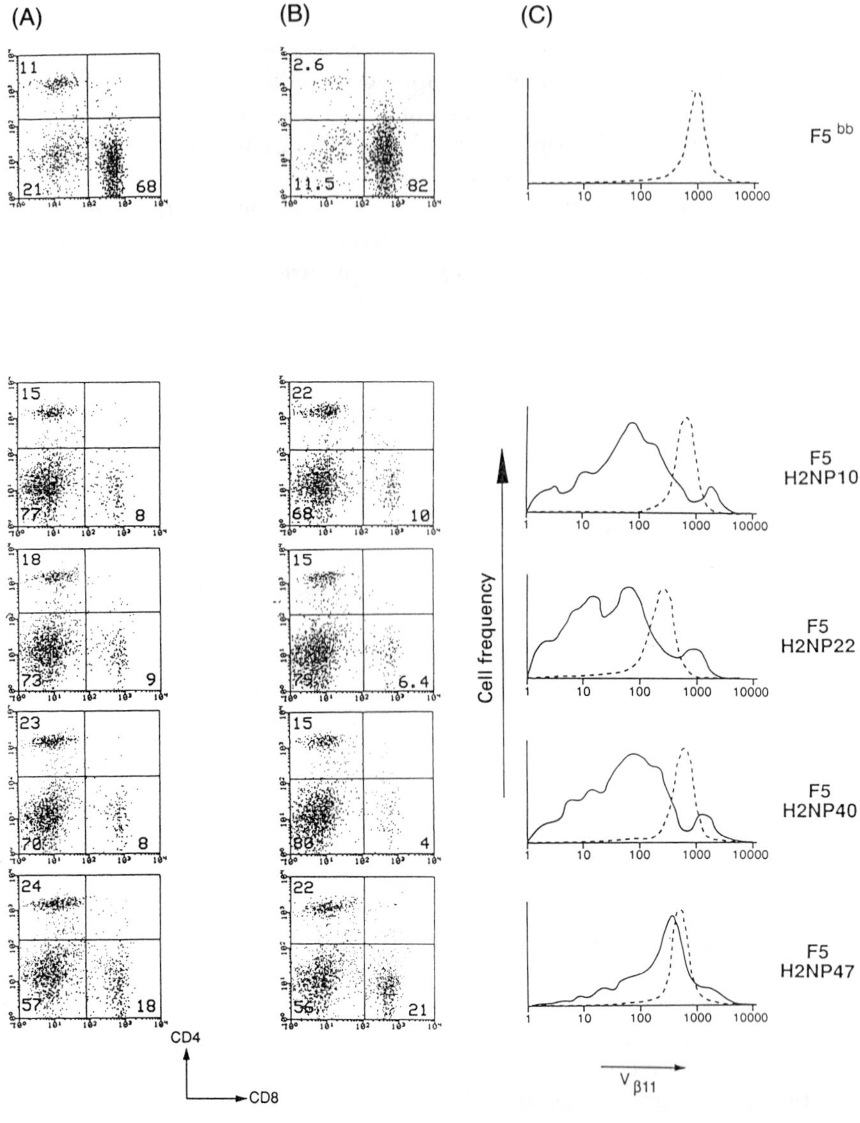

Fig. 3.2 Double transgenic mice with reduced numbers of CD8$^+$ peripheral T cells and low levels of TCR. Lymph node cells from TCR single transgenic or TCR/NP double transgenic mice were stained for CD4, CD8 and the transgenic Vβ11 TCR as described in methods before (A) or after (B) intraperitoneal treatment for 4 days with 50 nmol of antigenic peptide. Dot blots represent two-colour analysis of cells stained with CD4 and CD8. (C) Three-parameter data files were software-gated to generate single-colour staining histograms of Vβ11 expression on CD8$^+$CD4$^-$ single positive cells from double transgenic mice (solid line) and F5 single transgenic control (dotted line).

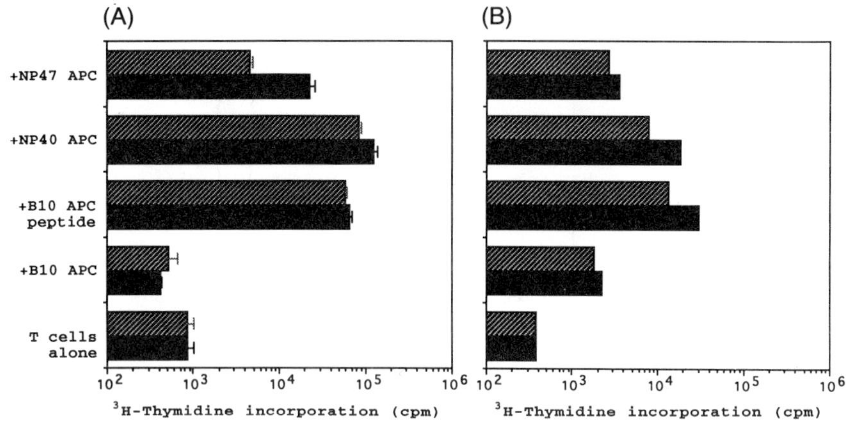

Fig. 3.3 F5/RAG$^{-/-}$ T-cell proliferation in vitro in the presence of NP macrophages and dendritic cells. F5/RAG$^{-/-}$ spleen T cells were stimulated in vitro by dendritic cells (DC) and macrophages (M) isolated from (A) spleens and (B) thymuses of NP40 and NP47 mice. B10 DC (black bars), and M from the same tissues (shaded bars) loaded with the antigenic peptide beforehand and then washed, were used as a positive control. Proliferation of the responders was measured by ^{3}H-thymidine incorporation.

Response of F5/NP transgenic mice to additional exposure to antigen

F5 TCR respond in vivo to four daily injections of 50 nmol of NP peptide by proliferation of the CD8$^+$ T cells and depletion of CD4$^+$8$^+$ thymocytes (14). They show a marked decrease (10–30-fold) of thymus cellularity. In contrast, F5/H2NP10, F5/H2NP22 and F5/H2NP40 show a decrease in the number of thymocytes of approximately 2–3-fold. The exception is F5/H2NP47 mouse which shows extensive thymic depletion similar to that seen in the F5 single transgenic control after peptide treatment. In the representative experiment shown in Fig. 3.1B the reduction in the proportion of double positive thymocytes in F5/NP mice treated with peptide was from 71% to 62% in F5/H2NP10, from 73% to 56% in F5/H2NP22, from 74% to 62% in F5/H2NP40, and from 86% to 12% in F5/H2NP47 mice. The proportion of CD8$^+$ T cells in the lymph nodes of F5/NP mice did not change upon exposure to antigenic peptide in vivo (Fig. 3.2B). No change was noted in the expression of Vβ11 on gated CD8$^+$ lymph node cells from F5/H2NP10, F5/H2NP22 and F5/H2NP40 double transgenic mice after administration of peptide (Fig. 3.4), presumably because most of these cells express endogenous α and/or β receptors. When F5/H2NP22/RAG-1$^{-/-}$ were treated with peptide, the transgenic TCR on the few circulating CD8$^+$ was further downmodulated. We conclude from those results that tolerance in most F5/NP mice involves the

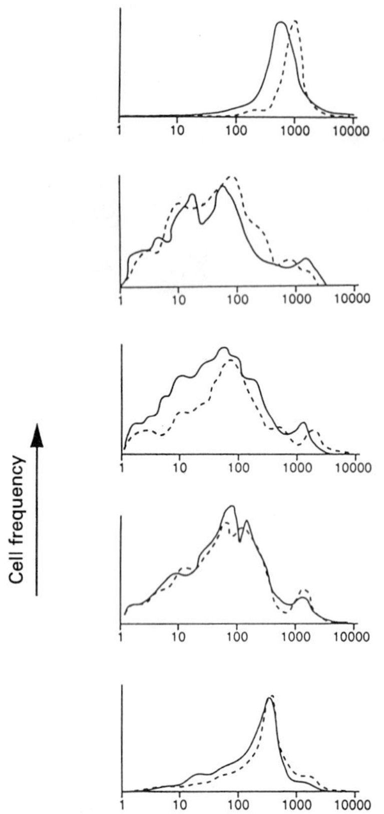

Fig. 3.4 Levels of TCR on peripheral $CD8^+$ T cells after treatment of double transgenic mice with antigen peptide. Three-parameter data files were software-gated to generate single-colour staining histograms of Vβ11 on $CD8^+CD4^-$ single-positive cells. Numbers indicate the mean fluorescence of Vβ11 staining in arbitrary units from single or double transgenic mice before (dotted line) or after (solid line) intraperitoneal treatment for 4 days with 50 nmol antigenic peptide.

$CD8^+$ population and is sufficient to protect the mice from autoimmunity due to low levels of TCR and coreceptor on these cells.

Functional analysis of T cells from double transgenic mice

Table 3.1 shows the results of exposing spleen cells from F5 and F5/NP double transgenic mice untreated or following peptide administration in vivo for 4 days, to H-2^b splenic APC, alone or peptide pulsed, in the presence of low concentrations rIL-2. Spleen cells from the F5 control mice made good peptide-specific proliferative responses before and after 4 days in vivo peptide

Table 3.1 Peptide-specific proliferative responses in vitro from spleen cells of F5 mice expressing cognate peptide from a transgene

Mouse	Peptide treatment	[^{3}H]-Proliferation (cpm)	
		+B10 APC (X ± SE)	+B10 APC^p (X ± SE)
F5	–	1326 ± 34	10314 ± 237
F5	4 days	1680 ± 43	88688 ± 447
F5/H2NP40	–	1607 ± 54	2085 ± 151
F5/H2NP40	4 days	1621 ± 59	2597 ± 212
F5/H2NP47	–	1264 ± 21	1695 ± 60
F5/H2NP47	4 days	1328 ± 32	1863 ± 79

administration. In contrast, none of the F5/NP mice made such a response, even after exposure to peptide in vivo. Peptide-specific cytotoxic T cells were found ex vivo in spleen cells from F5 mice following peptide administration but never in untreated mice, nor in any of the F5/NP double transgenic mice, whether or not given peptide in vivo (data not shown). In contrast, spleen cells from all F5/NP mice could develop cytotoxic effector cells after culture in vitro for 3 or 4 days in the presence of 20 IU/ml rIL-2.

DISCUSSION

We studied the forms of negative selection and tolerance induction caused in F5 TCR transgenic mice by nominal antigen when the latter is expressed in the form of a transgene. In the thymus of F5/NP double transgenic mice a complete absence of F5 TCR^{hi} thymocytes is observed. The CD8$^+$ peripheral mature population, on the other hand, is affected both in numbers and in the levels of Vβ11 expressed. The majority of these CD8$^+$ cells probably express endogenous α and/or β chains and this may be the reason they are positively selected and released in the periphery. It is possible that because of the presence of the antigen, these cells down-regulate the transgenic receptor causing upregulation of recombination machinery and consequently increased rearrangement of the endogenous TCR gene loci. This would be analogous to experiments describing receptor editing in self reactive B cells (20,21). We conclude from these findings that in F5 TCR mice negative selection of self reactive thymocytes to nucleoprotein occurs at the transition from CD4$^+$8$^+$ TCR^{lo} to CD4$^+$8$^+$ TCR^{hi}. It is unclear at the moment whether this involves elimination of developing thymocytes at the point of up-regulation of the receptor or arrest of these thymocytes at the TCR^{lo} stage due to the presence of the antigen. F5/NP47 mice present an interesting marginal situation. In these mice we also observe a reduction in the number of $CD8^+$ cells and most of these cells express the transgenic receptor, albeit at levels lower than those seen in F5 single transgenic mice. They respond to peptide treatment by deleting the double positive thymocytes. The picture in F5/NP mice strongly resembles that developing in F5 single transgenic mice treated with cognate peptide long term. In the treated mice thymus contains $CD4^+8^+$ cells bearing low levels of TCR and the peripheral lymphoid organs contain very few $CD8^+$ T cells with low levels of transgenic TCR (15). Thus, chronic exposure to cognate antigen leads to a situation similar to tolerance towards self antigen.

Additional exposure of tolerant T cells to high levels of antigen in other experimental models has led to further tolerization of these cells by down-modulation of the TCR and/or the coreceptor (22). Further antigenic exposure of T cells from F5/NP mice did not enhance their tolerization, judging from the levels of TCR and coreceptor: these remained unchanged after treatment with the antigenic peptide. When we repeated this experiment using RAG-$1^{-/-}$ the few $CD8^+$ $F5TCR^{lo}$ cells present in the periphery did down-regulate their receptor and coreceptor even further upon exposure to higher levels of antigen given as exogenously administered peptide. This is in agreement with evidence from an alloreactive transgenic TCR model (22), and confirms that although tolerance induced in double transgenic mice is sufficient for the levels of nucleoprotein transgene expressed, when higher levels of antigen are introduced, reactivity is avoided by down-regulating the TCR even further.

Despite unresponsiveness in vivo, stimulation of T cells from double transgenic mice was possible in vivo. Peripheral splenic T cells from them can generate peptide-specific cytotoxicity after in vitro culture 72–96 h in the presence of 20 IU/ml rIL-2. This shows that apparently anergic phenotype manifest in vivo can be converted to activation in the presence of IL-2. On the other hand, the proliferative capacity of these anergic T cells is severely compromised, suggesting that although terminal differentiation into effector cells is still possible, clonal expansion is not. The extent to which F5 T cells are restrained in vivo in the continuous presence of potentially activating antigen is a measure of the capacity of the organism to control autoreactivity. The fail-safe mechanism could clearly involve down-regulation of TCR and/or accessory molecules, as documented in this paper, but the ubiquitous presence of antigen on non-professional APC cells in the periphery could also have an inhibitory effect on the activation cascade via molecular interactions at present poorly understood.

CONCLUSION

Results in this and previous published reports indicate that negative selection in the thymus can take place at different stages of thymocyte development with ultimate result the absence of mature TCR^{hi} self reactive T cells. This can be accomplished as early as during the transition from $CD4^-CD8^-TCR^-$ to $CD4^+8^+TCR^{lo}$ (23,24) or later during the transition from $CD4^+8^+TCR^{lo}$ to $CD4^+8^+TCR^{hi}$ (F5/NP mice).

REFERENCES

1. Kappler, J. W., N. Roehm and Ph. Marrack. 1987. T-cell tolerance by clonal elimination in the thymus. *Cell* **49**:273–80.
2. MacDonald, H. R., R. Schleider, R. K. Lees *et al.* 1988. T cell receptor Vβ use predicts reactivity and tolerance to MIs^a-encoded antigens. *Nature* **332**:40–5.
3. Webb, S., C. Morris and J. Sprent. 1990. Extrathymic tolerance of mature T cells: clonal elimination as a consequence of immunity. *Cell* **63**:1249–56.
4. Jones, L. A., L. T. Chin, D. L. Longo and A. M. Kruisbeek. 1990. Peripheral clonal elimination of functional T cells. *Science* **250**:1726–32.
5. Kawabe, Y. and A. Ochi. 1991. Programmed cell death and extrathymic reduction of $V\beta11^+CD4^+$ T cells in mice tolerant to Staphylococcus aureus enterotoxin B. *Nature* **349**:245–8.
6. Rocha, B., P. Vassalli and D. Guy-Grand. 1992. The extrathymic T cell development pathway. *Immunol. Today* **13**:449–54.
7. Blackman, M., J. Kappler and Ph. Marrack. 1990. The role of the T cell receptor in positive and negative selection of developing T cells. *Science* **248**:1335–41.
8. Schwartz, R. H. 1989. Acquisition of Immunologic self-tolerance. *Cell* **57**: 1073–80.
9. Ramsdell, F. and B. J. Fowlkes. 1990. Clonal deletion versus clonal anergy: the role of the thymus in inducing self tolerance. *Science* **248**:1342–8.
10. Schonrich, G., U. Kallinke, F. Momburg *et al.* 1991. Down-regulation of T cell receptors on self-reactive T cells as a novel mechanism for extrathymic tolerance induction. *Cell* **65**:293–304.
11. Mueller, D. L., M. K. Jenkins and R. H. Schwartz. 1989. Clonal expansion versus functional clonal inactivation: a costimulatory signalling pathway determines the outcome of T cell antigen receptor occupancy. *Ann. Rev. Immunol.* **7**:445–80.
12. Townsend, A. R. M., J. Rothbard, F. M. Gotch *et al.* 1986. The epitopes of influenza nucleoprotein recognized by cytotoxic lymphocytes can be defined with short synthetic peptides. *Cell* **44**:959–68.
13. Mamalaki, C., T. Elliott, T. Norton *et al.* 1993. Positive and negative selection in transgenic mice expressing a T cell receptor specific for influenza nucleoprotein and endogenous superantigen. *Dev. Immunol.* **3**:159–74.
14. Mamalaki, C., T. Norton, Y. Tanaka *et al.* 1992. Thymic depletion and peripheral activation of Class I Major Histocompatibility Complex-restricted T cells by soluble peptide in T cell receptor transgenic mice. *Proc. Natl. Acad. Sci. USA* **89**:11 342–6.
15. Mamalaki, C., Y. Tanaka, P. Corbella *et al.* 1993. T cell deletion follows chronic antigen specific T cell activation in vivo. *Int. Immunol.* **5**:1285–92.
16. Lang, G., D. Wotton, M. J. Owen *et al.* 1988. The structure of the human CD2 gene and its expression in transgenic mice. *EMBO J.* **7**:1675–82.
17. Tomonary, K. and E. Lovering. 1988. T cell receptor specific antibodies against a Vβ11-positive mouse T cell clone. *Immunogenetics* **28**:445–51.
18. Stockinger, B. and B. Hausmann. 1994. Functional recognition of in vivo processed self antigen. *Int. Immunol.* **6**:247–53.

19. Spanopoulou, E., C. A. J. Roman, L. M. Corcoran *et al.* 1994. Functional immunoglobulin transgenes guide ordered B-cell differentiation in RAG-1 deficient mice. *Genes Dev.* **8**:1030–40.
20. Gay, G., T. Saunders, S. Camper and M. Weigert. 1993. Receptor editing: an approach by autoreactive B cells to escape tolerance. *J. Exp. Med.* **177**: 999–1008.
21. Tiegs, S. L., D. M. Russell and D. Nemazee. 1993. Receptor editing in self-reactive bone marrow B cells. *J. Exp. Med.* **177**:1009–20.
22. Hammerling, G. J., G. Schonrich, F. Momburg *et al.* 1991. Non-deletional mechanisms of peripheral and central tolerance: studies with transgenic mice with tissue specific expression of a foreign MHC class I antigen. *Immunol. Rev.* **122**:47–67.
23. Kisielow, P., H. Bluthman, U. D. Staerz *et al.* 1988. Tolerance in T cell receptor transgenic mice involves deletion of non mature $CD4^{+}8^{+}$ thymocytes. *Nature* **333**:742–5.
24. Berg, L. J., B. Fasekas de St. Groth, A. M. Pullen and M. M. Davis. 1989. Phenotypic differences between $\alpha\beta$ versus β T cell receptor transgenic mice undergoing negative selection. *Nature* **340**:559–63.

4

Thymus-targeted Oncogene Expression in TCR Transgenic Mice

Marianna Murdjeva, Yujiro Tanaka, Trisha Norton and Dimitris Kioussis

In studies of cellular and molecular biology when a large number of homogeneous populations of cells are required, the availability of immortalized cell lines is often of central importance. Since overexpression of c-*myc* proto-oncogene is one of the most common genetic abnormalities associated with T cell leukaemia (1–3), it may be possible to immortalize T cells in vivo by targeting the expression of the c-*myc* to the T cell lineage in transgenic mice. To this end, T-cell specific Thy-1 gene promoter sequences were used to direct the expression of c-*myc* in transgenic mice (4). Thy-1/c-myc (TM) transgenic mice developed thymic tumours from which cell lines of both non-adherent (thymocytes) and adherent (epithelial cells) phenotypes were established. All thymocyte cell lines were double positive (DP) – $CD4^+CD8^+$ and oligoclonal in origin. It was suggested that neoplastic transformation of thymocytes in TM mice occurs at a double positive stage in a stochastic manner. In an attempt to generate a better-defined system with which we could study cell differentiation events, we bred TM mice with mice transgenic for an $\alpha\beta$ TCR (F5) which recognizes a peptide from influenza virus nucleoprotein in the context of class I H-$2D^b$ (5,6). Subsequently we established double positive T cell lines expressing the transgenic TCR and studied their function in vitro.

MATERIALS AND METHODS

Animals

Thy-1/c-myc (4) and F5 TCR (6) transgenic mice were generated at the Laboratory of Molecular Immunology, NIMR, London. RAG-$1^{-/-}$ were a kind gift from Dr E. Spanopoulou (7). All mice including inbred C57BL/10 (B10) strain were maintained in colonies at the institute.

Immunoregulation in Health and Disease
ISBN 0–12–459460–3

Flow cytometry

Thymic tumour cells, cell lines and control F5 thymocytes were stained with antibodies against CD4 (PE-conjugated, Boeringer-Manheim), CD8 (FITC-conjugated YTS169.4, ATCC), Vβ11 (transgenic TCR) – biotinylated KT11, gift from Dr Tomonary), HSA (biotinylated M1/114, ATCC), CD3ε (biotinylated 2C11-145, ATCC), Thy-1.2 (biotinylated HO134, ATCC), streptavidin-tricolour (CALTAG, California) and streptavidin phycoerythrin (Biogenesis). Samples were analysed on FACScan (Becton Dickinson) using Lysis II software.

Tissue culture

Thymic tumours were mechanically disrupted and thymocytes were cultured in 12-well plates (Nunc) in RPMI 1640 (Gibco) supplemented with 10% (v/v) heat inactivated fetal calf serum (Globepharm), 0.06 g/l penicillin, 0.1 g/l streptomycin and 10 mM HEPES. Cells were incubated at 37°C in a humidified chamber with 5% carbon dioxide. A clone, designated F5.TM25.1.2 (abbreviated 25.1.2) was obtained by limiting dilution at 0.5 cells/well.

For analysis of programmed cell death, 25.1.2 cells were treated with 1×10^{-6} M hydrocortisone (Sigma) for 12 h. Total DNA was extracted from 25.1.2 cells and was run in 2% agarose gel containing ethidium bromide as described before (8).

Peritoneal macrophages from C57BL10 mice were prepared according to Morikawa *et al.* (9). Then macrophages were incubated with different concentrations of the 1968 NP peptide (synthesized at the National Institute for Medical Research, London, UK) for 90 min prior to coculture with 25.1.2 cells. 2×10^5 macrophages were cultured with 5×10^5 25.1.2 cells for 12 h. Viable cell numbers of lymphoid cells were counted by the trypan blue dye exclusion method and cells were stained for CD4, CD8, and Vβ11. Thymocytes from adult F5 transgenic mice were used as a control.

25.1.2 cells were cocultured with J774A.1 macrophage cell line (TIB 67, ATCC) in the presence or absence of anti-CD3 antibody (2C11.145) at 0.07 or 10 μg/ml. After 12 h culture cells were FACS analyzed as described above. Also fragmentation of DNA in 25.1.2 cells was analyzed as above after CD3 cross-linking.

RNA-PCR analysis of TCR gene transcripts

Total RNA was extracted from 25.1.2 cells by the guanidine thiocyanate method (10) and was reverse-transcribed (RT) by Moloney murine leukaemia virus reverse transcriptase (Promega) using oligo dT primers (Promega). One sixth of the RT product was amplified by PCR in 1.5 mM $MgCl_2$, 60 mM KCl,

15 mM Tris-HCl (pH 8.3), 6.75% glycerol, and 2U Taq polymerase (Perkin-Elmer) in thermal cycler (Hybaid).

Sense primers for TCR α constant region have been described previously (11). Also, primers specific for transgenic F5 TCR were used, synthesized in our institute:

Vα4: ACCAGACAAGCTTCACCTGCCAAGATAT,
Vα4′: CAGTATCCCGGAGAAGGTC,
Vβ11: CAAGCTCCTATAGATGATTC
hCD2: TCAAAATCAGAAGGAAGCTGG,
cβ: CCTTGGGTGGAGTCACATTTC.

PCR products were analysed in 2% agarose gels with ethidium bromide. A molecular size marker consisting of multimers of 123 bp DNA fragments (Pharmacia) was used.

RESULTS AND DISCUSSION

Generation of $CD4^+CD8^+$ double positive cell lines from a F5.TM25 double transgenic mouse

In an attempt to obtain thymic tumours and immortalized cell lines of immature phenotype, the TM25 line which produced HSA^{high} cell lines at a high frequency (4) was bred with F5 mouse. The F5/TM25.1 mouse developed a thymic tumour which consisted mostly of $CD4^+CD8^+$ cells (76.7%) (Fig. 4.1) and expressed high levels of Vβ11 (Fig. 4.1d, solid line), comparable to single positive F5 thymocytes (broken line). They were HSA^{high} (Fig. 4.1e, solid line) and $CD3^{low}$ (Fig. 4.1c, solid line). These data suggest that immature DP thymocytes expressing high levels of transgenic TCR were transformed in F5.TM25.1 mouse.

Several thymocyte lines were derived from a thymic tumour of the F5.TM25.1 mouse. All these lines were $CD4^+CD8^+$. However, the levels of HSA and Vβ11 expression varied among cell lines. Figure 4.2 shows an example of a 25.1.2 cell line which is DP (Fig. 4.2a) and expresses a high level HSA (Fig. 4.2d) and lower levels of CD3 and Vβ11. Since cultured cells have a larger cell size and thus an increased autofluorescence, it is difficult to compare directly the levels of CD3 (Fig. 4.2b) and TCR (Fig. 4.2c) between F5/TM25.1 cell lines and normal F5 thymocytes. Nevertheless, 25.1.2 cells seem to express lower Vβ11 than thymocytes in F5 mice (dashed line) or in the original F5/TM25.1. thymic tumour.

In order to examine if the transgenic TCR is expressed in 25.1.2 cell line, we analyzed transcription products of the transgene. Total RNA extracted from 25.1.2 cells was reverse transcribed and then amplified by PCR using primer sets specific for the transgenic TCR α and β chains (Vα4-hCD2 and

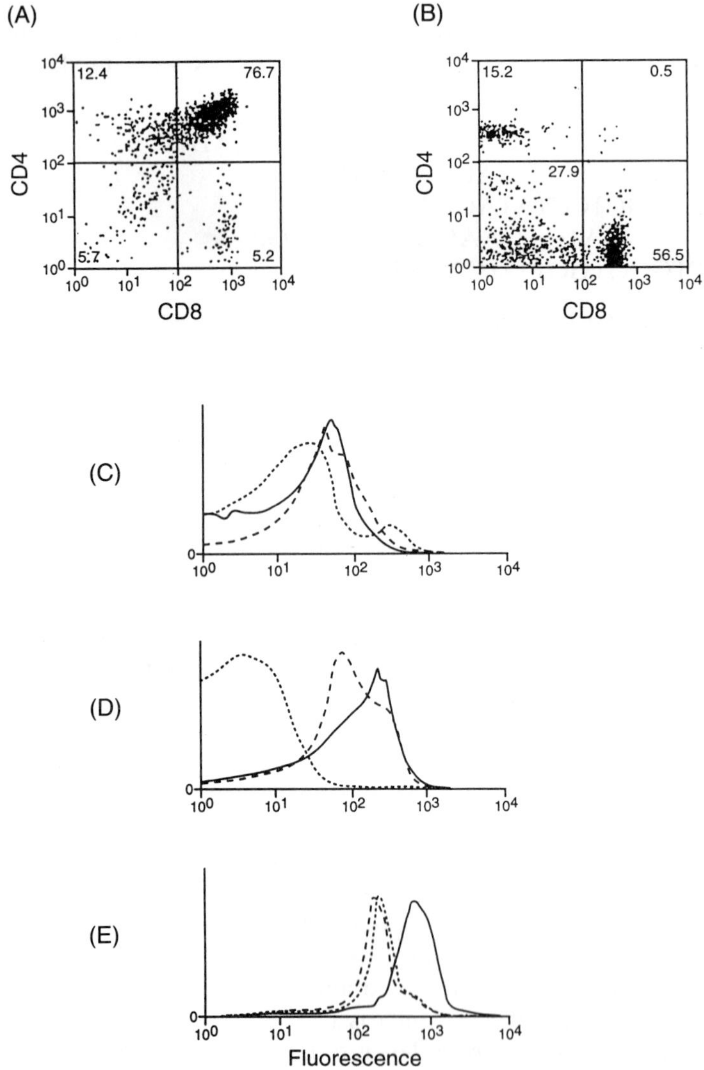

Fig. 4.1 Phenotype of T cells in the thymus and periphery of F5.TM25.1.2 mouse. (a) Expression of CD4 and CD8 on thymic tumour cells in F5.TM25.1 mouse. Proportion of CD8 single positive cells is significantly reduced compared with normal F5 mouse. (b) Expression of CD4 and CD8 on lymph node cells in F5.TM25.1 mouse. (c,d,e) Histograms showing levels of CD3 (c), Vβ11 (d) and HSA (e) on thymic tumour cells (solid lines). Dotted and broken lines in each histogram represent non-transgenic and adult F5 thymocytes respectively.

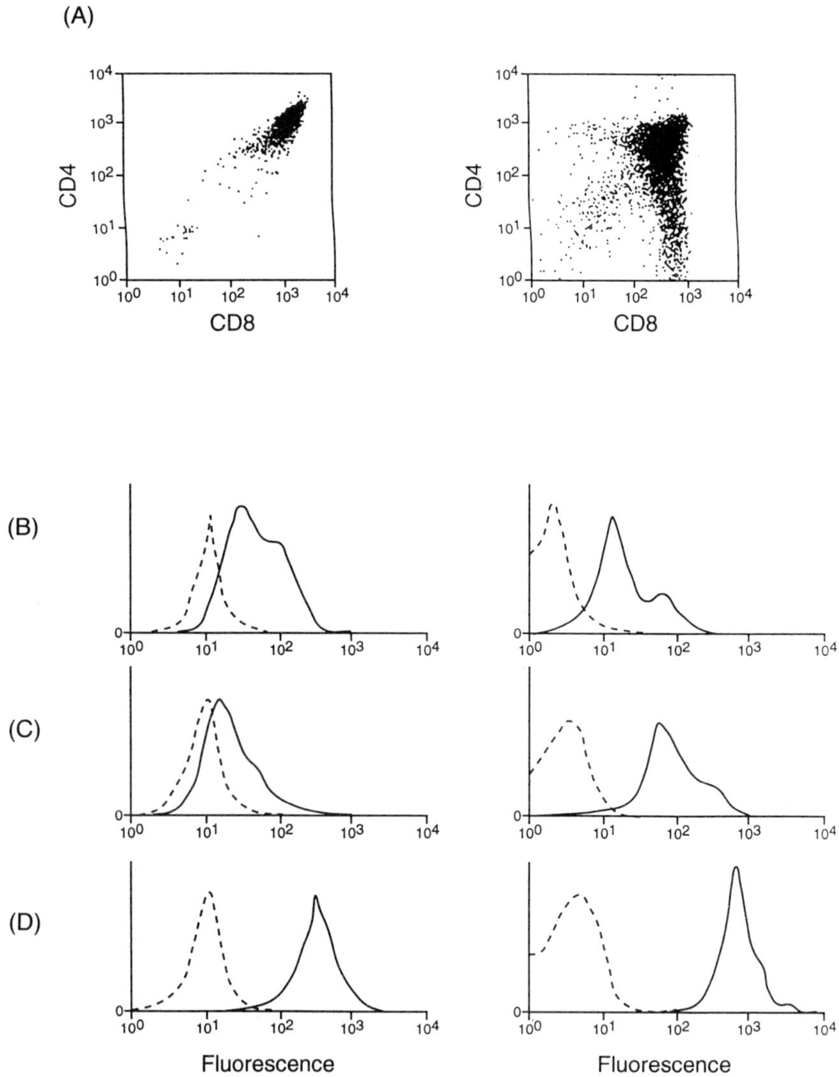

Fig. 4.2. Phenotype of F5.TM25.1.2 cell line. (a) Expression of CD4 and CD8 on 25.1.2 cells and F5 thymocytes. (b,c,d) Histograms illustrating expression of CD3 (b), Vβ11 (c) and HSA (d). Left panels and right panels represent 25.1.2 and control F5 thymocytes respectively. Dotted lines in histograms are unstained controls.

Vβ11-hCD2 or cβ). Figure 4.3 provides evidence that this cell line transcribes both α and β TCR transgenes which are seen as discrete bands of predicted sizes (Fig. 4.3a). In addition, RNA-PCR analysis using panels of different Vα and Vβ primer sets revealed that 25.1.2 cells transcribe rearranged endogenous Vα8(Fig. 4.3b) and Vβ5 (Fig. 4.3c). Although the presence of transcription products from endogenous α and β TCR genes does not mean they are expressed as proteins on the cell surface, the finding that endogenous chains are also expressed in these cells is consistent with the observation of higher stoichiometry of CD3 over Vβ11.

It is generally accepted that allelic exclusion of TCR β genes is strict and introduction of rearranged TCR β genes in transgenic mice prohibits thymocytes from rearranging their endogenous TCR β genes. The fact that mRNA for endogenous rearranged TCR genes was found in the 25.1.2 cells could be due to allelic inclusion in F5 TCR transgenic mice. However, it has also been shown that immortalized thymocytes tend to rearrange TCR genes (12). Allelic exclusion of dual TCR α chains has been demonstrated in normal T cells (13). Our data on rearrangement of endogenous TCR genes in F5 TCR transgenic 25.1.2 cell line support the hypothesis that immortalized immature T cells have defects in stopping TCR gene rearrangement.

The programmed cell death of F5/TM25.1.2 cell line

Treatment of 25.1.2 cells for 12 h with 1×10^{-6} M hydrocortisone, a known steroid inducer of programmed cell death in immature thymocytes (14), proved that these cells retained characteristics of immature double positive thymocytes. Total DNA was extracted after treatment and was analyzed in an agarose gel. As shown in Fig. 4.4a, the steroid-induced cell death (apoptosis) in the 25.1.2 cell line produces a prominent ladder of fragmented DNA.

NP peptide has been shown to induce deletion of DP F5 thymocytes when injected into adult F5 mice (15). Figure 4.4b shows the number of viable cells in 25.1.2 cells and control F5 thymocytes after culture with various concentrations of the 1968 NP. Normal F5 thymocytes were deleted by as

---

Fig. 4.3. RNA–PCR analysis of TCR gene transcripts. (a) Transgenic TCR products were detected using sense primers for Vα4 and Vβ11 in combination with anti-sense primers for a part of the vector (hCD2) or the constant region of β chain. mRNA from 25.1.2 cells was used, except for one sample in which the mRNA was isolated from parental 25.1 cell line (*). (b) Expression of rearranged endogenous TCR α loci. A Vα4 specific band could be derived either from transgenic or endogenous α chains, whereas a product for Vα8 could only originate from endogenous α gene. (c) Rearrangement of endogenous TCR β genes. A band for Vβ11 could be due to mRNA from either the transgenic or an endogenous gene.

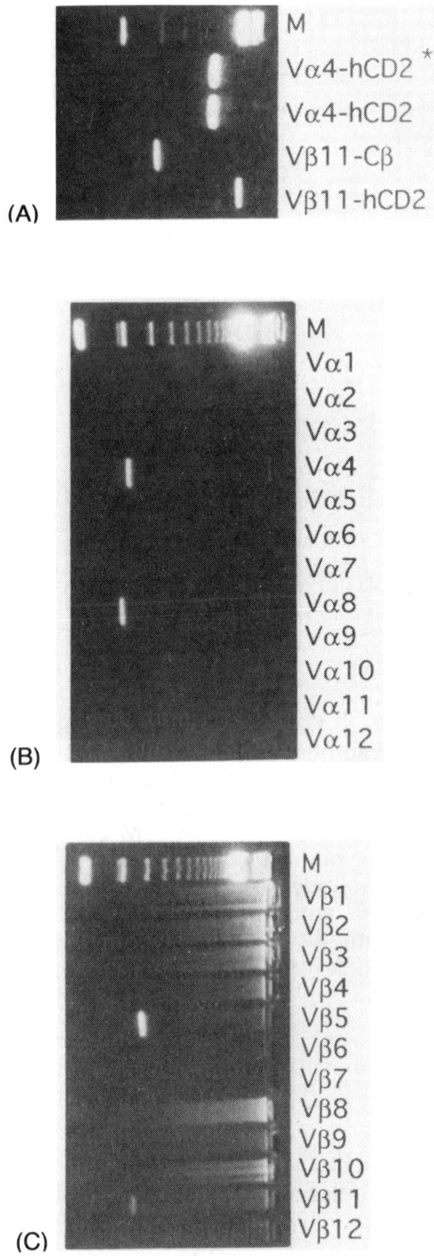
(A)
M
Vα4-hCD2 *
Vα4-hCD2
Vβ11-Cβ
Vβ11-hCD2
(B)
M
Vα1
Vα2
Vα3
Vα4
Vα5
Vα6
Vα7
Vα8
Vα9
Vα10
Vα11
Vα12
(C)
M
Vβ1
Vβ2
Vβ3
Vβ4
Vβ5
Vβ6
Vβ7
Vβ8
Vβ9
Vβ10
Vβ11
Vβ12

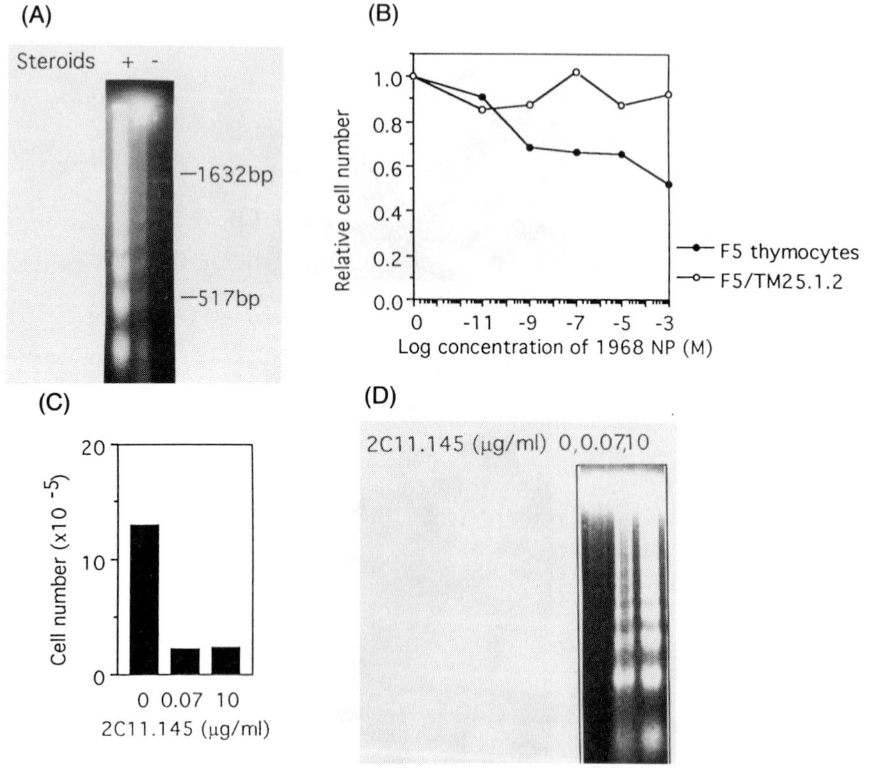

Fig. 4.4 Responses of 25.1.2 cells to steroid, peptide and CD3 cross-linking treatments. (a) DNA fragmentation in 25.1.2 cells induced by hydrocortisone. (b) Survival of 25.1.2 cells (closed circles) and F5 thymocytes (open circles) after culture in different concentrations of 1968 nucleoprotein peptide. NP caused deletion of F5 thymocytes at 10^{-9} M concentration, but did not affect 25.1.2 cells even at the highest concentration. (c,d) Cross-linking of CD3 on 25.1.2 cells by 2C11 antibody bound to Fc receptors on macrophage cell line J774A.1. The anti-CD3 antibody caused deletion of 25.1.2 cells (c) by programmed cell death as shown by characteristic DNA ladders (d) at concentrations of 70 ng/ml or 10 μg/ml.

little as 1×10^{-12} M concentration of the peptide, whereas 25.1.2 cells were not affected even by 1×10^{-6} M peptide. Also 25.1.2 cells did not change their $CD4^+CD8^+$ double positive phenotype. In line with these data, primary cultures of F5/TM25.1 thymic tumour cells in the presence of the cognate peptide did not cause deletion of DP cells, in spite of the fact that Vβ11 on DP cells was slightly down-regulated (data not shown). Taken together, DP thymocytes transformed in the F5/TM25.1 mouse appear to be resistant to clonal deletion by the cognate peptide. It could be argued that 25.1.2 cell line do not express transgenic TCR $\alpha\beta$ heterodimers at a high level enough to respond to the cognate peptide, given the fact they can rearrange endogenous TCR α and β. Alternatively, if 25.1.2 cells express the F5 TCR, albeit at a lower level, it could be either that TCR of 25.1.2 cells are uncoupled with intracellular signal transduction machineries or that there are defects in the downstream signalling system in these cells.

In order to examine the signalling capability of TCR in 25.1.2 cells, we cross-linked their CD3 molecules with an anti-CD3ε antibody (2C11.145), presented by Fc receptors on a macrophage cell line J774. Although J774 cells are derived from a CBA (H-2^k) mouse, which carry the endogenous mammary tumour virus that may delete V$\beta 11^+$ thymocytes, coculture of 25.1.2 cells with J774 did not cause deletion of 25.1.2 cells, probably because J774 cells do not express the superantigen. On the other hand the presence of anti-CD3 antibody in these cultures at 70 ng/ml or 10 μg/ml concentration dramatically reduced the number of viable cells (Fig. 4.4c) and induced DNA fragmentation of 25.1.2 cells as shown in Fig. 4.4d. These data demonstrate that the 25.1.2 cell line has an intact CD3-linked signal transduction mechanism, suggesting that the resistance of 25.1.2 cells to peptide-mediated deletion is due to either low levels of TCR expression or uncoupling of TCR $\alpha\beta$ with the CD3 complex.

F5/Thy-myc mice which do not rearrange endogenous TCR

In order to avoid the complications of endogenous T cell receptors being expressed during thymic development of F5/Thy-myc double transgenic mice, these mice were generated in RAG-$1^{-/-}$ background. They are deficient in the recombination activating gene (*RAG-1*) (6). In RAG-$1^{-/-}$ mice thymocyte development is arrested at the double negative $CD4^-8^-$ stage. If such mice are crossed to transgenic, carrying an already rearranged β chain transgene they proceed to the DP ($CD4^+8^+$) stage (16) and only the transgenic F5 TCR can be expressed on T cells.

Thymic tumour cells from F5/TM/RAG-$1^{-/-}$ mice were stained for CD4, CD8, Vβ11 (transgenic) and HSA and analysed on a FACS. Cell lines were isolated from these tumours and were analysed for expression of CD4, CD8, Vβ11, and HSA. However, in culture F5/TM/$RAG^{-/-}$ cell lines gradually down-regulate the expression of the transgenic TCR.

RAG-$1^{-/-}$ Thy-1-myc mice do not develop thymic tumours

Over 30 Thy-1-myc/RAG-$1^{-/-}$ mice at ages from 3 months to 1 year were examined and none of them developed thymic tumours, although in $RAG^{-/-}$ mice Thy-1 promoter is active in the double negative ($CD4^-8^-$) thymocytes thus excluding the possibility of transcriptional inactivity of the *myc* transgene. In contrast, most of the F5/Thy-1-myc/RAG-$1^{-/-}$ mice developed tumours. This shows that in order for the Thy-myc thymocytes to be transformed they have to proceed to the double positive stage in development.

CONCLUSIONS

The unique immature thymocyte cell line 25.1.2, transgenic for an $\alpha\beta$ TCR and the c-*myc* oncogene, is sensitive to steroid-induced apoptosis but did not respond to cognate peptide. This could be due to insufficient levels of expression of the F5 TCR or uncoupling to the CD3 complex. In addition, this line had rearranged and transcribed endogenous TCR α and β genes, in spite of the fact that transgenic α and β genes were also expressed.

F5/Thy-myc/RAG-1$^{-/-}$ mice developed thymic tumours, thus excluding the possibility that endogenous receptor expression (and signalling) were necessary for transformation of thymocytes.

Transformation of thymocytes in Thy-myc mice is a rare event and needs, in addition to the *myc* gene, a secondary event that occurs at the double positive stage.

REFERENCES

1. Gauwerky, C. and C. Croce. 1993. Chromosomal transolactions in leukaemia. *Semin. Cancer Biol.* **4**:333–40.
2. Casares, S., J. M. Rodriguez, A. Martin and A. Parrado. 1993. Rearrangement of c-*myc* and c-*abl* genes in tumour cells in Burkitt's lymphoma. *J. Clin. Pathol.* **46**:778–9.
3. Stephenson, J., R. Akdag, N. Ozbek and G. J. Mufti. 1993. Methylation status within exon 3 of the c-*myc* gene as a prognostic marker in myeloma and leukaemia. *Leuk. Res.* **17**:291–3.
4. Spanopoulou, E., A. Early, J. Elliot *et al.* 1989. Complex lymphoid and epithelial thymic tumours in *Thy-1/myc* transgenic mice. *Nature* **342**:185–9.
5. Townsend, A. R. M., J. Rothbard, F. M. Gotch *et al.* 1886. The epitopes of influenza nucleoprotein recognized by cytotoxic lymphocytes can be defined with short synthetic peptides. *Cell* **44**:959–67.
6. Mamalaki, C., T. Elliott, T. Norton *et al.* 1993. Positive and negative selection in transgenic mice expressing a T-cell receptor specific for influenza nucleoprotein and endogenous superantigen. *Dev. Immunol.* **3**:159–74.
7. Spanopoulou, E., A. J. Roman, L. M. Corcoran *et al.* 1994. Functional immunoglobulin transgenes guide ordered B-cell differentiation in RAG-1 deficient mice. *Genes & Dev.* **8**:1030–40.
8. Kawabe, Y. and A. Ochi. 1992. Programmed cell death and extrathymic reduction of Vβ8$^+$CD4$^+$ T cells in mice tolerant to *Staphylococcus aureus* enterotoxin B. *Nature* **349**:245–8.
9. Morikawa, Y., M. Furotani, N. Matsuura and K. Kakudo. 1993. The role of antigen-presenting cells in the regulation of delayed-type hypersensitivity. *Cell. Immunol.* **152**:200–10.
10. Sambrook, J., E. F. Fritsch and T. Maniatis. 1989. Extraction of RNA with

guanidinium thiocyanate followed by centrifugation in cesium chloride solutions. In: *Molecular Cloning. A Laboratory Manual* 7. 19–7.22. Cold Spring Harbor Laboratory Press, New York.

11. Casanova, J. L., P. Romero, C. Widmann *et al.* 1991. T cell receptor genes in a series of class I major histocompatibility complex-restricted T lymphocyte clones specific for a *Plasmodium berghei* nonapeptides: implications for T cell allelic exclusion and antigen-specific repertoire. *J. Exp. Med.* **174**:1371–83.
12. Malissen, M., J. Trucy, E. Jouvin-Marche *et al.* 1992. Regulation of TCR α and β gene allelic exclusion during T-cell development. Immunol. Today **13**:315–22.
13. Padovan, E., G. Casorati, P. Dellabona *et al.* 1993. Expression of two T cell receptor alpha chains:dual receptor T cells. *Science* **262**:422–4.
14. Wyllie, A. H. 1980. Glucocorticoid-induced thymocyte apoptosis is associated with endogenous endonuclease activation. *Nature* **284**:555–6.
15. Mamalaki, C., T. Norton, Y. Tanaka *et al.* 1992. Thymic depletion and peripheral activation of Class I major histocompatibility complex-restricted T cells by soluble peptide in T cell receptor transgenic mice. *Proc. Natl. Acad. Sci. USA* **89**:11342–6.
16. Mombaerts, P., A. R. Clarke, M. A. Rudnicki *et al.* 1992. Mutations in T-cell antigen genes α and β block thymocyte development at different stages. *Nature* **360**:225–31.

5

Effects of a Unique Adhesion-promoting Anti-rat CD45 Monoclonal Antibody on T-cell Activation

Miloš D. Pavlović and Miodrag Čolić

The leukocyte common antigen (CD45) is an abundant cell surface glycoprotein that is expressed on all nucleated cells of haematopoietic origin (reviewed in 1). It is a member of the transmembrane protein tyrosine phosphatase (PTP) family and plays an important role in the T-cell signal transduction (2,3). The extracellular portion of CD45 is generated by alternative splicing of a common mRNA giving rise to at least eight isoforms and further heterogeneity is introduced by post-translational glycosylation specific to cell and cell proliferation states (1,4). Despite considerable research efforts, natural ligands for CD45 have not been conclusively defined. A number of *cis*-interactions with other membrane molecules has been shown (reviewed in 1,3). Other candidate ligands in *trans* reported so far are CD22 on B cells and heparan sulfate on bone marrow stromal cells (5,6). Nevertheless, CD45 has been shown to exert a profound influence upon the activation, differentiation, apoptosis, and adhesion of T cells (1,7–9).

Recently we have generated a monoclonal antibody (mAb), G3C5, reactive with the framework region of rat CD45 (see materials and methods section). The mAb has a capacity to promote strong homotypic adhesion of rat leukocytes. The prevailing pathway of the adhesion is LFA-1-independent and can be completely blocked by an inhibitor of protein kinase (PK) A/PKG (HA1004) (manuscript in preparation). Along with this adhesion-promoting effect, G3C5 exerts a profound influence on T-cell proliferation and tyrosine phosphorylation. Here we show that G3C5 has a positive regulatory role in T-cell mitogenesis independent of its pro-aggregatory features, and influences both proximal and distal signal transduction cascades in T cells.

Immunoregulation in Health and Disease
ISBN 0-12-459460-3

MATERIALS AND METHODS

Animals

AO ($RT1^u$) and DA ($RT1^a$) female rats, 8–10 weeks old, were bred and maintained in the animal facility of the Institute of Medical Research, MMA, Belgrade.

Monoclonal antibodies and reagents

G3C5 mAb was produced at the IMR, MMA, Belgrade, Briefly, fusion was performed with P3X-Ag.8 myeloma cells and splenocytes of a BALB/c mouse immunized with rat granulocytes. The mAb (IgM) was purified by salt fractionation. In western blot, G3C5 reacted with molecules of 175, 185, and 220 kDa from thymocyte lysates and immunoprecipitation studies on biotin-labelled thymocytes and lymph node (LN) cells confirmed that G3C5 recognizes an epitope of the framework domain of CD45. Flow cytometric (FCM) analysis showed that the G3C5 epitope is expressed on all rat leukocytes but not on cells of epithelial origin.

Other mAb used were WT.1 (CD11a, IgG2a), WT.3 (CD18, IgG1) and 1A29 (CD54, IgG1) (a generous gift of Dr M. Miyasaka, Metropolitan Institute of Medical Science, Tokyo, Japan); OX-1 (CD45, IgG1), OX-22 (CD45RC, IgG1), W3/25 (CD4, IgG1), OX-8 (CD8, IgG1) and R73 ($\alpha\beta$TCR, IgG1) were purchased from Serotec. 8B12 (reactive with rat leukocytes, IgM) was produced at the IMR, MMA, Belgrade, Yugoslavia.

The reagents used were phorbol myristate acetate (PMA), A23187, phytohaemagglutinin (PHA), mitomycin C (Sigma), and concanavalin A (Con A) (Pharmacia LKB).

Cell preparation

Thymocytes, spleen, and LN cells were isolated from thymuses, spleens, and axillar LN respectively, by teasing the organs against a steel mesh to obtain a single-cell suspension as previously described (10). T cells were purified from these suspensions by passage over a nylon wool column. Spleen T cells were further separated into $CD4^+$ and $CD8^+$ subsets. $CD8^+$ and $CD4^+$ T-cell populations were produced by panning on plastic Petri dishes coated with W3/25 (CD4) and OX-8 (CD8) mAb, respectively. FCM analysis was employed to check the purity of the resulting cell population, which was always greater than 93%.

Proliferation assays

Stimulations were carried out in 96-well microtitre plates (200 μl final volume) in triplicate and quantified by filter mat harvesting and scintillation counting as described previously (11). In some experiments with purified T-cell populations, mitomycin C-treated syngeneic splenocytes were added to the wells (2.5×10^6 cells/ml). Where indicated, culture wells were coated overnight with 5 μg/ml R73 and 2 μg/ml G3C5, OX-1, or 8B12 mAb diluted in 0.1 M TRIS buffer pH 9.6. The wells were washed three times before T cells were added. After 54 h in culture, 1 μCi of [^{3}H]-thymidine was added to each well and thymidine incorporation was quantified following an additional 18 h of culture. For MLR assays, splenocytes were isolated from AO rats and treated with mitomycin C (50 μg/ml, 30 min at 37°C). Varying numbers of splenic stimulators were added to 1×10^6 LN T cells/ml (DA rats). After 4, 5, or 6 days in culture, an 18 h pulse of 1 μCi of [^{3}H]-thymidine was added to each well. Cell culturing was done in RPMI-1640 medium supplemented with 10% FCS, 10^{-4} M 2-mercaptoethanol, 2 mM glutamine, 200 U/ml penicillin and 60 U/ml streptomycin.

Phosphotyrosine analyses

Thymocytes (8×10^6 cells per sample) were suspended in 50 μl of RPMI-1640 supplemented with 10^{-4} M 2-ME, 2 mM glutamine, 200 U/ml penicillin, and 60 U/ml streptomycin and incubated at 37°C. Stimulations were initiated immediately by addition of 10 μl of G3C5 (1.5 μg/ml). Reactions proceeded for the indicated times and were terminated by addition of 15 μl of ice-cold 5 × TNT buffer: 5% Triton X-100, 750 mM NaCl, 250 mM TRIS (pH 7.5), 5 mM sodium orthovanadate, and 10 μg/ml of aprotinin, iodoacetamide, and leupeptin. Insoluble material and nuclei were removed with a 5 min microcentrifuge spin (12 000 g) at 4°C. Supernatants were added to SDS–PAGE sample buffer, boiled for 5 min, resolved on 10% SDS–PAGE and transferred to nitrocellulose. Detection of phosphotyrosine containing proteins was accomplished using a mouse monoclonal anti-phosphotyrosine antibody (PY20, ICN) followed by a peroxidase-conjugated secondary antibody. Visualization was performed using chemiluminescence (Amersham).

RESULTS AND DISCUSSION

G3C5 strongly augments mitogen-induced proliferation of T cells

A number of mAb directed to CD45 have been shown to either inhibit or, less frequently, stimulate T-cell proliferation induced by polyclonal mitogens (1,3). In our experiments we used both soluble G3C5 and G3C5 immobilized to plastic, chiefly in order to disclose any effect of the intercellular

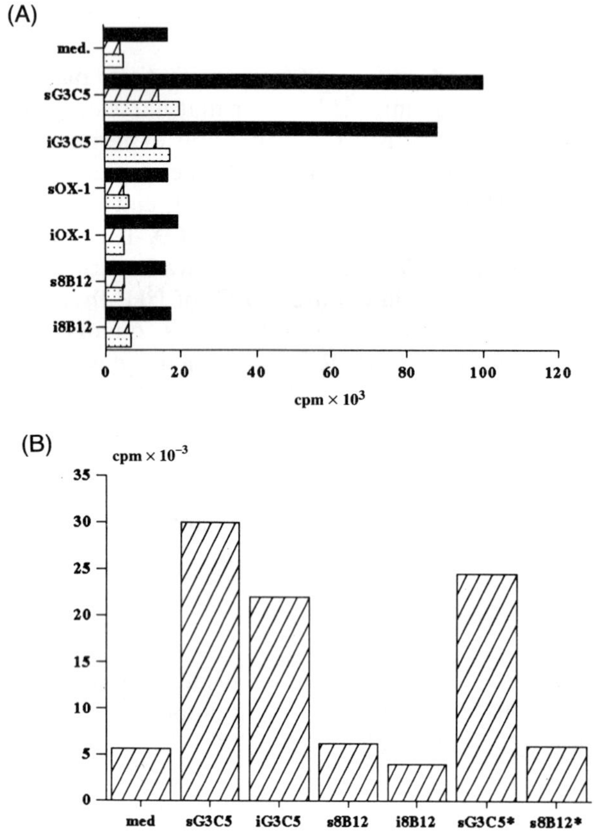

Fig. 5.1 G3C5 enhances proliferation of different T-cell populations and whole spleen cells stimulated by various mitogens. A: whole thymocytes (2.5×10^6 cells/ml) were incubated with 0.6 μg/ml Con A (black bars) or 50 μg/ml PHA (hatched bars) or R73 ascites (1:100) (dotted bars) without or with the addition of 1.5 μg/ml G3C5, OX-1 or 8B12 mAb or culture wells were coated with these mAb as described in materials and methods. B: spleen T cells (1×10^6 cells/ml) were mixed with mitomycin-C-treated syngeneic splenocytes (2.5×10^6 cells/ml) and cultivate with 0.6 μg/mL Con A and, where indicated, 1.5 μg/ml G3C5 or 8B12 mAb were added to the culture wells immediately or 24 h later (*). Some culture wells were coated with these mAb (see above) C: Spleen cells were cultured with a combination of 20 ng/ml PMA and 0.5 μM A23187 without or with the addition of 1.5 μg/ml G3C5 or 8B12 mAb or culture wells were coated with these mAb as described. D: $CD4^+$ (black bars) or $CD8^+$ (hatched bars) T cells (1×10^6 cells/ml) were mixed with mitomycin-C-treated syngeneic splenocytes (2.5×10^6 cells/ml) and stimulated with 0.6 μg/ml Con A and the mAbs as indicated. The cells were cultivated for 3 days and [^{3}H]-thymidine incorporation was measured as described in materials and methods. Triplicate variations were less than 5–15%. s, soluble; i, immobilized.

(C)

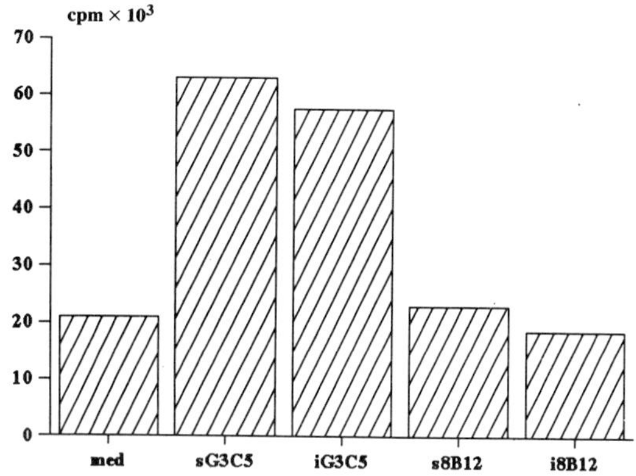

(D)

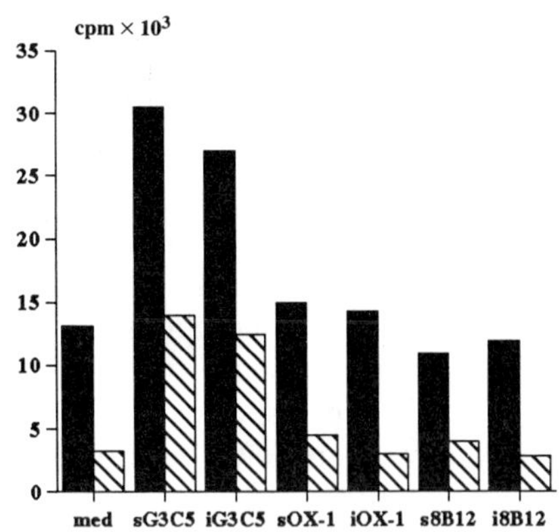

Fig. 5.1 continued

aggregation elicited by soluble G3C5. In all the experiments described below both soluble and immobilized antibody exerted similar effects, hence excluding a significant contribution of the adhesion process. As seen in Fig. 5.1A, G3C5 strongly stimulates proliferation of whole thymocytes induced by Con A, PHA, and R73. Similar results were obtained when spleen T cells were stimulated with Con A and LN T cells with R73 (Fig. 5.1B and not shown). Previous reports brought rather conflicting results while studying the influence of anti-CD45 mAb on lectin- or anti-CD3-stimulated T cells (1). However, these and the following results are interesting bearing in mind the adhesion-promoting features of G3C5. Lorenz *et al.* described an anti-CD45 mAb (NIH 45-2) which induces heterotypic T-cell/monocyte aggregation (LFA-1-dependent) and strongly inhibits CD3-driven T-cell proliferation (12,13). Moreover this mAb, and probably G3C5, increase intracellular cyclic adenosine monophosphate (cAMP) levels (12, manuscript in preparation).

Thus although G3C5 activates T-cell adhesion molecules by elevating cAMP, it simultaneously promotes mitogenic signals transduced via T-cell receptor (TCR). It is well known that CD45 impinges upon the most proximal signal transduction events in T cells, specifically protein tyrosine kinase (PTK) activation (2,3). Hence we have tested whether it might influence more distal signalling pathways. First, spleen T cells were stimulated with Con A and G3C5 was added to culture immediately or 24 h later (Fig. 5.1B). Second, G3C5 was added to spleen cells induced to proliferate by PMA and A23187 (Fig. 5.1C). In both cases G3C5 significantly enhanced the mitogenesis. A similar conclusion was drawn from a recent study but the authors used a Th2 clone instead of primary T cells, and the use of pharmacologic agents in our experiments is a more direct way of substantiating such a role of CD45 since these agents circumvent the initial signalling cascade (14). The results well complement the fact that the peak PTPase activity of CD45 occurs in late mitosis or in cytokinesis (15). There is a marked difference in response of $CD4^+$ and $CD8^+$ primary T cells stimulated via TCR to the inhibitory or stimulatory effect of anti-CD45 mAb (16–18). Thus we then tested the influence of G3C5 on T cells separated according to the expression of the CD4, CD8, and CD45RC antigens (Fig. 5.1D and not shown). Both $CD4^+$ and $CD8^+$ T cells stimulated by Con A increased their proliferation rate in the presence of G3C5 though the response of the latter was proportionally higher. It seems that G3C5 in a way compensates for the low proliferative response of $CD8^+$ T cells in the presence of Con A (Fig. 5.1D). We could not observe any difference in the response of $CD4^+CD45RC^+$ and $CD4^+$ $CD45RC^-$ T cells to Con A when G3C5 was present (data not shown).

G3C5 enhances allogeneic mixed lymphocyte reaction

Anti-CD45 or CD45R mAb reported thus far invariably display an inhibitory effect upon the allogeneic MLR (19). As seen in Fig. 5.2A, G3C5 augments MLR responsiveness particularly at suboptimal responder/stimulator ratios, whereas another anti-CD45 (OX-1, not shown) and isotype-matched control antibodies have no effect. Additionally, if G3C5 is added with a delay of 14 h, it shifts a peak of maximal proliferation for approximately one day in comparison to medium (Fig. 5.2B). The positive effect of G3C5 on MLR is in line with the fact that it stimulates proliferation of rat thymocytes cultured with thymic dendritic cells (M. Čolić, unpublished observations). In contrast, Prickett *et al.* found that a number of anti-CD45 mAb blocked the stimulation of human $CD4^+$ and $CD8^+$ T cells by dendritic cells (20).

G3C5 alters phosphotyrosine pattern in thymocytes

Finally, we studied the alterations in cellular phosphotyrosine induced by G3C5 since CD45 has an intrinsic phosphotyrosine phosphatase activity (1).

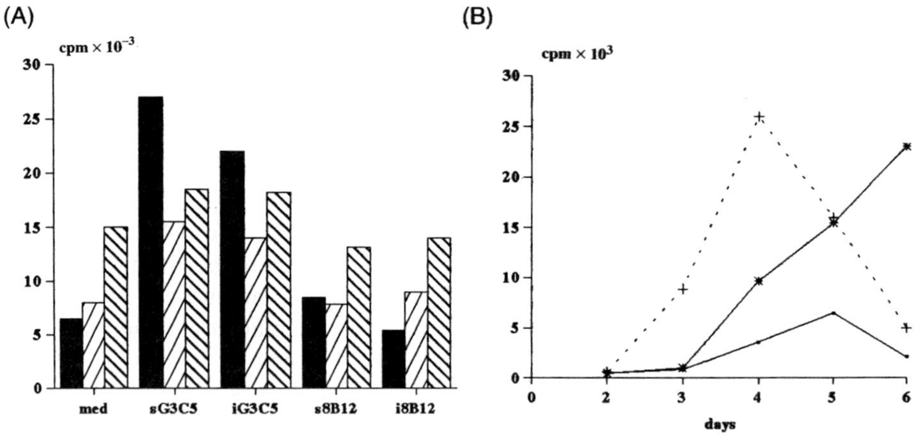

Fig. 5.2 G3C5 stimulates allogeneic mixed lymphocyte reaction. A: LN T cells of DA rats (1×10^6 cells/mL) were mixed with a varying number of mitomycin-C-treated splenocytes of AO rats without or with 1.5 μg/ml of soluble or immobilized G3C5 and 8B12 mAb. The cells were cultivated for 5 days at 37°C and [^{3}H]-thymidine was added as an 18 h pulse. B: The same as in A except that, as denoted, soluble G3C5 mAb was added to the culture immediately or 14 h later and [^{3}H]-thymidine incorporation was assessed after 2, 3, 4, 5 or 6 days of culture. Triplicate variations were less than 5–15%.

As shown in Fig. 5.3 the most prominent change is appearance of a phosphotyrosine protein of 100–110 kDa at 8 min and its complete absence at 30 min of incubation. Hyper- or dephosphorylation of a number of other substrates can be observed as well. At present we do not know the identity of the 100–110 kDa molecule, though the molecular weight could correspond to the catalytic subunit of phosphatidylinositol-3 kinase (p110), an enzyme known to occupy an important position in signal transduction cascade in T cells (21). Nevertheless, these results indicate that, by engaging CD45, G3C5 alters its enzymatic activity. It is noteworthy that sodium orthovanadate (a PTP inhibitor) does not block the adhesion induced by G3C5, again supporting the dichotomy in its influence on adhesion and proliferation of T cells (manuscript in preparation).

CONCLUSIONS

We have described some functional properties of an adhesion-promoting anti-rat CD45 mAb. It generally stimulates T-cell proliferation, affecting early as well as late signal transduction events, enhances allogeneic MLR, and alters thyrosine phosphorylation of cellular proteins. Together the

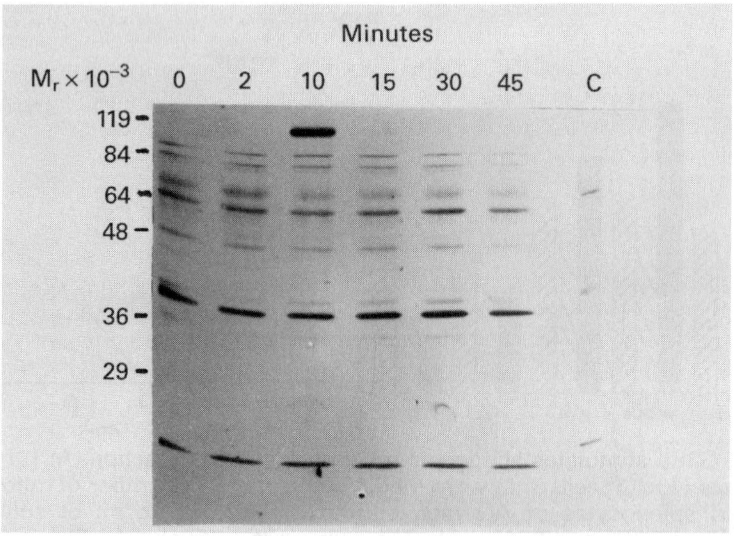

Fig. 5.3 G3C5 alters tyrosine phosphorylation in thymocytes. The cells were stimulated with 1.5 μg/ml G3C5 mAb and the reactions were terminated after different times as indicated. The cells were solubilized, supernatants were mixed with SDS–PAGE sample buffer, boiled for 5 min, resolved on 10% SDS–PAGE and transferred to nitrocellulose. Detection of phosphotyrosines was performed with PY20 mAb and peroxidase-conjugated secondary antibody and visualized by chemiluminescence, essentially as described in materials and methods.

described features make G3C5 unique among other anti-CD45 mAb examined so far.

REFERENCES

1. Trowbridge, I. S., M. L. Thomas. 1994. CD45: an emerging role as a protein tyrosine phosphatase required for lymphocyte activation and development. *Annu. Rev. Immunol.* **12**:85–116.
2. McFarland, E. C., E. Flores, R. J. Matthews and M. L. Thomas. 1994. Protein tyrosine phosphatases involved in lymphocyte signal transduction. *Chem. Immunol.* **59**:40–61.
3. Chan, A. C., D. M. Desai and A. Weiss. 1994. The role of protein tyrosine kinases and protein tyrosine phosphatases in T cell antigen receptor signal transduction. *Ann. Rev. Immunol.* **12**:555–92.
4. Ohta, T., K. Kitamura, A. L. Maizel and A. Takeda. 1994. Alterations in CD45 glycoprotein pattern accompanying different cell proliferation states. *Biochem. Biophys. Res. Commun.* **200**:1283–9.
5. Sgroi, D., G. A. Koretzky and I. Stamenkovic. 1995. Regulation of CD45 engagement by the B-cell receptor CD22. *Proc. Natl. Acad. Sci. USA* **92**: 4026–30.

6. Coombe, D. R., S. M. Watt and C. R. Parish. 1994. Mac-1 (CD11b/CD18) and CD45 mediate adhesion of hematopoietic progenitor cells to stromal cell elements via recognition of stromal heparan sulfate. *Blood* **84**:739–52.
7. Pilarski, L. M. 1993. Adhesive interactions in thymic development: Does selective expression of CD45 isoforms promote stage-specific microclustering in the assembly of functional adhesive complexes on differentiating T lineage lymphocytes? *Immunol. Cell Biol.* **71**:59–69.
8. Ong, C. J., D. Chui, H.-S. Teh and J. D. Marth. 1994. Thymic CD45 tyrosine phosphatase regulates apoptosis and MHC-restricted negative selection. *J. Immunol.* **152**:3793–805.
9. Spertini, F., A. V. T. Wang, T. Chatila and R. S. Geha. 1994. Engagement of the common leukocyte antigen CD45 induces homotypic adhesion of activated human T cells. *J. Immunol.* **153**:1593–602.
10. Pavlović, M. D., M. Čolić, N. Pejnović *et al.* 1994. Anti-rat CD18 monoclonal antibody triggers lymphocyte homotypic aggregation and granulocyte adhesion to plastic: Different intracellular signaling pathways in resting vs. activated thymocytes. *Eur. J. Immunol.* **24**: 1640–8.
11. Pavlović, M. D., M. Čolić, T. Tamatani *et al.* 1994. An adhesion promoting anti-rat CD18 monoclonal antibody differentially alters thymocyte responses to various mitogens. *Thymus* **23**:71–82.
12. Lorenz, H. M., T. Harrer, A. S. Lagoo *et al.* 1993. CD45 mAb induces cell adhesion in peripheral blood mononuclear cells via lymphocyte function-associated antigen-1 (LFA-1) and intercellular cell adhesion molecule 1 (ICAM-1). *Cell Immunol.* **147**:110–28.
13. Lorenz, H. M., A. S. Lagoo, S. Lagoo-Deenadayalan and K. J. Hardy. 1993. On the mode of action of CD45: Signals through different CD45 epitopes induce different intracellular signals. *J. Immunol.* **151**:111A, 623, Abstract.
14. Wolff, H. and C. Janeway Jr. 1994. Anti-CD45 augments response of a Th2 clone to TCR cross-linking. *Scand. J. Immunol.* **40**:22–5.
15. Melkerson-Watson, L. J., M. E. Waldmann, A. D. Gunter *et al.* 1994. Elevation of lymphocyte CD45 tyrosine phosphatase activity during mitosis. *J. Immunol.* **153**:2004–13.
16. Maroun, C. R. and M. Julius. 1994. Distinct involvement of CD45 in antigen receptor signalling in $CD4^+$ and $CD8^+$ primary T cells. *Eur. J. Immunol.* **24**:967–73.
17. Martorell, J., R. Vilella, L. Borche *et al.* 1987. A second signal for T cell mitogenesis provided by monoclonal antibodies to CD45 (T200). *Eur. J. Immunol.* **17**:1447–51.
18. Marvel J., G. Rimon, P. Tathamn and S. Cockcroft. 1991. Evidence that the CD45 phosphatase regulates the activity of the phospholipase C in mouse T lymphocytes. *Eur. J. Immunol.* **21**:195–201.
19. Lazarovits A. I., S. Poppema, M. J. White and J. Karsh. 1992. Inhibition of alloreactivity in vitro by monoclonal antibodies directed against restricted isoforms of the leukocyte-common antigen (CD45). *Transplantation* **54**:724–9.
20. Prickett T. C. R. and D. N. J. Hart. 1990. Anti-leukocyte common antigen (CD45) antibodies inhibit dendritic cell stimulation of CD4 and CD8 T lymphocyte proliferation. *Immunology* **69**:250–7.
21. Ward S. G., C. H. June and D. Olive. 1996. PI 3-kinase: a pivotal pathway in T-cell activation? *Immunol. Today* **17**:187–97.

6

Phenotype Characteristics of NKR-P1$^+$ Cells in Rats:

correlation between presence of NKR-P1$^+$/TCRα, β^- (NK) and NKR-P1$^+$/TCRα, β^+ (NT) cells with Th-cell response

Vladimir Badovinac, Vladimir Trajković, Duško Kosec, Nikola L. Vujanović and Marija Mostarica Stojković

T-cell dependent immune responses may be polarized by the activation of different CD4$^+$ Th cells, which produce distinct patterns of cytokines (1). Th1 cells secrete IL-2 and IFNγ, and predominate in cell-mediated immune (CMI) responses, particularly during intracellular infections (2). Conversely, Th2 cells produce IL-4, IL-5, IL-6, and IL-10, which help antibody production (3), and play a prominent role in antihelminth and allergic responses.

The nature of adaptive CD4$^+$ T-cell dependent responses may be determined by the earliest contact between a pathogen and components of the primitive, non-specific, immune defence system such as macrophages and NK cells (4). These events then provide a microenvironment that favours either Th1 or Th2 responses. It is now widely accepted that the presence of IFNγ, which is enhanced by IL-12, and the subsequent downregulation of IL-4, promotes the development of CD4$^+$ T cells secreting a Th1 pattern of cytokines. On the other hand, early secretion of IL-4 leads to polarization towards Th2 differentiation, both via autocrine production of IL-4 by Th2 cells and by secretion of IL-10, which down-regulates Th1 responses by suppressing the production of macrophage-derived IL-12 (reviewed in 5).

Two inbred strain of rats, AO and DA, differ in the production of Th1 cytokines (IFNγ and IL-2) and also in susceptibility to induction of experimental autoimmune encephalomyelitis (EAE) and multiple low dose streptozotocin (MLD-STZ)-induced diabetes. DA rats are highly susceptible to the induction of Th1 organ-specific autoimmune diseases and are 'high' producers of IFNγ and IL-2, whereas AO rats are relatively resistant to the induction of EAE and MLD-STZ-induced diabetes and are 'low' producers of IFNγ and IL-2 (6,7). Moreover, DA rats have significantly higher

Immunoregulation in Health and Disease
ISBN 0-12-459460-3

percentage of macrophages compared to AO rats (8). Since DA rats have a higher percentage of macrophages, which are, in turn, capable of producing substantial amounts of IL-12, a logical link between production of IL-12, IFNγ, and susceptibility to the induction of Th1 organ-specific autoimmune diseases is established. The situation for the Th2 mediated immune response is less clear since the inducer and the product are the same (9). Results of Yoshimoto and Paul[10] suggest the possibility that rare population of murine NK1.1$^+$(NKR-P1C$^+$)/CD4$^+$ population of T cells which produce IL-4 promptly after the injection of αCD3 antibodies, may be, at least in part, a source of IL-4 to favour the development of Th2 IL-4-producing cells.

The aim of this study was to investigate whether there is a rat equivalent of mouse NK1.1$^+$ (NKR-P1C$^+$) T cells and to analyse such a subset in rat strains with defined pattern of cytokine production and immune responsiveness.

Results presented here indicate a correlation between presence of minor populations of T cells that coexpressed NKR-P1 molecule on its surface, dominant cytokine profile, and Th cell response in AO and DA rats.

MATERIALS AND METHODS

Animals

Male and female Albino Oxford (AO) and Dark August (DA) 10–16-week-old rats, obtained from the animal colony maintained at the Institute for Biological Research, Belgrade, Yugoslavia, were used in the experiments.

Cell separation

Mononuclear cells (MNC) were isolated from spleen and separated by density centrifugation. Spleen MNC were passaged over the nylon wool column and CD8 depleted as previously described (11).

Monoclonal antibodies

Murine monoclonal antibodies specific for rat T lymphocytes were kindly provided by D. Mason (Sir William Dunn School of Pathology, Oxford, UK). They were OX-8 (αCD8) and W3/25 (αCD4). αCD3 (IF4, Serotec, Washington, DC, USA) and αTCRα,β (R7.3, a generous gift from M. Čolič, Institute of Medical Research, MMA, Belgrade, Yugoslavia) were also used in experiments. FITC-conjugated F(ab$'$)$_2$ fragments of goat anti-mouse IgG were purchased from INEP (Zemun, Yugoslavia). For detection of NKR-P1$^+$ cells, biotinylated αNKR-P1 (3.2.3, originating from Pittsburgh Cancer Institute, University of Pittsburgh, Pennsylvania, USA) and PE-labelled avidin were used.

Immunofluorescent analysis

Fluorescence staining was performed at 4°C in 100 μl containing 5–10 × 10^6 spleen mononuclear cells (MNC), nylon wool (NW) non-adherent spleen MNC, or CD8 depleted NW non-adherent spleen MNC. Cells were stained with biotinylated αNKR-P1 PE-labelled avidin in combination with FITC αCD3, αTCRα,β, αCD4, or αCD8 mAbs in PBS containing 2% FCS. After the staining, cells were fixed in 0.5 ml 1% paraformaldehyde. Fluorescence analysis was carried out with a FACScan Flow Cytometer (Becton Dickinson, Mountain View, USA).

RESULTS

Two-colour flow cytometric analysis using mAb 3.2.3 (αNKR-P1; PE/FL1) and αCD3 (FITC/FL2) reveals two distinct subsets of rat splenic mononuclear cells expressing variable levels of NKR-P1. Figure 6.1A,B illustrates that NKR-P1 is expressed at high levels on a subset of CD3$^-$ cells (quadrant 1). However, NKR-P1 is also expressed at lower levels on a clearly defined population of cells expressing CD3 molecule (Fig. 6.1A,B, quadrant 2).

In repetitive experiments, the NKR-P1$^+$/CD3$^+$ subset ranged from 4 to 11% of splenic MNC from AO rats (Fig. 6.1A, quadrant 2) or from 3 to 6.5% from DA rats (Fig. 6.1B, quadrant 2) indicating a higher percentage of T cells with NKR-P1 molecule in AO compared to DA rats. On contrary, DA having a higher percentage of NKR-P1^{high+} cells (NK cells) with the higher expression of these molecule per cell compared to AO strain (quadrant 1, Fig. 6.1A and B).

To further investigate the lineage of the NKR-P1$^+$/CD3$^+$ subset of cells, we performed two-colour analysis with αNKR-P1 (mAb 3.2.3), αTCRα,β (mAb R7.3), or αCD4 (mAb w3/25). As demonstrated in Fig. 6.2, the NKR-P1$^+$/TCR$^+$ subset expresses CD4 molecule on the surface in the less than 0.5% (Fig. 6.2B) of splenic MNC derived from AO rats.

The expression of TCRα,β and CD8 molecule on NKR-P1$^+$ cells were analysed on nylon wool (NW) non-adherent AO splenic MNC. We found that cells that expressed NKR-P1 molecule could be divided into a subset that was TCRα,β^- (Fig. 6.3A2, quadrant 1) and another containing ~30% of NKR-P1$^+$ cells that coexpressed TCRα,β (Fig. 6.3A2, quadrant 2). More than 90% of NKR-P1$^+$ cells coexpressed CD8 (Fig. 6.3A3, quadrant 2).

After in vitro depletion of CD8 (approximately 96% of depletion, Fig. 6.3B) in NW non-adherent AO splenic MNC, two-colour cytometric analysis reveals that NKR-P1$^+$ could be subdivided into a subset expressing NKR-P1$^+$/TCRα,β^-/CD8$^-$ (NK) (Fig. 6.3C1 and 3C3, quadrant 1) as well as, from comparison between Fig. 6.3C2, quadrant 2 and C3 quadrant 2, a minor subset (less than 1%) expressing NKR-P1$^+$/TCRα,β^+/CD8$^-$.

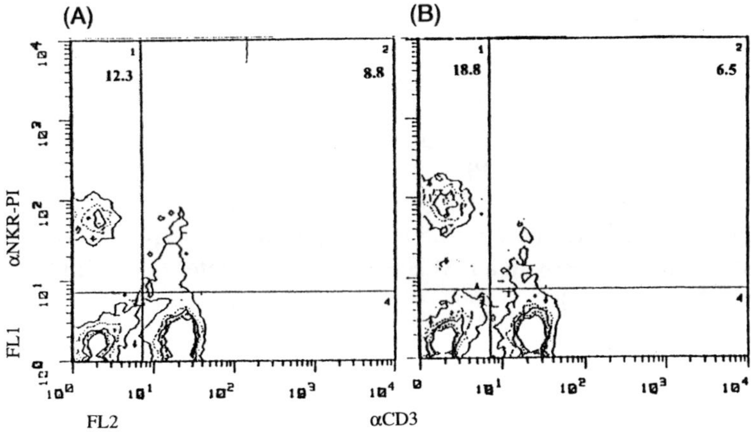

Fig. 6.1 Expression of NKR-P1 vs CD3 on AO (A) and DA (B) rat spleen MNC. Mononuclear cells were indirectly stained with biotinylated αNKR-P1 PE-labelled avidin mAb (FL1) in combination with αCD3 mAb plus FITC-conjugated $F(ab')_2$ fragments of goat anti-mouse IgG Ab (FL2). The numbers in the panels indicate the percentage of positive cells. Cells were analysed on FACStar Cytometer (Becton Dickinson). The data are representative of four different experiments.

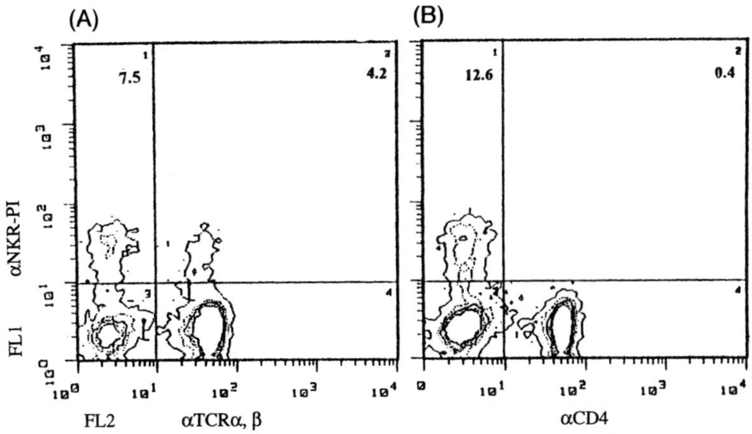

Fig. 6.2 Expression of NKR-P1 vs TCRα,β (A), or CD4 (B) on AO spleen MNC. Mononuclear cells were indirectly stained with biotinylated αNKR-P1 PE-labelled avidin mAb (FL1) in combination with αTCRα,β or αCD4 mAbs plus FITC-conjugated $F(ab')_2$ fragments of goat anti-mouse IgG Ab (FL2). The numbers in the panels indicate the percentage of positive cells.

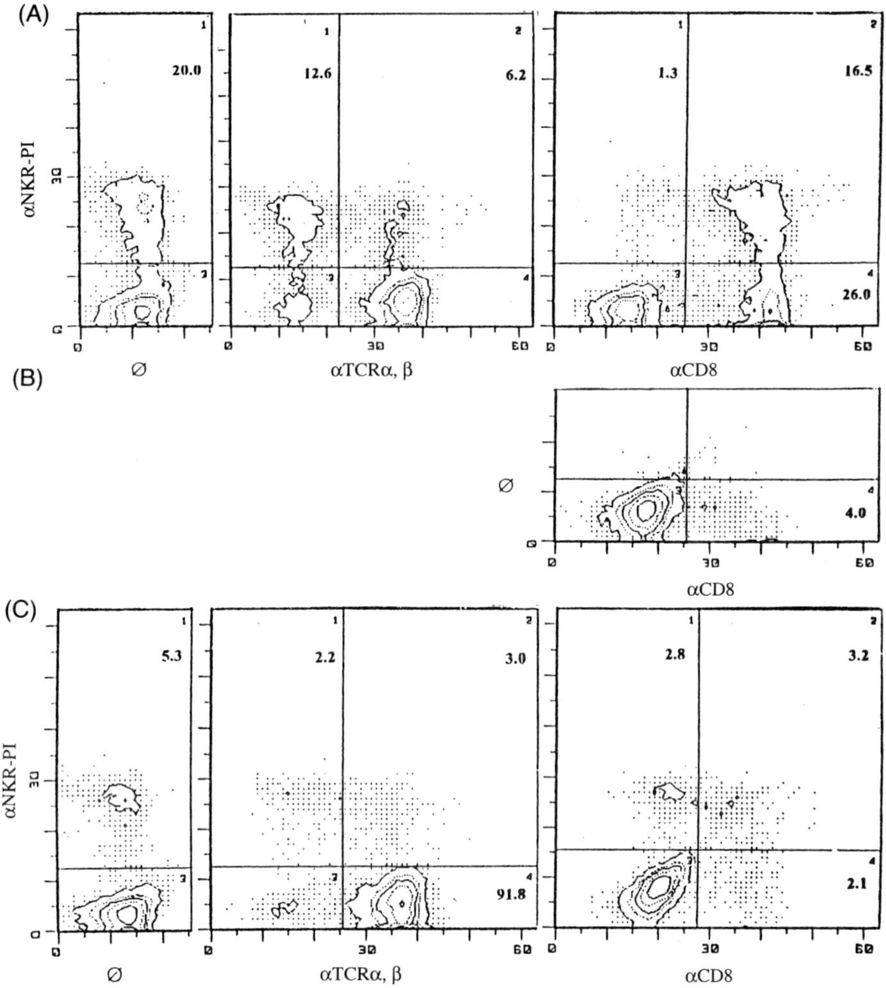

Fig. 6.3 Expression of NKR-P1 vs TCRα,β or CD8 on AO nylon wool (NW) non-adherent spleen MNC (A) or CD8 depleted NW non-adherent spleen MNC (B, C). Cells were stained with NKR-P1 mAb alone or in combination with αTCRα,β, or αCD8 Abs. After the CD8 depletion the percentage of CD8$^+$ was less than 5% (B). The numbers in the panels indicate the percentage of positive cells.

DISCUSSION

In this report we present the evidence for the expression of NKR-P1 on at least four subsets of normal rat spleen MNC including NKR-P1$^+$/TCRα,β^-/CD8$^+$, NKR-P1$^+$/TCRα,β^-/CD8$^-$ (NK) and NKR-P1$^+$/TCRα,β^+/CD8$^+$, NKR-P1$^+$/TCRα,β^+/CD8$^-$(NT) (Figs 6.1–6.3). DA rats have a higher percentage of NKR-P1^{high+} cells (NK cells) while AO rats, despite a lower percentage of NK cells, have a higher percentage of cells that coexpressed NKR-P1 and TCRα,β (or CD3) molecule on its surface.

Chambers *et al.* (12) produced mAb (3.2.3) which recognized NK cell activation receptor (NKR-P1). It has been shown that NKR-P1 is a receptor responsible for natural killing by binding carbohydrate ligands to NK-sensitive targets and by triggering NK cell activation (13). As well as their effector function, NK cells are regulatory, producing IFNγ and other cytokines, and it was shown that IFNγ can promote the development of CD4$^+$ T cells secreting a Th1 pattern of cytokines (14). Our previous results, showing that CD4$^+$ T cells derived from DA rats produce more IL-2 and IFNγ in contrast to lower production in AO rats (6,7), strongly correlate with functional analysis showing better killing capacity of DA MNC compared to AO MNC (8) and with obtained experimental data that DA rats have a significantly higher percentage of NK cells with higher expression of NKR-P1 molecule per cell, in blood (data not shown) and spleen MNC compared to AO rats (Fig. 6.1).

On the other hand, AO rats have higher percentage of NKR-P1$^+$ cells that expressed TCRα,β and/or CD3 (Fig. 6.1). The presence of TCRα,β on subsets of NKR-P1$^+$ cells demonstrates that these are T cells (newly assigned natural T (NT) cells (15)). It has been shown that cells of similar phenotype exist in Fisher 344 (F 344) rats (16) but there are no data concerning their possible immunoregulatory role. NT cells may be capable, as was shown in mice (10), of secreting IL-4 at the outset of immune responses and thus may act to regulate the pattern of priming of naive T cells, by providing a source of IL-4 to favour the development of Th2 IL-4-producing cells. Phenotype analysis of mouse NT cells has shown that these cells are NKR-P1$^+$ TCRα,β^+ CD4$^+$CD8$^-$ or NKR-P1$^+$ TCRα,β^+ CD4$^-$CD8$^-$ (DN NT). The existence of CD8 was not shown on mouse NK cells or on NT cells. On the other hand, more than 90% of rat-derived NKR-P1$^+$ cells coexpressed the CD8 molecule (Fig. 6.3A), as has been shown for rat large granular cells (LGL) in general (17), and for F 344 rat NKR-P1$^+$ cells (16).

Therefore, 'high' IFNγ production and susceptibility to Th1 organ-specific autoimmune diseases in DA rats compared to 'low' IFNγ production and susceptibility to Th2 organ-specific diseases in AO rats correlate with the percentage of NK as well as NT cells in these two strains. DA rats have a higher percentage of macrophages (8) and NK cells, cells that are capable of producing substantial amounts of IL-12 and IFNγ, whereas AO rats, despite a lower percentage of macrophages and NK cells, have a significantly higher percentage of NT cells. Subsequent study will clarify whether these cells, with a phenotype distinct from mouse NT cells, are capable of substantial production of IL-4.

CONCLUSION

To determine whether genetically determined differences in the production of Th1 cytokines are, at least in part, dependent on cells of non-specific immunity, we found that susceptible DA rats have a higher percentage of macrophages and NK cells. On the other hand, AO rats, despite a lower percentage of NKR-P1^{+} cells, have a higher percentage of NT cells. Further analysis will show whether these cells, as in mice, are capable of substantial IL-4 production and may be, at least in part, responsible for favouring the development of Th2-like IL-4 producing cells.

REFERENCES

1. Mosmann, T. R., H. Cherwinski, M. W. Bond *et al.* 1986. Two types of murine helper T cell clones. I. Definition according to profiles of lymphokine activities and secreted proteins. *J. Immunol.* **136**:2348–57.
2. Cher, J. D. and R. T. Mosmann. 1987. Two types of murine helper T cell clone. *J. Immunol.* **138**:3688–94.
3. Mosmann, R. T. and R. I. Coffman. 1989. Different patterns of lymphokine secretion leads to different functional properties. *Annu. Rev. Immunol.* **7**: 145–73.
4. Garside, P. and A. M. Mowat. 1995. Polarization of Th-cell responses: a phylogenic consequence of nonspecific immune defense? *Immunol. Today* **5**:220–3.
5. Reiner, L. S. and A. R. Seder. 1995. T helper cell differentiation in immune response. *Curr. Opin. Immunol.* **7**:360–6.
6. Vukmanović, S., M. Mostarica Stojković and M. L. Lukić. 1989. Experimental autoimmune encephalomyelitis in 'low' and 'high' Interleukin-2 producer rats. *Cell. Immunol.* **121**:238–46.
7. Arsov, I., V. Pravica, V. Badovinac *et al.* 1995. Selection for the susceptibility to experimental allergic encephalomyelitis also selects for high IFN-γ production. *Transplant. Proc.* **27**:1537–8.
8. Badovinac, V., V. Pravica, V. Trajković *et al.* 1996. Correlation between number of NK (NKR-P1^{+}) cells and production of cytokines in inbred AO and DA rats. *Microbiology* **33**: 45–52.
9. Seder, R. A., W. E. Paul, M. M. Davis and Fazekas de St. Groth. 1992. The presence of interleukin 4 during in vitro priming determines the lymphokine-producing potential of CD4^{+} T cells from T cell receptor transgenic mice. *J. Exp. Med.* **176**:1091–8.
10. Yoshimoto, T. and W. E. Paul. 1994. CD4^{pos}, NK1.1^{pos} T cells promptly produce interleukin 4 in response to in vivo challenge with anti-CD3. *J. Exp. Med.* **179**:1285–95.
11. Wysocki, L. J. and V. L. Sato. 1978. 'Panning' for lymphocytes: A method for cell selection. *Proc. Natl. Acad. Sci. USA* **75**:2844–8.
12. Chambers, H. W., N. L. Vujanović, A. B. DeLeo *et al.* 1989. Monoclonal antibody to a triggering structure expressed on rat natural killer cells and adherent lymphokine activated killer cells. *J. Exp. Med.* **19**:1373–89.
13. Bezouska, K., C. T. Yuen, J. O'Brien *et al.* 1994. Oligosaccharide ligands for NKR-P1 protein activate NK cells and cytotoxicity. *Nature* **372**:150–7.

14. Seder, R. A., R. Gazzinelli, A. Sher and W. E. Paul. 1993. IL-12 acts directly on $CD4^+$ T cells to enhance priming for IFN-γ production and diminishes IL-4 inhibition of such priming. *Proc. Natl. Acad. Sci. USA* **90**: 10 188–92.
15. Bix, M. and R. M. Locksley. 1995. Natural T cells. Cells that co-express NKR-P1 and TCR. *J. Immunol.* **155**:1020–2.
16. Brissette-Storkus, C., C. L. Kaufman, L. Pasewicz *et al.* 1994. Characterization and function of the NKR-$P1^{dim}$/T cell receptor α,β subset of rat T cells. *J. Immunol.* **152**:388–96.
17. Reynolds, C. W., S. O. Sharrow, J. R. Ortaldo and R. B. Herberman. 1981. Natural killer (NK) cell activity in the rat. II. Analysis of surface antigens on LGL by flow cytometry. *J. Immunol.* **127**:2204–8.

7

LFA-1/ICAM-1 Adhesion Pathway is Involved in Both Apoptosis and Proliferation of Thymocytes Induced by Thymic Dendritic Cells

Vesna Tadić, Miodrag Čolić, Masayuki Miyasaka and Vesna Ilić

Thymic dendritic cells (TDC) represent a small but functionally significant population of thymic non-lymphoid cells. Like other members of the DC family, they are bone marrow-derived cells of the monocyte–macrophage lineage, which efficiently present antigens to lymphocytes (1,2,3). Recent experiments in mice have revealed, however, that TDC may develop from an intrathymic precursor population, but its nature is unknown (4). TDC express MHC class I and II molecules, various adhesion molecules, and certain markers common to thymocytes (5,6). It seems that they are phenotypically heterogeneous, owing to either the existence of functionally distinct TDC subpopulations or different developmental stages along a maturation pathway (5,6).

It is believed that TDC have self antigen-presenting capacity, thus playing a key role in clonal deletion (apoptosis) of autoreactive immature thymocytes (7,8), but also in the proliferation and clonal amplification of a subset of mature medullary thymocytes (9). However, the mechanisms involved in these processes are poorly understood. In this work we demonstrate that purified rat TDC promote thymocyte apoptosis in vitro and also stimulate thymocyte proliferation. In both processes, the LFA-1/ICAM-1 adhesion pathway is involved.

Immunoregulation in Health and Disease
ISBN 0–12–459460–3

MATERIALS AND METHODS

Cell preparation

Thymocyte suspension was obtained by teasing thymuses of adult (8–10 weeks old) AO rats against a steel mesh using RPMI medium with 10% FCS. TDC were isolated from the obtained thymocyte suspension as low-density cells after centrifugation over a Nycodenz gradient (density 1.078 g/cm^3, osmolarity 390 mOsm) (Nycomed, Oslo, Norway) as described (6). After washing, the cells from the interface zone were cultivated for 1 h at 37°C in an incubator with 5% carbon dioxide. Non-adherent cells were discarded and adherent cells, containing predominantly macrophages and DC, were further cultivated for an additional 18 h. During this culture period the TDC became non-adherent. They were collected and again purified over the same gradient. The purity of such prepared TDC was usually more than 80%.

Flow cytometry

TDC or thymocytes were stained in suspension with WT.1 (anti-rat CD11a), WT.3 (anti-rat CD18) and 1A29 (anti-rat ICAM-1) monoclonal antibodies (mAbs) as previously described (6). Stained cells were analysed on a FACScan flow cytometer (Becton-Dickinson) after appropriate cell gating (6).

Rosette assay for TDC-thymocyte binding

Purified TDC (1×10^4) were mixed with 2×10^5 thymocytes in 20 μl of RPMI/10% FCS medium in Terasaki microwell plates and then cultivated in hanging drops at 37°C for 30 min. For blocking experiments, thymocytes were preincubated with WT.1 and WT.3 or an irrelevant IgG1 mAb (BH1), whereas TDC were preincubated with 1A29 or BH1 mAbs (all at 10 μg/ml) for 30 min before cell mixing. TDC that bound four or more thymocytes were scored as rosettes. The results were presented as:

% relative binding = number of rosettes with mAb/number of rosettes without mAb × 100.

For statistical analysis (Student's t test) the percentage of relative binding in the presence of specific mAb was calculated and compared to that using control, irrelevant mAb.

Thymocyte apoptosis

Suspensions of TDC and thymocytes (ratio 1 : 5) were cultivated for 24 h at 37°C in quadruplicate in 96-well round plates. After that, the cells were washed, fixed overnight in 4% formaline dissolved in ethanol, stained with haematoxylin, and examined under a light microscope. The percentage of apoptotic thymocytes (thymocytes with pyknotic nuclei) was determined on the basis of 400 calculated thymocytes per each sample.

Thymocyte proliferation assay

The proliferation of thymocytes in the presence of TDC was measured as previously described (6) using a [^{3}H]-thymidine incorporation assay. The following stimuli were used: R.73 (anti-rat $\alpha\beta$ TCR mAb) at concentration of 10 μg/ml; recombinant human IL-2 (Genzyme) (10 U/ml); PMA (Sigma) (20 ng/ml); calcium ionophore, A 23187 (Sigma) (0.5 μM). Monoclonal antibodies WT.1, WT.3, and 1A29 were continuously present during the culture period of 72 h.

RESULTS AND DISCUSSION

TDC potentiate thymocyte apoptosis in vitro

During the maturation and differentiation in the thymus autoreactive thymocytes are deleted by apoptosis, especially at the stage of double positive (DP) $CD4^+CD8^+$ cells (7–9). Experiments with superantigens and transgenic animals showed that deletion of thymocytes is mediated by various types of thymic non-lymphoid cells, but it is believed that TDC are the most potent ones (7,10). This process is a consequence of interactions between TCR on immature autoreactive thymocytes with self peptides associated with self MHC molecules displayed on TDC. Isolated thymocytes die spontaneously in culture by apoptosis. This process is significantly potentiated by cross-linking of TCR complexes by mAbs. Activation-induced apoptosis by mAbs to the TCR complex might mimic in vivo thymocyte negative selection (7). Little is known, however, whether TDC in vitro have similar effect on thymocyte apoptosis.

In our previous work (6; Čolić *et al.* submitted) we used a modified method for isolation of almost pure population of rat TDC. It was demonstrated that in culture with purified TDC a significantly higher number of apoptotic cells (studied by morphological criteria) in 24 h cultures of thymocytes with TDC (58.3 $\pm$ 4.8) was observed than in cultures without TDC (44.2 $\pm$ 5.1) ($p < 0.001$). Soluble products of TDC were inefficient, indicating that direct TDC/thymocyte contacts are necessary for apoptosis induction. Similar results were obtained by measuring apoptosis using propidium iodide or merocyanine 540 staining by flow cytometry.

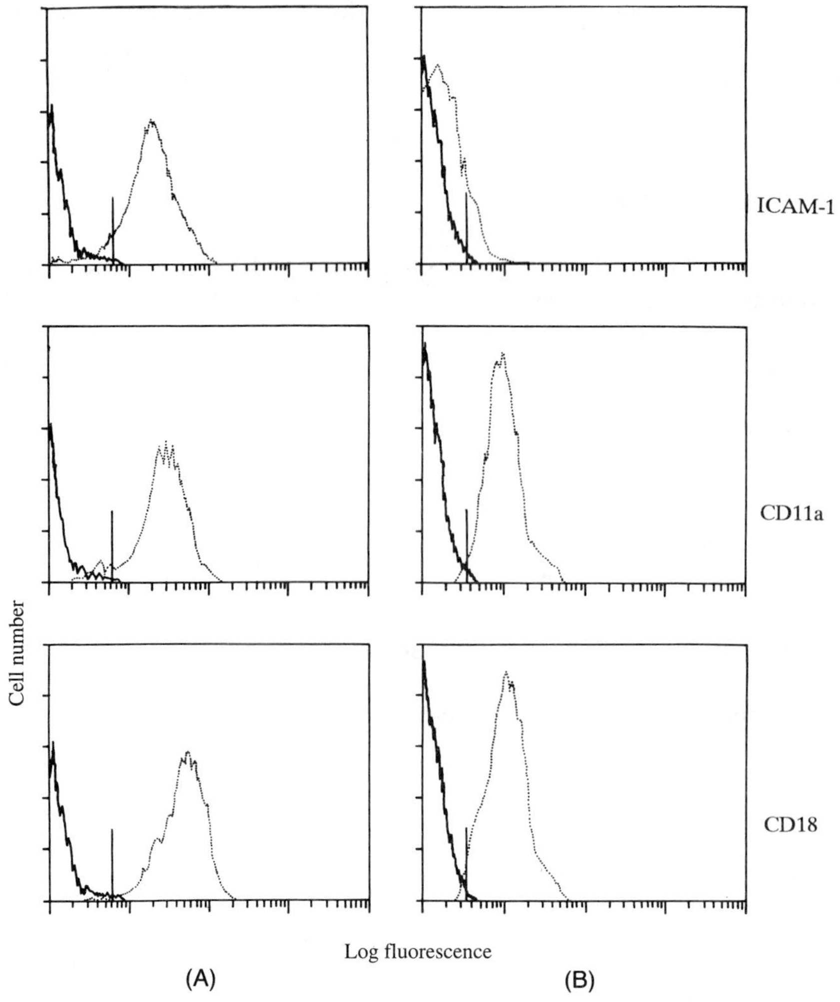

Fig. 7.1 Flow cytometric analysis of (A) purified TDC and (B) thymocytes stained by 1A29 (anti-ICAM-1), WT.1 (anti-CD11a) and WT.3 (anti-CD18) mAbs. Histograms of fluorescences are presented as dotted lines. Vertical bars on histograms represent the levels of non-specific staining using PBS and secondary antibody as control (solid line).

Role of LFA-1/ICAM-1 interactions in thymocyte apoptosis induced by TDC

The interaction of LFA-1 with its ligands (ICAM-1,2, and 3) is known to play a crucial role in the adhesive interactions of the immune cells and the effective functioning of the immune system (11,12). Previous studies

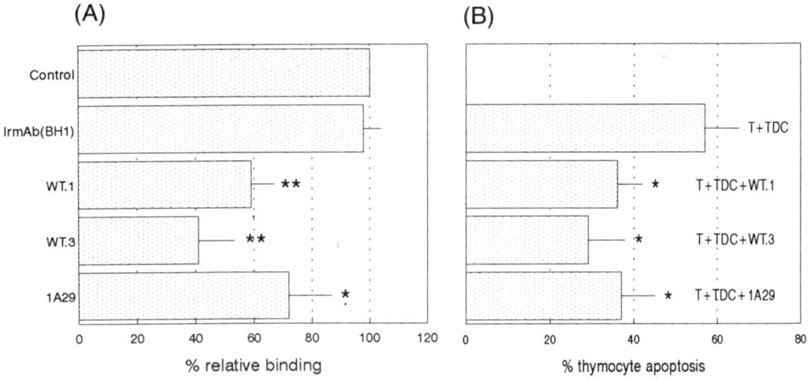

Fig. 7.2 (A) MAbs to LFA-1 and ICAM-1 inhibit thymocyte binding to rat TDC. The binding of thymocytes to TDC was determined after cell incubation for 30 min at 37°C as described in the materials and methods section. Values are given as the percentage of relative binding in the presence of mAbs (mean ± SD from three different experiments) in comparison to controls (samples without mAbs) used as 100%. * $= p < 0.05$; ** $= p < 0.005$ compared to the relevant mAb (BH1). (B) MAbs to LFA-1 and ICAM-1 inhibit thymocyte apoptosis induced by TDC. TDC-induced thymocyte apoptosis was determined by morphological analysis of pyknotic nuclei of thymocytes as described in the Materials and methods section. Values are given as mean ± SD from three different experiments. * $= p < 0.05$ in comparison to control (samples without mAbs).

demonstrated that the LFA-1/ICAM-1 interaction is important for thymocyte binding to thymic non-lymphoid cells and for the development of mature T cells (13). We therefore wanted to study whether this receptor–ligand pair is also involved in the TDC-induced thymocyte apoptosis.

The results presented in Fig. 7.1 show that almost all purified rat TDC and thymocytes express LFA-1 as demonstrated by WT.1 (anti-CD11a) and WT.3 (anti-CD18) mAbs. In contrast, 1A29 (anti ICAM-1) mAb binds to most TDC, but only to a subset (approximately 15%) of thymocytes.

All these mAbs significantly inhibited apoptosis of thymocytes induced by TDC (Fig. 7.2A). Among them, anti-ICAM-1 mAb had the most potent anti-apoptotic effect. These results are in accordance with inhibitory effects of the mAbs on the rosette formation between thymocytes and TDC (Fig. 7.2B). Since stronger inhibitory effect was obtained using anti-LFA-1 mAbs (especially WT.3) it can be hypothesized that LFA-1 might bind to other ligands such as ICAM-2 or ICAM-3 (14).

Up to now, few data have been published about the role of LFA-1/ICAM-1 interaction in negative selection and apoptosis of thymocytes. Previous results demonstrated that mAbs to LFA-1 and ICAM-1 blocked antigen-dependent deletion of DP thymocytes from mice that are transgenic for class I MHC restricted T-cell receptors (10,15). However, some in vitro studies suggest that the deletion of superantigen-specific human $CD4^+$ T cells can be blocked by antibodies directed against CD11a/CD18 but not ICAM-1 or ICAM-2 (16). Recent findings by Gonzalo *et al.* (17) also showed that in mice genetically deficient in ICAM-1, in vivo treated with *Staphylococcus aureus* enterotoxin (SEB), cellular interactions mediated by ICAM-1 are not essential for the induction of deletion or anergy of the SEB-reactive $V\beta8^+$ T cells in the periphery. On the other hand, ICAM-1 is required for proliferation of these T lymphocytes. However, the authors did not study whether similar mechanisms are operative in the thymus.

Role of LFA-1/ICAM-1 interactions in thymocyte proliferation induced by TDC

Another postulated role of TDC is the induction of proliferation of mature medullary thymocytes (9). It is known that T cell proliferation depends on signalling through the TCR complex but also on other cell-surface molecules that promote adhesion between T cells and DC, many of them displaying a costimulatory role. Among these molecules, the LFA-1/ICAM-1 interaction is very important (8,14).

Thymocytes respond poorly by proliferation in the presence of DC without additional stimuli. However, in our experiments we demonstrated (Fig. 7.3) that purified TDC are capable of inducing a substantial rate of thymocyte proliferation even without other stimuli. The TDC-induced thymocyte proliferation was significantly potentiated in the presence of r-IL-2, calcium ionophore, PMA, or an anti-$\alpha\beta$ TCR mAb (R7.3). Under all conditions anti-CD18 mAb inhibited thymocyte proliferation, whereas, unexpectedly, WT.1 (anti-CD11a) mAb significantly stimulated thymocyte proliferation. Anti-ICAM-1 mAb showed various effects depending on applied stimuli. It inhibited the TDC-induced thymocyte proliferation in the presence of r-IL-2, stimulated the process in the presence of PMA or was without any detectable effect when other agents (calcium ionophore, R7.3) were added.

It is known that blocking of interactions between LFA-1 and its counter-receptors by mAbs suppresses allo- and xenogeneic mixed lymphocyte reaction (MLR), antigen-specific, and Con A-induced T cell proliferation and T cell dependent antibody responses (12,14). This was also demonstrated for thymocytes using various mitogens (18). However, little information is available when purified, short-term cultivated TDC were used, such as the cells in our experiments. The finding that anti-CD-18 mAb blocks thymocyte proliferation indicates that a costimulatory signal through β_2 integrins is necessary for optimal proliferation of these cells in the presence of TDC. However, the stimulatory effect of WT.1 antibody was an unexpected phenomenon. WT.1 recognizes an 'inhibitory' epitope of the α chain of LFA-1 and, as demonstrated (Fig. 7.2A), inhibits thymocyte binding to TDC.

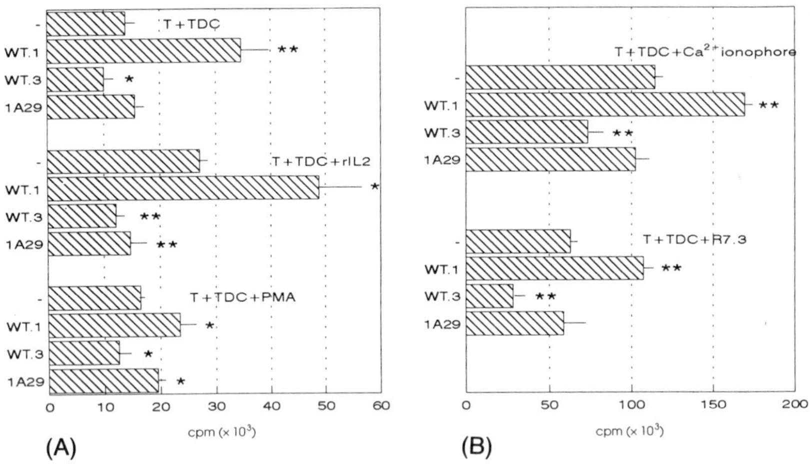

Fig. 7.3 Effect of mAbs to LFA-1 (WT1 and WT3) and ICAM-1 (1A29) on thymocyte proliferation induced by TDC in the presence of (A) IL-2 or PMA and (B) Ca^{2+} ionophore or R73 mAb. TDC-induced thymocyte proliferation was measured using a ^{3}H-thymidine uptake assay as described in the materials and methods section. Values are given as cpm (mean of triplicates) from three different experiments. $* = p < 0.05$; $**p < 0.001$ compared to corresponding controls.

In addition, WT.1 also partly inhibited the proliferation of unpurified thymocytes in the presence of Con A (data not shown).

It is known that β_2 integrins can exist in different activation states, but only some of them are able to bind ligands (14,19). Cross-linking of the T-cell receptors and some other cell-surface accessory molecules increases LFA-1-mediated adhesion, inducing the conformational changes of the integrin and increasing its affinity, but without increasing the surface expression of LFA-1. The affinity changes associated with LFA-1 activation are not a simple on/off switch, but a more complex series of changes with at least three detectable conformational changes (14). These are related to interactions with different members of the ICAM family. Some anti-LFA-1 mAbs are able to block binding to ICAM-3 but not to ICAM-1, and vice versa. Antibody-blocking studies indicate that in our experiments (depending on the applied stimuli) LFA-1 might use different ligands. This could be the reason why anti-ICAM-1 antibody in our experiments exerted different effects on thymocyte proliferation. However, it is not clear what are the signals that regulate affinity states of particular epitopes on LFA-1, what is the order of their involvement in the binding, and what are the functional consequences of these different ligand-binding interactions. One possible explanation for stimulatory effect of WT.1 antibody could be that blocking of the WT.1 epitope increases binding of LFA-1 for ligands other than ICAM-1, since anti-ICAM-1 mAb did not inhibit TDC-induced thymocyte proliferation in the presence of WT.1 mAb (data not shown). However, so far the human equivalents of ICAM-2 and ICAM-3 have not been discovered in the rat. In our system LFA-1 is expressed on both thymocytes and TDC, suggesting bidirectional binding of the integrin with its ligands which could additionally multiplicate these interactions. It is also possible that blocking of WT.1 epitopes increases the interactions of other adhesion molecules involved in signal transduction such as CD28/CTL4 on thymocytes and their ligands, the B.7 family of co-stimulatory molecules expressed on TDC (20). All these hypotheses are attractive subjects for further study.

CONCLUSION

Rat TDC promote thymocyte apoptosis in vitro. The apoptosis is inhibited by mAbs to LFA-1 (CD11a and CD18) and ICAM-1. The effect might be a consequence of inhibition of thymocyte binding to TDC, as demonstrated using a rosette assay. TDC also stimulate the proliferation of thymocytes without any additional stimuli. This process was potentiated using IL-2, anti-$\alpha\beta$ TCR (R-73), PMA or a calcium ionophore. The TDC-induced proliferation was inhibited by anti-CD18 mAb and stimulated by anti-CD11a mAb. In contrast, anti-ICAM-1 mAb shows differential effect on thymocyte proliferation, depending on applied stimuli.

REFERENCES

1. O'Heill, H. C. 1994. The lineage relationship of dendritic cells with other haematpoietic cells. *Scand. J. Immunol.* **39**:513–16.
2. Steimann, R. M. 1991. The dendritic cell system and its role in immunogenicity. *Annu. Rev. Inununol.* **9**:271–96.
3. Hsiao, L., K. Takahashi, M. Takeya and T. Arao. 1991. Differentiation and maturation of macrophages into interdigitating cells and their multicellular complex formation in the fetal and postnatal rat thymus. *Thymus* **17**:219–35.
4. Ardavin, C., L. Wu, C.-L. Li and K. Shortman, 1993. Thymic dendritic cells and T cells develop simultaneously in the thymus from a common precursor population. *Nature* **362**:761–3.
5. Banuls, M. P., A. Alvarez, I. Ferrero *et al.* 1993. Cell-surface markers of rat thymic dendritic cells. *Immunology* **79**:298–304.
6. Ilić, V., M. Čolić and D. Kosec. 1995. Isolation, cultivation and phenotypic characterisation of rat thymic dendritic cells. *Thymus* **24**:9–28.
7. Ramsdell, F. and B. J. Fowlkes. 1990. Clonal deletion versus clonal anergy: The role of the thymus in inducing self tolerance. *Science* **248**:1342–8.
8. Kyewski, B. 1988. Unrevealing the complexity of intrathymic cell-cell interaction. *Acta Pathologica Microbiologica and Immunologica Scandinavia* **96**:1049–60.
9. Landry, D., L. Doyon, J. Poudrier *et al.* 1990. Accessory function of human thymic dendritic cells in Con A-induced proliferation of autologous thymocyte subsets. *J. Immunol.* **144**:836–43.

10. Pircher, H., K. Brduscha, U. Steinhoff *et al.* 1993. Tolerance induction by clonal deletion of $CD4^+CD8^+$ thymocytes in vitro does not require dedicated antigen-presenting cells. *Eur. J. Immunol.* **23**:669–74.
11. Springer, T. A. 1990. Adhesion receptors of the immune system. *Nature* **346**:425–34.
12. Arnaout, M. A. 1990. Structure and function of leukocyte adhesion molecules CD11/CD18. *Blood* **75**:1037–50.
13. Fine, J. S. and A. M. Kruisbeek. 1991. The role of LFA-1/ICAM-1 interactions during murine T lymphocyte development. *J. Immunol.* **147**:2852–9.
14. Lub, M., Y. van Kooyk and C. G. Figdor. 1995. Ins and outs of LFA-1. *Immunol. Today* **16**:479–83.
15. Carlow, D. A., N. S. van Oers, S. J. Teh and H. S. Teh. 1992. Deletion of antigen specific thymocytes by dendritic cells requires LFA-1/ICAM-1 interactions. *J. Immunol.* **148**:1595–603.
16. Damle, N. K., G. Leytze, K. Klussman and J. A. Ledbetter. 1993. Activation with superantigens induces programmed death in antigen-primed $CD4^+$ class II^+ major histocompatibility complex T lymphocytes via a CD11a/CD18-dependent mechanism. *Eur. J. Immunol.* **23**:1513–19.
17. Gonzalo, J. A., C. A. Martinez, A. T. Springer and J. C. Gutierrez-Ramos. 1995. ICAM-1 is required for T cell proliferation but not for anergy or apoptosis induced by *Staphylococcus aureus* enterotoxin B in vivo. *Internat. Immunol.* **7**:1691–8.
18. Pavlović, M. D., M. Čolić, T. Tamatani *et al.* 1994. An adhesion-promoting anti-rat CD18 monoclonal antibody differentially alters thymocyte responses to various mitogens. *Thymus* **23**:71–82.
19. Ortlepp, S., P. E. Stephens, N. Hogg *et al.* 1995. Antibodies that activate $\beta 2$ integrins can generate different ligand binding states. *Eur. J. Immunol.* **25**:637–643.
20. Caux, C., B. Vanbervliet, C. Massacrier *et al.* 1994. B70/B7-2 is identical to CD86 and is the major functional ligand for CD28 expressed on human dendritic cells. *J. Exp. Med.* **180**:1841–7.

8

Apoptosis Induced by Microtubular Poisons in Thymocytes

Vladimir Bumbaširević, Andjelija Škaro-Milić, Aleksandar Mirčić and Bogdan Djuričić

Prominent cell and nuclear changes that occur during apoptosis, a type of programmed cell death, are a consequence of an extensive rearrangement of the cytoskeleton, including microtubules (1,2). Apoptosis occurs during various physiological and pathological conditions, when cells die in a controlled manner, following an intrinsic programme that is still not well understood, undergoing a series of morphological and biochemical changes (3). This process can be also induced by a number of agents (1–3), including microtubule disrupting drugs, MDD (4–6), drugs widely used in the treatment of various human cancers; however, the precise mechanism of their action has not been clearly established. The widely held view (7) that the main action of MDD is the blockade of mitosis has now been largely modified by the results of apoptosis induction in normal and malignant cell types by MDD (4–6).

To obtain more insight into the role of microtubules during the apoptotic process, we treated isolated thymocytes both with MDD and with a microtubule stabilizing agent (MSA), paclitaxel, for 1–24 h.

MATERIALS AND METHODS

Cell preparation and culture

Suspensions of thymocytes were obtained from male C57BL mice, 4–5 weeks old (6). A Trypan blue exclusion test showed more than 97% viable thymocytes after isolation. Cell suspensions were incubated in RPMI 1640 medium, supplemented with 10% fetal calf serum in a humidified atmosphere of 5% carbon dioxide in air, for 1–24 h.

Cells were incubated with or without microtubular poisons, 2 μM of

Immunoregulation in Health and Disease
ISBN 0-12-459460-3

colchicine, 2.5 μM of nocodazole, or 10 μM of paclitaxel (Taxol). In separate experiments, (Na,K)ATPase inhibitors, ouabain (3 mM), or vanadate (3 mM), were added together with MDD, in order to evaluate the role of the ionic pump in the apoptotic process. Induction of apoptosis by MDD was also tested by inhibition of protein synthesis by 50 μM cycloheximide, chelation of extracellular calcium by 5 mM etyleneglycol-bis-(β-aminoethyl ether)*N*,*N*,*N*′,*N*′-tetraacetic acid (EGTA), and by inhibition of apoptotic nuclease by 5 mM zinc sulphate.

Morphological studies

Following incubation, cells were washed and routinely processed to embedding in Epon. The percentage of apoptotic and mitotic cells was determined on toluidine blue stained semi-thin sections, as described previously (6), and ultrathin sections stained with uranyl acetate and lead citrate were examined in a Phillips EM 300 electron microscope.

DNA extraction and electrophoresis

Fragmentation of DNA was determined as previously described (5, 6). DNA (3 μg/per lane) was electrophoresed in 1.5% agarose gel, and photographed under ultraviolet light after staining with ethidium bromide.

RESULTS AND DISCUSSION

Exposure of thymocytes to both types of microtubular poisons, MDD or MSA, caused an increase in mitotic index (Fig. 8.1a and b). This was a consequence of mitotic blockade due to the absence of mitotic spindles, as confirmed by electron microscopy. Colchicine and nocodazole produced the disappearance of microtubules in both interphase and mitotic thymocytes (Fig. 1.1c), whereas cells incubated with paclitaxel displayed prominent

---

Fig. 8.1 (a) Light microscopic appearance of thymocytes incubated 4 h with colchicine. Note numerous apoptotic thymocytes (arrowheads) and mitotically arrested cells (arrows). Toluidine blue stained 1 μm section. Bar = 10 μm. (b) Apoptotic (AI) and mitotic (MI) indexes (mean values ± standard deviation) of thymocytes incubated for 4 h without drugs (con), with 2 μM colchicine (col), 2.5 μM nocodazole (noc), and 10 μM taxol (tax). (c) Mitotically arrested thymocyte showing absence of spindle microtubules and unusual position of centrioles (arrowheads); 2 h after incubation with 2 μM colchicine; Ch, chromosomes. Bar = 1 μm. (d) Microtubular 'bundle' (arrows) in the cytoplasm of a thymocyte incubated with 10 μM taxol for 4 h. Bar = 0.5 μm.

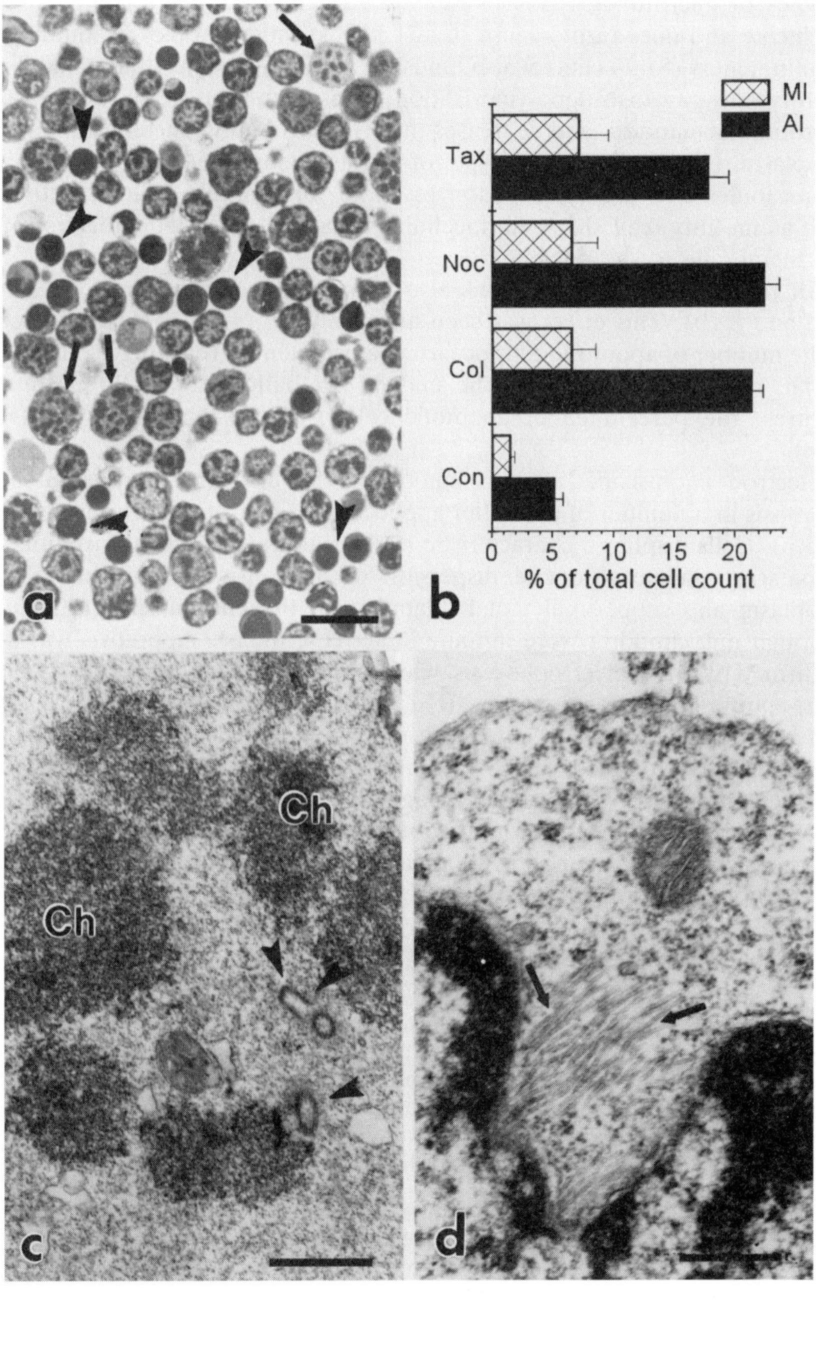
a
b
MI
AI
Tax
Noc
Col
Con
0 5 10 15 20
% of total cell count
Ch
Ch
c
d

bundles of microtubules (Fig. 8.1d). It is widely accepted that the MDD colchicine and nocodazole cause disassembly of microtubules by binding to tubulin dimers (8). Paclitaxel also binds to tubulin molecules, but it stabilizes microtubules against depolymerization, causes formation of cytoplasmic microtubular bundles, and decreases the critical tubulin concentration in the cytoplasm (9,10). So, both type of drugs disturb normal function of microtubules and the cytoskeleton essential for multiple cellular activities such as motility, cell shape, intracellular transport, and signalling from the cell membrane to the nucleus (8).

All three microtubular poisons also induced thymocyte apoptosis (Figs. 8.1a and 8.2b). This effect was seen after only 1 h, while a steady increase in the number of apoptotic cells occurred subsequently, reaching around 20% at 4 h, and close to 90% by the end of incubation (24 h). In untreated cultures, the percentage of apoptotic cells was substantially lower (Fig. 8.1b).

Electron microscopic analysis confirmed the ultrastructural features of apoptosis in a number of cells after application of microtubular poisons (Fig. 8.2a,b). Cells displayed characteristic nuclear alterations, such as peripheral chromatin condensation and dispersion of nucleoli, condensation of the cytoplasm and subplasmalemmal dilatation of the endoplasmic reticulum, although mitochondria were initially intact (Fig. 8.2b). Apoptosis was also confirmed by DNA electrophoresis, which showed the typical 'ladder' pattern of apoptotic DNA fragmentation (Fig. 8.2c).

It had been generally accepted that the arrest of cells in metaphase is the dominant effect of these drugs (7), but it has also been shown that they enhance apoptosis in normal and malignant cells (4–6). The apoptotic effect of MDD, as we have shown previously (4, 6), was mostly directed to interphase thymocytes, and it was apparently unrelated to the ability of these drugs to block mitosis, as most thymocytes are not cycling, and it is unlikely

---

Fig. 8.2 (a) Electron microscopic appearance of untreated thymocytes incubated 4 h (control). Bar = 2 μm. (b) Thymocyte with early (arrow) and advanced apoptotic changes (arrowheads), 4 h incubation in the presence of 10 μM taxol. Note the characteristic condensation of the nuclear chromatin, and the loss of the cell volume. Subplasmalemmal dilatation of endoplasmic reticulum is indicated by open arrows. Bar = 2 μm. (c) DNA electrophoresis in 1.5% agarose. DNA was extracted from thymocytes incubated for 4 h without drugs (lane 1), with 10 μM methylprednisolone (lane 2), 2 μM colchicine (lane 3), and 10 μM taxol (lane 4). Following lanes represent DNA from thymocytes incubated with colchicine in addition to 5 nM EGTA (lane 5), 5 mM $ZnSO_4$ (lane 6), 3 mM ouabain (lane 7), or 3 mM vanadate (lane 8). (d) Inhibitory effects of 50 μM cycloheximide (CHX), 5 mM EGTA, 5 mM $ZnSO_4$ and 3 mM ouabain (Oub) on induction of apoptosis by 2 μM colchicine (4 h incubation). Each bar represents mean value of at least three separate experiments.

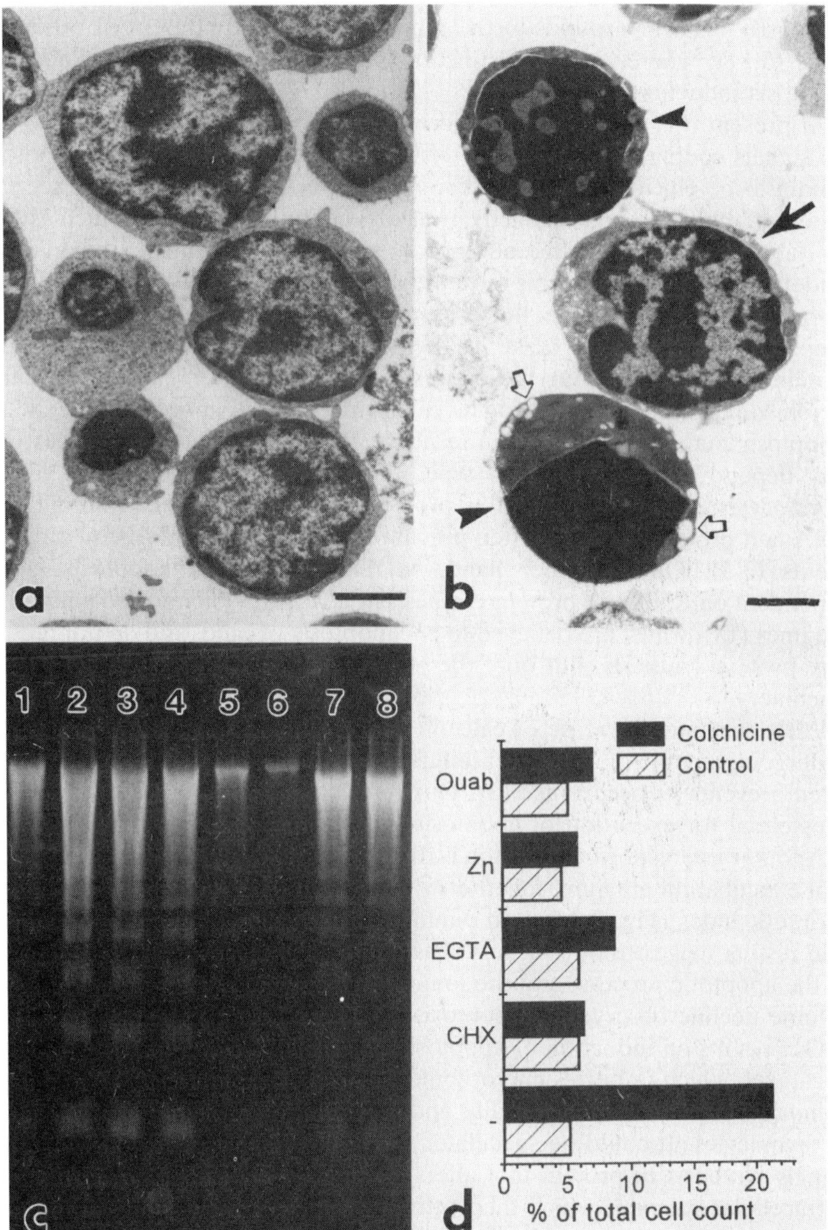
a
b
1 2 3 4 5 6 7 8
c
Colchicine
Control
Ouab
Zn
EGTA
CHX
-
0 5 10 15 20
% of total cell count
d

that during the first few hours of incubation mitotic block could precede apoptosis. This corresponds to the reports on MDD treatment of other cell types (5,11), where a clear distinction between the mitotic blockade and apoptosis induction is shown.

At present it is not clear how microtubular poisons induce apoptosis, and the signals coupling microtubular dysfunction to the induction of apoptosis remain to be elucidated. The occurrence of DNA fragmentation as seen by gel electrophoresis suggests activation of apoptotic nuclease, which is also substantiated by the fact that addition of zinc ions, or aurintricarboxylic acid (widely used inhibitors of this nuclease) prevented full spectrum of apoptotic morphology (Fig. 8.2d) in the presence of MDD (6). Also, induction of apoptosis by MDD, at least in thymocytes, is dependent on de novo protein synthesis, and on the presence of extracellular calcium, because cycloheximide and EGTA abrogate colchicine-induced apoptosis (Fig. 8.2d). Apoptosis may or may not require active RNA and protein synthesis: this may depend more on the cell type, than on the inducing agent (3,12). Thymocytes can be considered as prototypes of cells in which inhibitors of RNA and protein synthesis often prevent induction of apoptosis by different agents (2,3). On the other hand, MDD induction of apoptosis is not dependent on RNA and protein synthesis in several leukaemic and lymphoma cell lines (13), which are believed to be 'apoptosis-primed' and do not require new protein synthesis, but only the activation of effectors of the apoptotic machinery.

Early sustained increase of calcium ions was observed in many cell types undergoing apoptosis, and extracellular or intracellular chelation of calcium often prevents its occurrence (3). Our results also confirm that calcium flux is essential for execution of apoptosis induced by MDD.

Another interesting observation is that the presence of ouabain or vanadate in the incubation medium, together with colchicine, significantly lowered the apoptotic index (Fig. 8.2d), and diminished DNA fragmentation (Fig. 8.2c). The results suggest that (Na,K)ATPase activity is necessary for propagation of the apoptotic process, and the ionic pump is probably involved in the cell volume decline observed in apoptosis (1–3).

Our results on induction of apoptosis by yet another microtubular poison, paclitaxel, which stabilizes microtubules (9,10), suggest that any perturbation of normal microtubular assembly and function is able to trigger apoptosis in thymocytes. It could be speculated that recognition of this type of injury signals synthesis of protein that alters permeability of plasma membrane to extracellular calcium, which then activates the apoptotic signalling cascade, including endonuclease activation and DNA fragmentation. The important role of microtubules in the apoptotic process is also confirmed by reports showing that disassembly of microtubules (14), or their specific reorganization (15), are common features of the apoptotic process induced by other drugs.

CONCLUSION

The present study shows that any disturbance of normal microtubule functions, by either MDD or MSD, induces apoptosis in thymocytes, and that this effect is not related to their action on mitotic blockade. Induction of thymocyte apoptosis by microtubular poisons is dependent on extracellular calcium and preservation of protein synthesis, and is inhibited by inhibitors of apoptotic nuclease, as well as by the inhibition of the ionic pump, (Na,K)ATPase.

REFERENCES

1. Wyllie, A. H., J. F. R. Kerr and A. R. Currie. 1980. Cell death: the significance of apoptosis. *Int. Rev. Cytol.* **68**:251–306.
2. Djuricic, B. and V. Bumbasirevic, 1994. Programmed cell death. *Iugoslav. Physiol. Pharmacol. Acta* **30**:169–87.
3. Schwartzman, R. A. and J. A. Cidlowski. 1993. Apoptosis: The biochemistry and molecular biology of programmed cell death. *Enocr. Rev.* **14**:133–51.
4. Bumbaširević, V., V. Lačković and M. Japundžić. 1985. Enhancement of apoptosis in lymphoid tissue by microtubule disrupting drugs. *IRCS Med. Sci. (Biochem)* **13**:1257–8.
5. Martin, S. J. and T. G. Cotter. 1990. Specific loss of microtubules in HL-60 cells leads to programmed cell death (apoptosis). *Biochem. Soc. Trans.* **18**:299–301.
6. Bumbaširević, V., A. Škaro-Milić, A. Mirčić and B. Djuričić. 1995. Apoptosis induced by microtubule disrupting drugs in normal murine thymocytes in vitro. *Scanning Microsc.* **9**:509–18.
7. Anilkumar, T. V., C. E. Sarraf, T. Hunt and M. R. Alison. 1992. The nature of cytotoxic drug-induced cell death in murine intestinal crypts. *Br. J. Cancer* **65**:552–8.
8. Mandelkow, E. and E.-M. Mandelkow. 1995. Microtubules and microtubule-associated proteins. *Curr. Opin. Cell Biol.* **7**:72–81.
9. Caplow, M., J. Shanks and R. Ruhlen. 1994. How taxol modulates microtubule disassembly. *J. Biol. Chem.* **269**:23399–402.
10. Rowinsky, E. K., L. A. Cazanave and R. C. Donnehower. 1990. Taxol: a novel investigational antimicrotubule agent. *J. Nat. Cancer Inst.* **82**:1247–59.
11. Harmon, B. V., Y. S. Takano, C. M. Winterford and C. S. Potten. 1992. Cell death induced by vincristine in the intestinal crypts of mice and in a human Burkitt's lymphoma cell line. *Cell Prolif.* **25**:523–36.
12. Martin, S. J. 1993. Apoptosis: suicide, execution or murder? *Trends Cell Biol.* **3**:141–4.
13. Takano, Y., M. Okudaira and B. V. Harmon. 1993. Apoptosis induced by microtubule disrupting drugs in cultured human lymphoma cells. Inhibitory effects of phorbol ester and zinc sulphate. *Path. Res. Pract.* **189**:197–203.
14. Bumbaširević, V., A. Škaro-Milić, A. Mirčić and B. Djuričić. 1992. Ultrastructural analysis of apoptosis induced by microtubule disrupting drugs on isolated murine thymocytes. In: *Electron Microscopy 92*, Vol. III (L. Megias-Megias, M. I. Rodriguez-Garcia, A. Rios and J. M. Arias, eds.) University of Granada Serv. Publ., Granada, pp. 813–15.
15. Ireland, C. M. and S. M. Pittman. 1995. Tubulin alterations in taxol-induced apoptosis parallel those observed with other drugs. *Biochem. Pharmacol.* **49**:1491–9.

9

A Monoclonal Antibody R-MC 46 Induces Homotypic Adhesion and Activation of Rat Peripheral Blood Neutrophils

Nada Pejnović, Miodrag Čolić, Biljana Drašković-Pavlović and Aleksandar Dujić

Polymorphonuclear leukocytes (PMN) are the first cells that migrate into tissues in response to invading pathogens, but may mediate serious tissue damage. Apart from phagocytosis, granulocytes are now known as cells which regulate both inflammatory and immune responses. Neutrophil 'priming', NADPH oxidase activation, release of reactive oxygen intermediates (ROI), lytic enzymes, cytokines and adhesion are regulated by the number of membrane receptors and surface antigens (1).

PMN exert most of their physiological functions while adherent to surfaces, rather than in suspension. On stimulation they adhere to other neutrophils, endothelium, and extracellular matrix proteins. Neutrophil aggregation is thought to play a role in a variety of microvascular pathologies associated with sepsis, acute respiratory distress syndrome, and ischemic diseases. Neutrophil adhesion is largely mediated by β_2 integrins (CD11a,b,c/CD18) and L-selectin (CD 62L) which are also intracellular signalling molecules (2). Activation of NADPH oxidase by cytokines, bacterial wall products, and complement components, and subsequent production of ROI in neutrophils, is a major mechanism of bacterial killing and tissue damage. A number of reports show that various monoclonal antibodies binding to membrane antigens could modulate granulocyte functions such as production of ROI, haemotaxis, and adhesion (3).

Homotypic adhesion, originally reported to be induced by phorbol esters, represents a suitable model for exploring mechanisms of leukocyte

Immunoregulation in Health and Disease
ISBN 0-12-459460-3

aggregation (4). In this study, using this model, we describe that R-MC 46 monoclonal antibody triggers homotypic granulocyte aggregation and enhances phorbol ester (PMA)-induced NADPH oxidase activity and hydrogen peroxide production.

MATERIALS AND METHODS

MAb and reagents

R-MC 46 mAb was produced at the Institute for Medical Research, MMA, Belgrade, Yugoslavia. A fusion was performed with P3X myeloma cells and splenocytes of mice immunized with rat thymic stroma. This mAb was purified using Protein A Sepharose (LKB Pharmacia, Sweden) and its isotype is IgG1. In western blot it reacted with a molecule of 5.5 kDa from granulocyte lysates. This molecule is expressed on the membrane of granulocytes, monocytes, a subset of lymphocytes, and some endothelial and epithelial cells (5). WT.3 mAb (anti-rat CD18;IgG1) and WT.1 (anti-rat CD11a;IgG2a), were kindly provided by Dr M. Miyasaka from the Department of Immunology, Metropolitan Institute of Medical Science, Tokyo, Japan. OX-42 (anti-rat CD11b/c;IgG2a) and OX-18 (anti-rat class I MHC:IgG1) were purchased from Serotec, GB. The reagents used were PMA (Sigma, St. Louis, MO, USA), nitroblue tetrazolium (NBT) (ICN Pharmaceuticals, USA), medium HBSS without calcium and magnesium (Sigma, St. Louis, MO).

Cell preparation

Female AO rats (12–16 weeks old) were used as a source of cells. Peripheral blood granulocytes were prepared by centrifugation on a gradient NycoPrep Animal 1007 (Nycomed AS, Oslo, Norway). Purity of cells showed >95% granulocytes.

Semiquantitative adhesion assay

To measure homotypic adhesion we read the wells of microtitre plates using a phase contrast microscope, and the results are presented as number of aggregates per well (4).

Colorimetric assay of granulocyte adherence to plastic

We used a modified assay initially described by Oez *et al.* (6). Briefly, peripheral blood granulocytes were seeded at 5×10^5 cells/well and the plates incubated at 37°C for 60 min. Non-adherent cells were removed, adherent cells stained with 0.1% methylene blue and the absorbance of dissolved colour measured using an ELISA reader (Behring ELISA Processor, Behring, FRG).

Assessment of PMN activation

Hydrogen peroxide production was measured by modified microassay as described by Pick and Mozel (7). The activation of PMNs was evaluated as the reduction of NBT expressed as absorbance at 570 nm (8) after various times of PMN cultivation.

RESULTS

R-MC 46 induce homotypic aggregation of neutrophils

R-MC 46 induced strong homotypic clustering of neutrophils, so that large number of very compact aggregates with more than 100 cells in association were observed (Fig. 9.1a). OX-18 mAb (anti-class I MHC) did not induce cell aggregation as well as another anti-rat granulocyte mAb R-MC 45 (Fig. 9.1b). Cell clustering was completely abrogated at 4°C and cells reaggregated when returned to 37°C. The PMN aggregation induced by R-MC 46 mAb was dose- and time-dependent. Evident clustering occurred with 1.5 μg/ml and was maximal at 5–10 μg/ml (more than 100 aggregates/well), started 2 h after addition of mAb, reached peak after 6–18 h and remained almost

(A) (B) (C)

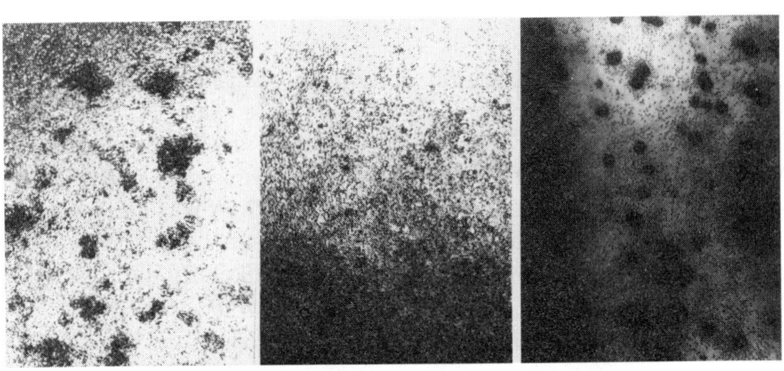

Fig. 9.1 Induction of neutrophil aggregation by R-MC 46 mAb. (a) R-MC 46 mAb; (b) OX-18 mAb; (c) PMA. Cells were plated at 5×10^5/well with R-MC 46 mAb (10 μg/ml), OX-18 (10 μg/ml), PMA (250 ng/ml) incubated at 37°C and photographed at 80× after 6 h of culture.

unchanged for the next 48 h. The kinetics and form of aggregates induced by mAb differed from those evoked by PMA (Fig. 9.1c). PMA induced smaller and looser aggregates which were visible after 30 min, reached a peak at 3–6 h (20–40 aggregates/well) and than deaggregated.

Role of divalent cations in R-MC 46 induced PMN aggregation

Granulocyte aggregation induced by R-MC 46 was fully prevented by incubating cells in calcium/magnesium-free medium. The addition of magnesium ions completely and calcium ions partially restored cell clustering induced by R-MC 46 (data not shown).

Role of the β_2 integrins in R-MC 46 induced PMN aggregation

MAb inhibition studies were done to identify potential adhesion molecules involved in R-MC 46-induced neutrophil aggregation. WT.3 (anti-CD18) and WT.1 (anti-CD11a) could not inhibit the mAb-evoked aggregation, while OX-42 (anti-CD11b/c) only partially blocked the cell clustering. In contrast, PMA-induced granulocyte aggregation was CD18 dependent and partially CD11a and CD11b/c dependent in our test system (data not shown).

R-MC 46 stimulates neutrophil adherence to plastic

Using a simple colorimetric assay, we showed that R-MC 46 had the ability to increase neutrophil adhesion to plastic to the same extent as that seen with PMA (medium 0.162, R-MC 46 0.300, PMA 0.328). WT.3 (anti-CD18) mAb completely blocked R-MC 46- and PMA-induced adhesion to plastic. OX-42 (anti-CD11b/CD11c) only slightly decreased adhesion with both agents (data not shown).

Effect of R-MC 46 in neutrophil activation

R-MC 46 did not trigger any NBT reduction by PMN, but enhanced PMA-induced dye reduction (Fig. 9.2a). Hydrogen peroxide release measured in the presence of the triggering agent PMA was increased 2–3-fold in R-MC 46 treated neutrophils in comparison with isotype-matched irrelevant antibody. R-MC 46 by itself did not evoke any hydrogen peroxide production (Fig. 9.2b).

DISCUSSION

The present study demonstrates that R-MC 46 monoclonal antibody induces homotypic adhesion of rat peripheral blood neutrophils and increased

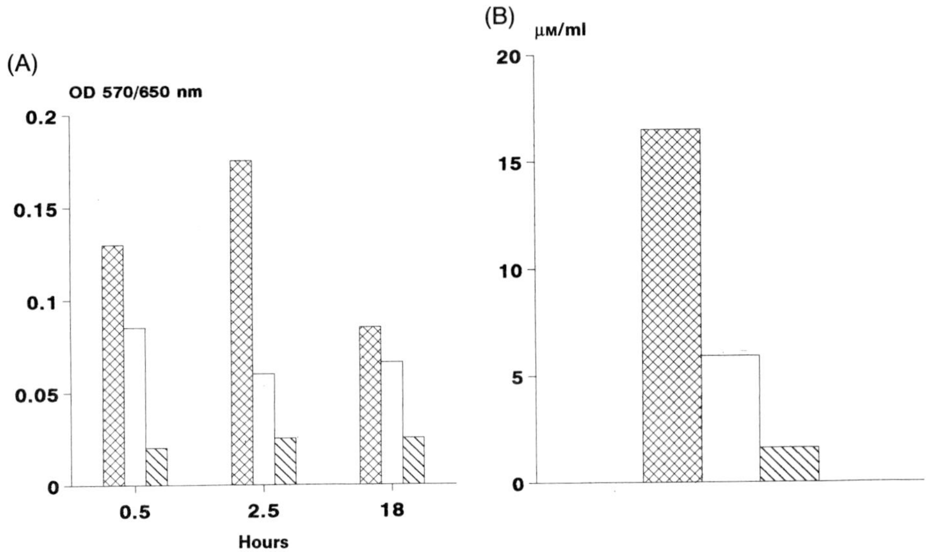

Fig. 9.2 Enhancement of neutrophil activation by R-MC 46 mAb. (a) NBT reduction; (b) hydrogen peroxide production. Cells were plated at 5×10^5/well with R-MC 46 (10 μg/ml) (hatched bars), PMA (125 ng/ml in NBT test or 10 ng/ml in hydrogen peroxide assay) (open bars) and R-MC 46 and PMA simultaneously (cross-hatched bars) added at the beginning of culture. The results represent the mean of triplicate of a representative of four separate experiments.

hydrogen peroxide-producing capacity and NBT reduction, two characteristics associated with the activated state of these cells. The requirement for magnesium and calcium ions and temperature dependence strongly indicates that R-MC 46-induced PMN aggregation is not a simple case of antibody crosslinking and that metabolically active cells were needed for this process to occur. The aggregation appeared to be morphologically and kinetically distinct from that induced by PMA. The finding that magnesium depletion abrogates, and magnesium reconstitution restores R-MC 46-induced PMN aggregation suggests the involvement of adhesion molecules of the integrin family. However, almost complete restoration of aggregation by addition of calcium suggests the involvement of other molecules. These findings are supported by mAbs blocking studies where anti-CD18 antibody could not prevent R-MC 46-induced cell clustering, while CD11b had a modest effect. Similar phenomena were seen with ED7 mAb which also induced CD18 independent aggregation of rat inflammatory granulocytes in the same test system (unpublished results). Most agents known to induce granulocyte aggregation such as C5a, PMA or anti-CD15 mAb mediate this effect by β_2 integrin molecules (9,10). There is a report which showed that formyl peptide (fMLP)-induced granulocyte aggregation was mediated by both CD18 and L-selectin molecules (3). It seems that initial increase of R-MC 46 adhesion shown as enhancement of PMN adhesiveness to plastic (which occurred in the first 60 min) was mediated by the CD18 molecule and partly by CD11b/CD18, and that subsequent aggregation involved other adhesion molecules or other epitopes of CD11/CD18 molecules which the mAbs used in our experiments do not detect. It is well documented that the adhesion of granulocytes to plastic is critically dependent on the function of CR3 (CD11b/CD18) (11). There are reports that anti-human CD18 mAb (KIM 127 and KIM 185) enhanced the adhesion of PMN to protein-coated glass or plastic by activating CR3 (12). Additionally, we recently reported that anti-rat CD18 mAb (NG2B12) induced granulocyte adhesion to plastic, but this effect was blocked by both anti-CD18 and OX-42 (anti-CD11b/CD18) (13).

Increase of ROI production by employing monoclonal antibodies to cell surface antigens has been reported. Anti-CD43 antibody was shown to increase hydrogen peroxide production in the presence of PMA in human monocytes (4). Anti-L-selectin mAb enhanced hydrogen peroxide production in subsequent response to FMPL and tumour necrosis factor (14) from human granulocytes. Two monoclonal antibodies which recognize antigens of high molecular weight were described to stimulate human PMN chemotaxis, superoxide anion production, and phagocytosis (3). It remains to be clarified whether the increased ROI production in our test system is mediated by signalling through adhesion molecules involved in increased adhesiveness of rat PMN or is mediated by direct signalling involving R-MC 46 antigen.

CONCLUSION

The control of granulocyte activity by particular cell surface antigens is essential for its normal functioning. Treatment of rat peripheral blood neutrophils by R-MC 46 mAb caused dramatic increase in aggregation which was only partly dependent on β_2 integrins and possibly involves other adhesion molecules. R-MC 46 two- to threefold enhanced the PMA-triggered hydrogen peroxide production and twofold enhanced NBT reduction capacity. These findings suggest that the surface molecule R-MC 46 is the novel receptor for an activation pathway that leads in neutrophils to activation.

REFERENCES

1. Cassatella, M. A. 1995. The production of cytokines by polymorphonuclear neutrophils. *Immunol. Today* **16**:21–6.

2. Simon, S. I., J. D. Chambers, E. Buthcer and L. A. Sidar. 1992. Neutrophil aggregation is beta-2 integrin and L-selectin-dependent in blood and isolated cells. *J. Immunol.* **149**:2765–71.
3. Laskin, L. D. and G. Rovera. 1985. Stimulation of human neutrophilic granulocyte chemotaxis by monoclonal antibodies. *J. Immunol.* **134**:1146–52.
4. Nong, Yu-Hua, E. Remold-O,Donnel, T. W. LeBien and H. G. Remold. 1989. A monoclonal antibody to sialophorin (CD43) induces homotypic adhesion and activation of human monocytes. *J. Exp. Med.* **170**:259–67.
5. Čolić, M., S. Gašić, L. J. Popović and A. Dujić. 1991. Identification of molecules shared between subcapsular/medullary epithelium, granulocytes, and a subset of macrophages in rat thymus. In: *Lymphatic tissues and in vivo immune responses.* (Imhof, A. B., S. Berrih-Aknin, S. Ezine eds.) Dekker, New York, pp. 61–73.
6. Oez, S., K. Welte, E. Platzer and J. R. Kalden. 1990. A simple assay for quantifying the inducible adherence of neutrophils. *Immunobiology* **180**: 308–15.
7. Pick, E. and D. Mozel. 1981. Rapid microassay for the measurement of superoxide and hydrogen peroxide production by macrophages in culture using an automatic enzyme immunoassay reader. *J. Immunol. Meth.* **46**:211–26.
8. Monboisse, J., R. Garnotel, A. Randoux *et al.* 1991. Adhesion of human neutrophils to and activation by type-I collagen involving a b2 integrin. *J. Leukoc. Biol.* **50**:373–80.
9. Anderson, C. D., L. J. Miller, F. C. Schmalstieg *et al.* 1986. Contributions of the Mac-1 glycoprotein family to adherence dependent granulocyte functions: structure-function assessments employing subunit-specific monoclonal antibodies. *J. Immunol.* **137**:15–27.
10. Kerr, A. M. and S. C. Stocks. 1991. The effect on neutrophil adhesion of antibodies against surface glycoproteins which express CD15 (3-fucosil-N-acetyllactosamine). *J. Leukoc. Biol.* **50**(supp.2):**36**.
11. Schleiffenbaum, B., R. Moser, M. Patarroyo and J. Fehr. 1989. The cell surface glycoprotein Mac-1 (CD11b/CD18) mediates neutrophil adhesion and modulates degranulation independently of its quantitative cell surface expression. *J. Immunol.* **142**:3537–45.
12. Robinson, K. M., D. Andrew, H. Rosen *et al.* 1992. Antibody against the Leu-CAM β-chain (CD18) promotes both LFA-1 and CR-3 dependent adhesion events. *J. Immunol.* **148**:1080–5.
13. Pavlović, M. D., M. Čolić, N. Pejnović *et al.* 1994: A novel anti-rat CD18 monoclonal antibody triggers lymphocyte homotypic aggregation and granulocyte adhesion to plastic: different intracellular signalling pathways in resting versus activated thymocytes. *Eur. J. Immunol.* **24**:1640–8.
14. Waddell, T. K., L. Fialkow, C. K. Chan *et al.* 1994. Potentiation of the oxidative burst of human neutrophils. A signaling role for L-selectin. *J. Biol. Chem.* **269**:18 485–91.

10

Microenvironment of the Rat Thymus after Cyclosporin Treatment

Novica M. Milićević, Vladimir Živanović and Živana Milićević

Cyclosporin (CS), a macrolide of fungal origin, has gained wide clinical application due to its immunomodulatory properties. Its effects on the peripheral lymphocyte pool have been well known for a longer time (1). It has also been demonstrated that CS blocks the maturation of thymocytes within the thymus at the double positive $CD4^{+}CD8^{+}$ stage, whereas autoreactive T lymphocytes are allowed to escape to the peripheral circulation (2,3). However, there are very few complete studies in the literature on the changes of thymic microenvironment after application of CS. Considering that the thymic microenvironment, which is composed of several types of non-lymphoid cells, is of the utmost significance for the process of thymocyte production, we considered it interesting to perform a comprehensive study, which was expected, on the one hand, to elucidate the changes of all types of thymic non-lymphoid cells induced by CS and, on the other hand, to indicate the functional roles of these cells in the process of thymocyte maturation, as well as the interplay between thymic lymphoid and non-lymphoid cells.

MATERIAL AND METHODS

Animals and treatment

Male 6-week-old Wistar rats, with an average body weight of 145 g at the beginning of the experiment (VMA Farm, Beograd), were used. The animals were given standard laboratory food and had free access to tap water. Cyclosporin ('Sandimmun', Basle, Switzerland) was daily administered orally, 30 mg kg of body weight, for 21 consecutive days. Five rats from the same litter receiving no CS served as controls. At the end of the experiment the animals were killed by exsanguination under ether anaesthesia.

Immunoregulation in Health and Disease
ISBN 0-12-459460-3

Demonstration of thymic epithelial cells

The changes of all types of thymic epithelial cells were studied after the application of CS using the immunohistochemical methods with the following panel of monoclonal antibodies: OX-6 (anti-Ia), KII, K8, K8.13 (panepithelial), K19, R-MC 20 (subcapsular/medullary epithelium), KL1 (subset of medullary epithelial cells). For further details see (4,5).

Demonstration of thymic macrophages and interdigitating cells

The following methods were used to study the changes of different kinds of thymic macrophages and interdigitating cells (IDC) after the application of CS: histochemistry – aldehyde fuchsin, Sudan black B, periodic acid–Schiff (PAS); enzymehistochemistry – acid phosphatase, non-specific esterase, succinic dehydrogenase, chloroacetate esterase; immunohistochemistry – using ED1, ED2, R-MC 41 monoclonal antibodies and rabbit polyclonal antisera to cyclo-oxygenase; electron microscopy. For further details see references 6–9.

RESULTS

Epithelial cells

In the untreated rats the epithelial network is very delicate in the cortex and slightly denser in the medulla. Three subtypes of epithelial cells may be distinguished according to morphological features and using monoclonal antibodies: cortical, subcapsulary/medullary, and Hassall's bodies.

After application of CS, subcapsular epithelial cells, although phenotypically similar to medullary epithelial cells, were changed in a similar manner to phenotypically distinct epithelial cells of the deep cortex. Both of these cell types became enlarged and stockier, whereas their cytoplasmic prolongations were thicker and coarser in comparison to control cells (Fig. 10.1a,b). Their number was not decreased. Due to these changes of subcapsular and cortical epithelial cells, the presentation of Ia antigens in the thymic microenvironment appeared increased. In contrast, the number of medullary epithelial cells in the remaining islands of medullary tissue was markedly reduced, whereby the cells with the most mature phenotype ($CK8^{+}10^{-}19^{-}$ and $CK8^{+}10^{+}19^{-}$) were the most prominently depleted (Table 10.1).

Macrophages and interdigitating cells

According to histochemical, enzymehistochemical, and ultrastructural features three types of mononuclear phagocytic cells may be distinguished within

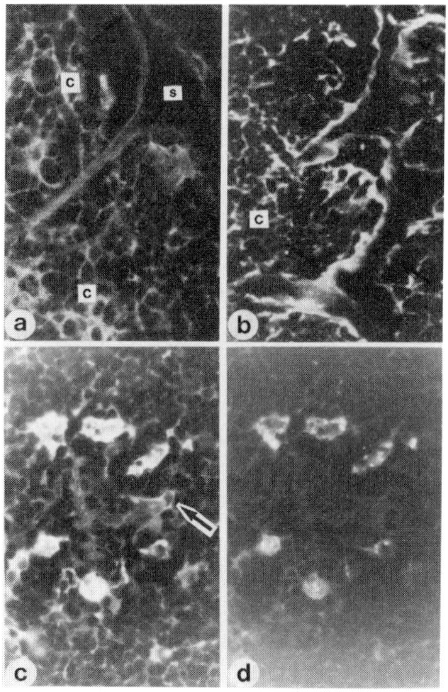

Fig. 10.1 (a) Control thymus. Epithelial cells in deep cortex (c) form a delicate web-like cytoreticulum. The flattened subcapsular epithelial cells with delicate, elongated processes (arrows) border the septal connective tissue(s). (b) Cyclosporin-treated thymus. Epithelial cells in deep cortex (c) are stockier, with thickened cytoplasmic prolongations. The epithelial meshwork is denser. The number of subcapsular epithelial cells (arrows) is not reduced, but these cells are also enlarged, stockier with thickened cellular processes. Immunofluorescence staining with anti-cytokeratin 8 monoclonal antibody. (c, d) Cyclosporin-treated thymus. Enlarged, rounded, double-positive macrophages in the cortex. Single-positive structure in 1c (arrow) is a capillary. Double immunofluorescence staining with anti-prostaglandin synthase and ED2 antibody, respectively. s = septum. (a, b) ×960 (modified from Milićević, Ž. *et al., J. Comp. Pathol.* **106**: 25–35, 1992) (c, d) × 1260 (modified from Milićević, N. M. *et al., Immunobiology* **190**:376–84, 1994). Copyright for Fig. 1a and b belongs to Academic Press (from Milićević, Ž. *et al., J. Comp. Pathol.* **106**:25–35, 1992). Copyright for Fig. 1c and d belongs to Gustav Fischer Verlag (from Milićević, N. M. *et al., Immunobiol.* **190**:376–84, 1994). Reprint permission requested.

the thymus: cortical macrophages, macrophages of the corticomedullary zone (CMZ), and IDCs of the thymic medulla (Table 10.2).

After application of CS the number of cortical macrophages and their phenotypic characteristics (detected by the use of monoclonal antibodies) did not change significantly. However, these cells became enlarged and rounded, and increased the activity of hydrolytic and respiratory enzymes, as well as the activity of prostaglandin synthase (cyclo-oxygenase, Fig. 10.1c,d).

Table 10.1 Phenotypic characteristics of epithelial cells in the normal rat thymus and after application of cyclosporin

	Normal				After CS			
	Appearance	Ia expression	Number	Maturity	Appearance	Ia expression	Number	Maturity
Subcapsular	Delicate	±	±	±	Coarse	+	±	±
Cortical	Delicate	±	±	±	Coarse	+	±	±
Medullary	Delicate	±	±	±	Delicate	±	−	−

− decreased; ± not changed; + increased; CS = cyclosporin

Table 10.2 Phenotypic characteristics of the macrophages in the normal rat thymus and of thymic cortical macrophages after application of cyclosporin

	Aldehyde fuchsin	Sudan Black B	Periodic acid–Schiff	Acid phos-phatase	Non-specific esterase	Succinic dehydro-genase	Chloro-acetate esterase	Prosta-glandin synthase	ED1	ED2	R-MC 41
Cortex	–	–	–	+	±	–	–	±	+	+	+
CMZ	+	+	+	+	+	+	+	+	+	+	+
Medulla	–	–	–	+	+	–	–	–	+	–	–
Cortex after CS	+	±	±	+	+	+	+	+	+	+	+

+cells are positive; ± some cells are weakly positive; – cells are negative; CMZ = cortico-medullary zone; CS = cyclosporin

Histochemical and ultrastructural features of cortical macrophages also became very similar to those of CMZ macrophages. The number of IDCs appeared decreased due to the decreased amount of medullary tissue, but these cells retained their usual phenotypic characteristics (Table 10.2).

DISCUSSION

Our studies document the prominent changes of thymic microenvironment after the application of CS. The subcapsular epithelial cells and medullary epithelial cells are differently affected by CS treatment, although these populations of thymic epithelial cells show great phenotypic similarity (10–13). The number of subcapsular epithelial cells is not decreased after application of CS, in contrast to medullary epithelial cells which are greatly reduced in number. Thus, it is very likely that there is a functional difference between thymic subcapsular and medullary epithelial cells in spite of their phenotypic resemblance. In addition, the morphology of subcapsular epithelial cells is markedly changed in comparison with control cells. In this respect the changes in subcapsular epithelial cells are similar to those of epithelial cells in deep thymus, which suggests that both of these subsets of cortical epithelial cells, although phenotypically different (10–13), might share some common function or functions. This study also shows not only that the number of medullary epithelial cells is decreased after the use of CS, but that the most mature medullary epithelial cells (with the most differentiated $CK8^{+}10^{+}19^{-}$ and $CK8^{+}10^{-}19^{-}$ phenotype) are even more profoundly depleted by CS than other subsets of medullary epithelium. Thus, it appears that CS may interfere with maturation of medullary epithelial cells. This is in agreement with the observed decrease in number of Hassall's bodies which we also noted. Our results show that after application of CS cortical macrophages become very similar to macrophages of the CMZ. It is possible that their morphological features reflect the increased production of arachidonic acid metabolites. It is very likely that in the normal thymus cortical macrophages accumulate enzymes necessary for prostaglandin production and upon their migration to CMZ, where the production of main quantity of prostaglandins may take place (according to the strongest expression of prostaglandin synthase in the normal thymus), acquire the specific morphological properties of CMZ macrophages. The results obtained after treatment with CS confirm this hypothesis. After application of CS, cortical macrophages develop morphological aspects, enzyme capacity, histochemical characteristics, and ultrastructural organization very similar to those of normal CMZ macrophages and show the abundance of prostaglandin synthase as well.

It is possible that CS exerts its effects directly on thymic non-lymphoid cells. However, it is even more likely that the changes of thymic non-lymphoid cells described here reflect the backward influences of thymic lymphoid cells, whose physiological life cycle has been disrupted after treatment with CS. It is known that not only are thymocytes dependent on signals delivered by thymic non-lymphoid cells to proceed through the process of maturation, but in turn the integrity of the latter also depends on thymic lymphoid population (14,15). CS affects the maturation of thymocytes at two levels: firstly, the development of double positive thymocytes and secondly, the generation of single positive thymocytes is blocked (16). Considering these facts it seems likely that the reduction of medullary epithelium, as well as retardation in maturation of these cells which we discussed above, is related to the reduction in number of mature medullary single positive thymocytes (17). The number of cortical double negative and double positive thymocytes is spared after CS treatment. Therefore, subcapsular and cortical epithelial cells remain preserved, in contrast to medullary epithelium. However, these cells also appear hypertrophied. The reason for such a reaction is unclear. It may be related to the block in maturation of thymocytes, which therefore might deliver abnormal signals to subcapsular and cortical epithelial cells. The direct action of CS on these cells cannot, however, be excluded because the proliferation of thymic epithelial cells in vitro under the influence of this agent has been recorded (18). Considering that the function of macrophages is heavily influenced by T lymphocytes (19), it seems very likely that similar mechanisms are operative in the control of thymocyte–macrophage interactions. This type of thymic cellular interplay is, however, much less studied than epithelial cell–thymocyte interactions, and undeniably warrants further attention.

CONCLUSION

Application of cyclosporin (CS) to rats induces prominent changes of all types of thymic non-lymphoid cells. Thymic cortical epithelial network becomes denser and coarser. Cortical epithelial cells become stocky with coarse cellular prolongations. Subcapsular epithelial cells, although phenotypically dissimilar from cortical epithelium, are changed in a very similar manner. The presentation of Ia antigens in the cortex thus appears increased. The number of medullary epithelial cells in the remaining islands of tissue is markedly reduced, whereby the cells with the most mature phenotype ($CK8^{+}10^{-}19^{-}$ and $CK8^{+}10^{+}19^{-}$) are the most prominently depleted. The number of Hassall's bodies is also decreased. Cortical macrophages become enlarged and rounded, but their number does not increase. Phenotypically they become similar to macrophages of the corticomedullary zone. Considering that after CS treatment the expression of prostaglandin synthase is increased, it is very likely that cortical macrophages become engaged in production of arachidonic acid metabolites, similarly to macrophages of the corticomedullary zone of the normal thymus. The number of interdigitating cells is decreased due to the reduction of thymic medulla, but phenotypically these cells do not change substantially. Although it is possible that CS directly affects thymic non-lymphoid cells, it is even more likely that the changes of thymic non-lymphoid cells reflect the backward influences of thymic lymphoid cells, whose physiological life cycle has been disrupted after treatment with CS.

REFERENCES

1. Hess, A. D. and P. N. Colombani. 1987. Cyclosporin-resistant and -sensitive T-lymphocyte subsets. *Ann. Inst. Pasteur (Immunol.)* **138**:606–11.
2. Gao, E.-K., D. Lo, R. Cheney *et al.* 1988. Abnormal differentiation of thymocytes in mice treated with cyclosporin A. *Nature* **336**:176–9.
3. Jenkins, M. K., R. H. Schwartz and D. M. Pardoll. 1988. Effects of Cyclosporine A on T cell development and clonal deletion. *Science* **241**:1655–8.
4. Milićević, Ž., M. Čolić and N. M. Milićević. 1991. Organization of thymic epithelial cells in cyclosporin-treated rats. Light microscopic immunohistochemical study. *Thymus* **17**:75–9.
5. Milićević, Ž., V. Živanović, V. Todorović *et al.* 1992. Differential effect of cyclosporin application on epithelial cells of the rat thymus. Immunohistochemical study. *J. Comp. Pathol.* **106**:25–35.
6. Milićević, N. M., Ž. Milićević and M. Čolić. 1989. Macrophages of the rat thymus after cyclosporin treatment. Histochemical, enzymehistochemical and immunohistochemical study. *Virchows Arch. B (Cell Pathol.)* **57**:237–44.
7. Milićević, N. M., Ž. Milićević, M. Čolić *et al.*, 1993. Ultrastructural study of macrophages of the rat thymus after cyclosporin treatment. *Thymus* **22**:35–44.
8. Milićević, N. M. and Ž. Milićević. 1993. Relationship between naphthol AS-D chloroacetate esterase and prostagladnin synthase. *Acta Histochem.* **95**:67–70.
9. Milićević, N. M., P. Appasamy, M. Čolić and Ž. Milićević. 1994. Immunocytochemical demonstration of prostaglandin synthase (cyclooxygenase) in thymic macrophages of normal and cyclosporin-treated rats. *Immunobiology* **190**:376–84.
10. Van Vliet, E., M. Melis and W. van Ewijk. 1984. Monoclonal antibodies to stromal cell types of the mouse thymus. *Eur. J. Immunol.* **14**:524–9.
11. De Maagd, R. A., W. A. Mackenzie, H.-J. Schuurman *et al.* 1985. The human thymus microenvironment: heterogeneity detected by monoclonal anti-epithelial cell antibodies. *Immunology* **54**:745–54.
12. von Gaudecker, B., G. G. Steinmann, M.-L. Hansmann *et al.* 1986. Immunohistochemical characterization of the thymic microenvironment. A light-microscopic and ultrastructural immunocytochemical study. *Cell Tiss. Res.* **244**:403–12.
13. Kampinga, J., F. G. M. Kroese, A. M. Duijvestijn *et al.* 1987. The rat thymus microenvironment: subsets of thymic epithelial cells defined by monoclonal antibodies. *Transplant. Proc.* **19**:3171–4.
14. Ritter, M. A. and R. L. Boyd. 1993. Development in the thymus: it takes two to tango. *Immunol. Today* **14**:462–9.
15. van Ewijk, W., E. W. Shores and A. Singer. 1994. Crosstalk in the mouse thymus. *Immunol. Today* **15**:214–17.
16. Kosugi, A., J. C. Zuniga-Pflucker, S. O. Sharrow *et al.* 1989. Effect of

Cyclosporin A on lymphopoiesis. II. Developmental defects of immature and mature thymocytes in fetal thymus organ cultures treated with Cyclosporin A. *J. Immunol.* **143**:3134–40.

17. Shores, E. W., W. van Ewijk and A. Singer. 1994. Maturation of medullary thymic epithelium requires thymocytes expressing fully assembled CD3–TCR complexes. *Internat. Immunol.* **6**:1393–402.
18. Dardenne, M., W. Savino, G. Feutren and J.-F. Bach. 1987. Stimulatory effects of cyclosporin A on human and mouse thymic epithelial cells. *Eur. J. Immunol.* **17**:275–9.
19. Doherty, T. M. 1995. T-cell regulation of macrophage function. *Curr. Opin. Immunol.* **7**:400–4.

Section 2

Molecular and cellular immunoregulatory mechanisms

11

Antibody and Protein Glycosylation in Health and Disease

Helen Arrol and Roy Jefferis

Glycoconjugates are amongst the most functionally and structurally diverse molecules in nature, and protein- and lipid-bound saccharides play essential roles in many molecular processes impacting eukaryotic biology and disease processes (1–3). Glycosylation of protein molecules represents an extensive post-translational modification that can influence biological activity, pharmokinetics, antigenicity, etc. Glycosylation may occur through attachment to the amide nitrogen atom of an asparagine residue (*N*-linked oligosaccharide) or the oxygen atom of serine or threonine residues (*O*-linked oligosaccharide). A prerequisite for *N*-linked glycosylation is the presence of the -Asn-X-Ser/Thr- motif (glycosylation sequon), where X can be any amino acid residue except proline. Although glycosylation takes place cotranslationally in the lumen of the endoplasmic reticulum (ER), secondary and tertiary structural features influence glycosylation such that potential glycosylation sites may not in fact be glycosylated. The primary *N*-glycosylation event is attachment of a high-mannose form of oligosaccharide, followed by a series of trimming and elongation reactions as the glycoprotein transits the Golgi apparatus (GA). The oligosaccharide may not be processed uniformly, so glycoprotein products may exhibit microheterogeneity (multiple glycoforms). Each glycoform is a structurally unique molecule and may be associated with unique or modulated function.

In this review we focus on the natural profile of glycoforms of protein molecules, particularly human IgG antibodies, and altered or abnormal glycoforms associated with disease. These associations have important implications for the biotechnology industry since control of the glycosylation of recombinant molecules produced in vitro and intended for therapeutic application in vivo, in humans is essential (1–5). It will be shown that this is particularly so for antibody molecules and for other molecules that are members of the Ig superfamily and account for around 70% of recombinant glycoproteins under development for in vivo therapeutic applications.

Immunoregulation in Health and Disease
ISBN 0-12-459460-3

GLYCOSYLATION IN THE IMMUNE SYSTEM

Glycosylation of the IgG antibody molecules: structural and functional significance

The IgG antibody molecule is a structural paradigm for molecules of the immunoglobulin supergene family. The intact IgG molecule comprises three globular protein moieties, two Fabs and an Fc fragment, linked through a flexible 'hinge' region. A conserved glycosylation site, at Asn 297 on the b4 bend of the Fx face, has been observed for all mammalian IgG molecules investigated. The oligosaccharide is of the complex type which has a minimal hexasaccharide core structure with variable attachment of outer arm sugar residues (Fig. 11.1). X-ray crystallographic analyses of Fc fragments allow resolution of an octasaccharide with a proximity to the protein structure to allow the possibility of a total of 85 contacts through 14 amino acid residues of the C_H2 domain (6–8).

Human IgG, Fc effector functions

The Fc region of the IgG molecule expresses multiple interaction sites for ligands (e.g. Fc receptors on leucocytes, C1q, rheumatoid factors). Employing site directed mutagenesis, we identified the sequence -Leu-Leu-Gly-Gly- as the optimal motif for recognition by FcγRI, FcγRII and FcγRIII (9,10). However, we also demonstrated that glycosylation, at Asn 297 in the C_H2 domain, is essential for expression of Fc mediated biological activities (11,12) and there is a consensus that Fcγ receptor recognition, C1q binding and C1 activation are compromised or abrogated for aglycosylated IgG (11–15). A detailed study of an aglycosylated chimeric human IgG3 anti-NP antibody demonstrated a reduction in affinity of two orders of magnitude for human FcγRI expressed on U937 cells (12) and a similar reduction in activation to superoxide production. This aglycosylated IgG3 protein was not able to activate biological responses through FcγRII or FcγRIII (9,10). The absolute requirement for glycosylation suggests that individual glycoforms may also differ in biological activities. Comparative studies of galactosylated and agalactosylated IgG have shown that the agalactosylated form has a reduced capacity to recognize Fcγ receptors and activate the classical complement cascade although increasing the capacity to bind and activate mannan binding protein (16–18). The proportion of human IgG molecules lacking galactose (Go-IgG) is increased in patients with rheumatoid arthritis and certain other chronic inflammatory diseases (19,20) and it has been suggested that Go-IgG (G0) may have a role in the pathogenesis of diseases in which its level is increased (20).

We have proposed that the conformation of the protein and oligosaccharide moieties are interdependent and generate a quaternary structure that

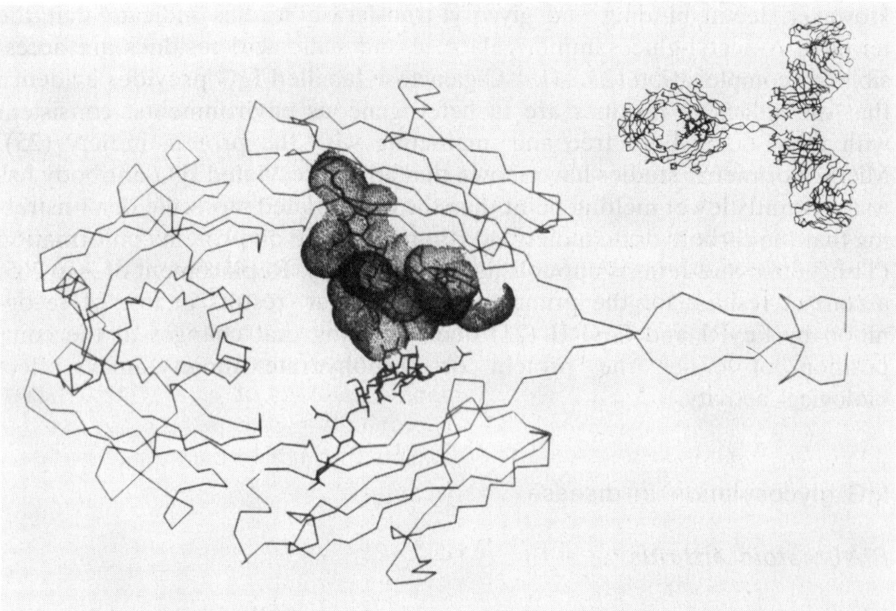

(B) (SA) - (G1) -(GN) - **M** (F)

\ |

(GN) - **M - GN - GN** - protein

/

(SA) - (G2) - **GN - M**

Fig. 11.1 (A) Alpha carbon backbone structures for the IgG molecule (inset) and the Fc region. The surface accessible to solvent is outlined for one oligosaccharide moiety. (B) The complex oligosaccharides that may be expressed within IgG molecules: The core oligosaccharide is in bold type and the outer arm sugars are bracketed. GN, *N*-acetylglucosamine; M, mannose; Gal, galactose; F, fucose; SA, sialic acid.

expresses ligand recognition motifs (21,22). However, outer arm sugars may modulate ligand recognition (specificity/affinity) and hence thresholds for biological activation (16–18,21). This postulate derives from the following observations: X-ray crystallographic studies have shown that the core oligosaccharide of an IgG molecule is sequestered within the protein quaternary structure and therefore not available for ligand binding (6–8).

However, lectin binding and glycosyl-transferase studies indicate that the terminal *N*-acetyl-glucosamine, galactose and sialic acid residues are accessible for complexation (23,24). ^{13}C-galactose-labelled IgG provides evidence that the galactose residues are in heterogeneous environments, consistent with them being both free and interacting with the protein moiety (25). Microcalorimetric studies have shown that an aglycosylated IgG antibody has a significantly lower melting point than the glycosylated molecule demonstrating that the carbohydrate moiety exerts an influence on protein conformation (Tishchenko and Jefferis unpublished observation). Replacement of Asp 265, a contact residue for the primary GlcNAc sugar, results in loss of recognition by FcγRI and FcγRII (21) demonstrating that changes in the composition of either the protein or carbohydrate moiety may affect biological activity.

IgG glycosylation in disease

Rheumatoid arthritis

An increase in agalactosyl glycoforms of the IgG molecules (G0) of all subclasses has been observed for patients with certain inflammatory diseases such as rheumatoid arthritis (RA), tuberculosis and Crohn's disease (3,19). The increased proportion of G0 IgG present in the serum has been shown to correlate with disease activity and clinical score (18,19). The proportion of G0 IgG present in the synovium is further increased, a finding that supports a hypothesis of intra-articular synthesis of G0 (19,26). This suggests that G0 IgG might be correlated with increased inflammation precipitated by immune complexes; however, it has been reported that agalactosylated IgG has a decreased ability to bind C1q and FcγRI and to activate C1 (16). The association of G0 IgG levels with disease activity is further demonstrated by pregnancy-induced remission seen in female patients with RA; the proportion of G0 IgG is reduced during gestation and increased following parturition, coinciding with remission and return to active disease (3,19).

The increase in G0 IgG in RA appears to be due to a defect in synthesis, rather than a degradative process, since decreased UDP β(1–4) galactosyltransferase (GTase) activity, the enzyme responsible for the addition of galactose onto the outer arms of the Fc carbohydrate, has been reported for peripheral blood B cells isolated from RA patients (19,27). Additionally, an increase in the level of IgG anti-GTase antibodies, but not IgM anti-GTase antibodies, has been reported (27). The activity of the enzyme increases in pregnancy and upon treatment with sulphasalazine, showing that its activity can be modulated in different physiological conditions (27). In addition, GTase activity has been shown to be depressed in T cells, which could potentially alter the glycosylation of the T cell receptor, and in major histocompatibility complex (MHC) and secreted lymphokines, which could also influence the defective immune function seen in this disease (27).

It is not known whether the increase in agalactosyl glycoforms is involved in the pathogenesis of the disease or occurs as a result. Many different hypotheses have been proposed for its role in the disease, some of which will be discussed here. The absence of galactose from the termini of the Fc carbohydrates leads to exposure of GlcNAc residues which could be recognized by the mannan binding protein (MBP) with consequent activation of complement via the classical pathway (3,18). Synovial fluid of RA patients has been found to contain MBP, and this combined with the increased G(0) found in the joint could result in chronic local inflammation, mediated through the sequelae of complement activation (19). Preferential incorporation of G0 IgG into immune complexes (ICs) present in synovial fluid further supports the association of decreased IgG galactosylation and disease activity in RA (28,29). The complexes could activate complement, leading to the accumulation of polymorphonuclear cells in the joint, which could then degranulate, releasing myeloperoxidase and kininogenases into the joint space, resulting in acute inflammation (26). IC formation could potentially result, in part at least, from reduced galactosylation of IgG in the following manner: absence of galactose could expose new antigenic determinants either in the carbohydrate or in the protein moiety of the antibody or secondly its absence could expose a lectin-like pocket into which the Fab carbohydrates could bind (3,19,28,29).

ICs are removed from the circulation by receptors in the liver which recognize galactose, thus the increase in G(0) could probably explain the decreased clearance rate. The complexes could be formed either by rheumatoid factor (RF – anti-IgG) binding to IgG or by antibodies becoming non-specifically trapped (26). The carbohydrate appears not to affect the binding, but the isotype does (23). However, IgG RFs (but not IgM RFs) have paradoxically been shown to bind best to Fcs where the carbohydrates are the most complete and complex (30). It has elsewhere been reported that high-affinity binding of IgG by IgM is associated with a decrease in galactose in IgG (29). Another potential mechanism for the involvement of G0 is in the regulation of TNF release from activated macrophages. This could be either by direct activation if their affinity was sufficient or via binding to FcγR or GlcNAc binding receptors. TNF is indeed found in the synovial fluid in RA and stimulates neovascularization and leucocyte infiltration (19).

The placenta transports galactosylated IgG more effectively than G(0), owing to the decreased affinity of G0 for FcγRn, and in fact the G0 in neonates is almost zero. The level then increases until about 6 months, when it starts to decrease again. However, in juvenile chronic arthritis levels remain elevated and correlate with the disease activity as in RA (19).

The increase in G0 has been shown to be valuable as a diagnostic and prognostic indicator in RA. Patients who show early agalactosylation show a more progressive disease and more bone erosions later on (19,20). In addition the decrease in galactose precedes the onset of RA and therefore has a predictive value (20). Early synovitis and increased G0 invariably leads to RA and can therefore be used in its differential diagnosis (19).

Other diseases associated with G(0)

Cystic fibrosis. Cystic fibrosis (CF) is a genetic disease affecting the lungs and digestive system and is due to an imbalance of ion and fluid transport resulting from a defect in a cAMP regulated chloride ion channel (31). A change in glycosylation of IgG has been observed in CF patients with a large proportion of structures lacking galactose and fucose (32). Thus the IgG glycosylation profile in CF is similar to that in RA. It is therefore interesting to note that there are some clinical similarities between the two diseases, with some CF patients manifesting early joint complications and some RA patients giving iontophoretic sweat test results similar to those of CF patients. In addition a high level of circulating ICs is seen in both diseases (32). The decrease in galactose content of IgG would cause a decrease in clearance rate and could be responsible for the raised levels of IgG and ICs seen in older CF patients (33).

Other glycoproteins have also been reported to show altered glycosylation profiles in CF. Perhaps most important is the membrane-associated glycoprotein CFTR (cystic fibrosis transmembrane conductance regulator) which is the product of the defective gene in this disease. In CF, this glycoprotein remains intracellular and is not expressed on the cell surface (34). There is evidence that CFTR is incompletely glycosylated in CF. This defect may cause the CFTR to be recognized as abnormal either preventing it from leaving the ER or directing it to lysosomes where it would be degraded (31,34).

Castleman's disease. This is a localized mediastinal lymph node hyperplasia characterised by plasma cell proliferation and polyclonal hypergammaglobulinemia. It has been proposed that IL6 may be involved in the pathogenesis of this disorder which is associated with an increase in G0. IL6 may also be implicated in RA, multiple myeloma (MM) and cardiac myxoma, which have all been associated with a change in the glycosylation patterns (35). However, IL6 is not increased in Crohn's disease or in TB so in these disorders the effect must either be local or mediated by some other mechanism.

IgG cryoglobulinemia. This condition is characterized by immunoglobulins undergoing reversible precipitation at low temperatures and is associated with a variety of diseases including multiple myeloma and autoimmune diseases such as RA and SLE. One such cryoglobulin was shown to be abnormally glycosylated in the first hypervariable region of its heavy chain. Cryoprecipitation of the intact IgG was inhibitable by glycosylated Fab but not by the aglycosylated fragment. Thus, for this protein at least the carbohydrate may be responsible for its abnormal cold insolubility (36).

Autoimmune haemolytic anaemia. The presence of IgG autoantibodies with a specificity for antigens on the patient's red blood cells (RBCs) results in FcγR-mediated recognition of sensitized cells by splenic macrophages and their destruction and/or removal from the circulation. Autoantibodies with a low G0 content have been found to have a greater lytic activity than those with high G0 content; thus the glycosylation profile of the antibodies could determine their pathogenicity (37).

The anti-gal antibody. It has been estimated that about 1% of circulating IgG recognizes the Gal(α1-3)gal epitope (38). This epitope is not found in humans, owing to a decrease in the activity of the α1-3 galactosyltransferase enzyme. Antibodies to this epitope are believed to be stimulated by bacteria in the gut. The repertoire of anti-gal antibodies is dependent on the ABO blood group of the individual. In individuals with blood group B or AB, tolerance prevents the production of anti-gal clones capable of recognizing fucosylated Gal-α(1-3)gal (the B antigen); however, blood groups O and A can produce antibodies with reactivity to both fucosylated and non-fucosylated antigen. In fact most anti-B antibody has anti-gal specificity. It appears that this antigen is present on RBCs in a cryptic form which becomes exposed on ageing of the RBC. The antigen can then be recognized by these antibodies and the RBC cleared by FCγR mediated phagocytosis, thus removing senescent RBCs from the circulation. One proposed mechanism for increased exposure is that ageing red cells lose water and thus become less deformable, causing them to be retained for longer in the sinuses of the RES where they are exposed to proteolytic enzymes which can then expose the antigen. In haemolytic disorders such as β-thalassemia and sickle cell anaemia there is premature exposure of the antigen with a resulting increase in extravascular lysis (38).

Anti-gal antibodies also appear to play a role in the hyperacute rejection of pig organs since the pre-existing complement fixing anti-gal antibodies will be reactive with the gal α(1-3)gal epitope expressed on this tissue. Thus removal or neutralization of anti-gal IgG could potentially suppress the hyperacute rejection (39).

Glycation of IgG in diabetes mellitus. Glycation is the covalent, non-enzymatic addition of glucose molecules to proteins. There is a correlation between the mean plasma glucose level and increased protein glycation. Prolonged hyperglycaemia would increase glycation in the immune system, possibly causing defective function. An increase in IgG glycation has been shown to increase its vascular clearance and its accumulation in the kidney, to decrease its ability to fix complement and to impair its binding to protein A. The dissociation of antigen–antibody complexes is increased and the affinity of the antibodies is decreased. Thus, glycation impairs both the Fc- and Fab-mediated functions of the antibodies. Together with the increased clearance of these antibodies this could explain the diminished immune response and the resulting increase in infections seen in diabetes mellitus (40,41).

Lymphocytes and lymphocyte activation

The glycosylation capacity of an individual cell is said to define its glycotype and may determine its structural and functional identity (32). For lymphocytes differential glycosylation capacities may define sub-populations of T and B cells or clonal individuality. The latter is evident from analysis of oligosaccharide profiles of monoclonal antibodies secreted by plasma cells. Many glycoproteins expressed on the cell surfaces of lymphocytes have been identified, structurally and antigenically, that when cross-linked or coligated result in lymphocyte activation. A requirement for their glycosylation has been demonstrated, e.g. in CD2. Numerous proteins expressed on lymphocyte cell surfaces contain one or more GlcNAc monosaccharide moieties, *O*-glycosidically linked to the peptide (OGlcNAc) (42). Previously it had been suggested that *O*-glycosylated proteins were mostly restricted to the nucleus and the cytoplasm (43).

Functionally distinct subsets of lymphocytes may be defined by the expression of unique membrane glycoproteins and different numbers of exogalactosylatable GlcNAc moieties (42,44). The saccharides on their surfaces confer different biological functions and specific binding properties which can be used for their isolation (42). Activation of lymphocytes results in a rapid but transient increase of OGlcNAc on the specific nuclear and cytoplasmic protein (44). Similarly, changes in oligosaccharide diversity and topography can be observed for lymphocyte surface glycoproteins (42), e.g. leukosialin (43).

Lectins and lymphocyte recirculation

Lectins are a class of non-enzymatic, non-immune proteins that bind to specific carbohydrates (45). Selectins are a family of integral membrane lectins, expressed on leucocytes and also transiently on activated endothelium (46), which aid in leucocyte binding to endothelium and to platelets during inflammation and clotting (45). Each selectin has a different role; L-selectin mediates adhesion of leucocytes to endothelial cells, E-selectin is responsible for recognition of leucocytes by stimulated or wounded endothelium and P-selectin is responsible for interactions between leucocytes and activated platelets or endothelium. The major carbohydrate ligand for selectins involved in neutrophil recirculation is the sialyl Lewis X oligosaccharide. These interactions slow the cells down to a slow roll, allowing integrin adhesion and extravasation to occur (46).

Kupffer cells, other macrophages and hepatic endothelial cells bear a lectin-like substance, the macrophage mannose receptor, which internalizes glycoproteins bearing terminal mannose, fucose or *N*-acetyglucosamine, resulting in their removal from the circulation. The structures recognized by this receptor are found on lysosomal enzymes, tPA and various pathogens (47). Thus, this receptor can prevent degradative enzymes from damaging the blood vessel lining and can aid the immune response against pathogens (47,48).

The mannose binding protein (MBP) is a C-type lectin secreted by hepatocytes and present in serum. It binds oligomannose or *N*-acetylglucosamine structures, such as those expressed on the surface of pathogens, and consequently opsonize it for recognition by the collectin receptor, expressed on the surface of phagocytes or through activation of the classical complement pathway (3,18,19,49).

Evidence for the role of selectins in lymphocyte recirculation comes from observations that when lymphocytes are treated with either exo-glycosidases or inhibitors of oligosaccharide-processing enzymes their migratory properties alter. Specific carbohydrate sequences, called addressins, are found on the target cell surface and are believed to mediate lymphocyte homing and other cellular targeting and adhesion processes (50). Individual lymphocytes have different migratory properties due to their specific binding properties with receptors on the high endothelial venules (HEV) of the target organ or tissue. Such specific migratory properties could be responsible for organ-specific immune responses to a common antigen and, where abnormal migration occurs, for autoimmune disease (32).

THE ROLE OF PROTEIN GLYCOSYLATION IN DISEASES EXCLUDING IgG

Introduction to protein glycosylation in disease

Altered glycosylation patterns of glycoproteins are observed in various disease states and can be either the cause or the result of the disease. They arise due to a defect in oligosaccharide processing or as a result of a change in the polypeptide structure. Many such diseases are caused by mutations in the genes for glycosidases, whilst a few are caused by defects in GTases (32). The glycoproteins can serve as ligands for blood group and tumour-associated antibodies and for cell attachment proteins of certain pathogens. Knowledge of the altered glycoprotein structure can be used to design therapies for these diseases; monoclonal antibodies to tumour-associated antigens may be used in diagnosis and therapy, and knowledge of the pathogen receptor specificity may allow design of prophylactic therapies inhibiting cellular adsorption (50).

In this section, the role of protein glycosylation in disease, in pathogenesis and determination of disease outcome and its implications for therapy, are considered.

Diseases associated with a change in protein glycosylation

Congenital dyserythropoietic anaemia type II/Hereditary erythroblast multinuclearity with positive acidified serum test (HEMPAS)

This anaemia, inherited in an autosomal recessive fashion, is due to an abnormal membrane organization in erythroid cells. It is characterized by hereditary erythroblast multinuclearity with positive acidified serum test (HEMPAS) and so is also known by this name. Patients with HEMPAS often have liver cirrhosis and haemosiderosis as well as other abnormalities including diabetes, gallstones and mental and sensory abnormalities. HEMPAS is a heterogeneous set of diseases resulting from defects in *N*-glycosylation pathways. Deficiencies have been found in *N*-acetylglucosaminyltransferase II (GnTII) in some patients, α-mannosidase II (α-manII) in others and a variant deficient in the membrane-bound form of galactosyltransferase has also been described.

In HEMPAS, serum glycoproteins such as transferrin are incompletely processed and so contain high mannose or hybrid instead of complex oligosaccharides. These serum proteins are recognized and trapped by receptors in the reticuloendothelial cells and the liver. Liver cirrhosis in HEMPAS may be caused by these huge amounts of abnormal glycoproteins saturating the receptors and exceeding the clearance capacity (51).

Wiskott–Aldrich syndrome (WAS)

This immunodeficiency, inherited in an X-linked recessive manner, is characterized by recurrent viral and bacterial infections, thrombocytopenia and eczema. The disorder affects B lymphocytes, T lymphocytes and platelets which show abnormal expression of two developmentally regulated GTases, suggesting that WAS may result from defective lymphocyte maturation. A primary defect in WAS is low core 2 GlcNAc transferase activity that may result in defective *O*-glycosylation. Altered glycosylation has been documented for both the CD23 and CD43 molecules. Patients show defective T-cell function with activated T lymphocytes being temporarily refractory to further stimulation through the T-cell antigen receptor. This unresponsiveness may indicate a state of pseudoactivation where specific T-cell responses are not possible (52–54).

Macular corneal dystrophy (MCD)

MCD is a progressive, inherited disorder where opaque deposits collect in the corneal stroma impairing vision which eventually requires corrective corneal transplantation. The defect in type 1 MCD is believed to be a fault in keratan sulfate synthesis caused by a defect in the sulfotransferase that usually sulfates lactosaminoglycans. This results in the proteoglycan not being processed properly. There is also a type II MCD where keratan sulfate proteoglycan is normal but dermatan sulfate proteoglycan is shorter and net synthesis of proteoglycans is much lower than normal (55).

Progeroid Syndrome

A progeroid syndrome was described in a 4-year-old child who had an aged appearance, delayed development and many connective tissue abnormalities. It was found that fibroblasts from this patient had a reduced ability to convert the core protein of small dermatan sulfate proteoglycan II into the mature proteoglycan-bearing glycosaminoglycans. Further investigation revealed the primary genetic defect in this patient to be a fibroblast deficiency of galactosyltransferase I. This enzyme usually catalyzes addition of galactose to xylose in the second glycosyl transfer in formation of the dermatan sulfate chain. How the clinical symptoms arise from this defect is uncertain, owing to a lack of knowledge of the function of this proteoglycan (56).

Carbohydrate-deficient glycoprotein syndrome (CDGS)

CDGS is an inherited, developmental disorder with multiple organ system involvement including the central and peripheral nervous systems, liver, bone, adipose tissue and the genital organs. A very high isoelectric point resulting in cathodal migration of serum transferrin is associated with this disease, believed to be due to a reduced sialylation, hence the disorder was originally called the disialotransferrin development deficiency syndrome. However, glycosylation deficiency affects many serum proteins in this disease. It appears that the *N*-linked glycans on proteins in CDGS have a normal structure but are somewhat reduced in number and so it is likely that the glycosylation defect is due to failure of saccharide attachment rather than a deficiency in processing enzymes. A defect in biosynthesis of the lipid-linked oligosaccharide precursor is more likely than defective biosynthesis of dolichyl phosphate or *N*-acetylglucosaminyl-pyrophosphoryl-dolichol. The underglycosylation that results could affect protein folding and function and ER–Golgi–plasma membrane secretion rates, and could alter processing of other oligosaccharide chains. Glycosylation deficiencies of certain proteins can explain individual symptoms, for example the hypogonadism seen in some patients could be due to underglycosylation of gonadotropic hormones converting them to antagonists (57).

Olivopontocerebellar atrophy of neonatal onset (OA)

OA shares many biochemical and clinical similarities with CDGS, suggesting that they may be different manifestations of a single genetic disease or may be closely related inborn errors of glycoprotein metabolism. The common clinical abnormalities include failure to thrive, hypotonia, delayed development, retinal abnormalities, joint restrictions, liver disease, pericardial effusion, diarrhoea and cerebellar atrophy. This is more severe than CDGS, with all reported cases dying before 2 years of age (58) whereas patients with CDGS have been reported at ages between 3 and 21 years (57). The abnormality in glycosylation and isoelectric point of serum transferrin in CDGS has also been seen in OA. Low serum concentrations of thyroid binding globulin and ceruloplasmin have also been observed, again implicating glycoproteins in the abnormality. The pathogenesis of the organ damage is unknown but the effects of such a disorder of metabolism are probably complex due to the roles of glycoproteins in cellular processes, cell–cell recognition and transport (58).

Nonthyroid illness (NTI)

Most illnesses and physiological stresses can induce changes in various aspects of the thyroid hormones. In NTI, patients usually have low serum T_3, free T_3, T_4 and free T_4 levels but a normal level of thyroid-stimulating hormone (TSH). This suggests that the TSH has a reduced biological activity which may be due to an altered glycosylation. This could be due to a deficiency in thyrotropin-releasing hormone (TRH) which is essential for key steps in TSH glycosylation (59).

Euthyroid, primary and central hypothyroid patients

Changes in the glycosylation of TSH have been observed in a variety of pathological and physiological states. In particular, sialylation has been found to influence the biological properties of such glycoprotein hormones. The degree of TSH sialylation is higher in patients with primary hypothyroidism (and increases with prolonged hypothyroidism) than in euthyroid patients. There is also a greater sialylation of TSH in primary hypothyroidism than in central hypothyroidism and no increase in sialylation was found in a patient with central hypothyroidism despite being in a clinical and biochemical hypothyroid state. This implies that TRH or other hypothalamic factors may influence TSH sialylation (60).

Hyperthyroidism in a TSH-secreting macroadenoma patient

Hyperthyroidism can result from TSH-secreting macroadenomas. Some such patients have hyperthyroidism with a normal TSH level suggesting the hyperthyroidism may be caused by increased secretion of a more bioactive TSH. Not all glycoforms of TSH will have the same bioactivity, so hyperthyroidism in these cases could be due to alteration in glycosylation profile of TSH. These patients can be treated with octreotide to attain a euthyroidal status; this drug lowers the serum TSH concentration and also alters glycosylation, suggesting the importance of TSH glycosylation in the disease (61).

von Willebrand disease (vWD)

von Willebrand disease results from an abnormality or defect in von Willebrand factor (vWF) and is usually characterized by mild mucocutaneous haemorrhage, a prolonged bleeding time and a decrease in factor VIIIc. vWF is the glycoprotein responsible for binding platelets to the subendothelium of blood vessels following injury and so is important in haemostasis. The glycosylation of this protein is crucial for its successful polymerization and subsequent secretion (32).

Gaucher disease

Gaucher disease is a lysosomal storage disease caused by a defect in the catalytic function, stability or post-translational processing of acid β-glucosidase (62).

Glanzmann's thrombasthenia and Bernard–Soulier syndrome

These are congenital bleeding disorders associated with abnormalities in platelet function. Glanzmann's thrombasthenia is inherited in an autosomal recessive manner with defects in clot retraction, platelet aggregation and a deficiency or defect in the platelet membrane GPIIb:GPIIIa complex. Bernard–Soulier syndrome is also inherited in an autosomal recessive manner, the primary abnormalities are a reduced vWF-mediated platelet adhesion, a reduced platelet survival time in the circulation, with a prolonged bleeding time tendency to bleed and a deficiency in glycoproteins Ib, Is, IX and V. In Bernard–Soulier syndrome, it is the GPIb and Is which are deficient. When functioning properly, GPIb and Is are involved in interaction between the vWF and platelet membrane during early phases of primary haemostasis. This deficiency can therefore explain the reduced vWF-mediated platelet adhesion and prolonged bleeding time. The glycoprotein abnormalities observed in these disorders is believed to be their underlying cause (63,64).

Paroxysmal nocturnal haemoglobinuria (PNH)

PNH is an acquired clonal disorder arising from a somatic mutation in a multipotential stem cell. It is characterized by the presence of RBCs abnormally susceptible to complement-mediated lysis causing chronic but episodic intravascular haemolysis. Cells other than RBCs may also be abnormal. The underlying cause is a deficiency of GPI-anchored glycoproteins. The defect is not absolute and there is either a hierarchy of access of different protein molecules to GPI anchors, distinct anchor biochemistries or differential regulation of protein–anchor assembly. These GPI-linked proteins include factors which regulate the complement cascade – decay accelerating factor, membrane inhibitor of reactive lysis and C8 binding protein – and thus their absence could be responsible for the enhanced susceptibility to complement-mediated lysis (65).

Haemophilia A (HA)

Haemophilia A (HA) is an X-linked recessive coagulation disorder with a frequency of 1 in 10 000 males. The disorder is due to a deficiency in factor VIII (an essential coagulation cofactor) procoagulant activity. The defects in factor VIII range from deletions, insertions and duplications to point mutations. Aly *et al.* have reported two cases where the defect is due to abnormal *N*-glycosylation blocking the factor VIII procoagulant activity and this is a mechanism for the pathogenesis of HA (66).

Osteogenesis imperfecta (OI)

Osteogenesis imperfecta (OI) is a heterogeneous group of genetic disorders characterized by bone fragility. There is evidence to suggest that the structure of type 1 procollagen is changed in some of these patients. Fibroblasts from a patient with OI were found to incorporate more [^{3}H]-mannose into the C-terminal of their type 1 procollagen. This could be due to incomplete trimming or to additional glycosylation sites being present in the C-terminal of the propeptide. This abnormal protein tends to form aggregates which could cause a loss of procollagen for synthesis of collagen fibrils. This may explain the clinical manifestations (67).

Hereditary angioneurotic edema (HANE)

HANE is an autosomal dominant disorder characterized by potentially life-threatening episodic angioedema of the skin and mucosa with manifestations such as severe abdominal pain (seen in gastrointestinal involvement) and airway obstruction (in respiratory-tract involvement). In type II HANE there is a decrease in C1 inhibitor activity. The DNA sequence coding for this protein in HANE was found to be a 3 bp deletion leading to creation of an *N*-linked glycosylation site. Thus, either the addition of the carbohydrate or the deletion of the amino acid interferes with the conformation and function of the protein either by steric hindrance or by an alteration in a secondary contact site for C1s (68).

Leucocyte adhesion deficiency (LAD)

LAD is an autosomal recessive trait in which neutrophils have severe adhesion and motility defects causing symptoms associated with a lack of adherence-dependent functions resulting in severe recurrent infections. Two types of LAD with different glycosylation defects have been described. Type 1 is due to a congenital defect in expression of glycoproteins LFA-1, Macl and p150,95 caused by defective biosynthesis of the β chain. Type 2 is also due to defective leucocyte adhesion molecules but is due to the absence of the carbohydrate sialyl-Lewis X ligand of E-selectin. Interactions involving selectins and sialyl Lewis X are required for slowing neutrophils down and for mediating their adhesion to the blood vessel wall and their extravasation out into the tissues; thus, where these molecules are deficient, neutrophils cannot be recruited to inflammatory sites and so patients suffer recurrent infections. The underlying cause may be defective fucose metabolism (69).

Viruses

The host cell's glycosylation machinery is used to glycosylate viral proteins so the virus becomes coated with glycoproteins indistinguishable from those of the host. The expression of host oligosaccharides allows the virus to evade immune surveillance and perhaps provide a way for the virus to attach to host cell receptors. An understanding of this interaction could pave the way for the development of oligosaccharides as anti-viral drugs (32).

Protozoa

Protozoa of the *Trypanosomatidae* family cause a variety of serious human diseases including South American Chagas disease and African sleeping sickness. Each stage of their life cycle is characterized by various changes including surface glycoconjugate expression. These may assist in evasion of the immune system, complement-resistance, host cell binding and also internalization and differentiation. These carbohydrate structures could be targeted in the development of drug therapies and vaccines (70).

Galactosaemia

Classic galactosaemia is a condition arising from a deficiency in galactose-1-phosphate uridyltransferase. It is treated by restricting galactose intake, which usually resolves the early, acute effects and the cataracts characteristic of the disorder but is less effective in the long-term outcome with many patients showing developmental delay, speech abnormalities and ovarian dysfunction. Two mechanisms have been proposed in the pathogenesis of this disorder; firstly, galactose-1-phosphate accumulation, mostly associated with the acute abnormalities and secondly, the synthesis of galactitol which may be involved in cataract formation (71).

Multiple sclerosis (MS)

The aetiology of MS is believed to involve both genetic and environmental factors which result in an immunologically mediated inflammatory response in the central nervous system (CNS). This disease occurs when there is a disruption of the myelin nerve sheath, caused for example by a fault in peripheral nerve myelin compaction. L2/HNK-1 is a carbohydrate epitope present on the myelin protein PO that is believed to have a role in peripheral nerve myelin compaction. Therefore any alteration in expression of this carbohydrate epitope could contribute to the pathogenesis of MS (32).

In experimental allergic encephalitis, an animal model for MS, the population of lymphocytes entering the CNS differs from the systemic population which suggests a role for abnormal lymphocyte migration in this disease. HNK-1, which is a neural adhesion molecule on lymphocytes, may be important for binding to HEVs and thus could also be a homing molecule (32).

I-cell disease and pseudo-Hurler polydystrophy

Fibroblasts from patients with I-cell disease (mucolipidosis type II) do not phosphorylate mannose residues on their lysosomal enzymes due to a deficiency of *N*-acetyl glucosamine 1-phosphotransferase caused by a decreased synthesis, stability or synthesis of a defective enzyme (72,73). The mannose-6-phosphate residues target the lysosomal enzymes to lysosomes and thus in its absence these enzymes are secreted into the culture medium or extracellular milieu. This causes the patients to be deficient in lysosomal enzymes. This can cause morphological alterations in many tissues. Patients with pseudo-Hurler polydystrophy have a low but present phosphorylation activity, which probably explains their milder clinical symptoms (72).

The Tn syndrome

This syndrome is characterized by persistent polyagglutination of red cells, on which the Tn antigen is exposed, by anti-Tn antibodies present in the blood. Normally, the Tn antigen, although expressed, is not exposed or accessible to antibody. In Tn disease the Tn antigen is exposed due to a deficiency in activity of UDPGal:GalNAc-α1-O-Ser/Thrβ1-3-D-galactosyltransferase, resulting in a failure to add galactose and, subsequently, terminal sialic acid to *O*-linked oligosaccharides. The abnormality is often only evident in a proportion of cells giving rise to mixed field polyagglutination. There is evidence that the abnormality also affects platelets, T cells, B cells and granulocytes. The Tn syndrome is an acquired myeloid dysplasia often found with anaemia, neutropenia and thrombocytopenia. A regulatory defect in the expression of the transferase has been shown to underlie altered antigen expression (74).

Diseases where glycosylation may determine the disease outcome or individual symptoms

Amenorrhoea in anorexia nervosa

Anorexia nervosa (AN) is an eating disorder where food intake is chronically and drastically reduced. Young females with the disorder frequently develop secondary amenorrhoea. Gonadotropin levels in the plasma of such patients suggests that the hypothalamus may be involved in the pathogenesis. The glycosylation of the gonadotropins can affect their bioactivity in different clinical conditions. Altered glycosylation of these hormones, especially FSH, was observed in a patient with psychogenic amenorrhoea which was improved by treatment with LH releasing hormone, implicating the qualitative and quantitative alterations of FSH molecular structure in the pathogenesis of stress-related amenorrhoea. There appears to be a change in glycosylation of the total gonadotropins in AN which may decrease their bioactivity and thus be responsible for the hypothalamic amenorrhoea observed in these patients (75).

Myocardial infarction

Myocardial infarction (MI) involves an acute necrosis of the muscular layer of the heart due to a sudden loss of blood supply to the affected tissue. The resulting ischaemia causes tissue damage resulting in local and systemic reactions which produce cytokines. These initiate the acute phase response which is characterized by increased concentrations of proteins called acute phase proteins, most of which are glycoproteins. The cytokines produced in the response can also cause changes in the glycosylation pattern and the concentration of the acute phase proteins. There is a clear relationship between glycoprotein concentrations such as α_1-acid glycoprotein (AGP) and the enzymatic myocardial infarction size. More recent evidence suggests that the glycosylation profile of α_1-antichymotrypsin, measured as the reactivity coefficient, correlates with the manifestation of acute heart failure in MI patients. Therefore, this may be used in evaluating the prognosis of MI patients, the reactivity coefficients being higher in those with heart failure (76).

Systemic lupus erythematosus (SLE)

This idiopathic chronic inflammatory disease may affect the skin, joints, kidneys, lungs, the nervous system, serous membranes and also other organs. It can be very difficult to differentiate between an exacerbation of SLE and an infection because fever can be symptomatic of both. It has been found that concanavalin A reactive glycoforms of AGP are increased in SLE patients with infections but not in those with increased disease activity and no infection. Therefore, it has been proposed that AGP microheterogeneity can be used to predict infection in SLE patients (77).

It is interesting to note that in both MI and SLE the change in glycosylation of cytokines is associated with predicting the patient's prognosis or disease status. It may be that the glycosylation profile of cytokines is also altered in other conditions and may prove to be a useful prognostic marker for a wide variety of diseases.

Sleep factor

The structure of sleep factor, which controls the balance of rapid eye movement (REM) and slow wave (SW) sleep, is similar to some peptidoglycan fragments from cell walls of Gram-negative bacteria which are somnogenic. Interleukin-1 may also contain similar structures and be somnogenic and pyrogenic and so contribute to the sleepiness often encountered in infectious disease. The balance of REM/SW sleep may influence the tendency to hallucinate (32).

Bee venom allergies

Antibodies of the IgE class with specificity terminal GlcNAc residues expressed on *N*-linked oligosaccharides present in bee venom have been detected in serum of allergic individuals, suggesting that oligosaccharide epitopes may contribute to the development of immediate type hypersensitivity (32).

Diseases due to defective lectin binding

Opsonic defect due to MBP deficiency

A common opsonic defect has been reported in 5–7% of the general population and has been found in many children with frequent unexplained infections, with chronic diarrhoea of infancy and with otitis media. This defect has been found to be associated with a low level of mannose-binding protein. An organism with many mannose groups on its cell wall can be bound by MBP, which then activates the classical complement pathway, aiding in its destruction. Thus a reduced MBP may explain the frequent infections which are seen in these children, especially between the time of maternal antibody depletion and attainment of a complete antibody repertoire (49).

Glycosylation in rheumatoid arthritis (excluding IgG)

Glycosylation of serum α_1-acid glycoprotein in rheumatoid arthritis

A change in glycosylation of acute phase proteins has been observed in this inflammatory reaction in RA. In particular, changes in fucosylation and sialylation have been seen, which can result in upregulation of sialyl Lewis X (SLEX) on these molecules; this structure can mediate the primary attachment to the inflamed endothelial cells allowing influx to inflammation sites. α_1-Acid glycoprotein (AGP) in RA sera is heavily fucosylated in a way that correlates with the disease activity. The increased SLEX on AGP may inhibit the influx of leucocytes to these areas, thus dampening the cellular inflammatory reaction. Methotrexate is often used in the treatment of RA. This drug has been found to decrease the degree of fucosylation, increase the sialylation and decrease the concentration of AGP. These effects may contribute to disease improvement (77).

Extravasation of lymphocytes in RA

In RA, HEV are induced in the synovium of the affected joints, causing extravasation of lymphocytes into the joint, and aberrant sequestration, causing the autoimmune disease (32). Thus, carbohydrates also affect lymphocyte migration in the disease.

Cancer

All human carcinomas manifest changes in cell surface carbohydrates, relative to their normal counterparts, and this offers a route to modifying tumour progression (78,79). Changes in carbohydrates may be secondary to a change in activity or concentration of GTases or glycosidases. Carbohydrates, including ECAMS, sialylated mucins, cell surface lactosamine and polylactosamine, have been implicated in tumour metastasis and location, with cell surface glycoproteins playing a role in blood-borne tumour cell implantation. It may be mediated by binding to lectins on endothelial cells, resulting in retention of blood-borne tumours, or through reduced binding to extracellular matrix proteins, contributing to tumour cell displacement. Tumours are heterogeneous for the metastatic phenotype, with subpopulations with a high density of metastatic glycoforms having a selective advantage over those with a lower density on their cell surface. NK cells can limit metastatic spread of cancer; this may be dependent on the density of specific oligosaccharides on the tumour cell surface because NK cells can recognize and lyse their targets according to the *N*-linked oligosaccharide type present (32).

Many clinical diagnostic procedures now utilize lectins to detect abnormal glycosylation on the malignant cell surface. Analysis of the glycoproteins can be used to indicate the lymph node stage, locoregional recurrence and survival, and the concentration of glycosylation enzymes can be used to monitor the success of therapy and disease stage for certain cancers (78,79).

CONCLUDING REMARKS

It will be evident that the addition of oligosaccharides to proteins and other matrices contributes to the generation of structural and functional diversity. Abnormal glycosylation patterns may therefore be of profound pathophysiological significance. There exists considerable potential, therefore, for the development of carbohydrate-based drugs and possible treatment of certain diseases by transfection of glycosidase or glycosytransferase genes. The technology to analyse and precisely characterize glycoconjugates has only recently become available to non-specialist laboratories and we may anticipate a virtual explosion of interest in this area. Natural and controlled glycosylation of recombinant proteins is a regulatory requirement for applications in human therapy.

REFERENCES

1. Varki, A. 1993. Biological roles of oligosaccharides: all the theories are correct. *Glycobiology* **3**:97–130.
2. Jenkins, N. and M. A. Curling. 1994. Glycosylation of recombinant proteins – problems and prospects. *Enzyme and Microbiol. Technol.* **16**:354–63.
3. Dwek, R. A. 1995. Glycobiology – towards an understanding of the function of sugars. *Biochem. Soc. Trans.* **23**:1–25.
4. Jefferis, R., J. Lund, H. Mizitani *et al.* 1990. A comparative study of the *N*-linked oligosaccharide structures of human IgG subclass proteins. *Biochem. J.* **268**:529–37.
5. Lund, J., N. Takahashi, H. Nakagawa *et al.* 1993. Control of IgG/Fc glycosylation: a comparison of oligosaccharides from chimeric human/mouse and mouse subclass immunoglobulin Gs. *Mol. Immunol.* **30**:741–8.
6. Deisenhofer, J. 1981. Crystallographic refinement and atomic models of a human Fc fragment and its complex with fragment B of protein A from *Staphylococcus aureus* at 2.9- and 2.8-Å resolution. *Biochemistry* **20**:2361–70.
7. Sutton, B. J. and D. C. Phillips. 1983. The three-dimensional structure of the carbohydrate within the Fc fragment of immunoglobulin G. *Biochem. Soc. Trans.* **11**:30–132.

8. Padlan, E. A. 1990. In: *Fc receptors and the action of antibodies* (H. Metger, ed.) American Society for Microbiology, Washington, pp. 12–30.
9. Lund, J., G. Winter, P. T. Jones *et al.* 1991. Human FcγRI and FcγRII interact with distinct but overlapping sites on human IgG. *J. Immunol.* **147**:2657–62.
10. Sarmay, G., J. Lund, J. Gergely *et al.* 1992. Mapping and comparison of the interaction sites on the Fc region of IgG responsible for triggering antibody dependent cellular cytotoxicity (ADCC) through different types of Fcγ receptor. *Mol. Immunol.* **29**:633–9.
11. Walker, M. R., J. Lund, K. M. Thompson *et al.* 1989. Aglycosylation of human IgG1 and IgG3 monoclonal antibodies eliminates recognition by human cells expressing FcγRI and/or FcγRII receptors. *Biochem. J.* **259**:1356–72.
12. Pound, J. D., J. Lund and R. Jefferis. 1993. Human FcγRI triggering of the mononuclear phagocyte respiratory burst. *Mol. Immunol.* **30**:469–75.
13. Leatherbarrow, R. J., T. W. Rademacher, R. A. Dwek *et al.* 1985. Effector functions of monoclonal aglycosylated mouse IgG2a: binding and activation of complement component C1 and interaction with human Fcγ receptor. *Mol. Immunol.* **22**:407–15.
14. Nose, M. and H. Wigzell. 1983. Biological significance of carbohydrate chains on monoclonal antibodies. *Proc. Natl. Acad. Sci. USA* **80**:6632–6.
15. Duncan, A. R. and G. Winter. 1988. The binding site for C1q on IgG. *Nature* **332**:738–40.
16. Tsuchiya, N., T. Endo, K. Matsuta *et al.* 1989. Effects of galactose depletion from oligosaccharide chains on immunological activities of human IgG. *J. Rheum.* **16**:285–90.
17. Boyd, P. N., A. C. Lines and A. K. Patel. 1995. The effect of removal of sialic acid, galactose and total carbohydrate on the functional activity of CAMPATH-1H. *Mol. Immunol.* **32**:1311–18.
18. Malhotra, R., M. R. Wormald, P. M. Rudd *et al.* 1995. Agalactosyl IgG activates complement via mannose-binding protein. *Nature Medicine* **1**:237–43.
19. Dwek, R. A., A. C. Lelloucj and M. R. Wormold 1995. Glycobiology: The function of sugar in the IgG molecule. *J. Anat.* **187**:279–92.
20. Vanzeben, D., G. A. W. Rook, J. M. W. Hazes *et al.* 1994. Early agalactosylation of IgG is associated with a more progressive disease course in patients with rheumatoid arthritis. *Br. J. Rheum.* **33**:36–43.
21. Lund, J., N. Takahashi, J. D. Pound *et al.* 1995. Oligosaccharide–protein interactions in IgG can modulate recognition by Fcγ receptors. *FASEB J.* **9**:115–19.
22. Lund, J., T. Tanaka, N. Takahashi *et al.* 1990. A protein structural change in aglycosylated IgG3 correlates with loss of huFcγR1 and huFcγ R111 binding and/or activation. *Mol. Immunol.* **27**:1145–54.
23. Newkirk, M. M., A. Lemmo and J. Rauch. 1990. Importance of IgG isotype, not state of glycosylation, in human rheumatoid factor binding. *Arthritis Rheum.* **33**:800–9.
24. Sumar, N., K. B. Bodman, T. W. Rademacher *et al.* 1990. Analysis of glycosylation changes in IgG using lectins. *J. Immunol. Meth.* **131**:127–36.
25. Gilhespy-Muskett, A. M., J. Partridge, R. Jefferis *et al.* 1994. A novel ^{13}C isotopic labelling strategy for probing the structure and dynamics of glycan chains *in situ* on glycoproteins. *J. Glycobiol.* **4**:485–90.
26. Leader, K. A., G. C. Lastra, J. R. Kirwan *et al.* 1996. Agalactosyl IgG in aggregates from the rheumatoid joint. *Br. J. Rheumatol.* **35**:335–41.
27. Axford, J. S., N. Sumar, A. Alavi *et al.* 1992. Changes in normal glycosylation mechanisms in autoimmune rheumatic disease. *J. Clin. Invest.* **89**:1021–31.

28. Bond, A., M. A. Kerr and F. C. Hay. 1995. Distinct oligosaccharide content of rheumatoid arthritis-derived immune complexes. *Arth. Rheum.* **38**:744–9.
29. Soltys, A. J., F. C. Hay, A. Bond *et al.* 1994. The binding of synovial tissue-derived human monoclonal immunoglobulin M rheumatoid factor to immunoglobulin G preparations of differing galactose content. *Scand. J. Immunol.* **40**:135–43.
30. Newkirk, M. M. and J. Rauch. 1993. Binding of human monoclonal IgG rheumatoid factors to Fc is influenced by carbohydrate. *J. Rheum.* **20**:776–80.
31. Cheng, S. H., R. J. Gregory, J. Marshall *et al.* 1990. Defective intracellular transport and processing of CFTR is the molecular basis of most cystic fibrosis. *Cell* **63**:827–34.
32. Rademacher, T. W., R. B. Parekh and R. A. Dwek. 1988. Glycobiology. *Ann. Rev. Biochem.* **57**:785–838.
33. Margolies, R. and T. F. Boat. 1983. The carbohydrate content of IgG from patients with cystic fibrosis. *Pediatr. Res.* **17**:931–5.
34. Parekh, R. B. 1991. Effects of glycosylation on protein function. *Curr. Op. Structural. Biol.* **1**:750–4.
35. Nakao, H., A. Nishikawa, T. Nishiura *et al.* 1991. Hypogalactosylation of immunoglobulin G sugar chains and elevated serum interleukin 6 in Castleman's disease. *Clin. Chim. Acta* **197**:221–8.
36. Middaugh, C. R. and G. W. Litman. 1987. Atypical glycosylation of an IgG monoclonal cryoimmunoglobulin. *J. Biol. Chem.* **262**:3671–3.
37. Hadley, A. G., B. Zupanska, B. M. Kumpel *et al.* 1995. The glycosylation of red cell autoantibodies affects their functional activity in vitro. *Br. J. Haematol.* **91**:587–94.
38. Galili, U. 1988. The natural anti-gal antibody, the B-like antigen, and human red cell aging. *Blood Cell* **14**:205–20.
39. Koren, E., M. Kujundzic, M. Koscec *et al.* 1994. Cytotoxic effects of human preformed anti-GAL IgG and complement on cultured pig cells. *Transplant. Prop.* **26**:1336–9.
40. Clements, G. B., D. N. Galbraith and K. W. Taylor. 1995. Coxsackie-B infection in childhood diabetes. *Lancet* **346**:221–3.
41. Kennedy, D. M., A. W. Skillen and C. H. Self. 1994. Glycation of monoclonal antibodies impairs their ability to bind antigen. *Clin. Exp. Immunol.* **98**: 245–51.
42. Torres, C. R. and G. W. Hart. 1984. Topography and polypeptide distribution of terminal *N*-acetylglucosamine residues on the surfaces of intact lymphocytes – evidence for *O*-linked GlcNAc. *J. Biol. Chem.* **259**:3308–17.
43. Jentoft, N. 1990. Why are proteins *O*-glycosylated? *TIBS* **15**:291–4.
44. Kearse, K. P. and G. W. Hart. 1991. Topology of *O*-linked *N*-acetylglucosamine in murine lymphocytes. *Arch. Biochem. Biophys.* **290**:543–8.
45. Drickamer, K. and M. E. Taylor. 1993. Biology of animal lectins. *Ann. Rev. Cell Biol.* **2**:237–64.
46. Hart, G. W. 1992. Glycosylation. *Curr. Op. Cell Biol.* **4**:1017–23.
47. Taylor, M. E. 1993. Recognition of complex carbohydrates by the macrophage mannose receptor. *Biochem. Soc. Trans.* **21**:468–73.
48. Hughes, R. C. and T. D. Butters. 1981. Glycosylation patterns in cells – an evolutionary marker. *TIBS* **6**:228–30.
49. Turner, M. W. 1994. Mannose binding protein. *Biochem. Soc. Trans.* **22**:88–94.
50. Paulson, J. C. 1989. Glycoproteins: What are the sugar chains for? *TIBS* **14**:272–6.

51. Marks, P. W. and A. J. Mitus. 1996. Congenital dyserythropoietic anemias. *Am. J. Hematol.* **51**:55–63.
52. Aspenstrom, P., U. Lindberg and A. Hall 1996. 2 GTPases, CD42 and RAC, bind directly to a protein implicated in the immuno-deficiency disorder Wiskott–Aldrich syndrome. *Curr. Biol.* **6**:70–5.
53. Piller, F., F. Ledeist, K. I. Weinberg *et al.* 1991. Altered *O*-glycan synthesis in lymphocytes from patients with Wiskott–Aldrich syndrome. *J. Exp. Med.* **173**:1501–10.
54. Remold-O'Donnell, E., F. S. Rosen and D. M. Kenney. 1996. Defects in Wiskott–Aldrich syndrome blood cells. *Blood* **87**:2621–31.
55. Midura, R. J., V. C. Hascall, D. K. Maccallum *et al.* 1990. Proteoglycan biosynthesis by human corneas from patients with type 1 and type 2 macular corneal dystrophy. *J. Biol. Chem.* **265**:15 947–55.
56. Quentin, E., A. Gladen, L. Roden *et al.* 1990. A genetic defect in the biosynthesis of dermatan sulfate proteoglycan-galactosyltransferase 1 deficiency in fibroblasts from a patient with a progeroid syndrome. *Proc. Natl. Acad. Sci. USA* **87**:1342–6.
57. Powell, L. D., K. Paneerselvam, V. Rohini *et al.* 1994. Carbohydrate-deficient glycoprotein syndrome – not an *N*-linked oligosaccharide processing defect, but an abnormality in lipid-linked oligosaccharide biosynthesis. *J. Clin. Invest.* **94**:1901–9.
58. Horslen, S. P., P. T. Clayton, B. N. Harding *et al.* 1991. Olivopontocerebellar atrophy of neonatal onset and disialotransferrin developmental deficiency syndrome. *Arch. Dis. Childhood* **66**:1027–32.
59. Lee, H. Y., J. Suhl, A. E. Pekary *et al.* 1987. Secretion of thyrotropin with reduced concanavalin-A binding activity in patients with severe nonthyroid illness. *J. Clin Endocrinol. Metab.* **65**:942–5.
60. Miura, Y., V. S. Perkel, K. A. Papenberg *et al.* 1989. Concanavalin-A, lentil and ricin lectin affinity binding characteristics of human thyrotropin: differences in the sialylation of thyrotropin in sera of euthyroid, primary, and central hypothyroid patients. *J. Clin. Endocrinol. Metab.* **69**:985–95.
61. Francis, T. B., R. C. Smallridge, J. Kane *et al.* 1993. Octreotide changes serum thyrotropin (TSH) glycoisomer distribution as assessed by lectin chromatography in a TSH macroadenoma patient. *J. Clin. Endocrinol. Metab.* **77**:183–7.
62. Grabowski, G. A. 1993. Gaucher disease – enzymology, genetics and treatment. *Adv. Hum. Genet.* **21**:377–441.
63. Lee, G. R., T. C. Bithell, J. Foerster *et al.* 1993. *Wintrobe's Clinical Haematology*, 9th edn. Lea & Febiger, Philadelphia.
64. Nurden, A. T. 1995. Polymorphism of human platelet glycoproteins – structure and clinical significance. *Thromb. Haemostasis* **74**:345–57.
65. Rosse, W. F. and R. E. Ware. 1995. The molecular basis of paroxysmal nocturnal hemoglobinuria. *Blood* **86**:3277–86.
66. Aly, A. M., M. Higuchi, C. K. Kasper *et al.* 1992. Hemophilia-A due to mutations that create new *N*-glycosylation sites. *Proc. Natl. Acad. Sci. USA* **89**:4933–7.
67. Peltonen, L., A. Palotie and D. J. Prockop. 1980. A defect in the structure of type I procollagen in a patient who had osteogenesis imperfecta: Excess mannose in the COOH-terminal propeptide. *Proc. Natl. Acad. Sci. USA* **77**:6179–83.
68. Parad, R. B., J. Kramer, R. C. Strunk *et al.* 1990. Dysfunctional C1 inhibitor Ta: Deletion of Lys-251 results in acquisition of an *N*-glycosylation site. *Proc. Natl. Acad. Sci. USA* **87**:6786–90.
69. Etzioni, A., M. Frydman, S. Pollack *et al.* 1992. Recurrent severe infections caused by a novel leukocyte adhesion deficiency. *N. Engl. J. Med.* **327**:1789–92.

70. Parodi, A. J. 1993. *N*-glycosylation in trypanosomatid protozoa. *Glycobiology* **3**:193–9.
71. Dunger, D. B. and J. B. Holton. 1994. Disorders of carbohydrate metabolism. In *The Inherited Metabolic Diseases* (J. B. Holton, ed.) Churchill Livingstone, Edinburgh, pp. 21–65.
72. von Figura, K. and A. Hasilik. 1986. Lysosomal enzymes and their receptors. *Ann. Rev. Biochem.* **55**:167–93.
73. Dicioccio, R. A. and A. L. Miller. 1993. Phosphorylation and subcellular localisation of α-L-fucosidase in lymphoid cells from patients with I-cell disease and pseudo-Hurler polydystrophy. *Glycobiology* **3**:489–95.
74. Thurnher, M., J. Fehr and E. G. Berger. 1994. Differences in regulation of specific glycosylation in the pathogenesis of paroxysmal-nocturnal hemglobinemia and the Tn syndrome. *Exp. Hematol.* **22**:267–71.
75. Tommaselli, A. P., R. Valentino, S. Savastano *et al.* 1995. Altered glycosylation of pituitary gonadotropins in anorexia nervosa: an alternative explanation for amenorrhea. *Eur. J. Endocrinol.* **132**:450–5.
76. Kazmierczak, M., M. Sobieska, K. Wiktorowicz *et al.* 1995. Changes of acute phase proteins glycosylation profile as a possible prognostic marker in myocardial infarction. *Int. J. Cardiol.* **49**:201–7.
77. van Dijk, W., G. A. Turner and A. Mackiewicz. 1994. Changes in glycosylation of acute-phase proteins in health and disease: occurrence, regulation and function. *Glycosylation & Disease* **1**:5–14.
78. Goss, P. E., M. A. Baker, J. P. Carver *et al.* 1995. Inhibitors of glycosylation: a new class of antitumor agent. *Clin. Cancer. Res.* **9**:935–44.
79. Jacobs, J. S. 1995. Glycosylation inhibitors in biology and medicine. *Curr. Op. Struct. Biol.* **5**:605–14.

12

Anti-DNA Antibodies: is DNA the Self Antigen or a Shelf Antigen, or are all Autoimmune Diseases Immunogen Driven?

Yehuda Shoenfeld

Do all autoimmune diseases behave according to accepted immunological rules? Are they all driven by autoantigen(s)? Is DNA, for instance, the immunogen for systemic lupus erythematosus (SLE)?

Two observations led me to suggest that at least in some autoimmune diseases there is no autoantigen that drives the immune system; the autoantigen identified by autoantibodies or autoreactive cells can be employed for diagnostic purposes, but this does not necessarily mean that the autoantigen is involved in the pathogenesis.

THE KALEIDOSCOPE OF AUTOIMMUNITY

Previously, we introduced the term 'mosaic of autoimmunity' to describe the diversity of the multifactorial aetiology of autoimmune diseases (1,2). Subsequently we developed the notion of a 'kaleidoscope of autoimmunity' (3) to denote the fact that a change in the immune system (e.g. thymectomy, splenectomy) may induce a remission or even a cure from one autoimmune disease, with the emergence of another. Two cases in point are:

- the development of aggressive SLE following thymectomy complicating myasthenia gravis (4,5)
- the induction of chronic active hepatitis following splenectomy performed for resistant autoimmune thrombocytopenic purpura (6).

Immunoregulation in Health and Disease
ISBN 0-12-459460-3

Table 12.1 Antigens that cross-react with anti-DNA antibodies

Synthetic nucleic acid polymers
poly (dT), poly (dC), poly (A), poly (I), poly (G), dsRNA, left-handed Z-DNA
Phospholipids
Cardiolipin
Phosphatidic acid
Phosphatidyl glycerol
Phosphatidyl serine
Phosphatidyl inositol
Cholesterol
Bacterial antigens
Pyruvylated galactose of *Klebsiella*
Capsular polysaccharides of group B meningococci and *E. coli*
Bacterial phospholipids
Cytoskeletal proteins
Raji cells
Platelets
Lymphocytotoxic reaction of antibodies
Proteoglycans
Hyaluronic acid
Chondriotin sulphate
Heparan sulfate
Synthetic polyanionic antigens
Dextran sulfate
Polyvinyl sulfate

Reproduced from reference 12 in which references are included.

In both examples the new emerging autoimmune condition cannot be attributed to a novel exposure to the presumed respective autoantigen of the disease. One has therefore to assume that just by perturbing the immune system, without any active intervention of an autoantigen, a variety of autoimmune diseases can be induced. Later on, I will support these clinical observations with experimental data.

IS DNA THE AUTOANTIGEN IN SLE?

Systemic lupus erythematosus represents the prototype of a multisystemic autoimmune disease. The organs and tissues afflicted in SLE include the joints, skin and hair, kidneys, nervous system, mucosa, haematopoietic system, heart valves, pericardium, myocardium and pleura. In addition to the great diversity of organ involvement, the disease is characterized by the longest list of autoantibodies (7) so far reported in any single autoimmune condition (Table 12.1). Yet, anti-dsDNA are believed to be the characteristic pathogenic autoantibodies in SLE.

It has been pointed out that when one steps into manure its adherence to shoes does not indicate the existence of manure receptors on shoes. Similarly, the fact that antibodies in sera of patients with SLE bind to DNA does not necessarily mean to say that DNA induced their generation.

In this paper I would like to propose that, despite the fact that the common autoantibodies in SLE do react with dsDNA on a solid phase (EIA, RIA) or in solution (Farr assay), this reaction is due merely to the fortuitous pick-up of DNA from the *shelf*, historically by four different groups (8–11), rather than an indication for DNA being the *self target antigen*.

A common notion regards DNA as the autoantigen in SLE (reviewed in (12)). Those who believe in this relationship designate anti-DNA antibodies (especially IgG, high-affinity anti-dsDNA with a basic isoelectrophoretic point, reviewed in 12) as the pathogenic autoantibodies in SLE (particularly, insult to kidneys) (reviewed in 12). Yet it is remarkable to note that human DNA is non-immunogenic; i.e. it fails to induce human anti-DNA antibodies upon active immunization (13).

Indeed, some anti-nucleic acid autoantibody specificities could be achieved by immunization of experimental animals with protein–nucleic acid complexes (reviewed in 14). It has been more difficult to obtain immunization-induced responses to dsDNA or ribosomal RNA or tRNA, unless certain dsDNA–protein combinations are used to yield antibody to dsDNA: e.g. bacterial DNA with methylated bovine serum albumin (BSA) (15); BK virus DNA with viral protein (16); and mammalian DNA with a peptide from a DNA-binding transcription factor (17).

Furthermore, most passive transfer experiments employing monoclonal and polyclonal anti-DNA antibodies failed to induce the panoply of SLE manifestations (18–21).

Let me begin by stressing that it is inconceivable that an autoantibody will be generated against the very substance of our genetic material. Needless to say, none of the organ involvements elsewhere in this article can logically be explained by the presence of anti-DNA antibodies. Even the kidney lesions in SLE, traditionally attributed to the deposition of anti-DNA in the glomeruli either as immune complexes (with DNA) or as binding to the solid phase of the glomerular basement membrane, are no longer accepted by most investigators as being the direct effect of anti-DNA antibodies (e.g. they are referred to as anti-heparan sulfate, anti-proteoglycans or anti-laminin) (22,23).

Interestingly enough, in 1983 we demonstrated that human monoclonal anti-DNA antibodies generated from SLE patients reacted with higher affinity with a synthetic polynucleotide (polydeoxythymidilic acid [poly (dT)], a *shelf* antigen), than with DNA (24,25). This observation had already been made by D. Stollar in 1966 for serum anti-DNA antibodies derived from patients with SLE (26).

These data stimulated me to raise the question whether DNA as an 'autoantigen' in SLE is really a *self* antigen or a *shelf* antigen. Is it possible that if the four groups defining anti-DNA antibodies in 1957 (8–11) had taken poly(dT) from the shelf, the classical autoantibodies determined in patients with SLE would have been referred to, nowadays, as poly(dT)? This would have obviated the need for so many articles indicating an aberrant surface presentation of *intracellular* autoantigens such as DNA or pyruvate dehydrogenase (the presumed mitochondrial autoantigen in primary biliary cirrhosis) in various diseases, or the need for evidence of transportation of an intracellular autoantigen to the surface of the cell tissue involved. Alternatively, we would not be compelled to show an intracellular penetration of autoantibodies into the cytoplasm or even into the nucleus of cells (27,28). Needless to say, the entry of the autoantibodies into the cytoplasm or even into the nucleus cannot explain the clinical findings.

These arguments do not exclude or lessen the enormously important roles of known autoantigens in other classical autoimmune diseases such as thyroglobulin in Hashimoto's disease, acetylcholine receptor in myasthenia gravis or glycoprotein IIb in autoimmune thrombocytopenia, especially since in some autoimmune diseases such as Hashimoto's thyroiditis the resection of the thyroid gland (target organ) may prevent the emergence of the disease (e.g. thyroiditis) (29,30).

CROSS-REACTIVITY OF ANTI-DNA ANTIBODIES

If DNA is not the self antigen, there must be other antigens imitating DNA in their epitopes. Therefore, it is not surprising that many groups have reported either on autoantigens cross-reacting with DNA (reviewed in 12), or on compounds that are combined with DNA to enhance the binding and to explain the pathogenic role (31). The list of cross-reacting antigens with DNA is summarized in Table 12.1, and the list shifts according to the fashion at a particular time. In the recent past it was popular to believe that the autoantigen of anti-DNA antibodies is the DNA–histone complex (nucleosomes) (32). Today it is fashionable to claim extracellular compounds such as heparan sulfate (33) and other proteoglycans such as laminin as the autoantigen (34). Furthermore, recently a new F_1 progeny of the cross between SWR and NZb mice (SNF_1) was reported (35). This strain develops severe immune complex glomerulonephritis, similar to that seen in human SLE. An idiotypically related family of nephritic antibodies (Id^{LN} F_1) has been shown to be important in the pathogenesis of autoimmune glomerulonephritis in these mice. Interestingly, the majority of Id^{LN} F_1^+ antibodies do not bind DNA (36). Treatment with antibody reactive with the nephritogenic Id suppressed its production and led to prolonged survival of NZB × SWR F_1 mice. Surprisingly, there was no difference in the incidence of anti-DNA antibody production between the treated and control SNF_1 mice. Thus these results support the hypothesis that dysregulation of pathogenic idiotypes, not confined to anti-DNA antibody idiotypes, may contribute to the development of SLE (37).

HYPOTHESIS

Is it possible that there is no autoantigen? Is it possible that as with the story of the existence of natural autoantibodies (38), we were misled by historical concept? For decades the autoimmune theories were blocked by Paul Ehrlich's 'horror autotoxicus'. For years, the existence of natural autoantibodies was dismissed by Burnet's 'forbidden clones' theory. Is it possible that because in the classical autoimmune diseases, such as autoimmune hymolytic anaemia, immune thrombocytopenic purpura, myasthenia gravis, Graves' disease, pemphigus, etc., there are well-defined autoantigens and the pathogenesis is well explained by the binding of the autoantibodies to the respective autoantigens, we believe that in *any* disease regarded as an 'autoimmune', one should find an autoantigen as the immunogen?

SCIENTIFIC SUPPORT FOR THE LACK OF AN INDUCING AUTOANTIGEN

The failure to induce SLE in naive mice by DNA immunization or passive infusion of anti-DNA antibodies led us to embark on a new approach to induce SLE. This approach involves *active* immunization of healthy strains of mice with the anti-DNA antibody emulsified in complete Freund's adjuvant. After 3–4 months from the boost the mice developed all the serological markers characteristic of SLE, associated with clinical findings including increased erythrocyte sedimentation rate (ESR), leukopenia, thrombocytopenia, and kidneys and CNS involvements (39–45). There were differences in the induction ability of SLE among the various strains of mice (45), and it seemed to be related to MHC-I (46).

Following immunization with Ab_1 (Id), the mice developed Ab_2 (anti-Id)

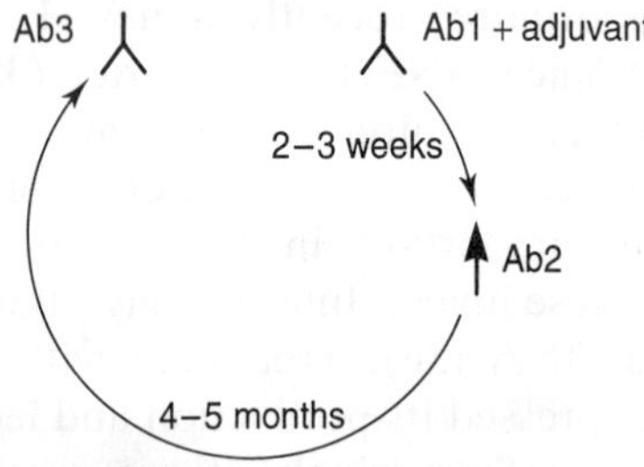

Fig. 12.1 Induction of autoimmune diseases by idiotypic dysregulation. Following immunization with the autoantibody (Ab_1) the animal develops anti-autoantibody (Ab_2) and anti-anti-autoantibody (Ab_3). Ab_3 has autoantibody characteristics and its appearance is associated with the respective clinical findings of the autoimmune condition.

and eventually Ab_3 which had autoantibody properties (Fig. 12.1). Our experiments may indicate that by idiotypic stimulation one can upregulate the production of (natural?) autoantibodies. It seems clear that the information required to produce these autoantibodies is inherent in our immune repertoire (e.g. the immunologic homunculus (47,48)). These stimulations are specific: when we immunize with anti-DNA, anti-La or anti-Sm antibodies, the mice develop the serological repertoire seen in patients with SLE (anti-DNA, RNP, Ro/La (39)). When immunized with anti-cardiolipin (49) or anti-phosphatidylserine (50), the mice developed anti-phospholipid antibodies including lupus anticoagulant, and when immunized with anti-proteinase-3 (Pr-3) (cANCA) they developed anti-PR-3 and anti-myeloperoxidase (MPO) antibodies (51). In all the above experiments the mice developed manifestations of the respective autoimmune disease. When they were immunized with anti-DNA antibodies, one could see increased ESR, leukopenia, thrombocytopenia, proteinuria, and immune complex deposition in the kidneys with mesangial deposition of the same idiotype employed at immunization (i.e. 16/6 Id), leading to glomerular atrophy. When immunized with anti-phospholipid antibodies the mice developed thrombocytopenia and thromboembolism. When they were mated they suffered from low fecundity rate and increased fetal loss. The most remarkable phenomenon observed entailed the generation by these naive mice of *all* the autoantibodies detected in the sera of *individuals* with SLE, including-anti-dsDNA, anti-histones, anti-cardiolipin, anti-Ro/La and even anti-Sm. Many of those antibodies were immortalized by the hybridoma technique (52), which was even used later on to induce a second generation of mice with the experimental model (52). Furthermore, the nucleotide sequence of some of the Abs-3 anti-DNA antibodies resembled the sequence of Ab-1 used for the first immunization (E. Mozes, personal communication). I would like to stress that the mice were not immunized with DNA, and we were dealing with completely healthy strains of mice that are not prone to autoimmunity (39–45,49,50). The latter experiment with cANCA teaches us much with regard to the necessity for an autoantigen in the induction of the autoimmune disease. Mice leucocytes (WBC) do not contain Pr-3r (A Wiik, personal communication). To confirm the production of anti-Pr-3 by the immunized BALB/c mice we had to use either human leucocytes or purified Pr-3 from human leucocytes as a substrate. When immunized with cANCA the mice developed sterile microabscesses, arteriolitis, granulomas, kidney involvement associated with mouse cANCA and anti-endothelial cell antibodies. Thus, we induced Wegener's granulomatosis (WG) in mice that do not have Pr-3. Furthermore, on some occasions the induction of the respective autoimmune condition was performed with autoantibodies derived from healthy subjects (e.g. natural autoantibodies). All these arguments are supported by several observations, suggesting the possibility that some autoimmune diseases may arise, not by autoantigen stimulation, but by some defects or destruction of natural serum inhibitors suppressing the effect of natural autoantibodies (53,54). Another possibility recently suggested is that some cross-reactive idiotypes are B-cell superantigens (55,56).

CONCLUSION

Thus, it seems conceivable, despite extensive and elaborate studies, that in several 'autoimmune diseases' in which the role of the presumed autoantigen was not clarified, we should abandon the idea that the autoantigen used for the detection of diagnostic autoantibodies is the inducing agent (immunogen) of the disease. This is especially true with SLE and DNA, but probably also holds true for Wegener's granulomatosis and Pr-3, primary biliary cirrhosis and the ubiquitous enzyme pyruvate dehydrogenase, as well as in the series of other autoimmune rheumatic diseases with *intracellular autoantigens*.

If this is so, how do we envisage that such autoimmune diseases are induced in patients? In the three experiments detailed above we have induced three autoimmune conditions – SLE, anti-phospholipid syndrome, and WG – following immunization in the footpads of naive healthy mice with the specific autoantibody emulsified in Freund's adjuvant. In all cases, the mice developed the disease-specific autoantibody (Ab_3 = anti-anti-autoantibody). We are aware that this experimental induction is dependent on the presence of adjuvant and intracutaneous (intrapedal) injection. We postulate that the 'natural' analogue of our experimental models resides in the induction of antibacterial antibodies carrying 'pathogenic' idiotypes in patients following infections. Indeed, we have already reported previously on the presence of increased titres of the 16/6 Id, a pathogenic idiotype of anti-DNA antibodies (summarized in 57), in the sera of patients infected with *Mycobacteria* (pulmonary tuberculosis) (58) and *Klebsiella* (pneumonia and urinary tract infections) and other Gram-negative bacterial infections (59,60). We recently summarized this relationship between infection and autoimmunity (61). Thus, it is conceivable that infection may trigger autoimmune diseases by inducing antibacterial antibodies carrying the pathogenic idiotypes of autoantibodies (Ab_1). In the presence of the adjuvant effect (or superantigen?) contributed by the various bacteria themselves, these antibodies (Ab_1) may initiate – in a subject with the 'proper' HLA and hormonal background (1,2) – the cascade of idiotypic dysregulation demonstrated by us in the experimental models, leading eventually to the generation of Ab_3, which may either by itself or via regulation lead to the overt clinical autoimmune condition. Our results support Cohen's 'immunological homunculus' (47,48) suggesting that even though any Ab_3 may be generated, we are aware of some selection that is responsible for the limited number of autoimmune diseases encountered in nature. Recently Pascual and Capra (55,56) raised the possibility that some cross-reactive idiotypes (e.g. 9G4) and specifically cold agglutinins utilizing the VH h-21 gene segments may react as B cell superantigens leading to upregulation of many B cells. Interestingly enough our 16/6 Id was sequenced recently, and found to be encoded by VH 4-21 (A. Weisman, Y. Shoenfeld, M. Blank, E. Mozes, submitted).

In many cases the disease emerges many months (or years) following the infection and, therefore, the relationship to the infection is remote. According to this theory, there is a group of autoimmune diseases in which, although there is a specific autoantibody and autoantigen(s), the autoantigen and/or the autoantibody are not necessarily directly implicated in the tissue damage. Thus, we do not have to explain how anti-DNA antibodies induce pleuritis or cognitive impairment, or how anti-cardiolipin leads to migraine and livedo reticularis, or how anti-proteinase-3 antibody causes glomerular lesion. Furthermore, we do not need to show the presence of *intracellular* autoantigens on the *surface* of some target cells as a prerequisite for pathogenicity of the respective autoantibody. The lesions in this group of diseases may be induced either by external antigen, or by some disequilibrium in the idiotypic network.

REFERENCES

1. Shoenfeld, Y. and D. A. Isenberg. 1989. *Immunol. Today* **10**:123–6.
2. Shoenfeld, Y. and D. A. Isenberg. 1988. The mosaic of autoimmunity. In: *The Factors Associated with Autoimmune Diseases*. Elsevier, Amsterdam, pp. 1–588.
3. Weiss, P. and Y. Shoenfeld. 1991. *Isr. J. Med. Sci.* **27**:216–17.
4. Alarcon-Segovia, D., R. F. Galbaith and J. E. Maldonado. 1963. *Lancet* **2**:662–5.
5. Calabreste, L. H., J. F. Bach and J. Cumie. 1981. *Arch. Int. Med.* **141**: 253–5.

6. Levene, N. A., D. Varon, N. Shtalrid and A. Berberi. 1991. *Isr. J. Med. Sci.* **27**:199–201.
7. Shoenfeld, Y., D. A. Isenberg, J. Rauch *et al.* 1983. *J. Exp. Med.* **158**:718–30.
8. Miescher, P. and R. Straassle. 1957. *Vox. Sang.* **2**:283–9.
9. Ceppellini, R., E. Polli and F. Celada. 1957. *Proc. Soc. Exp. Biol. Med.* **96**:572–81.
10. Robbins, W. C., H. R. Holman, H. Deicher *et al.* 1957. *Proc. Soc. Exp. Biol. Med.* **96**:575–83.
11. Seligmann, M. 1957. *C. R. Acad. Sci. Paris* **245**:243–56.
12. Buskila, D. and Y. Shoenfeld. 1992. Anti-DNA antibodies. Chapter 9 in: *Systemic Lupus Erythematosus*, 2nd edn. (R. G. Lahita, ed.). Churchill Livingstone, New York, pp. 205–36.
13. Plescia, O. J., W. Braun and N. C. Palczuk. 1964. *Proc. Natl. Acad. Sci. USA* **52**:279–83.
14. Stollar, B. D. 1992. *Prog. Nucl. Acid. Res. Mol. Biol.* **42**:39–77.
15. Gilkeson, G. S., J. P. Grudier, D. G. Karounos and D. S. Pisetsky. 1989. *J. Immunol.* **142**:1482–6.
16. Fredriksen, K., T. Traavik and O. P. Rekvig. 1990. *Scand. J. Immunol.* **32**:197–203.
17. Desai, D. D., R. M. Krishnan, J. T. Swindle and T. N. Marion. 1993. *J. Immunol.* **151**:1614–26.
18. Edberg, J. C., L. Tosic and R. P. Taylor. 1985. *Clin. Immunol. Immunopathol.* **51**:118–32.
19. Gavalchin, J. and S. K. Datta. 1987. *J. Immunol.* **138**:138–45.
20. Vlahakos, D. V., M. H. Foster, S. Adams *et al.* 1992. *Kidney Int.* **41**:1690–6.
21. Tsao, B. P., F. M. Ebling, C. Roman *et al.* 1990. *J. Clin. Invest.* **85**:530–8.
22. Faaber, P., P. J. A. Capel, G. P. M. Rijke *et al.* 1984. *Clin. Exp. Immunol.* **55**:502–8.
23. Berden, J. H. M., R. M. Termaat, K. Brinkman *et al.* 1982. *Neurologie* **10**:127–32.
24. Shoenfeld, Y., S. C. Hsu-Lin, J. E. Gabriel *et al.* 1982. *J. Clin. Invest.* **70**:205–8.
25. Shoenfeld, Y., J. Rauch, H. Massicotte *et al.* 1983. *New Engl. J. Med.* **308**:414–20.
26. Stollar, D., L. Levine and J. Marmur. 1962. *Biochim. Biophys. Acta* **61**:7–18.
27. Alarcon Segovia, D., A. Ruiz-Arguella and L. Lorente. 1979. *J. Immunol.* **122**:1855–62.
28. Vlahakos, D. V., M. H. Foster, A. A. Ucci *et al.* 1992. *J. Am. Soc. Nephrol.* **2**:1345–54.
29. Neu, N., K. Hala, H. Dietrich and G. Wick. 1985. *Clin. Immunol. Immunopathol.* **37**:397–405.
30. Wick, G., J. Most, K. Schauenstein *et al.* 1985. *Immunol. Today* **6**:359–64.
31. Naparstek, Y., A. Ben-Yehuda, M. P. Madaio *et al.* 1990. *Arthritis Rheum.* **33**:1554–61.
32. Mohan, C., S. Adams, V. Stanik and S. K. Datta. 1993. *J. Exp. Med.* **177**:1367–81.
33. Termat, R. M., K. Brinkman, E. Van. Gomple *et al.* 1990. *J. Autoimmun.* **3**:531–7.
34. Foster, M. H., J. Sabbage, S. R. Line *et al.* 1993. *J. Immunol.* **151**:814–24.
35. Uner, A. H., C. J. Knupp, A. H. Tatum and J. Gavalchin. 1994. *J. Autoimmun.* **7**:27–44.

36. Gavalchin, J., J. A. Nicklas, J. W. Eastcott *et al.* 1985. *J. Immunol.* **134**:885–94.
37. Uner, A. H., C. J. Knupp, A. H. Tatum and J. Gavalchin. 1994. *J. Autoimmun.* **7**:27–44.
38. Grabar, P. 1983. *Immunol. Today* **4**:337–40.
39. Mendlovic, S., S. Brocke, Y. Shoenfeld *et al.* 1988. *Proc. Natl. Acad. Sci. USA* **85**:2260–4.
40. Blank, M., S. Mendlovic, E. Mozes and Y. Shoenfeld. 1988. *J. Autoimmun.* **1**:683–91.
41. Mendlovic, S., H. Fricke, Y. Shoenfeld and E. Mozes. 1989. *Eur. J. Immunol.* **19**:729–34.
42. Shoenfeld, Y. 1989. *Curr. Opin. Rheumatol.* **1**:360–8.
43. Mozes, E., S. Brocke, Y. Shoenfeld and S. Mendlovic. 1989. *J. Cell. Biochem.* **40**:173–81.
44. Blank, M., M. Krup, S. Mendlovic *et al.* 1990. *Scand. J. Immunol.* **31**:45–52.
45. Mendlovic, S., S. Brocke, H. Fricke *et al.* 1990. *Immunology* **69**:228–36.
46. Mozes, E., L. D. Kohn, F. Hakim and D. S. Singer. 1993. *Science* **261**:91–3.
47. Cohen, J. R. 1992. *Immunol. Today* **13**:441–6.
48. Cohen, J. R. 1992. *Immunol. Today* **13**:490–4.
49. Bakimer, R., P. Fishman, M. Blank. 1992. *J. Clin. Invest.* **89**:1558–663.
50. Blank, M., A. Tincani and Y. Shoenfeld. 1994. *J. Rheumatol.* **21**:100–4.
51. Blank, M., Y. Tomer, M. Stein *et al.* 1995. *Clin. Exp. Immunol.* **102**:120–30.
52. Blank, M., I. Krause, M. Ben-Bassat, Y. Shoenfeld. 1992. *J. Autoimmunit.* **5**:495–509.
53. Kra-Oz, I., M. Lorber and Y. Shoenfeld. 1993. *Clin. Exp. Immunol.* **93**:265–8.
54. Cheng, H. M. 1991. *Immunol. Today* **12**:96–8.
55. Pascual, V. and J. D. Capra. 1991. *Curr. Biol.* **1**:315–17.
56. Cross-reactive idiotope and B-cell superantigens. 1994. *Clin. Immunol.* **10**:6–13.
57. Shoenfeld, Y. and E. Mozes. 1990. *FASEB J.* **4**:2646–51.
58. Sela, O., A. El-Roeiy, D. A. Isenberg *et al.* 1987. *Arthritis Rheumat.* **30**:50–5.
59. El-Roeiy, A., O. Sela, D. A. Isenberg, R. L. Kennedy and Y. Shoenfeld. 1987. *Clin. Exp. Immunol.* **67**:507–15.
60. Shoenfeld, Y. and I. R. Cohen. 1987. Infection and autoimmunity. In: *The Antigens* (M. Sela, ed.) Boca Raton, FL, Academic Press, pp. 307–25.
61. Abu-Shakra, M. and Y. Shoenfeld. 1991. *Autoimmunity* **9**:337–44.

13

Pathophysiology of Th1 and Th2 Responses in Humans

Ljiljana Tomašević, Enrico Maggi and Sergio Romagnani

The protective value of immune responses depends on the pattern of cytokines produced by T cells involved. In 1986 two distinct subsets of murine $CD4^+$ Th cell clones showing different patterns of cytokine production and effector functions were identified (1). Th1 cells secrete interleukin (IL)-2, tumour necrosis factor (TNF)β and interferon (IFN)γ and are the principal effector of cell-mediated immunity against intracellular microbes and of delayed-type hypersensitivity reactions. Murine Th1 cells can also stimulate production of antibodies of the IgG2a class which are effective at activating complement and opsonizing antigens for phagocytosis. Th2 cells produce IL-4, which stimulates IgE and IgG1 antibody production, and IL-5, IL-10 and IL-13, which together with IL-4 inhibit macrophage functions. Th1 cells trigger phagocyte-mediated host defence, and infections with intracellular microbes tend to induce Th1-type responses, whereas the Th2 subset is mainly involved in phagocyte-independent host defence which is mediated by IgE and eosinophils (2). In the absence of polarizing signals, $CD4^+$ Th cell subsets with a less differentiated cytokine profile than Th1 or Th2 cells, designated Th0, usually arise (3).

For about 5 years such a dichotomic and cross-regulatory system was not found in humans. Then, we and others generated clones specific for particular antigens or derived them from patients who had various diseases; most $CD4^+$ Th cell clones specific for helminth antigens (namely secretory/excretory antigens from the nematode *Toxocara canis*) or for allergens exhibited a Th2 profile of cytokine secretion, whereas the great majority of Th cell clones specific for the endocellular pathogens (such as purified protein derivative PPD from *Mycobacterium tuberculosis* or streptokinase) derived from the same donors showed a Th1 profile (4,5). As we will describe later, accumulation of Th1 cells has been found in target organs in Basedow's disease, Crohn's disease, ulcerative cholitis, chronic hepatitis, Sjögren's syndrome, rheumathoid arthritis and nickel dermatitis. Th2 cells are

Immunoregulation in Health and Disease
ISBN 0-12-459460-3

mainly present in Omenn's syndrome, measles infection, systemic lupus erythematosus, helminth infestations, HIV infection and phologistic infiltrates of allergic diseases (6).

Thus, although in humans the expression of some cytokines, such as IL-2, IL-6, IL-10 and IL-13, appears to be less restricted (7,8), there is now general consensus for the existence of human $CD4^+$ Th cells with cytokine patterns and functions that are comparable to murine Th1 and Th2 cells. However, it is important to remember that the Th cell-mediated effector response is much more complex than Th1 and Th2, which have to be considered as two polarized forms of functional T cells due to chronic antigenic stimulation. Accordingly, we can hypothesize that they probably play a pathogenetic role mainly in the chronic inflammatory diseases.

FUNCTIONAL ACTIVITIES OF HUMAN Th1 AND Th2 CELLS

Human Th1 and Th2 cells differ in their responsiveness to exogenous cytokines. Both Th1 and Th2 cells proliferate in response to IL-2, but Th2 are much more responsive to IL-4 than Th1 (9). IFNγ plays a selective inhibitory effect on the proliferative response of Th2 cells (9). Human Th1 and Th2 cells were found to differ in their cytolytic potential and helper function for B cell antibody synthesis. Th2 cells, which usually have no cytolytic potential, induced IgM, IgG, IgA, and IgE synthesis by autologous B cells in the presence of the specific antigen in a dose–response fashion proportional to the T/B cell ratio (10). In contrast, Th1 clones, which are cytolytic, provided B-cell help for IgM, IgG, and IgA (but not IgE) synthesis, but their helper activity is inversely related to the T/B cell ratio of the culture; in other words they exert a strong cytolytic activity against autologous antigen-presenting B-cell targets (10). This probably represents an important down-regulatory mechanism of antibody responses in vivo (11). Finally, these functional subsets also differ for their activity on cells of monocyte/macrophage lineages. Th1, but not Th2, clones induced both procoagulant activity by monocytes and their synthesis of tissue factor (TF), by acting through both physical cell–cell interaction and release of soluble mediators (12). The induction of TF production by monocytes appears to be, at least partially, mediated by IFNγ released by Th1 clones, whereas both Th2-type cytokines (mainly IL-4 and IL-10) exert inhibitory effect on Th1-induced TF production (12).

Th1- AND Th2-ASSOCIATED MOLECULES

In the last few years, the possibility that the Th1 or Th2 pattern of cytokine production could be associated with the expression of peculiar membrane molecules has also been extensively investigated. Among possible candidates, we considered CD30, a member of the tumour necrosis factor (TNF)/nerve growth factor (NGF) receptor superfamily (13,14). CD30 was described as a surface molecule recognized by the Ki-1 monoclonal antibody (mAb) on Hodgkin's and Reed–Sternberg (H-RS) cells of Hodgkin's disease (HD) (15) and in the neoplastic cells of certain types of non-Hodgkin's lymphomas, such as $CD30^+$ anaplastic large cell lymphoma (ALCL), angioimmunoblastic-like lymphoma, and human T-cell lymphotropic virus (HTLV)-1^+ adult T-cell-leukaemia/lymphoma (ATLL) (16). In healthy people there are no $CD30^+$ cells in the blood. In vitro, CD30 antigen expression is inducible on lectin-stimulated blood T- and B-cell blasts, on virally (HTLV-1/2, Epstein–Barr virus) transformed T and B cells (17,18). When we analyse the molecule on established T cell clones, Th1 clones resulted negative, whereas CD30 was strongly expressed by most T-cell blasts from all Th2 clones; noticeable proportions of T-cell blasts from the majority of Th0 clones also showed expression of membrane CD30 (19). Analysis of CD30 mRNA expression by some T-cell clones and measurement of soluble CD30 (sCD30) in their supernatants confirmed the preferential association between CD30 expression/sCD30 release and production of Th2-type cytokines (19). The kinetics of CD30 expression by T cells activated in vitro with the allergens or helminth antigens suggests a temporal relationship between the expression of CD30 antigen and beginning of Th2-type cytokine production (19).

The preferential association in T cells between the expression of CD30 antigen and the production of Th2-type cytokines is also observed in $CD8^+$ T-cell clones. Indeed, the great majority of $CD8^+$ T-cells, which usually exhibit a Th1-like cytokine profile, did not express membrane CD30 (20). However, a few $CD8^+$ clones able to produce IL-4 and IL-5 in addition to IFNγ, which could be generated from healthy donors, were $CD30^+$ (20). Furthermore, high numbers of $CD8^+$ clones exhibiting a Th2-like profile of cytokine secretion, which were generated from the peripheral blood or the skin of patients with the acquired immune deficiency syndrome (21), showed expression of membrane CD30 and released detectable amounts of sCD30 in the supernatants (20).

On the whole, these data strongly support the concept that CD30 is preferentially expressed on, and sCD30 released by, cells (both $CD4^+$ and $CD8^+$) producing IL-4 and IL-5. This finding may have potential importance in detecting pathophysiological conditions characterized by CD30 overexpression in lymphoid tissues and/or by enhanced levels of sCD30 in biological fluids. It is important also to establish whether CD30 may represent a marker for the detection of Th2-type responses occurring in vivo. Besides the CD30 expression by H-RS cells in Hodgkin's lymphoma, in anaplastic large cell lymphoma and occasionally in other non-Hodgkin's lymphomas (15,16), several $CD30^+$ activated T cells were observed in lymph node involved by infectious mononucleosis. In normal lymphoid tissue CD30 is detectable only on a small population of large mononuclear cells with evident nucleolus, mainly grouped around B-cell follicles, and to a minor degree, at the edge of germinal centres (22). There are no extra-lymphohaemopoietic CD30-expressing cells in human body, with the exception of exocrine pancreatic cells and decidual cells (23). We know that Th2-type responses against common environmental allergens play a critical triggering role in the pathogenesis of atopic disorders (24). We have therefore looked at the presence of $CD30^+$ circulating T cells in atopic patients. Virtually no $CD4^+CD30^+$ cells were detected in the blood of grass-sensitive atopic donors examined before the grass pollination season; however, the majority of grass-sensitive subjects examined during the season showed small numbers of $CD4^+CD30^+$ cells in their circulation (from 0.08 to 0.3%) (19). If circulating $CD4^+$ T cells were fractionated into $CD30^+$ and $CD30^-$ cells and expanded in IL-2, only $CD4^+CD30^+$ cells proliferated in response to Lol p 1 and exhibited the ability to produce IL-4 and IL-5 (production of both IFNγ and TNFβ was predominant in $CD30^-$ cells) (19), thus suggesting that $CD4^+CD30^+$ Th2-like cells can circulate in the peripheral blood of sensitive patients only during in vivo exposure to grass pollen allergens. The definitive proof that, even in vivo, $CD30^+$ cells are associated with Th2 responses, was provided by results obtained on the Omenn's syndrome, a rare congenital immunodeficiency disorder due to abnormal Th2-like cells. High proportions of $CD30^+$ T cells (>10%) were observed in the lymph node and PBL from children with Omenn's syndrome and T cell clones established from them exhibited a Th2-type profile (25). More recent data also provide evidence that sCD30 is elevated in the sera of patients with atopic dermatitis and systemic sclerosis and that several $CD30^+CD4^+$ IL-4-producing cells are infiltrating lesional skin (Del Prete *et al.* personal communication, Mavilia *et al.* personal communication).

A molecule which can be considered associated to IFNγ-producing T cells is the antigen encoded by the lymphocyte activation gene (*LAG*)-3, a member of the immunoglobulin superfamily, that was found in human activated $CD4^+$, $CD8^+$ and NK cells (26). The compared exon/intron organization and the chromosomal localization display that LAG-3 is closely related to CD4 (26). Even though LAG-3 and CD4 share the same ligand, i.e. MHC class II molecules (26), however, LAG-3 does not bind the human immunodeficiency virus gp120 (26). In vivo, LAG-3 expression was found neither in primary nor in secondary lymphoid organs. However, it was readily detected in inflamed tonsils, or lymph nodes with follicular hyperplasia, thus proving that even in vivo LAG-3 is expressed following activation (27). The physiological role of encoded LAG-3 protein is still unclear: antigen-specific stimulation of T-cell clones in the presence of anti-LAG-3 monoclonal antibody (mAb) led to increased thymidine incorporation, higher expression of activation marker CD25 and enhanced cytokine production (28). Accordingly, addition of a soluble recombinant form of LAG-3 inhibited antigen-specific T-cell proliferation suggesting a regulatory role of LAG-3 in $CD4^+$

T-lymphocyte activation (29). Studies of human $CD4^+$ T cell clones have shown that expression of LAG-3, like CD30, was preferentially related to one or another phenotype of cytokine secretion. Results demonstrate that LAG-3 correlated with IFNγ, but not IL-4, production in antigen-stimulated T cells and it was up-regulated by IL-12 addition in bulk culture. Moreover, most Th1 and Th0 clones expressed membrane LAG-3 and released detectable amounts of soluble LAG-3, whereas only a few Th2 clones showed LAG-3 expression and release (30).

MECHANISMS INVOLVED IN THE REGULATION OF Th DEVELOPMENT

Even though it was suggested that Th1 and Th2 cells might arise from distinct precursors, experiments with homogeneous populations of cells from T-cell receptor (TCR) transgenic mice support the concept that a single precursor can differentiate into either a Th1 or a Th2 phenotype (31). Reiner and colleagues (32) show that T cells from mice infected with *Leishmania major* express a restricted TCR repertoire in both progressive infection and protective immunity, regardless of histocompatibility haplotypes, further supporting this possibility. Naive Th precursor (Thp) cells mainly produce IL-2 and progress into early-memory Th0 effector cells following a first activation by the specific antigen (33); these cells would then terminally differentiate into Th1 or Th2 cells upon repeated antigen stimulations (34). However, the mechanisms responsible for the differentiation of naive Th cells into the Th1 or Th2 phenotype have not yet been completely clarified. Besides the genetic background, attention has been focused on the possible role of type of antigen-presenting cells (APC), nature of antigenic determinants, T cell repertoire and soluble factors present in the microenvironment at the time of allergen presentation.

Genetic factors influencing Th differentiation

Very little information is at present available on the genetic factors influencing Th1/Th2 differentiation. Some new data concern mainly genetic mechanisms in atopic diseases, where, traditionally, the immunogenetic of high IgE response can be divided into antigen-specific and non-antigen-specific ones (35). The former is strongly influenced by HLA-D-encoded, major histocompatibility complex (MHC) class II genes and involves cognate T–B cell interaction. The latter, non-cognate regulation of IgE, could involve primarily mast cells, basophils, and possibly other FcεRI+ cells, and obviously Th2 cells (35). Recent evidence for a linkage of overall IgE to markers in chromosome 5q31.1, especially to the IL-4 gene, has been provided (36), suggesting that one or more polymorphisms exist in a coding region or, more probably, a regulatory region of the IL-4 gene. Transcription of IL-4 gene is stringently regulated by multiple promoter elements acting together (36,37). Other genes map within 5q31.1, including several other candidates which might influence IgE production such as IL-13, IRF1 (whose gene product up-regulates IFNα) (37) and IL-12B (which encodes the β chain of IL-12, a cytokine down-regulating Th2 development) (37,38). Thus, alterations of molecular mechanisms directly involved in the regulation of IL-4 gene expression, as well as deficient regulatory activity of cytokines responsible for inhibition of Th2-cell development (such as IFNα and IL-12), or both, may account for the preferential Th2-type response towards environmental allergens in atopic people (38,39).

APC, antigen and T-cell repertoire triad

As far as the APC is concerned, very little is known on the monocyte/macrophage potential to respond to different antigens, in terms of expression of costimulatory molecules and production of soluble cytokines.

Langerhans' cells (LC) in the skin, as well as dendritic cells (DC) localized in the respiratory tract, represent the primary contact site between the immune system and allergens. These cells carry allergen to regional lymph nodes where allergen presentation to specific CD4$^+$ T cells occurs. Some data suggest that asthmatic patients have higher numbers of intraepithelial DC than non-asthmatic subjects and that these cells in the presence of allergen molecules can induce T cell activation and release of IL-4 and IL-5 (40). However, the role played by professional APC in driving the development of allergen-reactive Th2-like cells remains to be elucidated. Recent studies have also shown that costimulatory signals (from APC to T cells) can modulate the Th1/Th2 differentiation; CD80–CD28 and CD86–CD28 interactions, for instance, seem to induce a Th1 and Th2 switch, respectively (41). Finally, CD30–CD30L interaction plays an important role in the differentiation of Th2 cells. In fact, costimulation of PBMC with the anti-CD30 mAb with agonistic activity synergized with the soluble antigen in inducing proliferative response and cytokine production by Th0/Th2 TCC, but not by Th1 cells. Moreover, anti-CD30 agonistic antibody (which mimics the CD30L/CD30 interaction) resulted in the preferential development of antigen-specific cell lines and clones showing the Th2-like profile of cytokine secretion. Conversely, early blockade in bulk culture of CD30 ligand (CD30L)/CD30 interaction shifted the development of antigen-specific T cells towards the opposite (Th1-type) phenotype (42).

The role of T cell repertoire in determining the development of Th1 or Th2-type responses is controversial. In mice infected with *Leishmania major* both Th1 and Th2 cells possessing the same repertoire and recognizing the same peptide have been demonstrated, suggesting that cells with identical T-cell receptor (TCR) can differentiate into either the Th1 or the Th2 phenotype (32). However, evidence for an important role of specific Vβ-expressing T cell subsets in the stimulation of IgE production and increased airways responsiveness induced by ragweed allergen has been reported (43). Thus, it cannot be excluded that the recognition of allergen by the TCR provides a signal or sets of signals that drive T cells to a defined direction, e.g. to produce IL-4 or, alternatively, IFNγ.

As far as the role of antigen is concerned, large panels of T cell clones have recently been generated from donors with low or high serum IgE levels specific for two non-apeptides (p92 and p96). Both p92- and p96-specific T-cell clones generated from 'high IgE' donors produced remarkable amounts of IL-4 and low IFNγ. In contrast, T-cell clones generated from 'low IgE' donors showed a clear-cut difference in their profile of cytokine production: the majority of those specific for p96 produced high amounts of both IL-4 and IFNγ, whereas most p92-specific T cell clones showed a Th1-like profile of cytokine production (high IFNγ and low IL-4) (Parronchi *et al.* personal communication). These data suggest that the nature and/or the intensity of TCR signalling provided by the allergen peptide ligand can influence the cytokine profile of Th cells. However, the data clearly indicate that altered regulation of IL-4 production is overwhelming the influence exerted by the allergen peptide ligand. With regard to the possibility that modulation of IL-4 production can be due to altered down-regulatory mechanisms, recent experiments suggest a possible role of allergen-specific $CD8^+$ T cells in controlling the Th response against allergens not only in experimental animals, but also in humans. First, the peptide 92 (see above) expanded higher numbers of $CD8^+$ cell clones in 'low' than in 'high' IgE producers. In addition, lactalbumin expanded higher numbers of $CD8^+$ T cell clones in non-atopic than in atopic milk-sensitive donors, suggesting that in non-atopic people allergen-specific $CD8^+$ T cells may play an important role (via IFNγ production?) in preventing the differentiation of $CD4^+$ Th cells to the same allergen towards the Th2 pathway (Parronchi unpublished).

Microenvironmental hormones

The presence in the microenvironment of hormones can promote the differentiation of Th cells: glucocorticoids enhance Th2 activity, and synergize with IL-4, whereas dehydroepiandrostenon sulfate enhances Th1 activity (44). Another major prohormone, 25-hydroxycholecalciferol (25-OH vitamin D_3) may have a reverse effect on the Th1/Th2 balance (45). More importantly, calcitriol analogues can rival cyclosporin A in its ability to prolong survival of skin grafts by inhibiting Th1 activity (45). Progesterone favours the in vitro development of human Th cells producing Th2-type cytokines and promotes both IL-4 production and membrane CD30 expression in established human Th1 clones (45). Conversely, relaxin, which is a hormone increased during pregnancy, has been seen to favour IFNγ and TNFβ production in Th2 clones (Piccinni, personal communication). The imbalance of these hormones may represent one of the mechanisms involved in the Th1/Th2 switch which has been hypothesized to occur at the maternal–fetal interface in order to improve fetal survival and promote successful pregnancy (46).

Microenvironmental cytokines

Attention has recently been focused on the possibility that the type of Th response is depending upon the factors produced by antigen-presenting cells (APC) or by other cell types during antigen exposure, in determining the development of the specific Th1 or Th2 response.

The factors that regulate the development of human Th1 and Th2 clones have extensively been investigated in our laboratory by using peripheral blood lymphocytes cultured with bacterial antigens and allergens in the presence or in the absence of exogenous cytokines or anti-cytokine antibody.

Soluble signals favouring the Th2 development

The effect of cytokines produced by macrophages and/or B cells on the development of Th2 cells seems to be less critical than for Th1 cells. IL-10 has been shown to favour the development of Th2 cells in both mouse and humans (31). IL-1 is a selective cofactor for the growth of some murine Th2 clones (47) and can favour the in vitro development of human Th2-like clones (48). However, in both murine and human systems, IL-4 appears to be the most dominant factor in determining the likelihood for Th2 polarization in cultured cells (37,49–52). Recently we have looked at both the cytokine profile of CD8$^+$ human T-cell clones and the mechanisms involved in their development. While the majority of CD8$^+$ T-cell clones derived from the peripheral blood of normal individuals showed the same cytokine profile as Th1-type CD4$^+$ T-cell clones, several CD8$^+$ T-cell clones exhibiting a Th0 profile, or even a clear-cut Th2 profile, could be derived from peripheral blood of patients with severe atopy, Kaposi's sarcoma skin lesions or unharmed skin of HIV-infected patients, and skin lesions of patients with lepromatous lepra. Furthermore, also for CD8$^+$ T cells IL-4 addition in bulk culture before cloning favours high proportions of CD8$^+$ T cells to shift from the Th1- to the Th0/Th2-like phenotype (Maggi *et al.* unpublished). Accordingly, IL-4-K.O. mice fail to generate mature Th2 cells in vivo and to produce IgE antibodies (53), suggesting that early IL-4 production by another cell type must be involved. Possible candidates include a still uncharacterized T cell subset (54), a double negative (CD4$^-$ CD8$^-$) $\alpha\beta$TCR early thymic circulating T-cell subset (55), as well as mast cells and basophils, releasing stored IL-4 in response to FcεR triggering (56–58). Since helminth antigens or allergens are unable to crosslink these receptors prior to a specific immune response eliciting specific IgG and IgE antibodies, and mast-cell-deficient mice develop normal Th2 responses (59), IL-4 production by mast cells may play a role only in amplifying secondary responses, not in inducing the Th2 development in primary immune responses. An alternative explanation is that some proteolytic enzymes, which are produced in large quantity by many helminth parasites, trigger mast cells to release IL-4 and other cytokines that induce a Th2 differentiation in the primary response. In fact some environmental allergens are proteases and the injection of papain into BALB/c mice resulted in 10–30-fold increases in IL-4 and IL-5 but not IFNγ or IL-2 in draining lymph nodes (60). However, allergens induce Th2-type responses only in selected people, and this suggests that atopic individuals would have genetic dysregulation in the production of IL-4 and/or of cytokines exerting regulatory effects on the development and/or function of Th2 cells (61).

Signals for the development of Th1-like response

The clearest examples of factors affecting the differentiation pathways of both murine and human Th1 cells appear to be cytokines released by APC and/or other cell types at the time of antigen presentation (6,62). Thus, IFNα, IL-12 and TGFβ produced by macrophages and B cells particularly in response to intracellular bacteria have been shown to play an important role in the induction of Th1 expansion in various systems (6,38).

In contrast, anti-IL-12 antibody favoured the differentiation of PPD-specific T cells into Th0 or Th2, instead of Th1, clones (6,38). The addition in bulk culture of IFNα and IFNγ not only favoured the development of allergen-specific T-cell clones showing both Th0/Th1 profile but also elicited a cytolytic activity (52). These data suggest that the development of $CD4^+$ T-cell clones with a given profile of cytokine production and the expression of cytolytic activity are similarly regulated. Besides the effects on the cytokine pattern and cytolytic activity, exogenous IFNα is able to modulate selectively the epitope specificity of T cells. Indeed, the study of fine specificity of Poa p 9-specific TCC derived in presence of IFNα suggests that it promoted a selective expansion of TCC specific for a single peptide (peptide 26) of the allergen molecule. Although a substantial proportion of both TCC generated in the presence or absence of IFNα expressed the Vβ2 element, IFNα favoured the expansion of Vβ2, Vβ17 and Vβ22 positive Poa p 9-specific T cells. These data clearly suggest that IFNα can both shift the cytokine profile of Vβ2 positive T cells and restrict their response to only one peptide. At present, the mechanisms by which IFNα can modulate the epitope specificity of allergen-specific T cells are unclear, but we favour the possibility that IFNα influences antigen presentation and/or processing by the APC (62). IFNα and

IL-12 are produced predominantly by macrophages, cells that have an important role in the presentation of antigen to Th cells.

Interestingly, allergen-specific T cell lines, grown in the presence of IFNα, of poly I:C (a synthetic double-stranded RNA contained in different viruses), or of influenza virus, contained significantly higher proportions of both CD3$^+$ CD8$^+$ and CD3$^-$ CD16$^+$ cells than T-cell lines grown in the presence of allergen alone. Moreover, the removal of either CD8$^+$ or CD16$^+$ cells from PBL populations reduced the capacity of poly I:C to shift the differentiation of allergen-specific T cells from the Th2 to the Th0 or Th1 profile. Finally, and more importantly, we recently demonstrated that poly I:C induces the production of IFNα and IL-12 directly by macrophages (63). Taken together, these data suggest that intracellular bacteria and viruses induce specific immune responses of Th1 type at least partly because they either directly stimulate CD8$^+$ T cells and NK cells to produce IFNγ, or because they induce macrophage production of IFNα and IL-12 which, in turn, stimulate NK cell growth and IFNγ production. However, the production of high concentrations of IFNγ by NK cells, although important, does not appear to be sufficient for the induction of Th1 responses. Indeed, the addition of anti-IFNγ antibody to bulk cultures does not prevent or reverse the inhibitory effect of poly I:C on the differentiation of allergen-specific T cells into Th2 clones. Likewise, blocking of IFNα or IL-12 alone with specific antibodies was ineffective. In contrast, the poly I:C-induced Th0 or Th1 differentiation of allergen-specific T cells could be driven to the Th2 profile by the simultaneous addition of IL-4 plus antibodies reactive with IFNγ, IFNα and IL-12 (6,63). Thus, it is possible that poly I:C interferes with IL-4 production by T cells. It can be concluded, therefore, that viruses and intracellular bacteria induce Th1 responses because the profile of the 'natural' immune response they evoke provides optimum conditions (high concentrations of IFNγ and absence of IL-4) for the development of Th1 cells.

Taken together, these findings support the notion that the cytokine profiles of memory CD4$^+$ cells are mutable, and are not fixed as had been suggested by previous studies of murine CD4$^+$ memory T cells. Therefore, it is likely that the results obtained in the human in vitro models reflect not only a selection process but, at least in part, even the shifting of a common memory CD4$^+$ T cell to one or another phenotype.

ROLE OF Th1 AND Th2 CELLS IN THE PATHOGENESIS OF HUMAN DISEASES: PERSPECTIVES FOR NEW THERAPEUTIC STRATEGIES

The two polarized forms of Th1 and Th2 responses are of great importance not only for the mechanisms of protection against exogenous offending agents, but also for the knowledge of the pathogenetic mechanisms of several human diseases. Several pathophysiological conditions have indeed been suspected to be the result of dominant Th1- and Th2-type responses. $CD4^+$ Th cells infiltrating the conjunctiva in patients with vernal conjunctivitis (64), as well as allergen-specific cells derived from the bronchial mucosa of patients with allergic asthma (65) prevalently showed a Th2 profile. In contrast, virtually all $CD4^+$ T cells derived from the thyroid gland cell infiltrates of patients with Hashimoto's thyroiditis had a clear-cut Th1 functional phenotype (6). Other laboratories derived Th2-like clones from the peripheral blood or the skin of patients with atopic dermatitis (66), as well as from the skin of patients with lepromatous (susceptible) leprosy (67). Th1-type cells appeared to predominate in the skin of patients with contact dermatitis (68) or tuberculoid (resistant) leprosy (67), as well as in the CSF of patients with multiple sclerosis (69) and in the synovial fluid of patients with Lyme's arthritis or reactive arthritis (70,71). By in situ hybridization, cells expressing mRNA for IL-4 and IL-5, but not for IL-2 and IFNγ, were found in the biopsy of bronchial mucosa and in the BAL of patients with allergic asthma (72,73), whereas IFNγ and/or TNFα predominated in multiple sclerosis lesions (69) and in the pancreas of patients with type I diabetes (74). Abnormal expression of Th2 cells is also involved in the pathogenesis of Omenn's syndrome (75) and evidence for excessive Th2 activity (76), as well as for monoclonal Th2-cell disease presenting as hypereosinophilic syndrome (77), has been reported.

Since the human specific immune response against offending agents is determined by the set of cytokines produced by Th cells, it is reasonable to suggest that the failure to control infectious diseases often results from inappropriate rather than insufficient immune responses. The best example is non-healing forms of murine and human leishmaniasis, which represent strong, but counterproductive, Th2-dominated responses (6).

Another example, even if more controversial, is HIV infection. In HIV-infected subjects a reduced ability of HIV-infected macrophages to produce IL-12, which is an important Th1-inducing cytokine, has been found (78). It has been also suggested that a switch from Th1 to Th2 may play a critical role in the progression of disease (79). More importantly, at least in vitro, Th2 clones appear to be more efficient supporters of HIV replication than Th1 cells (80). In this regard, of note is the recent demonstration in our laboratory that HIV infection can favour CD30 expression in $CD4^+$ T cells (81), and that CD30 triggering by $CD8^+$ T cells expressing the natural CD30 ligand enhances HIV replication in HIV-infected $CD4^+$ T cells (81). Thus, immunotherapeutic strategies devoted to potentiating the development of Th1 cells and/or their effector function or to antagonizing CD30 expression and/or triggering might be of value in the fight against HIV infection.

If Th1 inflammatory responses to several pathogenic micro-organisms are protective, such responses to self-antigens are usually deleterious. Some animal models of inflammatory autoimmune diseases (82,83), as well as in vitro and in vivo studies in patients suffering from organ-specific autoimmunity (6,69,74), suggest that preferential activation of Th1 responses is central in the pathogenesis of these disorders. Inhibition of autoantigen-specific Th1 responses or administration of Th1-inhibiting cytokines (IL-4 and IL-10) may be beneficial in the prevention or treatment of these disorders. In contrast, a prevalent Th2 response seems to be involved in the immunopathogenesis of systemic lupus erythematosus (SLE). A Th2-type immune response has been clearly demonstrated to be pathogenic in experimental SLE induced by allogeneic stimulation or chemicals (84). Moreover, a recent study in patients with SLE showed significantly elevated values of sCD30 in their serum (85) and this parameter directly correlated with clinical features of SLE activity, suggesting an abnormal Th2-type cell function in vivo (74). Similarly $CD30^{+}CD4^{+}$ T cells have been found in the skin of patients with systemic sclerosis; in these patients the presence of high serum levels of sCD30, IgE and IL-4 strongly suggests that also in such disease Th2 response may be involved (Mavilia *et al.* personal communication).

The new insights in the pathogenesis of allergic disorders provide novel opportunities for the development of immunomodulatory regimens in allergic diseases. Essentially two new approaches to allergen-specific immunotherapy regimens can be hypothesized: induction of T cell anergy with allergen-derived peptides (86), and induction of T-cell class switch (from Th2 to Th0/Th1). A first possibility is to down-regulate established allergen-specific Th2 responses, i.e. by acting at level of memory T cells. Down-regulation of Th2 cells may result from either induction of tolerance, as well as by selective manipulation of cytokine secretion patterns (reduction of IL-4 production and increase in IFNγ production). However, a potentially more successful approach should be the up-regulation of allergen-specific Th1 responses, which is directed to prime naive T cells in manner which selects for prevalent Th1 phenotype. In vitro, substantial alterations of the allergen-specific Th subset balance have been accomplished by antigen stimulation of Th cells in the presence of IL-12, IL-1Ra, IFNγ or IFNα and/or anti-IL-4 antibodies (6). Furthermore, IL-4 production by T cells from atopic patients can be considerably reduced by specific immunotherapy (87). More recently, a strong Th1-inducing effect was also obtained with poly I:C, that appeared to be capable of inducing high production of both IFNα and IL-12 by macrophages (63). As we have previously described, IFNα was not only found to be able to modulate the cytokine profile of allergen-specific T cells, but also to affect their TCR repertoire (62). These data suggest that the injection of selected allergen peptides in combination with Th1-inducing cytokines may represent the basis for a novel immunotherapeutic strategy in allergic disorders. Thus, new therapy with modified forms of allergen capable of shifting the Th2 responses to less pathogenic Th0 or Th1 responses could be hypothesized (24).

Finally, the new information on the two subsets of $CD4^{+}$ T cells and on mechanisms influencing their development can be directly applied to vaccine development (for example, the use of IL-12 as adjuvant). Our knowledge will become more powerful when we succeed in identifying the source of the IL-4 that drives Th2 differentiation, or better defining the factors responsible for the induction of cytokines, such as IL-10, which inhibit Th1 differentiation and in determining mechanisms by which pathogens can selectively stimulate IL-12 or IL-4 production.

ACKNOWLEDGEMENTS

The experiments reported in this paper have been performed by grants provided in part by the AIRC, in part by the Istituto Superiore di Sanità (AIDS and MS Projects), in part by CNR (ACRO Project) and in part by EC Biotech and FAIR Projects.

REFERENCES

1. Mosmann, T. R., H. Chervinski, M. W. Bond *et al.* 1986. Two types of murine helper T-cell-clone. I. Definition according to profiles of lymphokine activities and secreted proteins. *J. Immunol.* **136**:2348–57.
2. Mosmann, T. R. and R. L. Coffman. 1989. TH1 and TH2 Cells: Different patterns of lymphokine secretion lead to different functional properties. *Annu. Rev. Immunol.* **7**:145–73.
3. Street, N. E., I. H. Schumacher, T. A. T. Fong *et al.* 1990. Heterogeneity of mouse helper T cells: Evidence from bulk cultures and limiting dilution cloning for precursors of Th1 and Th2 cells. *J. Immunol.* **144**:1629–39.
4. Del Prete, G. F., M. De Carli, C. Mastromauro *et al.* 1991. Purified protein derivative of *Mycobacterium tuberculosis* and excretory-secretory antigen(s) of *Toxocara canis* expand in vitro human T cells with stable and opposite (type 1 T helper or type 2 T helper) profile of cytokine production. *J. Clin. Invest.* **88**:346–50.
5. Parronchi, P., D. Macchia, M.-P. Piccinni *et al.* 1991. Allergen- and bacterial antigen-specific T-cell clones established from atopic donors show a different profile of cytokine production. *Proc. Natl. Acad. Sci. USA* **88**:4538–42.
6. Romagnani, S. 1994. Lymphokine production by human T cells in disease states. *Annu. Rev. Immunol.* **12**:227–57.
7. Del Prete, G. F., M. De Carli, F. Almerigogna *et al.* 1993. Human IL-10 is produced by both type 1 helper (Th1) and type 2 helper (Th2) T cell clones and inhibits their antigen-specific proliferation and cytokine production. *J. Immunol.* **150**:1–8.
8. Romagnani, S. 1994. Th1 and Th2 subsets of CD4+ T lymphocytes. *Scient. Amer. Science & Medicine* **1**:68–77.
9. Romagnani, S. 1994. Human Th1 and Th2 subsets: 'Eppur si muove!' *Eur. Cyt. Netw.* **5**:7–12.
10. Del Prete, G. F., M. De Carli, M. Ricci and S. Romagnani. 1991. Helper activity for immunoglobulin synthesis of TH1 and TH2 human T cell clones: the help of Th1 clones is limited by their cytolytic capacity. *J. Exp. Med.* **174**:809–13.

11. Romagnani, S. 1991. Human T_H1 and T_H2: Doubt no more. *Immunol. Today* **12**:256–7.
12. Del Prete, G. F., M. De Carli, R. Lammel *et al.* 1995. Th1 and Th2 T helper cells exert opposite regulatory effects on procoagulant activity and tissue factor production by human monocytes. *Blood* **86**:250–7.
13. Smith, C., T. Davis, D. Anderson *et al.* 1990. A receptor for tumor necrosis factor defines an unusual family of cellular and viral proteins. *Science* **248**:1019–23.
14. Smith, C. A., H.-J. Gruss, T. Davis *et al.* 1993. CD30 antigen, a marker for Hodgkin's lymphoma, is a receptor whose ligand defines an emerging family of cytokines with homology to TNF. *Cell* **73**:1349–60.
15. Schwab, U., H. Stein, J. Gerde *et al.* 1982. Production of a monoclonal antibody specific for Hodgkin's and Sternberg–Reed cells of Hodgkin's disease and a subset of normal lymphoid cells. *Nature* **299**:65–7.
16. Stein, H., D. Y. Mason, J. Gerdes *et al.* 1985. The expression of Hodgkin's disease associated antigen Ki-1 in reactive and neoplastic lymphoid tissue: Evidence that the Reed Sternberg cells and histocytic malignancies are derived from activated lymphoid cells. *Blood* **66**:848–58.
17. Andreesen, R., J. Osterholz, G. W. Lohr and K. J. Bross. 1984. A Hodgkin cell-specific antigen is expressed on a subset of auto- and alloactivated T (helper) lymphoblasts. *Blood* **63**:1299–302.
18. Ellis, T. M., P. E. Simms, D. J. Slivnick *et al.* 1993. CD30 is a signal-transducing molecule that defines a subset of human activated $CD45RO^+$ T cells. *J. Immunol.* **151**:2380–9.
19. Del Prete, G. F., M. De Carli, F. Almerigogna *et al.* 1995. Preferential expression of CD30 by human CD4+ T cells producing Th2-type cytokines. *FASEB J.* **9**:81–6.
20. Manetti, R., F. Annunziato, R. Biagiotti *et al.* 1994. CD30 expression by CD8+ T cells producing Th2-type cytokines. Evidence for large numbers of CD8+CD30+ T cell clones in human immunodeficiency virus (HIV) infection. *J. Exp. Med.* **180**:2407–11.
21. Maggi, E., M. G. Giudizi, R. Biagiotti *et al.* 1994. Th2-like CD8+ T cells showing B cell helper function and reduced cytolytic activity in human immunodeficiency virus type 1 infection. *J. Exp. Med.* **180**:489–96.
22. Farrah, T. and C. Smith. 1992. An emerging cytokine family. *Nature* **358**:26–9.
23. Ito, K., T. Watanabe, R. Horie *et al.* 1994. High expression of the CD30 molecule in human decidual cells. *Am. J. Pathol.* **145**:276–80.
24. Romagnani, S., 1994. Regulation of Th2 development in allergy. *Curr. Opin. Immunol.* **6**:838–46.
25. Chilosi, M., F. Facchetti, L. Notarangelo *et al.* 1996. CD30 cell expression and abnormal soluble CD30 serum accumulation in Omenn's syndrome: evidence for a T helper 2-mediated condition. *Eur. J. Immunol.* **26**:1180–6.
26. Triebel., F., S. Jitsukawa, E. Baixeras *et al.* 1990. LAG-3, a novel lymphocyte activation gene closely related to CD4. *J. Exp. Med.* **171**:1393–405.
27. Huard, B., P. Gaulard, F. Faure and F. Triebel. 1994. Cellular expression and tissue distribution of the human LAG-3-encoded protein, an MHC class II ligand. *Immunogenetics* **39**:213–17.
28. Huard, B., M. Tournier, T. Hercend *et al.* 1994. Lymphocyte-activation gene 3/major histocompatibility complex class II interaction modulates the antigenic response of CD4+ T lymphocytes. *Eur. J. Immunol.* **24**:3216–21.
29. Huard, B., P. Prigent, F. Pagès *et al.* 1996. T cell MHC class II molecules downregulate T cell proliferation following LAG-3 binding. *Eur. J. Immunol.* **26**: 1180-6.

30. Annunziato, F., R. Manetti, Lj. Tomasévic *et al.* 1996. Expression and release of LAG-3-associated protein by human CD4+ T cells are associated with IFN-γ. *FASEB J.* **10**:769–75.
31. Hsieh, C.-S., A. B. Heimberger, J. S. Gold *et al.* 1992. Differential regulation of T helper phenotype development by IL-4 and IL-10 in an ab-transgenic system. *Proc. Natl. Acad. Sci. USA* **89**:6065–9.
32. Reiner, S. L., Z.-E. Wang, F. Hatam *et al.* 1993. Th1 and Th2 cell antigen receptors in experimental leishmaniasis. *Science* **259**:1457–60.
33. Swain, S. L. 1991. Regulation of the development of distinct subsets of CD4+ T cells. *Immunol. Res.* **142**:14–18.
34. Coffman, R. L., R. Chatelain, L. M. C. C. Leal and K. Varkila. 1991. Leishmania major infection in mice: a model system for the study of CD4+ T-cell subset differentiation. *Res. Immunol.* **142**:36–9.
35. Lack, G., H. Renz, J. Saloga *et al.* 1994. Nebulized but not parenteral IFN-γ decreases IgE production and normalizes airways function in a murine model of allergen sensitization. *J. Immunol.* **152**:2546–54.
36. Marsh, D. G., J. D. Neely, D. R. Breazeale *et al.* 1994. Linkage analysis of IL-4 and other chromosome 5q31.1 markers and total serum immunoglobulin E concentrations. *Science* **264**:1152–6.
37. Murphy, K. M., T. L. Murphy, J. S. Gold and S. J. Szabo. 1993. Current understanding of IL-4 gene regulation in T cells. *Res. Immunol.* **144**:575–8.
38. Manetti, R., P. Parronchi, M. G. Giudizi *et al.* 1993. Natural killer cell stimulatory factor (interleukin 12) induces T helper type 1 (Th1)-specific immune responses and inhibits the development of IL-4-producing Th cells. *J. Exp. Med.* **177**:1199–1204.
39. Hsieh, C.-S., S. E. Macatonia, C. S. Tripp *et al.* 1993. Development of Th1 CD4+ T cells through IL-12 produced by listeria-induced macrophages. *Science* **260**:547–9.
40. Schon-Hegrad, M. A., J. Oliver, P. G. McMenamin and P. G. Holt. 1991. Studies on the density, distribution and surface phenotype of intraepithelial class II MHC (Ia) antigen-bearing dendritic cells in the conductive airways. *J. Exp. Med.* **173**:1345–56.
41. Kuchroo, V. K., M. Prahbu Das, J. A. Brown *et al.* 1995. B7-1 and B7-2 costimulatory molecules activate differentially the Th1/Th2 development pathways: application to autoimmune disease therapy. *Cell* **80**:707–18.
42. Del Prete, G. F., M. De Carli, M. M. D'Elios *et al.* 1995. CD30-mediated signalling promotes the development of human Th2-like T cells. *J. Exp. Med.* **185**:1–7.
43. Renz, H., J. Saloga, K. L. Bradley *et al.* 1993. Specific Vβ T cell subsets mediate the immediate hypersensitivity response to ragweed allergen. *J. Immunol.* **151**:1907–17.
44. Rook, G. A. W., R. Hernandez-Pando and S. L. Lightman. 1994. Hormones, peripherally activated prohormones and regulation of the Th1/Th2 balance. *Immunol. Today* **15**:301–3.
45. Piccinni, M.-P., M.-G. Giudizi, R. Biagiotti *et al.* 1995. Progesterone favors the development of human T helper (Th) cells producing Th2-type cytokines and promotes both IL-4 production and membrane CD30 expression in established Th1 clones. *J. Immunol.* **155**:128–33.
46. Wegmann, T. G., H. Lin, L. Guilbert and T. R. Mosmann. 1993. Bidirectional cytokine interactions in the maternal-fetal relationship: is successful pregnancy a Th2 phenomenon? *Immunol. Today* **14**:353–6.
47. Williams, M. E., T. L. Chang, S. K. Burke *et al.* 1991. Activation of functionally

distinct subsets of CD4+ T lymphocytes. *Res. Immunol.* **142**:23–7.

48. Manetti, R., V. Barak, M.-P. Piccinni *et al.* 1994. Interleukin 1 favors the in vitro development of type 2 helper (Th2) human T cell clones. *Res. Immunol.* **145**:93–100.
49. Swain, S. L. 1993. IL-4 dictates T-cell differentiation. *Res. Immunol.* **144**:616–20.
50. Maggi, E., P. Parronchi, R. Manetti *et al.* 1992. Reciprocal regulatory role of IFN-γ and IL-4 on the in vitro development of human T_H1 and T_H2 clones. *J. Immunol.* **148**:2142–8.
51. Seder, R. A., W. E. Paul, M. M. Davis and B. Fazekas de St. Groth. 1992. The presence of interleukin 4 during in vitro priming determines the lymphocyte-producing potential of CD4+ T cells from T cell receptor transgenic mice. *J. Exp. Med.* **176**:1091–8.
52. Parronchi. P., M. De Carli, M.-P. Piccinni *et al.* 1992. IL-4 and IFNs exert opposite regulatory effects on the development of cytolytic potential by T_H1 or T_H2 human T cell clones. *J. Immunol.* **149**:2977–83.
53. Kopf, M., G. Le Gros, M. Bachmann *et al.* 1993. Disruption of the murine IL-4 gene blocks Th2 cytokine responses. *Nature* **362**:245–8.
54. Yashimoto, T. and W. E. Paul. 1994. $CD4^{pos}$, $NK1.1^{pos}$ T cells promptly produce interleukin 4 in response to in vivo challenge with anti-CD3. *J. Exp. Med.* **179**:1285–95.
55. Zlotnik, A. and A. G. D. Bean. 1993. Production of IL-4 by non-Th2-cell subsets: possible role of CD4-CD8-$\alpha\beta$TCR+ and CD4 subset T cells in T helper subset regulation. *Res. Immunol.* **144**:608–9.
56. Bradding, P., I. H. Feather, P. H. Howarth *et al.* 1992. Interleukin 4 is localized and released by human mast cells. *J. Exp. Med.* **176**:1381–6.
57. Brunner, T., C. H. Heusser and C. A. Dahinden. 1993. Human peripheral blood basophils primed by interleukin 3 (IL-3) produce IL-4 in response to immunoglobulin E receptor stimulation. *J. Exp. Med.* **177**:605–11.
58. Piccinni, M. P., D. Macchia, P. Parronchi *et al.* 1991. Human bone marrow non-B, non-T cells produce interleukin 4 in response to cross-linkage of Fcε and Fcγ receptors. *Proc. Natl. Acad. Sci. USA* **88**:8656–60.
59. Wershil, B. K., C. M. Theodos, S. J. Galli and R. G. Titus. 1994. Mast cells augment lesion size and persistence during experimental Leishmania major infection in the mouse. *J. Immunol.* **152**:4563–71.
60. Finkelman, F. D. and J. F. Urban. 1992. Cytokines: making the right choice. *Parasitol. Today* **8**:311–14.
61. McMenamin, C. and P. G. Holt. 1993. The natural immune response to inhaled soluble protein antigens involves major histocompatibility complex (MHC) class I-restricted CD8+ T cell-mediated but not MHC class-II-restricted CD4+ of T cell-dependent immune deviation resulting in selective suppression of immunoglobulin E production. *J. Exp. Med.* **178**:889–99.
62. Parronchi, P., S. Mohapatra, S. Sampognaro *et al.* 1996. Effects of IFN-α on cytokine profile T cell receptor repertoire and peptide reactivity of human allergen-specific T cells. *Eur. J. Immunol.* **26**:697–703.
63. Manetti, R., F. Annunziato, Lj. Tomasévic *et al.* 1995. Polynosinic acid: polycitidylic acid (poly I:C) promotes T helper type 1 (Th1)-specific immune responses by stimulating macrophage production of interferon (IFN)-α and interleukin (IL)-12. *Eur. J. Immunol.* **25**:2656–60.
64. Maggi, E., P. Biswas, G. F. Del Prete *et al.* 1991. Accumulation of Th2-like helper T cells in the conjunctiva of patients with vernal conjunctivitis. *J. Immunol.* **146**:1169–74.

65. Del Prete, G. F., M. De Carli, M. M. D'Elios *et al.* 1993. Allergen exposure induces the activation of allergen-specific Th2 cells in the airway mucosa of patients with allergic respiratory disorders. *Eur J. Immunol.* **23**:1445–9.
66. van der Heijden, F. L., E. A. Wierenga, J. D. Bos and M. L. Kapsenberg. 1991. High frequency of IL-4-producing CD4+ allergen-specific T lymphocytes in atopic dermatitis lesional skin. *J. Invest. Dermatol.* **97**:389–94.
67. Brod, S. A., D. Benjamin and D. A. Hafler. 1991. Restricted T cell expression of IL-2/IFN-γ mRNA in human inflammatory diseases. *J. Immunol.* **147**:810–15.
68. Kapsenberg, M. L., E. A. Wierenga, J. D. Bos and H. M. Jansen. 1991. Functional subsets of allergen-reactive human CD4+ T cells. *Immunol. Today* **12**:392–5.
69. Selmaj, K., C. S. Raine, B. Cannella and C. F. Brosnan. 1991. Identification of lymphotoxin and tumor necrosis factor in multiple sclerosis lesions. *J. Clin. Invest.* **87**:949–54.
70. Yssel, H., M. C. Shanafelt, C. Soderberg *et al.* 1991. *Borrelia burgdorferi* activates a T helper type 1-like T cell subset in Lyme arthritis. *J. Exp. Med.* **174**:593–601.
71. Schlaak, J., E. Hermann, M. Ringhoffer *et al.* 1992. Predominance of Th1-type T cells in synovial fluid of patients with *Yersinia enterocolitica* reactive arthritis. *Eur. J. Immunol.* **22**:2771–6.
72. Hamid, Q., M. Azzawi, S. Ying *et al.* 1991. Expression of mRNA for interleukin-5 in mucosal bronchial biopsies from asthma. *J. Clin. Invest.* **87**:1541–6.
73. Robinson, D. S., Q. Hamid, S. Ying *et al.* 1992. Predominant Th2-like bronchoalveolar T-lymphocyte population in atopic asthma. *New Engl. J. Med.* **326**:295–304.
74. Foulis, A. K., M. McGil and M. A. Farquharson. 1991. Insulitis in type I (insulin-dependent) diabetes mellitus in man – macrophages, lymphocytes, and interferon-γ containing cells. *J. Pathol.* **165**:97–102.
75. Schandené, L., A. Ferster, F. Mascart-Lemone *et al.* 1993. T helper type 2-like cells and therapeutic effects of interferon-γ in combined immunodeficiency with hypereosoniphilia (Omenn's syndrome). *Eur. J. Immunol.* **23**:56–60.
76. Field, E. H., R. J. Noelle, T. Rouse *et al.* 1991. Evidence for excessive Th2 CD4+ subset activity in vivo. *J. Immunol.* **151**:48–59.
77. Cogan, E., L. Schandané, A. Crusiaux *et al.* 1994. A TH2 clonal disease presenting as hypereosinophilic syndrome. *New Engl. J. Med.* **330**:535–8.
78. Chehimi, J., S. E. Starr, I. Frank *et al.* 1994. Impaired interleukin-12 production in HIV-Infected patients. *J. Exp. Med.* **179**:1361–6.
79. Clerici, M. and G. M. Shearer. 1993. A Th1 to Th2 switch is a critical step in the etiology of HIV infection. *Immunol. Today* **14**:107–11.
80. Maggi, E., M. Mazzetti, A. Ravina *et al.* 1994. Ability of HIV to promote a Th1 to Th0 shift and to replicate preferentially in Th2 and Th0 cells. *Science* **265**:244–8.
81. Maggi, E., F. Annunziato, R. Manetti *et al.* 1995. Activation of HIV expression by CD30 triggering in CD4+ T cells from HIV-infected individuals. *Immunity* **3**:251–5.
82. Khoury, S. J., W. W. Hancock and H. L. Weiner. 1992. Oral tolerance to myelic basic protein and natural recovery from experimental autoimmune encephalomyelitis are associated with downregulation of inflammatory cytokines and differential upregulation of transforming growth factor β, interleukin 4, and prostaglandin E expression in the brain. *J. Exp. Med.* **176**:1355–65.
83. Campbell, I., T. W. Kay, L. Oxbrow and L. C. Harrison. 1991. Essential role

for interferon-γ and interleukin-6 in autoimmune insulin-dependent diabetes in NOD/Wehi mice. *J. Clin. Invest.* **87**:739–45.

84. Goldmanm, M., P. Druet and E. Gleichmann. 1991. Th2 cells in systemic autoimmunity: insights from allogeneic diseases and chemically-induced autoimmunity. *Immunol. Today* **12**:223–7.
85. Caligaris Cappio, F., T. Bertero, M. Converso *et al.* 1995. Circulating levels of soluble CD30, a marker of cells producing Th2 type cytokines, are increased in patients with systemic lupus erythematosus and correlate with disease activity. *Clin. Exp. Rheumatol.* **13**:339–43.
86. Yssel, H., S. Fasler, J. Lamb and J. De Vries. 1994. Induction of non-responsiveness in human allergen-specific type 2 helper cells. *Curr. Opin. Immunol.* **6**:847–52.
87. Secrist, H., C. J. Chelen, Y. Went *et al.* 1993. Allergen immunotherapy decreases interleukin 4 production in CD4+ T cells from allergic individuals. *J. Exp. Med.* **178**:2123–30.

14

Monoclonal Antibodies Against Idiotypes of Human Anti-insulin Antibodies

Maria Stamenova, Vanya Manolova, Ivan Kehayov and Stanimir Kyurkchiev

Type 1 insulin-dependent diabetes results from a progressive autoimmune response which specifically and selectively destroys the insulin-producing beta cells of Langerhans (1–3). Autoimmunity to the beta cells or beta cell products in insulin-dependent diabetes is clearly both humoral (4,5) and cell-mediated (6,7). Humoral immunity is characterized by the appearance of autoantibodies to beta-cell membranes, beta-cell contents or beta-cell secretory products – anti-insulin autoantibodies.

Knowledge of the antigenic determinants of anti-insulin autoantibodies might be of great importance in understanding the nature of the immune response to self antigens, whether the autoantibodies are products of germline genes or somatically mutated ones.

In the present chapter, the results of a study on the immunogenicity of the epitopes of human anti-insulin autoantibodies are reported. The aim of this investigation was to obtain a panel of antibodies reacting specifically with patients' anti-insulin autoantibodies.

MATERIALS AND METHODS

Sera were obtained from 247 patients with type 1 insulin-dependent diabetes and tested for anti-insulin antibodies by ELISA.

Positively reacting sera (OD 0.346 ± 0.042) against insulin were pooled and used for isolation of specific anti-insulin autoantibodies by affinity chromatography on CNBr-activated sepharose 4B (Sigma, USA) coupled with insulin. Chromatographic fractions were tested against insulin by ELISA, and homogeneity was proved by SDS-electrophoresis. The fraction of anti-insulin antibodies was used for immunization. BALB/c mice (about 20 g) were

Immunoregulation in Health and Disease
ISBN 0-12-459460-3

injected subcutaneously with 20 μg purified anti-insulin autoantibodies emulsified in complete Freund's adjuvant (Difco, USA) for the first injection or in incomplete Freund's adjuvant for the subsequent injections, done at 15-day intervals. After the third injection mice were bled and the sera were tested for the presence of anti-anti-insulin antibodies (IAA). Mice with the highest antibody titre were boosted by intraperitoneal injection with 20 μg purified anti-insulin autoantibodies.

Splenocytes from the immune animal were fused with mouse myeloma P3 × 63.Ag8.653 cells, following the protocol generally used in our laboratory (8). Briefly, after washing in serum-free RPMI 1640 medium the pooled splenocytes and myeloma cells were treated with polyethylene glycol (Serva, Germany) for 8 min at room temperature, washed again and resuspended in RPMI 1640 medium supplemented with 10% fetal bovine serum, L-glutamine, sodium pyruvate and antibiotics. Hypoxanthine, aminopterine and thymidine were added to this medium as selective agents. Cells were distributed in microtitre 96-well plates (Costar) at a concentration of 3×10^5 cells per well and incubated at 37°C in 5% carbon dioxide. About 10–12 days after fusion wells with growing hybridomas were tested and those reacting positively were cloned by limiting dilutions. Hybridomas were grown in mass cultures and frozen or used to induce ascites in BALB/c mice.

Tissue culture medium, fetal bovine serum and all additives for cell cultures were purchased from Sigma Co. (USA).

An indirect enzyme-linked immunoassay (ELISA) was used to screen for hybridomas secreting anti-idiotypic antibodies. Wells of polyvinylchloride (PVC) plates were coated with 50 μl/well of purified auto anti-insulin antibodies in carbonate–bicarbonate buffer pH 9.3 by incubation overnight at 4°C. After extensive washing with phosphate buffered saline (PBS) containing 0.05% Tween 20 (T-PBS) and blocking with 10% inactivated calf serum in 0.1 M TRIS-HCl buffer, pH 8.3, supernatants from wells with growing hybridomas were added and incubated for 2 h at RT. Plates were washed again and porcine anti-mouse Ig conjugated with peroxidase and diluted 1/2000 in blocking buffer was added to each well for 1 h at room temperature. Bound enzyme activity was developed with 0.4 mg/ml *ortho*-phenilenediamine (Sigma, USA) in citrate buffer containing 0.05% hydrogen peroxide for 5 min in the dark. Sulfuric acid (4N solution) was added to stop the colour reaction and the optical density was read on a Micro-ELISA reader (Dynatech, USA) at 492 nm.

Purified human auto anti-insulin antibodies were run on SDS–electrophoresis in 10% polyacrylamide gel as described by Laemmli (9).

RESULTS

Only 54 of 247 diabetic sera were positive for insulin autoantibodies (IAA). The positive sera were pooled, purified by precipitation with ammonium

Table 14.1 Screening of monoclonal antibodies against individual IAA (+) human sera

IAA (+) sera No	Positively reacting hybridoma
27	2F10; 4E5
28	2F10; 4E5; 4C10
29	2F10; 4E5; 4C10
43	2F10; 4E5; 4C10; 1A2; 2C1
57	2F10; 4E5; 2C1
58	2F10; 2C1; 4E5
108	4C10; 4E5
110	2F10; 4C10; 4E5
111	2F10; 4E5
113	1A2; 4E5
115	1A2; 2C1; 4C10; 4E5
118	2C1; 4C10;4E5
124	2A4; 2F10; 4E5
188	2A4; 2F10; 4C10; 4E5

Table 14.2 Specificity of selected monoclonal antibodies

mAb/ Antigen	Ins	Coll	Hem	HSA	dsDNA	Cr	Hu IgG	+K
1A2	++	−	+++	+	++	++	++	+++
2A4	−	−	−	−	−	−	+	+
2C1	++	+	+++	+	++	++	+++	+++
2F10	−	−	+	+++	−	−	+	+++
4C10	−	−	−	−	−	−	+	+++
4E5	−	−	−	−	−	−	+	++

Ins, insulin (4 mg/ml); Coll, collagen (30 mg/ml); Hem, hemoglobin (32 mg/ml); HSA, human serum albumin (1 μg/ml); Cr, crystalin (human, 100 μg/ml); Hu IgG, human immunoglobulin G (39 μg/ml); +K, human sera, containing IAA, reacting in strongest way with respective mAb; (−), denotes negative reaction in ELISA; (+), denotes positive reaction (absorption at 492 nm below 0.1); (++), positive reaction (absorption 0.1–0.2); (+++), positive reaction (absorption above 0.3).

sulfate and subsequently subjected to affinity chromatography on a CNBr-Sepharose column. The homogeneity of anti-insulin antibodies was proved by SDS–electrophoresis. The fraction of anti-insulin antibodies was used to immunize mice. After the immune response was developed, the mice were bled and the sera were tested against human sera, containing anti-insulin antibodies and sera negative with reference to insulin. Splenocytes from immunized mice were used for fusion. As result of the hybridization 32 cell clones were obtained which reacted positively with pooled sera containing anti-insulin antibodies. Of these, clones were selected to produce monoclonal

Table 14.3 Distribution of IAA epitopes recognized by the monoclonal antibodies in IDDM patient's sera

Monoclonal antibodies	Number of positively reacting IAA (+) human sera
2A4; 4C10; 4E5	9
2A4; 4E5	8
4C10; 4E5	9
4C10; 2A4	0
4E5	6
4C10	0
2A4	0

antibodies reacting with all or with part of individual human anti-insulin sera. Monoclonal antibodies designated Mab 1A2, Mab 2C1, Mab 2F10, Mab 2A4, Mab 4C10, Mab 4E5 were selected (Table 14.1). The specificity of monoclonal antibodies was tested against different antigens: insulin, collagen, haemoglobin, human serum albumin, double-strained DNA, crystallin and human immunoglobulin (Table 14.2). The results presented in Table 14.2 suggest dividing the monoclonal antibodies into two groups:

- mouse monoclonal antibodies (1A2, 2C1, 2F10), reacting with epitopes on human immunoglobulins and other antigens
- mouse monoclonal antibodies (2A4, 4C10, 4E5), reacting only with human immunoglobulins.

The monoclonal antibodies of the second group were tested by ELISA against individual human sera, containing anti-insulin antibodies and sera without these antibodies. The reactivity of each monoclonal antibody is shown in Table 14.3. The results showed that Mab 2A4 reacted with 13 human sera, containing anti-insulin antibodies, Mab 4C10 with 26, and Mab 4E5 with 39 of all tested sera. The three monoclonal antibodies reacted simultaneously with nine human sera. Monoclonal antibodies 4E5 reacted positively with six of the sera (39, 43, 113, 124, 274, 282), which reacted negative with the other two (2A4 and 4C10).

DISCUSSION

Antibodies are usually characterized by their antigenic specificity and their isotype. The characterization of human autoantibodies by their idiotypes is of great importance in understanding the nature of pathogenic autoreactivity. It is well known that during the normal development of immune response auto-anti-idiotypes are generated. The auto-anti-idiotypes play a major role in regulation by either enhancing or suppressing idiotype formation. Anti-idiotypes not only regulate autoimmune reactions, but also can induce de novo autoimmunity (10). On the other hand, anti-idiotypes can suppress the autoimmune reaction by active immunization with a pathological idiotype (11). Knowledge of the origin of pathological idiotypes yields useful information for understanding the pathogenesis of autoimmune disorders. The results presented here show that discrete epitopes of anti-insulin antibodies can be characterized with monoclonal antibodies raised against pooled affinity purified sera of patients with diabetes type 1. Monoclonal antibodies are useful tools in investigating the versatility and distribution of anti-insulin autoantibodies in patient's sera. The discrete character of recognized epitopes could be explained by the somatic mutation origin of anti-insulin antibodies (12). We failed to find major cross-reactive idiotypes among IAA and the results are consistent with the idea that anti-insulin antibodies are produced by memory B cells and the primary immune response is mounted early in life.

CONCLUSIONS

1. The immunosorbent assay used for detecting anti-insulin antibodies is a convenient method and could be applied for both purified IAA and human sera.
2. The immunization of animals with an affinity-purified IAA fraction results in generation of antibodies, reacting with discrete epitopes of IAA from individual patient's sera.
3. The monoclonal antibodies produced revealed the presence of at least three discrete antigenic determinants.
4. Cross-reactive idiotypes were not detected among human IAA.
5. These results demonstrate the somatic-mutation origin of human IAA and are consistent with the idea that IAA are produced by memory B cells.

REFERENCES

1. Gepts, W. and P. Lecompte. 1981. The pancreatic islets in diabetes. *Am. J. Med.* **70**:105–15.
2. Foulis, A. K. and J. A. Stewari. 1984. The pancreas in recent-onset Type 1 (insulin-dependent) diabetes mellitus: insulin content of islets, insulitis and associated changes in the exocrine acinar tissue. *Diabetologia* **26**:456–61.
3. Eisenbarth, G. S. 1986. Type 1 diabetes mellitus, a chronic autoimmune disease. *N. Engl. J. Med.* **314**:1360–6.
4. Cahill, G. F. and H. O. McDevit. 1981. Insulin-dependent diabetes mellitus: the initial lesion. *N. Engl. J. Med.* **304**:1454–65.

5. Baekkeskov, S., J. H. Nielson, B. Marner *et al.* 1982. Autoantibodies in newly diagnosed diabetic children immunoprecipitate human pancreatic islet cell proteins. *Nature* **298**:167–9.
6. Wang, Y., L. Hao, R. G. Gill and K. J. Lafferty. 1987. Autoimmune diabetes in NOD mouse is L3T4 T-lymphocyte dependent. *Diabetes* **36**:535–8.
7. Bendelac, A., C. Carnaud, C. Boitard and J. F. Bach. 1987. Syngeneic transfer of autoimmune diabetes from diabetic NOD mice to healthy neonates. *J. Exp. Med.* **166**:823–32.
8. Kyurkchiev, S., Ts. Surneva-Nakova, M. Ivanova *et al.* 1988. Monoclonal antibodies to porcine zona pellucida that block the initial stages of fertilization. *J. Reprod. Immunol. Microbiol.* **18**:11–16.
9. Laemmli, U. V. 1970. Cleavage of structural during the assembly of the head of bacteriophage T4. *Nature* **227**:680–5.
10. Shoenfeld, Y., Amital, H., Ferrone, S. and Kennedy, R. C. 1994. Anti-idiotypes and their application under autoimmune, neoplastic and infectious conditions. *Arch. Allergy Immunol.* **105**:211–23.
11. Zouali, M., M. Jolivet, C. Leclerc *et al.* 1985. Suppression of murine lupus autoantibodies to DNA by administration of muramyl dipeptide and syngenic anti-DNA IgG. *J. Immunol.* **135**:1091–9.
12. Poskitt, D. C., M. J. B. Jean-Francois, S. Turnbull *et al.* 1991. The nature of immunoglobulin idiotypes and idiotype-anti-idiotype interactions in immunological networks. *Immunol. Cell Biol.* **69**:61–70.

15

Effects of Amyotrophic Lateral Sclerosis IgGs on Calcium Homeostasis in Neural Cells

Pavle R. Andjus, Leonard Khiroug, Andrea Nistri and Enrico Cherubini

The most frequently encountered primary form of progressive motoneuron disease is amyotrophic lateral sclerosis (ALS), a devastating neurological disorder affecting upper and lower motoneurons. Passive transfer of disease occurs when immunoglobulins (IgGs) from ALS patients are injected into experimental animals (1). Neuronal death due to excitotoxicity has been suggested to contribute to ALS aetiopathogenesis. Excitotoxicity might be produced by abnormally high levels of glutamate released by nerve terminals following increased intracellular free calcium ($[Ca^{2+}]_i$) through an action of ALS IgGs on ligand and/or voltage-gated calcium ion channels, thus suggesting an autoimmune process involved in this disease. Electrophysiological evidence for ALS IgGs modulation of voltage-activated calcium ion currents of central neurons has, however, provided contrasting results ranging from depression (2) to potentiation (3). In the present experiments, a non-invasive study of the effects of ALS IgGs on changes in $[Ca^{2+}]_i$ was performed using confocal laser scanning microscopy. To this end rat hippocampal pyramidal neurons in culture were employed as a convenient model of identified central neurons endowed with various classes of calcium ion channel (4).

MATERIALS AND METHODS

Hippocampal cell cultures were prepared from 2–4-day-old rats (5). Pyramidal neurons (5–15 days in culture) were preincubated (45–60 min; 37°C) with the calcium fluorescent probe fluo-3 (2 μM) in standard experimental solution (SES, in mM: 3.5 KCl, 132 NaCl, 1 $MgCl_2$, 2 $CaCl_2$,

Immunoregulation in Health and Disease
ISBN 0–12–459460–3

10 glucose, 10 Hepes, pH 7.4), supplemented with 0.5% BSA and 0.05% Pluronic-F127. Measurements on single cells were performed in the presence of 1 μM tetrodotoxin (to block sodium ion currents) by eliciting calcium ion transients with 100–500 ms pressure pulses of 0.1–0.2 M KCl (in sodium-free SES) from a glass pipette (o.d. 3–5 μm) at 50–100 μm distance from the pyramidal cell. Fluorescence signals were analysed using confocal laser scanning microscopy (MultiProbe 2001, Molecular Dynamics) over the area of the whole pericaryon central optical section of a single cell, in the 32-line rapid scan mode (temporal resolution of 320 ms per section). Maximal amplitude (ΔF) and area (A) under the signal peak were measured and expressed as percentage of control. The data are presented as mean values ± SEM and are statistically analysed by paired *t*-test or ANOVA analysis of variance for grouped data. In situ calibration experiments (6) showed that intracellular calcium ion concentration ranged from 41 ± 5 nM ($n = 5$) at rest to 296 ± 96 nM at the peak of the response. Preliminary measurements were also performed on clusters of cells by scanning larger pixel arrays with 4 s per section time resolution. Calcium ion transients were elicited in the absence of tetrodotoxin, with 1 s pressure pulses of 1 M KCl from 200–300 μm distance. In all of the above experiments cells were continuously superfused (1–2 ml/min) with SES.

Three female ALS patients (aged 70.7 ± 5.4; 1.2 ± 0.2 y illness duration; one had been treated with intravenous TRH) and three healthy donors (two males and one female; aged 55.3 ± 2.7 y) provided the sera from which IgGs were obtained using affinity chromatography (protein A-sepharose) as previously reported (2). Aliquots of IgGs (0.1 mg/ml in SES), kept frozen until use, were applied by pressure (10–20 s or 1 s duration for single or cell clusters, respectively) through a pipette 50–100 or 200–300 μm from the cell soma or cell cluster, respectively. Drugs were either bath-applied or delivered by a pressure pipette.

RESULTS

The transient rise in $[Ca^{2+}]_i$ elicited by potassium chloride was abolished by calcium-free medium or reduced by cadmium (0.1–0.2 mM) to 44 ± 4% and 34 ± 4% of control ΔF and A values, respectively ($n = 14$, $p < 0.01$, paired *t*-test applied to raw data Fig. 15.1 A,B). These data suggest that the potassium chloride-induced rise in $[Ca^{2+}]_i$ was dependent on influx through voltage-activated calcium ion channels. In the presence of cadmium the residual response was fully blocked by the ionotropic glutamate receptor antagonist CNQX (20 μM; $n = 4$; Fig. 15.1B), indicating that endogenous glutamate released by KCl participated in the rise in $[Ca^{2+}O]_i$. One approach of the present study was to eliminate such an indirect effect by applying the glutamate receptor antagonists CNQX (10 μM) or kynurenic acid (1 mM). The

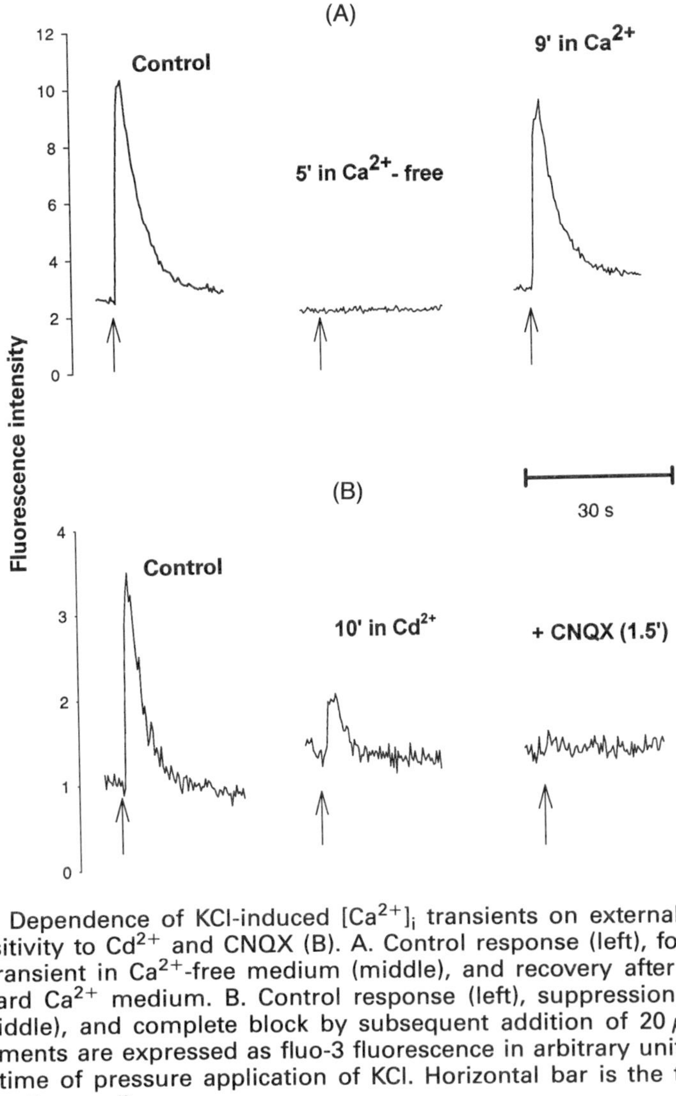

Fig. 15.1 Dependence of KCl-induced $[Ca^{2+}]_i$ transients on external Ca^{2+} (A) and sensitivity to Cd^{2+} and CNQX (B). A. Control response (left), followed by lack of transient in Ca^{2+}-free medium (middle), and recovery after returning to standard Ca^{2+} medium. B. Control response (left), suppression by 50 μM Cd^{2+} (middle), and complete block by subsequent addition of 20 μM CNQX. Measurements are expressed as fluo-3 fluorescence in arbitrary units. Arrows indicate time of pressure application of KCl. Horizontal bar is the time scale (30 s) for all recordings.

relative contribution of different types of calcium ion channel (4,7) to the potassium chloride-induced $[Ca^{2+}]_i$ rise was then dissected out by applying blockers selective for the L, N or P/Q type of channel (nifedipine, ω-conotoxin GVIA or ω-agatoxin IVA, respectively). As shown by the histograms (open columns) in Fig. 15.2 (top and bottom), nifedipine (10 μM) ω-conotoxin GVIA (5 μM) and ω-agatoxin IVA (200 nM) reduced ΔF to

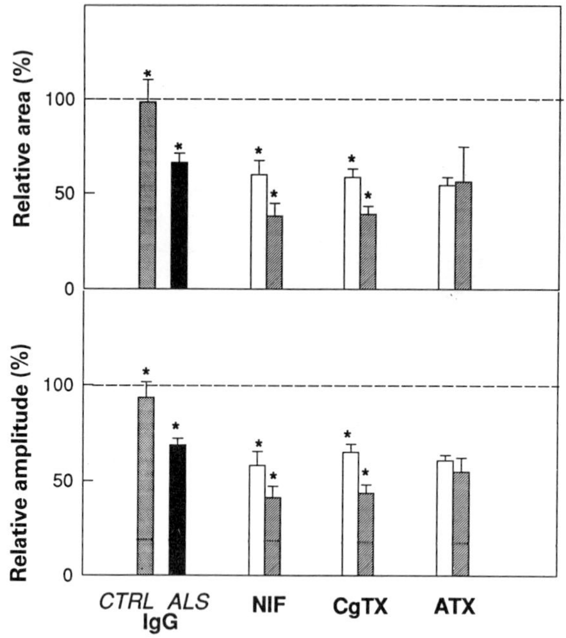

Fig. 15.2 Effects of IgGs from healthy (control) donors or from ALS patients on KCl-induced responses and the effect of selective blockers of voltage-activated Ca^{2+} channels. Each bar represents the mean relative area (*A*, top graph) or amplitude (ΔF, bottom graph) of response obtained 3–5 min after 10–20 s pulse application of IgGs. CTRL is the mean from three control subjects (n = 15 where n indicates the number of cells tested) while ALS is from three ALS patients (n = 33), obtained for responses in 1 mM kynurenic acid (n = 44) or in 10 μM CNQX (n = 4; ALS IgG treated) solution. Open bars: response mean after action of selective blockers of voltage-activated Ca^{2+} channels, namely nifedipine (NIF), ω-conotoxin GVIA (CgTX) and ω-agatoxin IVA (AgTX); hatched bars: effect of ALS IgGs on cells pretreated with Ca^{2+} blockers (n = 7, 11, and 6, respectively). Error bars are SEM. Asterisks indicate significantly different pairs of mean values (Student's t-test $p < 0.01$). Responses were normalized with respect to control data taken as 100% (dashed horizontal line).

58 ± 7, 67 ± 5 and 62 ± 4%, respectively (n = 8–13). Corresponding *A* values were 60 ± 7, 60 ± 5 and 54 ± 6%.

Unlike the ineffective IgGs from healthy donors, ALS IgGs, applied 3–5 min before potassium chloride, irreversibly reduced $[Ca^{2+}]_i$ transients by about 30% ($\Delta F = 68 \pm 3\%$. $A = 66 \pm 5\%$; n = 33; Fig. 15.2). In order to assess if any particular calcium ion channel was the target of ALS IgGs, the calcium ion channel blockers listed above were applied prior to ALS IgGs. ALS IgGs still reduced calcium ion transients in cells pretreated with 5 μM ω-conotoxin GVIA or 10 μM nifedipine ($\Delta F = 69 \pm 6\%$, $A = 68 \pm 8\%$,

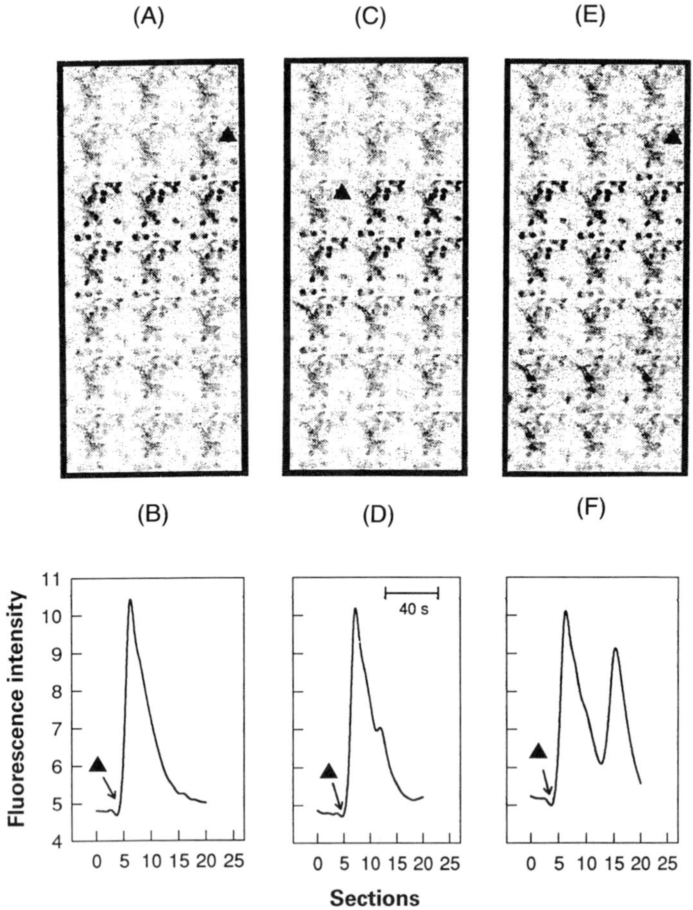

Fig. 15.3 Delayed response to KCl in a cell cluster after ALS IgG application. Top (A, C, E): Serial display (in a rastered fashion) of confocal sections (from left to right, starting from top left) each taken every 4 s. Bottom (B, D, F): response curves obtained by measuring the fluorescence intensity (arbitrary units) over the whole area of each section (abscissa) from the corresponding series above (40 s bar in D indicates the time scaling). A, B: control response; C, D: response 6 min after pressure application (1 s) of ALS IgGs; E, F: response after 6 min of subsequent application (3 s) of ALS IgGs. Black triangles indicate time points of KCl pressure application (1 s).

$n = 11$ or $\Delta F = 58 \pm 7\%$, $A = 60 \pm 7\%$, $n = 8$, respectively) although they failed to do so in those superfused with ω-agatoxin IVA ($\Delta F = 89 \pm 9\%$, $A = 98 \pm 25\%$, $n = 6$; compare open and hatched columns in Fig. 15.2). The effect of ω-agatoxin IVA on neurons already pretreated with ALS IgGs was also tested and found to be absent (amplitude of the response normalized to the response after ALS IgG treatment was $97 \pm 5\%$, $n = 3$; not shown).

Preliminary experiments were also performed with cell clusters without adding tetrodotoxin or ionotropic glutamate receptor antagonists. An example of such an experiment is shown in Fig. 15.3. Each image section (whose intensity was measured over the whole section area of the cell group) was obtained after a 4 s scanning period and repeated for about 80 s, as shown by the rastered display of the fluorescence signal as depicted in Fig. 15.3 A,C,E. It can be seen that after 1 s pressure application of potassium chloride some cells within the group responded with a transient rise in $[Ca^{2+}]_i$ (Fig. 15.3 A,B). After 1 s application of ALS IgGs, potassium chloride induced a similar transient response in the same cells but a later response was also recorded in another subgroup of cells (Fig. 15.13 C) giving rise to a hump in the recovery phase of the $[Ca^{2+}]_i$ transient curve (Fig. 15.3 D). Subsequent pressure application of ALS IgGs for 3 s recruited even more cells for the delayed response which thus became more apparent (Fig. 15.3 E,F).

DISCUSSION

The principal finding of the present study is that ALS IgGs reduced potassium chloride-induced $[Ca^{2+}]_i$ transients by an apparently selective action on the P/Q type of voltage-activated calcium ion channels. This effect developed with a delay as short as the one reported for the action of ALS IgGs on L-type calcium ion channels reconstituted in artificial bilayers (8) presumably because of a relatively unrestricted access of focally applied IgGs to their target. The present data accord with previous electrophysiological studies demonstrating a strong depression of high-voltage activated calcium ion channels in central neurons (2) or skeletal muscle (8,9) and provide pharmacological characterization of the subtype of calcium ion channel involved in the effect on neurons. Unlike the present data, ALS IgGs were found to enhance the P type of calcium ion channel in cerebellar Purkinje cells (3). This discrepancy might be due to different methodologies – whole cell patch clamp recording rather than imaging of intact cells – or by the use of barium instead of calcium as a charge carrier. Furthermore, changes in subunit composition of calcium ion channels between Purkinje and pyramidal neurons may also account for this difference (10). ALS IgG-induced fall in somatic $[Ca^{2+}]_i$ transients may not be incompatible with the excitotoxicity theory. In fact, blocking of calcium ion influx through voltage-dependent channels, such as the P type, is expected to enhance the action of glutamate on central neurons by suppressing the $[Ca^{2+}]_i$-dependent desensitization of NMDA receptors which normally limits excitability (11–13). This phenomenon might largely amplify glutamate responses up to excitotoxicity and neuronal death. Moreover, in a set of experiments on cell clusters it was observed that ALS IgGs induce a delayed response to potassium chloride in previously unresponsive cells. Since these experiments were not done with antagonists of glutamate receptors, the delay in the ALS IgG-induced response to potassium chloride may indicate that these cells were actually sensitized to endogenously released glutamate. This hypothesis is further underlined by the observation that in some cultured cells treatment with ALS IgGs induced sensitization of the response to exogenously applied glutamate (5 mM, 100–500 ms pressure application, from 200 μm above the cells; not shown). These preliminary results on cell clusters justify further studies which should be aimed at the precise identification of responsive cells, and at the specificity of this effect by testing IgGs from healthy donors or from patients with motoneuron pathologies other than ALS.

CONCLUSIONS

Confocal laser scanning microscopy (with the fluorescent calcium dye fluo-3) was used to test the involvement of ALS IgGs in $[Ca^{2+}]_i$ changes induced by potassium chloride on rat hippocampal neurons in culture. Potassium chloride-induced transient $[Ca^{2+}]_i$ rise was partially blocked (60% of response) by cadmium and was completely abolished in calcium-free medium. In presence of an inhibitor of ionotropic glutamate receptors (CNQX or kynurenic acid) the potassium chloride-induced response was affected by specific blockers of L-, N- or P/Q-type voltage-gated calcium ion channels (nifedipine, ω-conotoxin GVIA or ω-agatoxin IVA, respectively) each suppressing the $[Ca^{2+}]_i$ transient by about 30–40%. In presence of CNQX or kynurenic acid, ALS IgGs evoked a depression of the potassium-induced response which did not occur with IgGs from healthy donors. This depression was prevented by the inhibitor of P/Q-type calcium ion channels, ω-agatoxin IVA, while inhibitors of L- or N-type channels were ineffective. In experiments on cell clusters it was observed that ALS IgGs induced a delayed response to potassium chloride in previously unresponsive cells. Since in these experiments glutamate receptors were not blocked, the delay in the ALS IgG-induced response to potassium chloride may indicate that these cells were actually sensitized to endogenously released glutamate.

ACKNOWLEDGEMENTS

This work was supported by a grant (n. 502) from the Telethon Foundation. IgGs from ALS patients were kindly provided by Dr P. Annunziata (Istituto di Scienze Neurologiche, Facoltá di Medicina e Chirurgía, Siena, Italy).

REFERENCES

1. Appel, S. H., J. I. Engelhardt, J. Garcia and E. Stefani. 1991. Immunoglobulins from animal models of motor neuron disease and from human amyotrophic lateral sclerosis patients passively transfer physiological abnormalities to the neuromuscular junction. *Proc. Natl. Acad. Sci. USA* **88**:647–51.
2. Zhainazarov, A. B., P. Annunziata, S. Toneatto *et al.* 1994. Serum fractions from amyotrophic lateral sclerosis patients depress voltage-activated Ca^{2+} currents of rat cerebellar granule cells in culture. *Neurosci. Lett.* **172**:111–4.
3. Llinas, R., M. Sugimori, B. D. Cherksey *et al.* 1993. IgG from amyotrophic lateral sclerosis patients increases current through P-type calcium channels in mammalian cerebellar Purkinje cells and in isolated channel protein in lipid bilayer. *Proc. Natl. Acad. Sci. USA* **90**:11743–7.
4. Mogul, D. J. and A. P. Fox. 1991. Evidence for multiple types of Ca^{2+} channels in acutely isolated hippocampal CA3 neurones of the guinea-pig. *J. Physiol.* **433**:259–81.
5. Malgaroli, A. and R. W. Tsien. 1992. Glutamate-induced long-term potentiation of the frequency of miniature synaptic currents in cultured hippocampal neurones. *Nature* **357**:134–9.
6. Kao, J. P. Y., A. T. Harootunian and R. Y. Tsien. 1989. Photochemically generated cytosolic calcium pulses and their detection by fluo-3. *J. Biol. Chem.* **264**:8179–84.
7. Brown, A. M., R. J. Sayer, P. C. Schwindt and W. E. Crill. 1994. P-type calcium channels in rat neocortical neurones. *J. Physiol.* **475**:197–205.
8. Magnelli, V., T. Sawada, O. Delbono *et al.* 1993. The action of amyotrophic lateral sclerosis immunoglobulins on mammalian single skeletal muscle Ca^{2+} channels. *J. Physiol.* **461**:103–18.
9. Delbono, O., J. Garcia, S. H. Appel and E. Stefani. 1991. IgG from amyotrophic lateral sclerosis affects tubular calcium channels of skeletal muscle. *Am. J. Physiol. Neurosci.* **260**:C1347–C1351.
10. Hofmann, F., M. Biel and V. Flockerzi. 1994. Molecular basis for Ca^{2+} channel diversity. *Annu. Rev Neurosci.* **17**:399–418.
11. Tong, G., D. Shepard and E. J. Craig. 1995. Synaptic desensitization of NMDA receptors by calcineurin. *Science* **267**:1510–12.
12. Medina, I., N. Filippova, G. Barbin *et al.* 1994. Kainate-induced inactivation of NMDA currents via an elevation of intracellular Ca^{2+} in hippocampal neurons. *J. Neurophysiol.* **72**:456–65.
13. Medina, I., N. Filippova, G. Charton *et al.* 1995. Calcium-dependent inactivation of heteromeric NMDA receptor-channels expressed in human embryonic kidney cells. *J. Physiol.* **482**:567–73.

16

Strain-dependent Induction and Modulation of Autoimmunity by Mercuric Chloride in Two Strains of Rats

Sanja Mijatović, Lota Ejdus, Vera Pravica,
Stanislava Stošić-Grujičić and Miodrag L. Lukić

Mercuric chloride induces an autoimmune syndrome in susceptible strains of experimental animals. Disease is characterized by the appearance of various autoantibodies such as anti-glomerular basal membrane (a-GBM) and non-organ specific anti-nuclear and anti-nucleolar antibodies (ANA) (1), followed by intensive proteinuria as a consequence of kidney tissue damage caused by anti-GBM antibodies and/or immune complex deposits (1). The cellular and molecular mechanisms by which mercuric chloride exerts its effects are not fully explained. The agent has a propensity to bind to sulfhydryl groups of proteins and non-protein tiols, modifying them.

It has been suggested that chemical modification of MHC class II molecules, T-cell receptors, autoantigenic peptides, or some other cell surface molecules result in formation of altered self structures, promoting autoreactive responses (2). Additionally, several lines of evidence suggest that mercuric chloride induces T-cell dependent polyclonal B-cell activation (3).

More recently, mercuric chloride-induced autoimmunity was related to the balance of different subpopulation of T helper (Th) cells. Two different $CD4^+$ T cell subsets, named Th1 and Th2, have been characterized in rodents (4) and humans (5). Th1 cells, responsible for cell-mediated immunity and complement activating antibodies, produce predominantly IL-2 and IFNγ, while Th2 cells produce mainly IL-4, IL-5, and IL-10 and are related to

Immunoregulation in Health and Disease
ISBN 0-12-459460-3

allergic and non-cytotoxic antibody production (4). We have previously shown that Albino Oxford (AO) rats are low producers of IFNγ and IL-2, and do not develop Th1 cytokine-mediated autoimmunity such as experimental allergic encephalomyelitis (EAE) (6) and chemically induced autoimmune diabetes (7). In contrast, Dark August (DA) rats are high producers of Th1 cytokines and they are susceptible to these autoimmune disorders (6,7). Bearing this in mind, one would expect that these two strains differ in susceptibility to Th2 mediated autoimmune diseases as well. We therefore examined the strain differences in susceptibility to mercuric chloride-induced autoimmune syndrome in AO and DA rats and possible mechanisms responsible for development and/or resistance to mercury disease.

MATERIALS AND METHODS

Animals

Inbred AO and DA male rats, 3–4 months old, were obtained from our own facilities.

Experimental protocol and determination of proteinuria

Mercuric chloride (Kemika, Zagreb, Yugoslavia) was administered subcutaneously at a dose of 1 mg/kg body weight over the 10-day period, at 2-day intervals. Twenty-four-hour urinary protein loss was measured at 7-day intervals by Bradford's method (8) and presented as protein/creatinin (PRT/Cre) index. At day 45, the animals were killed and the renal tissue snap-frozen in liquid nitrogen.

Immunofluorescence analysis

The presence of immune complexes (IC) in kidney tissue was evaluated by indirect immunofluorescence analysis. Mouse anti-rat κ-chain (OX-12) mAb (Serotec, UK) was used as primary antibody followed by rabbit anti-mouse IgG conjugated with FITC (INEP, Zemun, Yugoslavia). Presence of ANA in animal sera was tested on frozen normal rat liver section, as described previously (9).

The percentage of $CD8^+$ cells in spleen mononuclear cell population was determined by indirect immunofluorescence and flow cytometry. Cells were incubated with mouse anti-rat CD8 (OX8, Serotec) mAb, or with an irrelevant mAb as a negative control. FITC-conjugated rabbit anti-mouse IgG was added as a second antibody. Cells were analysed on an Epics flow cytometer (Coulter Corp.).

Mixed leukocyte reactions

Non-adherent lymph node cells (5×10^6) were cultured in RPMI 1640 with 5% FCS (Flow, Scotland) in flat-bottom microculture plates (Falcon, 3040 Microtest IL, USA) with mitomycin C (Sigma, USA)-inactivated (50 μg/ml) syngeneic thymocytes (5×10^6) as stimulatory cells in a volume of 200 μl. After 6 days of incubation at 37°C in humidified atmosphere with 5% carbon dioxide cells were pulsed with 1 μCi of ^{3}H-thymidine (^{3}H-TdR, Amersham) for 18 h before harvesting.

Measurement of IFNγ and IL-2

Production of IFNγ and IL-2 was determined in supernatants of Con A-stimulated (5 μg/ml) mononuclear spleen cells (5×10^6) cultured for 2 days in 1 ml volume. An enzyme-linked immunosorbent assay (ELISA) was performed for detection of IFNγ using an ELISA kit specific for rat IFNγ (Holland Biotechnology). Determination of IL-2 was performed by using a CTLL cell bioassay (10).

Quantification of blood eosinophils

The relative number of eosinophils was determined in the blood smears. Samples were stained by Giemsa May–Grunwald and the number of eosinophils was presented as the percentage of eosinophils in the total leukocyte population.

Induction of experimental autoimmune diabetes

Diabetes was induced by multiple low doses (MLD) of streptozotocin (SZ, Sigma, 20 mg/kg body weight, given intraperitoneally for 5 consecutive days). In order to evaluate possible modulatory effects of mercuric chloride, rats were treated with the agent at 2-day intervals given subcutaneously in 3–5 consecutive doses of 1 mg/kg per day. The treatment with mercuric chloride started either concomitantly with MLD-SZ treatment, or on day 10 after the first SZ injection. The development of the disease was determined by measuring plasma glucose level at 7-day intervals, using the glucose oxidase technique.

RESULTS AND DISCUSSION

AO and DA rats, characterized as 'low' and 'high' producers of Th1 cytokines respectively, differ in susceptibility to Th1 cytokines dependent autoimmunity (6,7). On the basis of these data we examined whether genetically determined high and low Th1 cytokine production influenced the susceptibility to autoimmune disorder induced by mercuric chloride. We examined production of different autoantibodies such as ANA, presence of IC in renal tissue and proteinuria after the induction of mercuric chloride-induced autoimmunity. In the sera obtained from AO rats treated with mercuric chloride, ANA were found in maximal titre from days 17 to 25 after the first injection of mercuric chloride (data not shown). The same treatment of DA rats did not provoke the production of ANA (not shown). Further, IC deposits were found in renal tissue in mercuric chloride-treated AO rats but not in DA rats (data not shown). We also analysed protein level in the urine. The treatment of AO rats with mercuric chloride induced transient proteinuria between the 4th and 5th weeks after induction of the disease, in comparison to their non-treated controls (data not shown). In contrast, the urine protein level of mercuric chloride-treated DA rats was normal, similar to non-treated DA rats. These results indicate that in response to mercuric chloride AO rats develop immunopathologic manifestations of Th2 cytokine-related systemic autoimmune diseases, such as production of various autoantibodies followed by renal tissue damages.

There is evidence that mercuric chloride induces T-cell mediated autoreactive response against MHC class II molecules (11). The presence of these autoreactive cells could be tested in syngeneic mixed lymphocyte culture. Mercuric chloride pretreatment significantly stimulated the proliferative response to the syngeneic inactivated host, the T cells derived from AO rats. On the other hand, there was no difference in proliferative response to self antigens between DA rats receiving mercuric chloride and non-treated animals. These differences were found on days 17, 21 (Fig. 16.1) and 39 after the first mercuric chloride injection. These results, thus, show the strain differences in autoreactivity after administration of mercuric chloride, with intensive autoreactive response detected in AO rats, in contrast to the DA strain.

In order to understand a possible mechanism responsible for the protection of DA rats against mercuric chloride-induced autoimmunity, we analysed production of the relevant cytokines following the induction of mercury disease. We found that 6 days after the first mercuric chloride injection, the spleen cells derived from DA rats produced twelvefold more IFNγ and threefold more IL-2 than a saline-treated control. However, mercuric chloride treatment did not affect the production of IFNγ and IL-2 in AO rats (data not shown). Bearing in mind that the Th1 and Th2 type cytokines are reciprocally regulated (5), our results may indicate that the resistance of DA rats to Th2-mediated mercuric chloride-induced autoimmunity is a consequence of higher production of Th1 cytokines, which in turn down-regulated Th2 cytokine production. Up-regulation of IFNγ production after mercuric chloride treatment in DA rats may be due to the increase of $CD8^{+}$ cells as IFNγ-producing cells in these animals, as already shown by others (12) and by us (13).

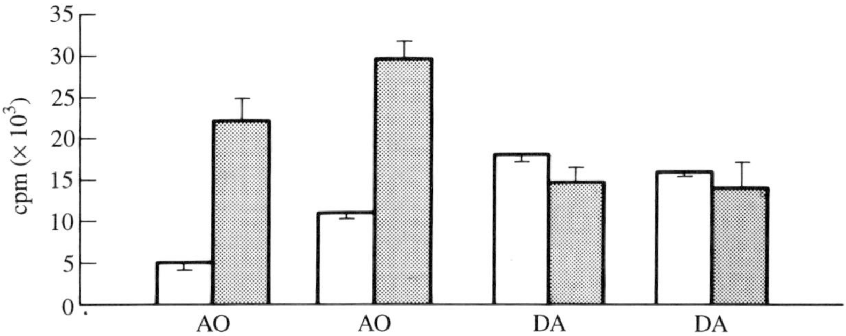

Fig. 16.1 Syngeneic mixed leukocyte reaction in AO and DA rats treated (white bars) and non-treated (dark bars) at day 21 after the first mercuric chloride injection. The results represent the values of two individual animals of each group.

Although mercuric chloride did not induce autoimmune manifestations in DA rats, it was of interest to find out whether it promoted any Th2-dependent activity. Knowing that proliferation and differentiation of eosinophils are IL-5 dependent (14), development of eosinophilia could be indirect proof for increased production of Th2 cytokines. Our results revealed that DA rats developed mild eosinophilia in response to mercuric chloride (Fig. 16.2). However, the number of eosinophils was significantly lower in these animals compared to mercuric chloride-treated AO rats, and the observed mild increase might be related to enhanced Th2 cell activity even in the DA strain, which is resistant to mercuric chloride-induced autoimmunity. In order to confirm this we designed another experimental approach, based on the fact that the Th1 and Th2 subpopulations are reciprocally regulated and that enhanced production of Th2 cytokines might inhibit the development of Th1-dependent autoimmune diseases as IDDM (15), or EAE (16). For this purpose, we used MLD-SZ-induced autoimmune diabetes as a Th1-associated disease (17). Administration of mercuric chloride during the induction of MLD-SZ diabetes in DA rats resulted in suppression of the disease development. Animals which received MLD-SZ only developed sustained hyperglycemia, but in mercuric chloride-treated animals the plasma glucose level was significantly lower. The protective effect of mercuric chloride was observed when the treatment started during the induction of diabetes with SZ (Fig. 16.3), and was even more pronounced if started 10 days later (not shown). These data suggest that mercuric chloride affects the autoimmune process rather than the initial SZ-induced damage of the islets. Mercury-induced suppression of diabetes in DA rats is another indirect proof for enhanced Th2 cell activity in this strain in response to mercuric chloride.

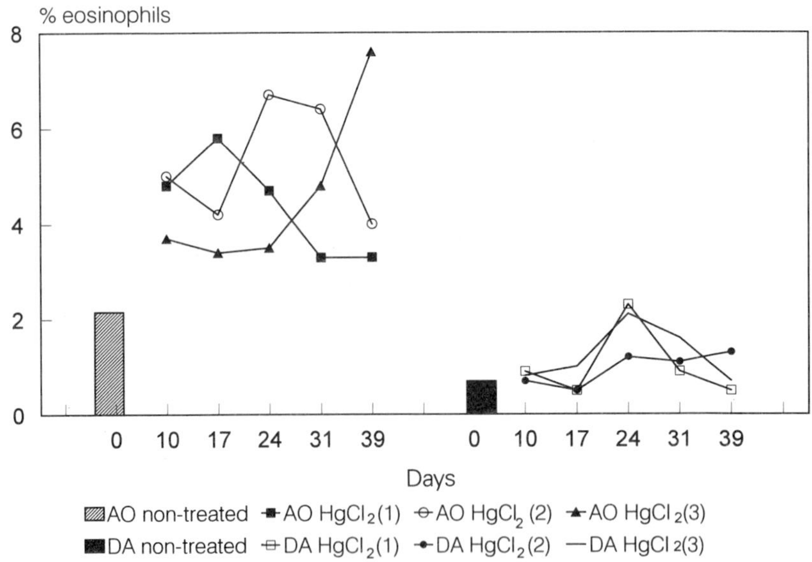

Fig. 16.2 Eosinophilia in AO and DA rats treated with mercuric chloride. Percentage of eosinophils was calculated in relation to total leukocyte number in peripheral blood.

It has to be assumed that the production of Th2 cytokine in DA rats was sufficient to down-regulate the T-cell–macrophage-mediated autoimmune process despite enhanced Th1 production. Conversely, enhanced IFNγ production in DA rats probably prevents the triggering of antibody-mediated autoaggression readily seen in IFNγ 'low' producer AO rats.

Taken together, results presented here and elsewhere illustrate that the pattern of chemically induced autoimmunity is dependent on the genetically determined pattern of cytokine production.

CONCLUSIONS

Multiple subtoxic doses of mercuric chloride have a potent effect on the immune system of rats and the outcome of this treatment is strain dependent. In the AO strain, resistant to Th1 type organ-specific autoimmune diseases, administration of mercuric chloride results in production of various autoantibodies, followed by systemic autoimmune disorders and causing renal tissue damages. Increased activity of the Th2 subset with corresponding cytokine production may be in the background of the autoimmune response. In contrast, the DA strain, susceptible to Th1-mediated autoimmune diseases, did not develop autoantibodies and related manifestations in

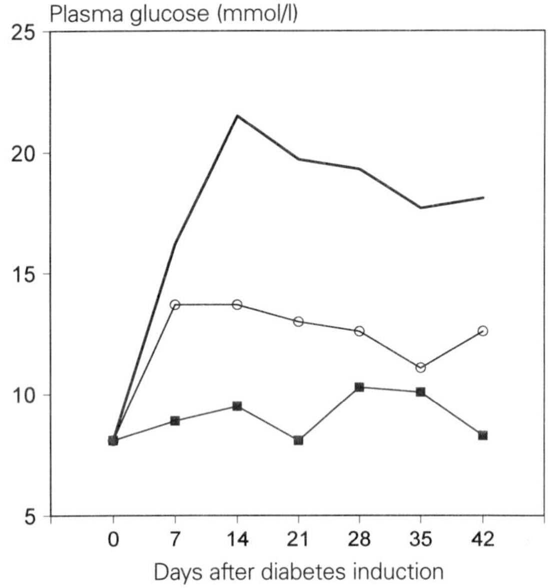

Fig. 16.3 Treatment with mercuric chloride has down-modulatory effect on MLD-SZ induced diabetes. Administration of mercuric chloride (1 mg/kg per day, at 2-day intervals) was from days 0 to +4 in relation to MLD-SZ treatment (20 mg/kg per day, 5 consecutive days). Bold line, SZ only; black squares, mercuric chloride only; white circles, SZ plus mercuric chloride.

response to mercuric chloride. Although in DA rats this treatment probably promoted Th2 cytokine synthesis, indirectly proved by eosinophilia and inhibition of autoimmune diabetes, as in Th1-mediated disease, the net effect could be down-modulation of Th2 response due to the overproduction of Th1 cytokines.

REFERENCES

1. Rossert, J., L. Pelletier, R. Pasqier and P. Druet. 1988. Autoreactive T cells in mercury induced autoimmunity. Demonstration by limiting dilution analysis. *Eur. J. Immunol.* **18**:1761–6.
2. Christopher, L. R. and D. O. Lucas. 1987. Heavy-metal mitogenesis: Zn^{++} and Hg^{++} induce cellular cytotoxicity and interferon production in murine T lymphocytes. *Immunobiology* **175**:455–69.
3. Goldman, M., P. Druet and E. Gleichmann. 1991. Th2 cells in systemic autoimmunity: insights from allogeneic diseases and chemically-induced autoimmunity. *Immunol. Today* **12**:223–7.
4. Mossman, T. R. and R. L. Coffman. 1989. Th1 and Th2 cells: different patterns

of lymphokine secretion lead to different functional properties. *Annu. Rev. Immunol.* **7**:145–51.

5. Haanen, J. B. A. G., R. De Waal Malefijt and P. C. M. Res. 1991. Selection of human T helper type 1-like T cell subset by mycobacteria. *J. Exp. Med.* **174**:583–92.
6. Vukmanović, S., M. Mostarica and M. L. Lukić. 1989. Experimental autoimmune encephalomyelitis in 'low' and 'high' interleukin-2 producer rats. *Cell. Immunol.* **121**:238–46.
7. Lukić, M. L., R. Al-Sharif, M. Mostarica *et al.* 1991. Immunological basis of the strain differences in susceptibility to low-dose streptozotocin-induced diabetes in rats. In: *Lymphatic Tissues and In Vivo Immune Response* (B. A. Imhof, S. Berrih-Aknin and S. Ezine, eds.) Marcel Dekker, New York, pp. 643–7.
8. Bradford, M. M. 1976. A rapid and sensitive method for the quantification of protein utilizing the principle of protein-Pyc binding. *Anal. Biochem.* **72**:248–54.
9. Fritzler, M. J. 1986. Immunofluorescent antinuclear antibody tests. In: *Manual of Clinical Laboratory Immunology* (Noel L. Rose, Hermnan Friedman, John L. Fahey, eds.) American Society for Microbiology, Washington, DC, pp. 733–40.
10. Hamblin, A. S. and A. O'Garra. 1987. Assay of IL-2 on CTLL cells. In: *Lymphocytes – A Practical Approach.* (G. G. B. Klaus, ed.) National Institute for Medical Research, London, p. 213.
11. Dubey, C., B. Bellon, F. Hirch *et al.* 1991. Increased expression of class II major histocompatibility complex molecules on B cells in rats susceptible or resistant to $HgCl_2$-induced autoimmunity. *Clin. Exp. Immunol.* **86**:118–23.
12. Castedo, M., L. Pelletier, J. Rossert *et al.* 1993. Mercury-induced autoreactive anti-class II T cell line protects from experimental autoimmune encephalomyelitis by the bias of $CD8^+$ antiergotypic cells in Lewis rats. *J. Exp. Med.* **177**:881–9.
13. Stošić-Grujićić, S., S. Mijatović, L. Ejdus, and M. L. Lukić. 1996. Enhancement of Th2 type activity down-regulated diabetes induction. *Trans. Proc.* **28**:3260.
14. Holgate, S. T. and M. K. Church. 1993. *Allergy*. Gower Medical Publishing, London, pp. 733–40.
15. Liblau, R. S., S. M. Singer and H. O. McDevitt. 1995. Thl and Th2 $CD4^+$ T cells in the pathogenesis of organ-specific autoimmune diseases. *Immunol. Today* **16**:34–8.
16. Racke, M. K., A. Bonomo, D. E. Scot *et al.* 1994. Cytokine-induced immune deviation as a therapy for inflammatory autoimmune disease. *J. Exp. Med.* **180**:1961–6.
17. Lukić, M. L., V. Pravica, S. Stošić and A. Shanin. 1995. Cytokine network determines susceptibility to low dose streptozotocin-induced diabetes. *Int. J. Diabetes* **3**:150–7.

17

An Excess of IL-6 Production in the Early Muscle Stage of *Trichinella spiralis* Infection in Mice is Associated with Strain Susceptibility to Infection

Ljiljana Sofronić-Milosavljević, Kosta Čuperlović, Nada Pejnović, Zorka Kukić and Aleksandar Dujić

The immune response elicited by *Trichinella spiralis* (TS) infection is very complex. This complexity is influenced particularly by the stage specificity of parasite antigens and different localization of each stage in the body (1). Therefore, infection with this nematode induces extensive tissue injury at different places in the organism depending on the stage of the life cycle (2,3). The immune response is characterized by elevated antibody levels of all isotypes and by marked immune-mediated inflammation with powerful immunopathological consequences for the host (4).

The pattern of cytokines secreted by T cells and other cells involved in the response to an infectious agent can determine the success with which the host fights the infection, but may also modify overall immune reactivity of the host (5,6). The TS–host relationship might result in a wide range of immune aberrations. These include suppression of the immune response to other T-dependent antigens (7), suppression of skin allograft rejection (8), increased susceptibility to other pathogens (9) and potentiation of the immune response to some bacterial infections or malignancies (10,11).

In addition to previously described alterations we provided evidence that

Immunoregulation in Health and Disease
ISBN 0-12-459460-3

TS infection may enhance autoreactivity. In two inbred mouse strains, BALB/c (H-2^d) and C57Bl/6 (H-2^b), we observed that the appearance of autoantibodies provoked by trauma in the C57Bl/6 strain was significantly amplified when the injury was combined with TS infection (12). It is suggested that increased IL-6 production can influence autoantibody synthesis through induction of polyclonal B-cell proliferation (13). In this study we investigated the difference in IL-6 production between the above-mentioned strains of mouse infected with TS. This study was performed 3 weeks after infection, e.g. when the phenomenon of autoantibody synthesis amplification was observed and when the final stage of parasite development commenced, accompanied by muscle inflammation.

MATERIALS AND METHODS

Mice

Female BALB/c and C57Bl/6 mice (8–10 weeks of age, 19–22 g body weight, bred in animal facilities of the Institute for Medical Research, MMA, Belgrade) were used in the experiments. Mice of each strain were randomly divided into 2 groups containing 10 animals per group. They were exposed to TS infection (group TS) and a control group (C) of non-treated mice. Mice were sacrificed on day 21 for the determination of muscle larva recovery, production of specific antibodies and analysis of IL-6 cytokine production.

Parasite

Trichinella spiralis, maintained by periodical passage in Wistar rats at INEP, was shown to belong to the T1 gene pool, by Dr. E. Pozio, Instituto Superiore di Sanità, Rome.

TS infection

Infectious L1 larvae were obtained by digestion of minced TS-infected rat carcasses in 1% pepsin-HCl for 4 h at 37°C. The mice were infected by oesophageal intubation with 200 L1 larvae each.

Muscle larva recovery

The number of developed L1 larvae in experimental mice was determined after enzymatic digestion of the mouse carcass and expressed as reproductive capacity index (RCI = larvae recovered/larvae administered).

L1 crude antigen preparation

L1 larvae were sonicated on ice until the cuticles were disrupted. The suspensions were centrifuged at $9000 \times g$ for 30 min, dialyzed against phosphate-buffered saline and stored at −80°C.

Enzyme-linked immunosorbent assay (ELISA)

Serum samples from each infected mouse were analysed for antibody production to TS L1 excretory-secretory (ES) antigens by enzyme linked immunosorbent assay (ELISA) (14). Isotype-specific analyses were done using polyclonal goat, biotin labelled, anti-mouse antibodies (anti IgG1, anti IgG2a and IgG2b) (Amersham International, Bucks, UK). Avidin-Peroxidase (Sigma, USA) and TMB (Sigma, USA) were applied in the test. The results of the ELISA were estimated by the reading of optical density (OD) at 450 nm. The cut-off value for each ELISA test was set at 0.1 OD. All negative control sera were below this value.

IL-6 cytokine production

Spleen cell suspensions were diluted to 5×10^6 cells/ml in RPMI 1640 (ICN, Flow) medium with 2% FCS (ICN, Flow), 5×10^{-5} M 2 ME and antibiotics and cultured in 24-well flat-bottomed culture plates. 1 ml of cell suspension was supplemented with 5 μg Con A (INEP, Zemun) or 100 μg L1 crude antigen preparations for 24 h at 37°C in a humidified atmosphere containing 5% carbon dioxide. Cells cultured in medium alone were used as controls. At the end of incubation, cell supernatants were collected and frozen at −20°C until tested.

Units of IL-6 were defined by their capacity to stimulate the hybridoma cell line B9. Briefly, 2.5×10^3 cells/well were cultured in 96-well plates for 66–68 h with different dilutions of the supernatants (four replicates per dilution). The number of cells was assessed by the MTT colorimetric test (reading at 570 nm). Cytokine activity is expressed as stimulatory units/ml (IU/ml) using human rIL-6 (Genzyme) as a standard. Values are expressed as mean ± SE. The sensitivity of the assay was 0.0025 IU/ml.

The data were analysed using Student's t test; p levels less than or equal to 0.05 were considered to be significant.

RESULTS AND DISCUSSION

Muscle larva recovery and detection of TS specific antibodies

The outcome of the infection with 200 L1 larvae in the two strains is presented in Fig. 17.1. BALB/c mice harboured approximately 50% fewer L1 larvae in their muscles than C57Bl/6 mice. This confirmed previous findings, since BALB/c mice are considered to be resistant and C57Bl/6 susceptible with respect to muscle larva burden (15). The lower larva burden in BALB/c mice correlated with the higher production, as evaluated by optical density and extended repertoire of the antibody response compared to C57Bl/6. IgG isotype analyses revealed that in BALB/c mice antibodies were IgG1, IgG2a and IgG2b while in C57Bl/6 only the IgG1 subclass was detected (Fig. 17.1). Sera of non-infected mice contained no detectable antibodies of any class to TS (data not shown). This confirmed the results of other authors (16), who observed that the TS-resistant AKR strain of mice produced more TS-specific IgG2a than susceptible B10.BR mice (both strains share the H-2^k haplotype).

IL-6 cytokine production

On Con A stimulation (Fig. 17.2), cell supernatants from control animals of both strains had almost the same amount of detected IL-6. On TS infection, IL-6 released in stimulated cultures increased in both strains. This increase, however, was much higher in susceptible C57Bl/6 animals. The main difference in the level of IL-6 production was obtained after antigenic

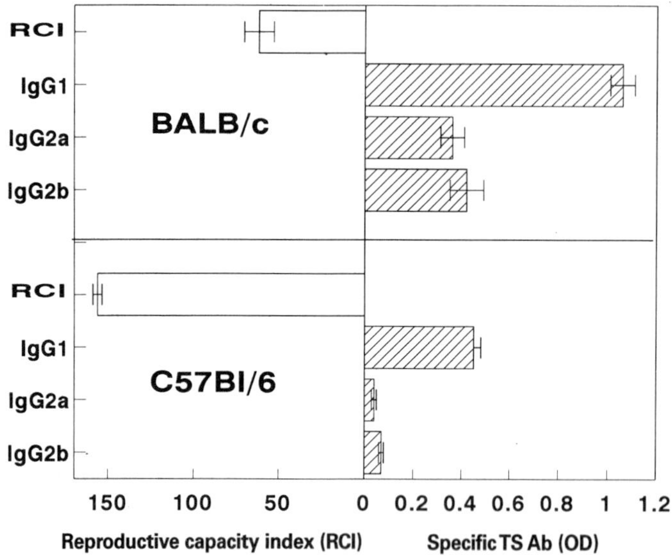

Fig. 17.1 Muscle larva burden and detection of specific antibodies in *T. spiralis* infection. Values are expressed as mean ± SE for RCI and ELISA (serum dilution 1:40).

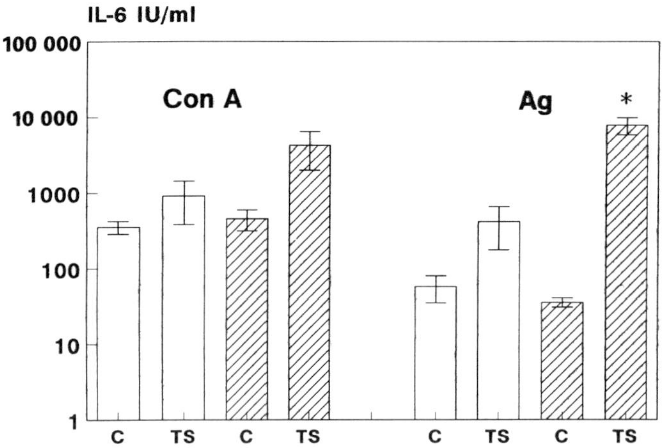

Fig. 17.2 IL-6 cytokine production after mitogen (Con A) and (Ag) stimulation of spleen cells from experimental mice. Light bars, BALB/c group; shaded bars, C57Bl/6 group. *, $p<0.05$ vs control.

stimulation of the spleen cells derived from susceptible C57Bl/6 mice. The total spleen cells population produced a significantly ($p<0.05$) higher quantity of IL 6 when compared with the controls. This enhancement was observed in relatively resistant BALB/c mice also, but the difference did not reach the level of statistical significance. Still, it should be stressed that cell cultures of C57Bl/6 strain secreted much higher amounts of IL-6 after antigen stimulation than did BALB/c mice.

IL-6 production in acute intestinal inflammation provoked by adult stage TS infection has already been investigated in rats (17). It was found that neither peritoneal macrophages nor cells from infected intestine secreted greater than normal amounts of IL-6, suggesting that these cells do not appear to be activated in vivo by TS. Our results indicate that acute muscle inflammation provoked by parasite invasion in the last stage of infection is capable of influencing IL-6 production.

IL-6 is known as pluripotent cytokine and influences many phases of the immune response, such as acceleration of B-cell differentiation (18), induction of cytotoxic T cells as killer helper factor (19) and production of acute phase protein in hepatocytes (20). IL-6 also participates in the pathogenesis of some autoimmune diseases (21) and if extensively produced in vivo it might enhance their progression (13).

Based on the results presented here we can conclude that TS infection in a susceptible strain of mice leads to the increase production of pleotropic cytokine IL-6. This finding may explain our previous data indicating that TS infection enhances autoantibody production (12). Thus, it appears that TS infection may lead to the disregulation of immunity mediated by inappropriate production of IL-6. The observed phenomenon therefore deserves more intensive study.

SUMMARY

The production of IL-6 has been investigated in the early muscle stage of *T. spiralis* infection in the two inbred strains of mouse, BALB/c and C57Bl/6, which differ in their response to the parasite. A significant increase of IL-6 production by the antigen-stimulated spleen cells was found in the *T. spiralis* susceptible C57Bl/6 mice. The increase of IL-6 production in resistant BALB/c mice did not reach statistical significance when compared to the controls, uninfected mice. We assume that previously reported stimulation of autoantibody production by TS infection may be related to the enhanced production of IL-6.

REFERENCES

1. Silberstain, D. S. and D. D. Despommier. 1985. Effects on *Trichinella spiralis* of host responses to purified antigens. *Science* **227**:948–50.
2. Ko, R. C., L. Fan, D. L. Lee and H. Compton. 1994. Changes in host muscles induced by excretory/secretory products of larval *Trichinella spiralis* and *Trichinella pseudospiralis*. *Parasitology* **108**:195–205.
3. Murrell, K. D. and F. Bruschi. 1994. Clinical trichinellosis. In: *Progress in Clinical Parasitology*, Vol. 4 (S. Tsieh, ed.) CRC Press, Inc., Boca Raton, FL, pp. 117–50.
4. Wakelin D. and D. A. Denham. 1983. The immune response. In: *Trichinella and Trichinosis* (W. C. Campbell, ed.) Plenum Press, New York, pp. 265–308.
5. Grencis, R. K., L. Hultner and J. K. Else. 1991. Host protective immunity to *Trichinella spiralis* in mice: activation of Th cell subsets and lymphokine secretion in mice expressing different response phenotypes. *Immunology* **74**:329–32.
6. Pond, L., D. L. Wassom and C. E Hayes. 1992. Influence of resistant and susceptible genotype, IL-1, and lymphoid organ on *Trichinella spiralis*-induced cytokine secretion. *J. Immunol.* **149**:957–65.
7. Faubert, G. and C. E. Tanner. 1971. *Trichinella spiralis*: Inhibition of sheep hemaglutinins in mice. *Exp. Parasitol.* **30**:120–3.
8. Svet-Moldavsky, G. J., G. S. Shaghijian, I. Y. Cheenyakhovskaya *et al.* 1970. Inhibition of skin allograft rejection in *Trichinella* infected mice. *Transplantation* **9**:69–70.
9. Lubiniecki, A. S. and R. H. Cypess. 1975. Immunological sequelae of *Trichinella spiralis* infection in mice: effect on the antibody responses to sheep erythrocytes and Japanese B encephalitis virus. *Infect. Immun.* **11**:1306–11.
10. Cypess, R. H., J. Molinari, J. L. Ebersole and A. S. Lubiniecki. 1974. Immunological sequelae of *Trichinella spiralis* infection in mice. II. Potentiation of cell-mediated response to BCG following infection with *Trichinella spiralis*. *Infect. Immun.* **10**:107–10.
11. Molinari, J. A. and J. R. Ebersole. 1977. Antineoplastic effects of long-term *Trichinella spiralis* infection on B-16 melanoma. *Int. Arch. Allergy Appl. Immunol.* **55**:444–8.

12. Sofronić-Milosavljeić, Lj., K. Čuperlović, A. Dujić and Č. Radojičić. 1990. Immunomodulatory factors during *T. spiralis* infection. *Period. Biol.* **92**(1): 36–7.
13. Kimura, T., K. Suzuki, S. Inada *et al.* 1994. Induction of autoimmune disease by graft-*versus*-host reaction across MHC class II difference: modification of the lesions in IL-6 transgenic mice. *Clin. Exp. Immunol.* **95**:525–9.
14. Gamble, H. R. 1985. *Trichinella spiralis*: Immunisation of mice using monoclonal affinity isolated antigens. *Exp. Parasitol.* **59**:398–404.
15. Wassom, D. L., C. S. David and G. J. Gleich 1979. Genes within the major histocompatibility complex influence susceptibility to *Trichinella spiralis* in the mouse. *Immunogenetics* **9**:491–6.
16. Pond, L., D. L. Wassom, and C. E. Hayes. 1989. Evidence for differential induction of helper T cell subsets during *Trichinella spiralis* infection. *J. Immunol.* **143**: 4232–7.
17. Stadnyk, A. W., H. Baumann, and J. Gauldie. 1990. The acute-phase protein response in parasite infection. *Nippostrongylus brasiliensis* and *Trichinella spiralis* in the rat. *Immunology* **69**:588–95.
18. Muraguchi, A., T. Hirano, B. Tang *et al.* 1988. The essential role of B cell stimulatory factor 2 (BSF-2/IL-6) for the terminal differentiation of B cells. *J. Exp. Med.* **167**:332–44.
19. Okada, M., M. Kitahara, S. Kishimoto *et al.* 1988. IL-6/BSF-2 functions as a killer helper factor in the in vitro induction of cytotoxic T cells. *J. Immunol.* **141**:1543–9.
20. Gauldie, J., C. Richards, D. Harnish *et al.* 1987. Interferon beta2/B-cell stimulatory factor type 2 shares identity with monocyte-derived hepatocyte-stimulating factor and regulates the major acute phase protein response in liver cell. *Proc. Natl. Acad. Sci. USA* **84**:7251–5.
21. Hirano, T., T. Matsuda and M. Turner. 1988. Excessive production of interleukin 6/B cell stimulatory factor-2 in rheumatoid arthritis. *Eur. J. Immunol.* **18**:1797–801.

18

Naturally Occurring Anti-peptide Antibodies in the Rat: anti-Met-Enk Antibodies

Jelena Radulović, Vesna Vujić, Stanislava Stanojević, Tatjana Vasiljević, Vesna Kovačević-Jovanović and Marko Radulović

It is well established that both B (1) and T lymphocytes (2) exert autonomous immunological activities before any experimental challenge with antigen. Natural IgM and IgG antibodies show specificity for a wide variety of self proteins, including structural as well as secretory molecules of the lymphoid cells and tissues (3). Several reports have demonstrated the presence of antibodies against neuropeptides, molecules known to influence numerous biological functions, including modulation of immunological responsiveness. Catalytic IgG autoantibodies to vasoactive intestinal peptide were recorded in some healthy human subjects and asthma patients (4). Increased level of anti-β-endorphin IgG antibodies was observed in human sera by enzyme-linked immunosorbent assay (ELISA) in individuals with major depression (5), but in this study little attention was given to the finding that normal human sera also exhibited some anti-β-endorphin activity. In our preliminary experiments we detected autoantibodies to several biologically active peptides, such as Met-Enk, leucine-enkephalin (Leu-Enk), cholecystokinin and neurotensin, in normal rat sera and sera of rats injected with complete Freund's adjuvant (CFA). The level of anti-Met-Enk antibodies was significantly higher in comparison with antibodies for other peptides.

Taking into account that Met-Enk is a biologically active peptide secreted by a wide variety of tissues, and that Met-Enk may exert numerous actions within the nervous, endocrine and immune systems (6), the aim of the present study was to characterize anti-Met-Enk antibodies in greater detail. For this purpose, specificity, affinity and stability of complexes formed between natural anti-Met-Enk antibodies and Met-Enk were investigated.

Immunoregulation in Health and Disease
ISBN 0–12–459460–3

MATERIALS AND METHODS

Animals

Twelve-week-old male Wistar rats were obtained from the Medical Military Academy (Belgrade). Animals were kept in plexiglass cages (4 rats per cage) and given food pellets and water *ad libitum*.

Generation of antisera

Antibodies to synthetic Met-Enk (Serva, Heidelberg) were obtained from 10 20-week-old Wistar rats, as previously described (7). Briefly, after coupling of Met-Enk to bovine serum albumin (BSA, Sigma, St. Louis) using the glutaraldehyde method, the conjugate was dialyzed against PBS, coupling efficiency checked spectrophotometrically, and water-in-oil emulsion prepared by mixing equal volumes of Met-Enk–BSA with complete Freund's adjuvant (CFA). Rats were immunized monthly by intradermal injections of 100 μl of the Met-Enk–BSA/CFA emulsion containing 100 μg of Met-Enk and 300 μg of *Mycobacterium tuberculosis* (Lederle Laboratories, Pearl River) per injection. Another group of 10 rats was injected identically with CFA. Two weeks after the third immunization, animals were sacrificed and exsanguinated, and sera pooled. Normal sera were obtained from age-matched non-immunized Wistar rats.

Met-Enk ELISA

Standardization of Met-Enk ELISA was performed using specific rat anti-Met-Enk serum and rabbit anti-Met-Enk serum (kindly provided by Professor A. E. Panerai and Dr. Paola Sacerdote, Department of Pharmacology, School of Medicine, Milan), previously characterized by competitive radioimmunoassay (8). Polystyrene 96-well plates (Nunc, Roskilde) were coated overnight at 4°C with 40 μg/ml of Met-Enk in 0.05 M carbonate buffer pH 9.6. In preliminary assays, this concentration produced coating saturation. Plates were washed with PBS containing 0.05% Tween-20, and antigen was fixed with 100% methanol for 5 min (9). Further steps were performed by conventional ELISA, using peroxidase-labelled antibodies and *o*-phenylenediamine (Sigma). Under these assay conditions, binding of sera for saturant was negligible. Binding of secondary antibody for Met-Enk (absorbance = 0.010–0.015) served as background control, and these values were subtracted from test sample absorbances.

Precipitation of immunoglobulins (Ig)

Ig fractions were obtained following precipitation with ammoniun sulfate (10) of pooled sera obtained from normal rats (normal rat Ig), sera of rats injected with CFA (Ig of rats given CFA) and specifically-induced anti-Met-Enk rat sera (Anti-Met-Enk) Ig. The IgG/IgM ratio was determined by gel filtration on a Superose-12 FPLC column (Pharmacia, LKB, Uppsala), and Ig content calculated on spectrophotometrical analysis at 280 nm. All samples were set up to 10 mg of Ig/ml.

Examination of the stability of antigen-antibody complexes in neutral 0.3–0.6 M NaCl

Stability of antigen–antibody complexes was checked in the presence of neutral 0.3, 0.4, 0.5 and 0.6 M NaCl by ELISA (11). Anti-Met-Enk rat Ig, Ig of rats given CFA and normal rat Ig were added as previously described. After incubation, separate wells were washed four times each with PBS alone or 0.3–0.6 M NaCl in PBS and then washed three times with PBS–0.05% Tween. Residual antibody was measured by conventional ELISA. The absorbance after washing with PBS without additional NaCl was considered to express 100% bound antibody.

Competition experiments

The specificity and cross-reactivity of CFA-induced antisera were determined by modified anti-Met-Enk ELISA : (a) using plates coated with conjugated peptide Met-Enk-BSA; antiserum was incubated with or without Met-Enk-BSA or Leu-Enk-BSA at 37°C for 2 h (b) by competition of rat antisera with specific anti-Met-Enk rabbit antisera for unconjugated plate-bound Met-Enk at 37°C or 2 h.

Separation of IgG and IgM fractions

IgM and IgG fractions, obtained from normal, CFA-induced and specific anti-Met-Enk rat sera, were separated on an FPLC gel-filtration chromatography column Superose-12 (Pharmacia) equilibrated with PBS. Sample volumes of 0.5 ml of sera, diluted 1/1 with PBS, were applied to the column. IgG and IgM contents were determined spectrophotometrically. Ig were stored at 4°C in 40% glycerol 0.05% azide prior to use in ELISA.

RESULTS AND DISCUSSION

Normal rat Ig exhibited low Met-Enk binding capacity, as determined by the titration curve in ELISA (Fig. 18.1A). In rats immunized with CFA alone, anti-Met-Enk antibody titre was markedly increased and slope of the titration curve was steeper in comparison to the normal rat Ig. These findings are in agreement with previous reports demonstrating that polyclonal stimulation

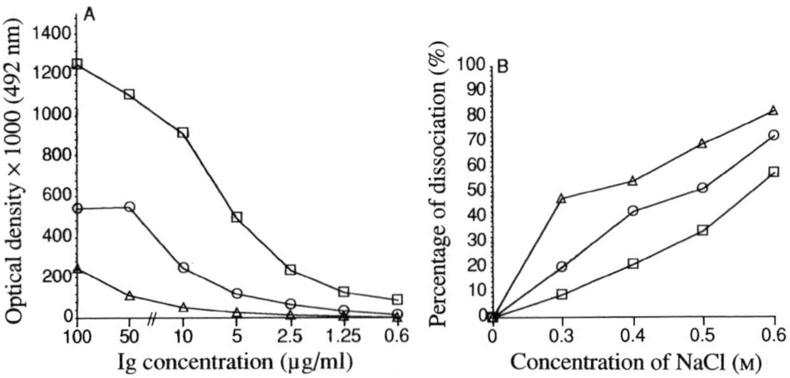

Fig. 18.1 A low, intermediate and high anti-Met-Enk antibody titre in normal rat Ig (triangles), Ig of rats given CFA (circles) and anti-Met-Enk Ig (squares), respectively. B. Low, intermediate and high stability of Ig-Met-Enk complexes in ELISA, following washing of normal rat Ig (triangles), Ig of rats given CFA (circles) and anti-Met-Enk rat Ig (squares), respectively, with different concentrations of sodium chloride in phosphate-buffered saline.

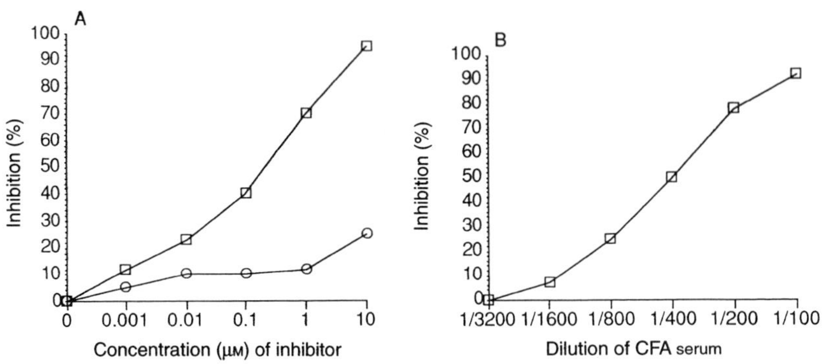

Fig. 18.2 Displacement curves established by ELISA tests from competition experiments between: A. Met-Enk coated at 100 μg/ml and increasing concentrations of Met-Enk-BSA (squares) or Leu-Enk-BSA (circles) previously incubated with CFA-induced serum; and B. Increasing concentrations of CFA-induced rat serum and specific rabbit anti-Met-Enk serum (dilution 1/8000 that exerts 50% binding to plate bound Met-Enk).

of the immune system due to administration of polyclonal B cell activators (12) or infections (13) is commonly accompanied by increased levels of natural antibodies. As shown in Fig. 18.1B, antibodies bound to Met-Enk were differentially dissociated by increasing concentrations of sodium chloride. Anti-Met-Enk Ig was slightly dissociated from Met-Enk at lower concentration of sodium chloride and maximal dissociation was up to 58%, whereas normal rat Ig markedly dissociated from Met-Enk even at a concentration of sodium chloride as low as 0.3 M, and over 80% at 0.6 M of

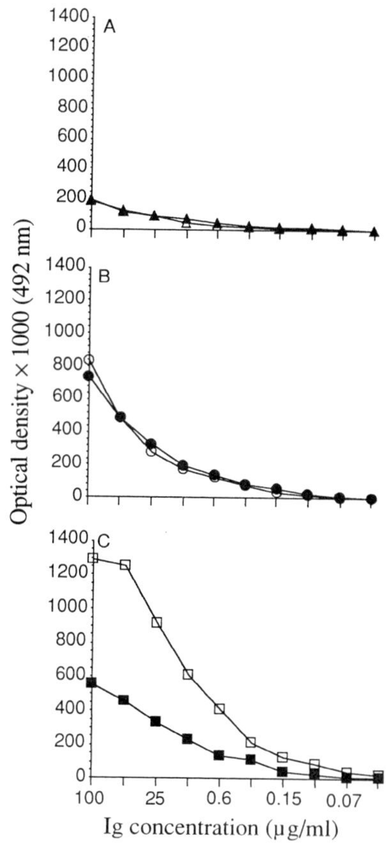

Fig. 18.3 Met-Enk binding capacity of IgG (open symbols) and IgM (black symbols) obtained from (A) normal; (B) CFA-induced; and (C) anti-Met-Enk rat sera.

sodium chloride. An intermediate dissociation curve was obtained from Ig of rats immunized with CFA. These findings imply that anti-Met-Enk antibodies have limited physiological relevance in neutralizing the activity of endogenous Met-Enk. It is possible, however, that these antibodies gain more significance under particular circumstances, such as polyclonal activation of the immune system, when the level of antibodies that show specificity for Met-Enk (Fig. 18.2A) and no cross-reactivity to Leu-Enk (Fig. 18.2B) markedly increases.

Separation of IgM and IgG fractions from non-immunized rat Ig revealed that both isotypes exhibited Met-Enk-binding properties (Fig. 18.2). Injections of CFA induced marked rise in IgM and IgG anti-Met-Enk antibodies, and the anti-Met-Enk activity of these fractions was similar with respect to their level and affinity for Met-Enk. These findings differed from results obtained with specifically produced anti-Met-Enk Ig, where IgG anti-Met-Enk antibodies largely exceeded IgM anti-Met-Enk antibodies in quantity and affinity. Analysis of titration curves showed that higher concentrations (100 and 50 μg/ml) of separated IgM and IgG from normal sera had more pronounced anti-Met-Enk activity than the same concentrations of unseparated Ig. At lower concentrations (10 μg/ml and below) these differences were not recorded. We assume that this finding may be due to idiotypic interactions between IgM and IgG (14) that prevent the binding of autoantibodies to Met-Enk up to a particular Ig dilution. A similar result was obtained with Ig derived from CFA injected rats. On the other hand, the use of specific anti-Met-Enk sera demonstrated similar anti-Met-Enk activity of total Ig and separated IgG. In this case, high affinity IgG most probably displaced lower affinity IgM anti-Met-Enk antibodies.

Modulation of immune responses by brain opioid peptides, including Met-Enk, is well established (6). In addition, several reports showed that the immune system affected the functioning of opioid peptides within the CNS. Immunosuppression induced by irradiation dramatically suppressed opioid-induced withdrawal symptoms in the rat (15). It was shown that a genetic defect in opioid-induced antinociception may be transferred to normal recipients by B cells and adherent accessory cells (16). These findings demonstrated that some components of the immune system counteract the activity of opioids within the nervous system. The presence of natural anti-Met-Enk antibodies and their increase due to polyclonal stimulation, as demonstrated in this study, may represent a mechanism by which the immune system influences the activity of Met-Enk.

SUMMARY

Anti-Met-Enk antibodies were detected in the sera of normal outbred Wistar rats by ELISA. Polyclonal activation, induced by repeated immunizations with CFA, produced a marked increase in the level of anti-Met-Enk antibodies accompanied by increased stability of the antibody-Met-Enk complexes. Specificity of binding to Met-Enk by sera from CFA-injected rats was shown in competition experiments with conjugated peptides and specific antisera. Separation of IgG and IgM fractions from sera of non-immunized and CFA injected rats revealed that both isotypes bound to a similar extent to Met-Enk.

REFERENCES

1. Portnoi, D., A. Freitas, D. Holmberg *et al.* 1986. Immunocompetent autoreactive B lymphocytes are activated cycling cells in normal mice. *J. Exp. Med.* **164**:25–35.

2. Pereira, P., E.-L. Larsson, L. Forni *et al.* 1985. Natural effector T lymphocytes in normal mice. *Proc. Natl. Acad. Sci. USA* **82**:7691–5.
3. Avrameas, S., G. Dighiero, P. Lymberi and B. Guilbert. 1983. Natural autoreactive B cells and autoantibodies: The 'Know thyself' of the immune system. *Ann. Immunol.* (*Inst. Pasteur*) **137**D:150–6.
4. Paul, S., S. I. Said, A. B. Thompson *et al.* 1989. Characterization of autoantibodies to vasoactive intestinal peptide in asthma. *J. Neuroimmunol.* **23**:133–42.
5. Roy, B. F., J. W. Rose, H. F. McFarland *et al.* 1986. Anti-β-endorphin immunoglobulin G in humans. *Proc. Natl. Acad. Sci. USA* **83**:8739–43.
6. Janković, B. D. and J. Radulović. 1992. Brain, enkephalins, and immunity: modulation of immune responses by methionine-enkephalin injected into lateral ventricles of the rat brain. *Int. J. Neurosci.* **67**:241–70.
7. Ogawa, N., A. E. Panerai, S. Lee *et al.* 1979. β-Endorphin concentration in the brain of intact and hypophysectomized rats. *Life Sci.* **25**:317–26.
8. Panerai, A. E., A. Martini, A. Di Giuglio *et al.* 1983. Plasma β-endorphin, β-lipotropin, and met-enkephalin concentrations during pregnancy in normal and drug-addicted women and their newborn. *J. Clin. Endocrinol. Metab.* **57**:537–43.
9. Green, N., H. Alexander, A. Olson *et al.* 1982. Immunogenic structure of the influenza hemagglutinin. *Cell* **28**:477–81.
10. Hudson, L. and F. C. Hay. 1980. *Practical Immunology* (2nd edn.) Blackwell Scientific, New York.
11. Kanai, Y. and T. Kubota. 1989. A novel trait of naturally occurring anti-DNA antibodies: dissociation from immune complexes in neutral 0.3–0.5 M NaCl. *Immunol. Lett.* **22**:293–300.
12. Primi, D., L. Hammarström, C. I. E. Smith and G. Möller. 1977. Characterization of self-reactive B cells by polyclonal B-cell activators. *J. Exp. Med.* **145**:21–30.
13. Ortiz-Ortiz, L., D. E. Parks, M. Rodriguez and W. O. Weigle. 1980. Polyclonal B lymphocyte activation during *Trypanosoma cruzi* infection. *J. Immunol.* **124**:121–6.
14. Adib, M., J. Ragimbeau, S. Avrameas and T. Ternynck. 1990. IgG autoantibody activity in normal mouse serum is controlled by IgM. *J. Immunol.* **145**:3807–13.
15. Beitner, D. B., K. Rasmussen, J. H. Krystal *et al.* 1989. Effects of opiate withdrawal on locus ceruleus neurons: behavioral, biochemical, and physiological correlates. *Soc. Neurosci. Abstr.* **15**:143.
16. Kimball, E. S. and R. B. Raffa. 1989. Obligatory role of B cells and adherent accessory cells in the transfer of a defect in morphine-mediated antinociception in C57BL/6J-bg/bg (beige J) mice. *J. Neuroimmunol.* **22**:185–92.

19

Expression of Y7 Idiotope on IgM Molecules from Cord Sera

Marko Radulović, Bogoljub Ćirić, Aleksandar Jurišić, Ratko Jankov, Slobodan Apostolski, Snežana Živančević-Simonović and Ljiljana Dimitrijević

Idiotypes were originally defined as antigenic determinants unique for the individual antibody clone (1). Later, it was found that idiotypes can also be shared between distinct antibody clones (2), and these are usually referred to as cross-reactive idiotypes (CRI). It is assumed that CRI have an important role in immunoregulation mediated through an idiotype network (3), and are encoded by germline, or minimally mutated germline gene segments (4). CRI have been studied mainly on immunoglobulins involved in immune response or disease (5). Less attention has been paid to idiotypes present on natural antibodies. It is widely accepted that natural antibodies are products of B cells stimulated by the organism's internal environment that includes self antigens and idiotypes, independently of any external antigenic challenge (3). Consequently, idiotopes found on natural antibodies are called natural idiotopes (6). We have previously defined the Y7 idiotopic determinant on human monoclonal IgM DJ derived from a patient with Waldenstrom macroglobulinemia (7). IgM DJ has been shown to possess all natural antibody characteristics: polyspecificity, autoreactivity and low affinity (submitted for publication). Therefore, in this study we wanted to examine whether the Y7 idiotope could also be detected on other natural antibodies. This idiotope showed 7% average cross-reactivity with immunoglobulins from normal adult sera in inverse solid phase RIA (8). It could not be ascertained whether this cross-reactivity was caused by natural antibodies, since sera obtained from healthy adults, besides large amount of natural antibodies, also contain antibodies produced as a result of previous stimulations by external antigens, or ongoing but not apparent infection. Accordingly, this work aimed to determine the expression of the Y7 idiotope

Immunoregulation in Health and Disease
ISBN 0-12-459460-3

on IgM from human cord sera. We have restricted it to the IgM isotype because cord blood IgM is entirely synthetized by the fetus as it is well established that IgM cannot cross the placenta (9), whereas IgG, on the contrary, is mainly of maternal origin. As the fetus has essentially never experienced challenge by exogenous antigen (with the exception of idiotypes present on maternal IgG), all cord blood IgM can be considered as a natural antibody pool. This was recently documented with studies of the antibody repertoire of fetal and cord B cells secreting IgM (10) where it was shown that almost all lymphocytes from fetal liver and cord blood secrete antibodies showing all characteristics of natural antibodies.

The present study provides a simple and convenient experimental model for definition and examination of natural idiotypes.

MATERIALS AND METHODS

Monoclonal antibodies

Production and characterization of the murine monoclonal antibody (mAb) 202 (IgG_{2a}), specific for the Fc fragment of human IgM polymer, was previously described (11). MAb 202 was purified from ascites as IgG_{2a} fraction on a protein A column (Pharmacia) by elution with 0.1 M citric buffer, pH 4.5. Murine monoclonal antibody Y7 (IgG_1) was also previously produced and characterized (7) as specific for the idiotopic determinant on human monoclonal IgM DJ. It was affinity purified on an IgM DJ–Sepharose 4B immunoaffinity column as described previously (7).

Human IgM DJ was used as a standard for the Y7 idiotope as well as total IgM quantification. It was isolated from serum of the patient D.J. with Waldenstrom macroglobulinemia by means of euglobulin precipitation followed by gel-exclusion chromatography on a Superose-6 column (FPLC system, Pharmacia). Concentration of IgM DJ standard was determined by Lowry. Standard IgM DJ solution was kept at 4°C at concentration of 0.5 mg/ml in 40% (v/v) glycerol/PBS with 0.1% sodium azide.

Cord blood sera

Sera were obtained from the Obstetric and Gynaecology Clinic, Narodni Front, Belgrade.

Two-site sandwich ELISA

Assays (12) were performed using two mAbs (mAb 202 and mAb Y7) directed towards two distinct epitopic determinants on the IgM DJ molecule. MAb 202 was used for capturing of cord serum IgM and quantification of total IgM, while mAb Y7 was used for quantification of the IgM-bearing Y7 idiotopic determinant. Briefly, wells of microtitre plates (E.I.A. II plus, Linbro, Flow) were coated for 1 h at 37°C with mAb 202 (50 μl, 5 μg/ml), and overcoated for 1 h at 37°C with 0.2% BSA. Subsequently, serial dilutions of IgM DJ standard (0.25–5μg/ml) for determination of total IgM and 0.75–100 ng/ml for Y7 idiotope determination were added to wells in PBS/0.2%BSA (BPBS). Cord sera diluted (1/70) in BPBS were tested in parallel with dilutions of IgM DJ standard. Four washes with PBS/Tween-20 were performed between each step. After 1 h incubation at room temperature, the plates were washed and 50 μl of biotin-labelled mAb 202 or biotin-labelled mAb Y7 (1 μg/ml) were added for determination of total IgM and Y7 idiotope respectively. Binding was detected in the presence of streptavidin-HRP and OPD as supstrate (492 nm microplate reader Titertek, Flow). Concentrations of total cord blood IgM and Y7 idiotope were calculated from standard calibration curves. Percentage of Y7-positive IgM was calculated by dividing Y7 idiotope concentration with concentration of total IgM, for every individual cord serum.

RESULTS AND DISCUSSION

The results have defined Y7 idiotope as a natural CRI, by showing a relatively high incidence of Y7 idiotope expression on IgM isotype in all cord sera tested. Calibration curves were obtained by quantitative sandwich ELISA (12) and plotted using mean values from four separate experiments for determination of total IgM (Fig. 19.1) and Y7 idiotope concentration (Fig. 19.2) in individual sera. Standard curves were linear at concentrations from 250 ng/ml to 5 μg/ml for total IgM (Fig. 19.1) and 6–100 ng/ml for IgM expressing Y7 idiotope (Fig. 19.2). Concentrations of total IgM calculated from standard curves (20–176 μg/ml) were in agreement with those already reported for IgM concentrations in cord blood sera (9).

The results show that incidence of Y7 idiotope expression was 2–13% of the total IgM population. The majority of sera (31/43 or 72%) showed Y7 positivity in the range of 3–6% (Fig. 19.3). It is important to note that such abundant Y7 idiotope expression was not due to rheumatoid factor activity of cord IgM towards Y7 anti-idiotopic antibody (IgG_1), since we have determined in a separate experiment that cord serum IgM (in the same dilution of cord sera used for sandwich assay) did not significantly bind unrelated murine mAb of the same isotype as Y7 (IgG_1), adsorbed to polystyrene. As Y7 idiotope was found to be expressed on a sizable portion of a cord blood IgM pool, which is by definition entirely composed of natural antibodies, it may be regarded as 'natural' CRI. We are not aware of other studies aimed to determine the expression of CRI on immunoglobulins from cord sera. Our results are comparable with recent studies of CRI expression

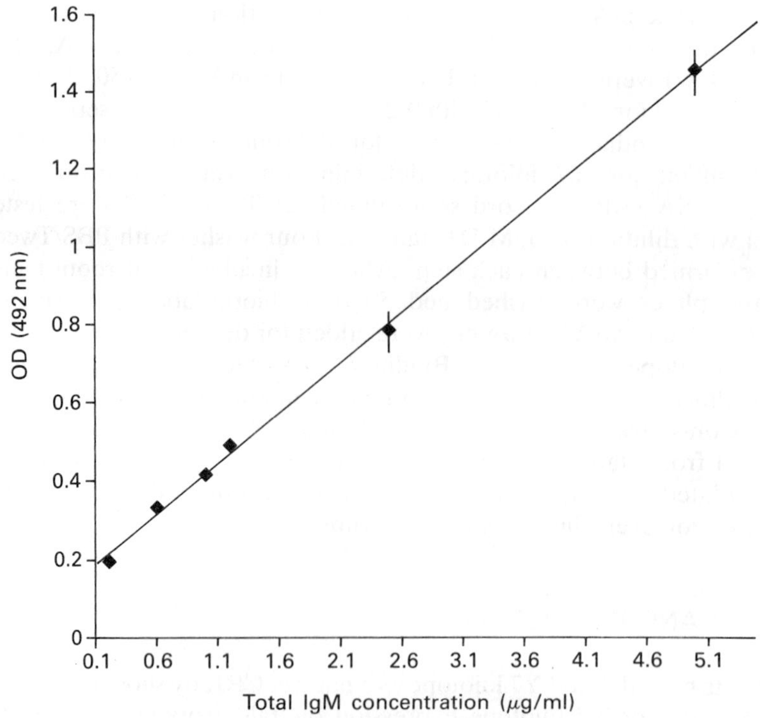

Fig. 19.1 Calibration curve for determination of total IgM concentrations in cord sera. MAb 202 specific for human IgM was adsorbed to polystyrene and used as a capture antibody. Amount of total captured IgM (during incubation with cord sera) was detected with biotin-labelled mAb 202 as a secondary reagent. Complete procedure is outlined in materials and methods section. Error bars shown in the figure for two highest optical densities represent SD. $y = 0.0258x + 0.1625$; $r = 0.9991$.

on the primary follicles of human fetal spleen (13), which also showed a high frequency of CRI expression. Unfortunately, these findings were not further extended to studies of CRI expression on free cord serum immunoglobulins. The incidence of expression in individual follicles was 5.5% for B6 CRI, 6.8% for 17.109 CRI, 6.9% for G6 CRI and 17% for Lc1 CRI. High incidence of CRI among fetal and neonatal membrane-bound and free immunoglobulins suggests that only a limited number of idiotopes are expressed at this stage of development. This observation was supported by experiments at the immunoglobulin gene level that show preferential use of certain V_H gene families among natural antibodies (14). Besides high frequencies of CRI expression, panels of monoclonal antibodies obtained from neonatal spleens also showed a very high degree of mutual idiotypic connectivity (25–28%) in a criss-cross test (15). It was proposed that high antibody connectivity in

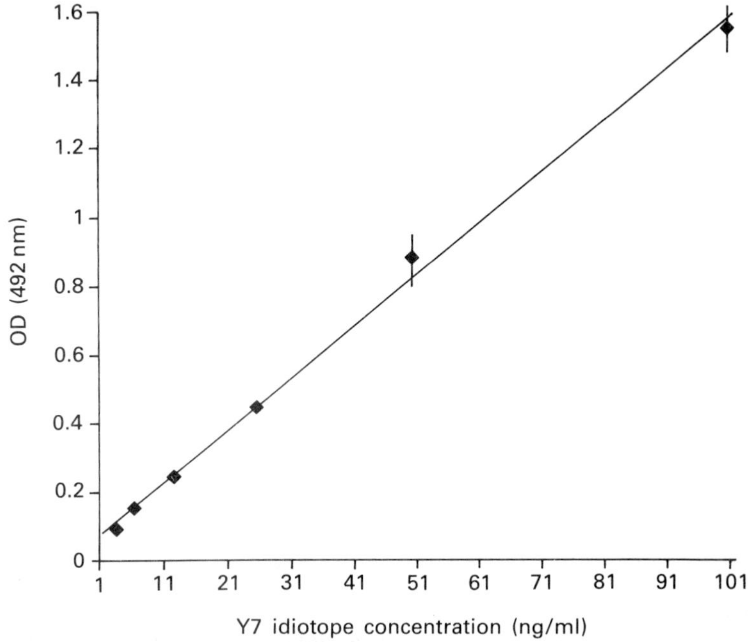

Fig. 19.2 Calibration curve for determination of Y7 idiotope concentration. MAb 202 specific for human IgM was adsorbed to polystyrene and used as a capture antibody. Captured IgM that expresses Y7 idiotope was quantitated by use of biotin-labelled anti-idiotopic MAb Y7 as a secondary reagent. Complete procedure is outlined in materials and methods. Error bars shown in the figure for two highest optical densities represent SD. $y = 0.0151x + 0.0701$; $r = 0.997$.

newborns is essential for the normal development of the immune system, mainly for the selection and establishment of the available repertoires (3). In recent studies a high degree of CRI expression was also shown in peripheral blood lymphocytes obtained from healthy human adults (16). The percentage of expression was 1.7% for G6 CRI, 3.2% for G8 CRI, 11% for B6 CRI and 19.5% for D12 CRI. Similarly, another group has studied a distribution of a panel of CRIs on normal lymphoid tissues (17). The percentage of expression was similar for tonsils, spleen, appendix and peripheral blood lymphocytes and varied from 0.2 to 9.1% for different CRIs. Taken together, these results imply that high incidence of CRI expression is not an exclusive property of early B cells as it is also found in similar percentages on B lymphocytes derived from adults. This is in agreement with our previous findings which showed 7% average cross-reactivity of the Y7 idiotope with normal adult sera (7).

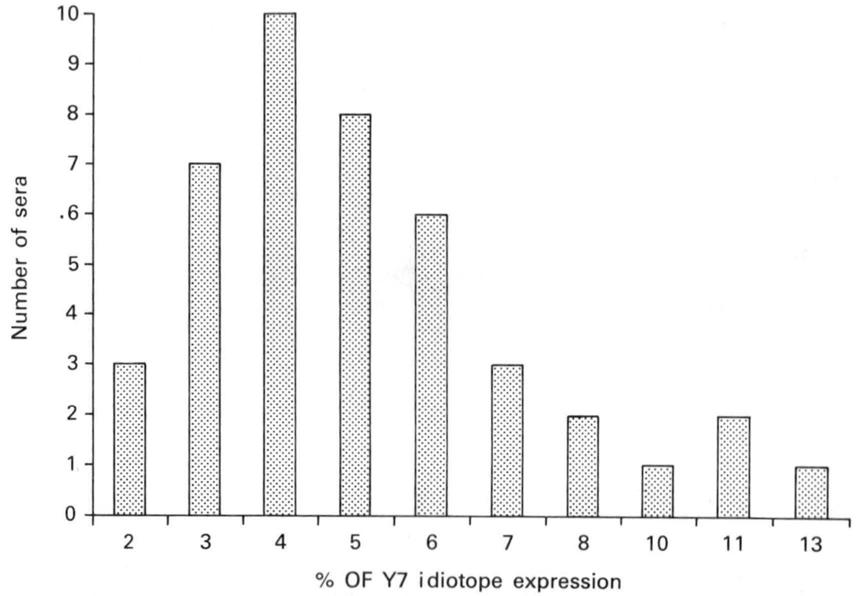

Fig 19.3 Percentage of Y7 idiotope expression within 43 cord sera tested. Data are presented as number of sera which express the same percentage of Y7 idiotope within cord sera IgM.

CONCLUSION

The Y7 idiotope was shown to be substantially expressed (2–13%) on cord sera IgM, in all individual sera tested. As cord IgM belongs entirely to the natural antibody pool, the Y7 idiotope can be defined as 'natural'. These results provide additional experimental support for the high frequency of CRI expression within neonatal immunoglobulins, which may represent a structural basis for high mutual idiotypic connectivity of newborn IgM.

REFERENCES

1. Kunkel, M., M. Mannik and R. C. Williams. 1963. Individual antigenic specificity of isolated antibodies. *Science* **140**: 1218–19.
2. Williams, R. C., H. G. Kunkel and J. D. Capra. 1968. Antigenic specificities related to the cold agglutinin activity of gamma M globulins. *Science* **161**: 379–81.
3. Coutinho, A. 1995. The network theory – 21 years later. *Scand. J. Immunol.* **42**: 3–8.
4. Goldfien, R. D., P. Chen, T. J. Kipps *et al.* 1987. Genetic analysis of human B cell hybridomas expressing a cross-reactive idiotype. *J. Immunol.* **138**: 940–4.

5. Waisman, A., Y. Shoenfeld, M. Blank *et al.* 1995. The pathogenic human monoclonal anti-DNA that induces experimental systemic lupus erythematosus in mice is encoded by a V(H)4 gene segment. *Int. Immunol.* **7**: 689–96.
6. Ehrenstein, M. R., B. Hartley, L. S. Wilkinson and D. A. Isenberg. 1994. Comparison of a monoclonal and polyclonal anti-idiotype against a human IgG anti-DNA antibody. *J. Autoimmunity* **7**: 349–67.
7. Dimitrijević, L., M. Radulović, B. Ćirić *et al.* 1992. Immunochemical characterization of a murine monoclonal anti-idiotypic antibody. *J. Immunoass.* **13**: 181–96.
8. Ivanović, V., L. Popović, K. Kovačina *et al.* 1990. Detection of a cross reactive idiotypes in sera of lymphoma patients by inverse monoclonal radioimmunoassay. *Acta Haematol.* **84**: 64–7.
9. Ailus, K. and T. Palosuo, 1995. IgM class autoantibodies in human cord serum. *J. Repr. Immunol.* **29**: 61–7.
10. Lydyard, P. M. R., B. Quartey-Papafio, L. Broker *et al.* 1990. The antibody repertoire of early human B cells I. High frequency of autoreactivity and polyreactivity. *Scand. J. Immunol.* **31**: 33–43.
11. Ćirić, B., M. Radulović, L. Dimitrijević and R. Jankov. 1995. Effect of valency on binding properties of the anti-human IgM monoclonal antibody. *Hybridoma* **14**: 537–44.
12. Fandeur, T., J. Gysin and J. M. Postal. 1989. A two site sandwich immunoradiometric assay of squirrel monkey (*Saimiri scireus*) IgM using monoclonal antibodies. *J. Immunol. Meth.* **118**: 109–17.
13. Kipps, T. J., B. A. Robbins and D. Carson. 1990. Uniform high frequency expression of autoantibody-associated crossreactive idiotypes in the primary B cell follicles of human fetal spleen. *J. Exp. Med.* **171**: 189–96.
14. Holmberg, D. 1987. High connectivity, natural antibodies preferentially use 7183 and QPC52 VH families. *Eur. J. Immunol.* **17**: 399–403.
15. Zoller, M. and M. Achtnich. 1991. Idiotypic profile of natural autoantibodies in newborn and young adult BALB/c mice. *Scand. J. Immunol.* **33**: 15–24.
16. Shokri, F., R. A. Mageed, P. Richardson and R. Jefferis. 1993. Modulation and high frequency expression of autoantibody-associated cross-reactive idiotypes linked to the V_H1 subgroup in CD5-expressing B lymphocytes from patients with chronic lymphocytic leukaemia (B-CLL). *Scand. J. Immunol.* **37**: 673–9.
17. Inghirami, G., D. R. Foitl, A. Sabichi, B. Ying Zhu and D. M. Knowles. 1991. Autoantibody-associated cross reactive idiotype-bearing human B lymphocytes: distribution and characterization, including Ig V_H gene and CD5 antigen expression. *Blood* **78**: 1503–15.

20

Alterations in Neonatal Sexual Differentiation Affect T-cell Maturation

Biljana Vidić Danković, Branka Karapetrović, Duško Kosec, Sandra Obradović and Gordana Leposavić

It is well known that application of sex hormones causes thymic involution (1), and that gonadectomy increases the thymic size in experimental animals (1, 2). It has also been shown that sex hormones influence the T-cell maturational sequence (3, 4) as well as that thymocyte phenotypic profile differs between male and female rats (4). Moreover, strict synchrony has been observed between the generation of immunocompetent cells and the development and organization of hypothalamic centres involved in the regulation of gonadal function, and a close ontogenical interdependence in the development of hypothalamo–pituitary–gonadal (HHG) and thymolymphatic systems has been suggested (5). On the other hand, it has been shown that gender differentiation of the hypothalamic–pituitary complex and normal development of the HHG axis in rodents are highly dependent on the presence or absence of testosterone during the early postnatal period (6). Bearing that in mind, to test the latter hypothesis neonatal female rats were injected with testosterone and the thymocyte composition defined by expression of CD4 and CD8 molecules and TCR$\alpha\beta$ was analysed.

MATERIALS AND METHODS

Animals

Ten pregnant AO rats were obtained from the vivarium at the Military Medical Academy, Belgrade. Parturition occurred on the 22nd day of gestation and litter size was equated to 8 animals by cross-fostering pups. Litters were assigned randomly to an experimental condition, 5 to oil and 5 to testosterone-acetate (TA) treatment.

Immunoregulation in Health and Disease
ISBN 0-12-459460-3

Neonatal injection

On the 2nd postpartum day, one group of female offspring was removed from their mothers and injected subcutaneously with 2.5 mg TA (Fluka AG, Buchs SG, Germany) in 50 μl vegetable oil. A control group of female littermates was administered an equivalent volume of the oil vehicle.

Vaginal opening

Daily examination of rats for vaginal opening began on day 28.

Preparation of cell suspensions

Androgenized and control animals either 30 or 75 days old were weighed and then decapitated. The thymuses were removed, weighed and then placed in ice-cold PBS. Thymocyte suspensions were prepared by grinding the thymic tissue between the frosted ends of microscope slides and passing the resultant suspension through a fine nylon mesh. The single-cell suspensions so obtained were washed three times in ice-cold PBS (pH 7.3) containing 2% fetal calf serum (Gibco, Grand Island, NY, USA) and 0.01% sodium azide (PS medium); then counted in a standard haemocytometer. The viability of such cell preparations, as determined by Trypan blue exclusion, was routinely greater than 95%.

Flow cytometry (FCA)

Immunofluorescence staining of thymocytes and splenic cells was performed using two independent systems: (a) direct two-colour staining with FITC-conjugated anti-CD4 (clone W3/25, Serotec, Oxford, UK) and phycoerythrin (PE)-conjugated anti-CD8 (clone MRC OX-8, Serotec) mAbs and (b) indirect one-colour staining with biotin-conjugated mAb, most likely directed at a constant determinant of the rat $\alpha\beta$ heterodimeric T-cell receptor (TCR) (clone R73, Serotec), as primary reagent followed by FITC-conjugated streptavidin (Becton Dickinson, Mountain View, CA, USA).

For direct two-colour FCA, the aliquots of 1×10^6 lymphoid cells were incubated for 30 min on ice with both mAbs simultaneously. For indirect one-colour FCA, aliquots of 1×10^6 lymphoid cells were incubated with the first reagent for 30 min on ice, washed three times in PS medium, and incubated for another 30 min on ice with the second reagent. Antibodies were previously titrated to optimal concentrations.

After labelling, the cells were washed in PBS and fixed in 0.5 ml 1% paraformaldehyde. All samples were analysed on the same day on a FACScan flow cytometer (Becton Dickinson). 10^4 flow cytometric events for the two-colour and 5×10^3 flow cytometric events for one-colour FCA were analysed. The analyses were carried out with Consort 30 and Lysis software (Becton Dickinson).

Determination of oestradiol and progesterone concentrations

After decapitation, trunk blood was collected, serum separated and stored at −20°C until radioimmunoassay (RIA) was performed. Oestradiol (E_2) and progesterone (P) concentrations were measured using the ESTR-CTRIA kit (CIS bio international, Gif-sur-Yvette, France) and the RIA Progesteron kit (INEP Dijagnostika, Zemun, Yugoslavia), respectively. The RIA procedures were carried out according to the guidelines provided by the kit producers.

Statistical analysis

Differences between groups were analysed by Student's *t* test.

RESULTS AND DISCUSSION

As expected (6), neonatal TA treatment produced long-lasting dysfunctions in the HHG axis. None of the TA-treated rats showed signs of vaginal opening on the day of sacrifice. The serum E_2 concentration was significantly ($p<0.01$) lower in both the TA-treated peripubertal (1.82 ± 0.6 vs. 18.2 ± 1.2 pmol/ml) and adult rats (7.5 ± 3.7 vs. 26.6 ± 1.4 pmol/ml) compared with the age-matched oil-treated controls. Similarly, the serum P concentration was significantly ($p<0.05$) reduced in both the neonatally androgenized peripubertal (48.95 ± 7.07 vs. 99.18 ± 25.30 nmol/l) and adult rats (99.53 ± 16.12 vs. 165.63 ± 18.87 nmol/l) over that value in the age-matched controls.

Irrespective of age, the thymic weight did not differ between TA-treated and control rats (Table 20.1). However, the total thymocyte yield was reduced in the androgenized compared with age-matched control rats (Table 20.1). Supporting these data is the finding that changes in HHG development evoked by the blockade of LHRH receptors during the first 5 days of life causes the complete suppression of thymocyte proliferation response at 7 days of age and inhibition of blastogenic potential maturation until 3 months of age (5). This effect can be related to alterations in the sex hormone secretion, but also to the phenomenon of hormonal imprinting (7). In other words, the absence or presence of sex hormones during the critical postnatal period is of decisive importance for the maturation of the hormonal receptors, and later, for the development of the normal response capability of the cells (7). The unaltered value of the thymic weight, coupled with the reduced size of

Table 20.1 Effects of the neonatal testosterone acetate (TA) treatment on the thymic weight, total thymocyte yield and absolute number of $CD4^-8^-$, $CD4^+8^+$, $CD4^+8^-$ and $CD4^-8^+$ thymocytes, as well as on the absolute number of the thymocytes with total, low and high expression of TCR$\alpha\beta$ in peripubertal and adult female rats.

	Peripubertal rats		Adult rats	
	Oil treated ($n = 5$)	TA treated ($n = 8$)	Oil treated ($n = 7$)	TA treated ($n = 9$)
Thymic weight (g)	0.26 ± 0.01	0.23 ± 0.01	0.38 ± 0.01	0.37 ± 0.02
Thymocyte yield ($\times 10^7$)	5.36 ± 0.31	$1.95 \pm 0.21^{**a}$	8.83 ± 0.92	$4.75 \pm 0.14^{**b}$
$CD4^-8^-$ ($\times 10^7$)	0.07 ± 0.01	0.05 ± 0.01	0.43 ± 0.21	0.11 ± 0.02
$CD4^+8^+$ ($\times 10^7$)	4.86 ± 0.27	$1.66 \pm 0.20^{**a}$	7.68 ± 0.09	$3.67 \pm 0.01^{**b}$
$CD4^+8^-$ ($\times 10^7$)	0.31 ± 0.02	$0.18 \pm 0.02^{**a}$	0.79 ± 0.01	$0.32 \pm 0.01^{**b}$
$CD4^-8^+$ ($\times 10^7$)	0.12 ± 0.01	$0.06 \pm 0.01^{**a}$	1.01 ± 0.24	$0.39 \pm 0.03^{*b}$
TCR$\alpha\beta$ total ($\times 10^7$)	3.88 ± 0.29	$1.45 \pm 0.13^{**a}$	6.66 ± 0.23	$3.03 \pm 0.07^{**b}$
TCR$\alpha\beta$ low ($\times 10^7$)	3.03 ± 0.23	$1.12 \pm 0.11^{**a}$	5.28 ± 0.26	$2.46 \pm 0.07^{**b}$
TCR$\alpha\beta$ high ($\times 10^7$)	0.85 ± 0.08	$0.33 \pm 0.04^{**a}$	1.38 ± 0.02	$0.57 \pm 0.01^{**b}$

[a]TA treated peripubertal rats vs. age-matched oil treated rats.
[b]TA treated adult rats vs. age-matched oil treated rats.
Each value represents mean ± SEM.
$^{**}p < 0.01$; $^{*}p < 0.05$.

thymocyte population in neonatally androgenized rats, suggests an enlargement in the non-lymphoid thymic component. In support of this assumption are findings showing that thymic epithelial cells (TEC) express receptors for both E_2 and P (8). Moreover, using a rat thymic epithelial cell line (IT-45R1) a strong inhibitory effect of E_2 on TEC proliferation has been shown (9). In addition, it has been demonstrated that P in vitro can generate a biphasic TEC proliferative response: an increase that reaches a peak at 3×10^{-10} mmol/l, and progressive loss of TEC yield at concentrations of above 3×10^{-9} mmol/l (9). In the same reference are findings in vivo showing that during pregnancy, when the placenta develops and produces high levels of sex steroids, TEC become crowded together and show signs of cell death (10).

In the peripubertal rats which were neonatally treated with TA the percentage of $CD4^+8^+$ double positive (DP) cells was reduced, while the percentages of $CD4^-8^-$ double negative (DN) and $CD4^+8^-$ single positive (SP) cells were increased (Fig. 20.1A). Since, in these rats, the percentage of thymocytes with high expression of TCR$\alpha\beta$ was also increased (Fig. 20.1B), it can be assumed that the subset of $CD4^+8^-$ SP cells was enlarged on account of the cells being in a final stage of maturation. This assumption is in keeping with the finding that E_2 alters the distribution of MHC class II molecules on TEC and reduces its expression (10).

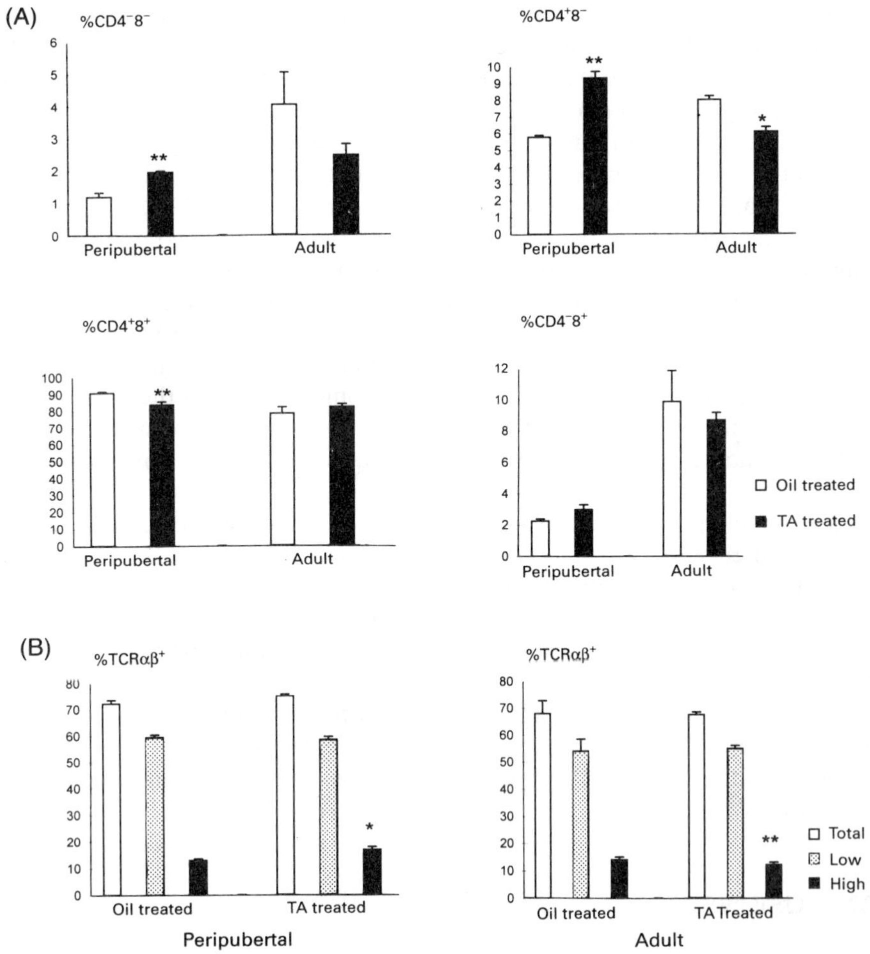

Fig. 20.1 Effects of neonatal androgenization induced by single injection of TA on the 2nd postnatal day on (A) the percentages of $CD4^-8^-$ DN, $CD4^+8^+$ DP, $CD4^-8^+$ SP and $CD4^+8^+$ SP thymocytes as well as (B) the percentage of cells expressing low and high levels of TCR$\alpha\beta$ in the thymus of the peripubertal and adult female rats. The percentage of thymocyte subsets was determined by direct two-colour and indirect one-colour FCA, respectively. Each value represents mean $\pm$ S.E.M. (n= 5–9). $^{**}p<0.01$; $^{*}p<0.05$.

Unlike the peripubertal rats, in the adult androgenized rats the percentages of $CD4^+8^-$ SP and TCR$\alpha\beta^+$ cells with high expression of this molecular complex were reduced (Fig. 20.1A, B). Taken together these findings suggest that the decrease in the percentage of cells bearing only a CD4 molecule was related to a reduction of the percentage of cells with more mature phenotype.

This observation is in agreement with previous data showing that the percentage of $CD4^+8^-$ thymocytes was significantly decreased in the adult rats neonatally treated with LHRH antagonists (3). It has also been shown that in adult female hypogonadal mice with a genetic deficiency of LHRH, the percentages of both single-stained $CD8^+$ and $CD4^+$ thymocytes were significantly reduced, whereas brain grafts containing LHRH cells were able to correct both the reproductive and the immune defects (11).

Differential effects of neonatal androgenization on the composition of thymocyte subsets in peripubertal and adult rats can be ascribed to the alterations in the sex steroid milieu related to maturation. The concentrations of both E and P differed significantly, not only between the androgenized and age-matched control rats, but also between androgenized rats of different ages. In other words, the results suggest that some changes in the HHG axis, as well as in the of intrathymic T-cell maturation, occurred during postnatal development, but their patterns were quite different from those in controls.

Since the thymocyte yield was significantly reduced in the androgenized peripubertal rats, the total number of thymocytes belonging to any of the analysed thymocyte subsets, except that of $CD4^-8^-$ DN cells, was decreased (Table 20.1). The similar pattern of changes in the absolute number of cells within the analysed subset was also found in adult androgenized rats (Table 20.1).

The results showed that changes in sexual differentiation of HHG function caused by injection of testosterone during early neonatal period can induce alterations in the thymic development and, consequently, T-cell maturation.

CONCLUSIONS

In female rats androgenized by a single injection of TA on the 2nd postnatal day and sacrificed at age either 30 or 75 days the thymic yield was significantly reduced compared with age-matched controls. In the peripubertal TA-treated rats the percentage of $CD4^+8^+$ DP cells was reduced, whereas the percentages of $CD4^-8^-$ DN and $CD4^+8^-$ SP cells were increased. These data, coupled with an increase in the percentage of cells with high expression of TCR$\alpha\beta$, implicate an increase in the percentage of $CD4^+8^-$ cells in a final stage of maturation. In adult TA-treated rats decrease in the percentages of both $CD4^+8^-$ cells and thymocytes with high expression of TCR$\alpha\beta^+$ was found. These findings suggest a reduction in the percentage of $CD4^+8^-$ cells in a final stage of maturation. The study showed that changes in the development of HHG axis can affect the process of intrathymic T-cell maturation.

REFERENCES

1. Martin, A., L. Alonso, M. Gomez del Moral and A. G. Zapata. 1994. Morphometrical changes in the rat thymic lymphoid cells after treatment with two different doses of estradiol benzoate. *Histol. Histopath.* **9**: 281–6.
2. Utsuyama, M. and K. Hirokawa. 1989. Hypertrophy of the thymus and restoration of immune functions in mice and rats by gonadectomy. *Mechanisms Ageing Dev.* **47**: 175–85.
3. Screpanti, I., S. Morrone, D. Meco *et al.* 1989. Steroid sensitivity of thymocyte subpopulations during intrathymic differentiation. *J. Immunol.* **142**: 3378–83.
4. Leposavić, G., B. Karapetrović, S. Obradović *et al.* 1996. Differential effects of gonadectomy on the thymocyte phenotypic profile in male and female rats. *Pharmacol. Biochem. Behav.* **54**: 269–76.
5. Morale, M. C., N. Batticane, G. Bartoloni *et al.* 1991. Blockade of central and peripheral luteinizing hormone-releasing hormone (LHRH) receptors in neonatal rats with a potent LHRH-antagonist inhibits the morphofunctional development of the thymus and maturation of the cell-mediated and humoral immune responses. *Endocrinology* **128**: 1073–85.
6. Barraclough, C. A. 1966. Modifications in the CNS regulation of reproduction after exposure of prepubertal rats to steroid hormones. *Rec. Prog. Horm. Res.* **22**: 503–29.
7. Csaba, G., O. Dobozy, A. Inczefi-Gonda and Sz. Szeberenyi. 1988. Effects of the absence of neonatal testosterone imprinting on the activity of microsomal enzyme system and on the dexamethason binding of the thymus in adulthood. *Acta Physiol. Hungar.* **71**: 421–7.
8. Kawashima, I., K. Sakabe, K. Seiki *et al.* 1991. Localization of sex steroid receptor cells, with special reference to thymulin (FTS)-producing cells in female rat thymus. *Thymus* **18**: 79–83.
9. Sakabe, K., I. Kawashima, R. Urano *et al.* 1994. Effects of sex steroids on the proliferation of thymic epithelial cells in a culture model: A role of protein kinase C. *Immunol. Cell. Biol.* **172**: 193–9.
10. Clarke, A. G. and M. D. Kendall. 1994. The thymus in pregnancy: the interplay of neural, endocrine and immune influences. *Immunol. Today* **15**: 545–51.
11. Moscovitz, H. C., S. Schmitt, G. J. Kokoris and I. Z. Leiderman. 1988. Thymocyte maturity in male and female hypogonadal mice and effect of preoptic area brain graft. *J. Reprod. Immunol.* **13**: 263–71.

21

A Study of Human Immunoglobulin (IgG and IgE) Glycosylation by Interaction with Lectins

Ljiljana Hajduković-Dragojlović, Milena Nešić, Margita Čuperlović, Miodrag Movsesijan, Nebojša Dovezenski, Nada Milošević-Jovčić and Lidija Jovanović

Glycosylation is a characteristic property of the class of immunoglobulins with regard to the type, number and composition of the oligosaccharide chains. Immunoglobulins IgG, IgM, IgA and IgE contain various numbers of oligosaccharides bound to the heavy chains, which can be N-type, O-type, complex or high-mannose type, differing also in the sequence of monosaccharide units (1).

The human serum IgG molecule contains two oligosaccharide chains located at the conserved glycosylation site of Asn 297 within CH2 domains of Fc fragments. Additional chains could be found in Fab fragments, in the variable regions of the light and heavy chains (2,3) as the consequence of variable region mutations (4). Thus, both the amount and the location of Fab-associated oligosaccharides are variable. Structural microheterogeneity of biantennary complex oligosaccharides of IgG is expressed by the content of sialic acid, the presence or absence of terminal galactose residues, and the presence or absence of fucose and bisecting *N*-acetyl glucosamine residues (5,6).

Despite the complex nature of IgG oligosaccharides, their composition in the IgG population from sera of healthy individuals is rather constant. Most of the sugar chains are fucosylated and non-bisected, and digalactosylated chains are prevalent among them (2). Fucosylated, non-bisected structures account for 65% of the oligosaccharide moieties, with preferred galactosylation on the Man (1–6) arm over the Man (1–3) arm (7). It might be expected, however, that a variety of other oligosaccharide patterns could be found in myeloma IgG (8). Analyses of monoclonal and myeloma antibodies showed

Immunoregulation in Health and Disease
ISBN 0-12-459460-3

in fact that each clone has a heterogeneous distribution of oligosaccharides (9). This unique glycosylation profile reflects the properties of the clone, which suggests that the profile observed for polyclonal IgG is the sum of all clones contributing to the IgG production (7).

Study of glycosylation of myeloma IgE revealed that there are three regular N-type oligosaccharide units per heavy chain which contain sialic acid, fucose, galactose, mannose and *N*-acetyl glucosamine in the molar ratio of 1 to 2:1:2:3:4 and one oligosaccharide unit per heavy chain containing only mannose and *N*-acetyl glucosamine (6:2) (10). It was pointed out that in the case of IgE there was no evidence of microheterogeneity, but more recent investigations revealed that different IgE glycoforms vary in their degree of sialylation (11). This insight into IgE microheterogeneity was enabled by a study of its interaction with an endogenous lectin.

Galectin-3, described also as an IgE binding protein, is the β-galactoside-binding lectin (12). It belongs to the galectin gene family and shares the characteristic galectin features: amino acid sequences, affinity for β-galactoside sugars and non-classical pathways of secretion (12). Galectin-3 is also characterized by an M_r of 26–35 kDa and is made up of two structural domains, an N-terminal domain containing short repeats rich in proline and glycine and a globular carbohydrate-binding C-terminal domain bearing a carbohydrate-binding motif homologous to the S-type lectin family (13).

The investigation of the interaction of galectin-3 with human IgE in vitro indicated that only a subpopulation of IgE reacts with galectin-3, with individual variations in the proportion of lectin recognized IgE from over 60% to barely detectable amounts, as a reflection of heterogeneous sialylation of IgE (11). This study was one of the relatively rare investigations of protein microheterogeneity based on interactions with an endogenous lectin which is or can be the natural ligand in vivo. Study of IgE glycosylation with plant lectins of various sugar specificity was less successful (14, our unpublished results). On the other hand, lectin-based studies of IgG microheterogeneity have generally been performed with lectins of plant origin (15).

Thus, the aim of this work was to examine glycosylation of myeloma IgG using five plant lectins and that of polyclonal hIgE using galectin-3. The applied methods were lectin crossed affinity immunoelectrophoresis (CAIE) and competitive enzyme–lectin binding assay (ELBA) for the study of IgG microheterogeneity, and IgE interaction with solid-phase bound galectin-3 and with galectin-3 exposed on the surface of elicited mouse macrophages.

MATERIALS AND METHODS

Samples

For IgG examinations serum samples were obtained from 12 healthy blood donors and 10 patients with multiple myeloma. IgG was isolated from pooled normal sera, and from each patient serum individually, so that 10 myeloma proteins were obtained including all four subclasses and both light chains.

Sera for IgE examination were obtained from atopic patients or from parasite-infected children and used without further purification.

Lectins

Galectin-3 was isolated from livers of immature Wistar rats (16). Lectin activity of the obtained preparation was tested by haemagglutination, laminin precipitation and the prepared solid-phase assay.

The applied plant lectins were isolated from the corresponding plant materials using standard procedures (17).

Lectin crossed affinity immunoelectrophoresis (CAIE)

Serum samples containing approximately 0.15 mg IgG were run on two-dimensional electrophoresis with (or without) lectin (0.5 mg/ml gel) in the first dimension and with anti-human IgG antibodies in the second dimension of the agarose gel. First-dimension electrophoresis was run at 10 V/cm for 2 h, and the second dimension at 2 V/cm for 18 h. The next day, gels were washed, pressed, dried and stained with Coomassie Brilliant Bue (18).

Competitive enzyme-lectin binding assay (ELBA)

Microtitre plates were coated with glycoproteins which are appropriate ligands for the applied plant lectins: ovalbumin for Con A, PSA, PHA-E and WGA and asialofetuin for PNA. Samples of IgG were added to the wells in serial dilution starting from 1 mg/ml, followed by lectin–HRPO conjugates. After 2 h incubation at room temperature, the wells were rinsed three times with PBS-Tween. Then substrate (urea peroxide) and chromogen (3,3′, 5,5′-tetramethylbenzidine) were added and the resulting colour measured at 450 nm (19).

Solid-phase competitive assay for galectin-3/IgE interaction

Galectin-3 isolated from the livers of immature rats was adsorbed to the surface of polystyrene test tubes. The coating solution contained 40 μg of lectin/ml and 0.1 ml of this solution was used for the adsorption. Laminin obtained from human placenta (20) was iodinated with ^{125}I using the chloramine T method (21). The dose-dependent interaction of insolubilized galectin-3 with ^{125}I-laminin was lactose inhibitable. The examined sera were diluted 10 000 times and 0.05 ml of each sample was incubated with 0.05 ml of ^{125}I-laminin galectin-coated tubes for 48 h at 4°C. The tubes were rinsed with PBS-Tween and bound radioactivity was counted.

Peritoneal macrophages

Female Balb/c mice were used at 7–8 weeks of age. Thioglycollate (TG)-elicited macrophages were obtained, as described by Woo *et al.* (22), from mice that had been injected 3–4 days before they were sacrificed with 1.5 ml of 4% (w/v) solution of thioglycollate broth (Torlak). This procedure yielded approximately 10^7 peritoneal cells per mouse.

Binding assays, unless otherwise specified, were performed with 10^6 cells per assay, in polystyrene tubes precoated with 0.5% BSA. The examined ligands, labelled by iodination, and in the presence or absence of inhibitory materials, were incubated with the cell suspension for 1 h at 4°C. Cells were washed in PBS and centrifuged to remove unbound radioactivity and finally the pellet was counted.

Haemagglutination assays

These were carried out with rabbit trypsin-treated erythrocytes (23). The cells were used as a 2% suspension in 0.9% NaCl. The assay was performed in glass tubes (0.7 × 5 cm); each tube contained 0.2 ml of cell suspension and 0.2 ml of the sample. The result was scored after 30 min incubation at room temperature. The inhibiting effect of lactose was examined by preincubating of the samples with sugar solution, followed by the haemagglutination assay.

RESULTS

Microheterogeneity of IgG as determined by using plant lectins

Crossed affinity immunoelectrophoresis

The affinity of the applied plant lectins for the examined IgG samples was expressed by the retardation or cathodic shift of the precipitation peaks, formed in the second dimension with anti-IgG antiserum. It was calculated as the retardation coefficient (R), defined as $R = l_0/l_r–1$, where l_0 and l_r are migration distances without or with lectin in the first-dimension gel, respectively (18).

The Con A reactivity with IgG from three sera (one from a blood donor and two from patients with multiple myeloma), as determined by CAIE, is shown in Fig. 21.1. IgG from normal serum formed one precipitation peak with specific anti-IgG antibodies (Fig. 21.1a). This peak was retarded if Con A was added to the first-dimension gel, and the retardation coefficient was 0.24 (Fig. 21.1A). IgG present in the sera of multiple myeloma patients, after reaction with anti-IgG antibodies, precipitated in two partially overlying

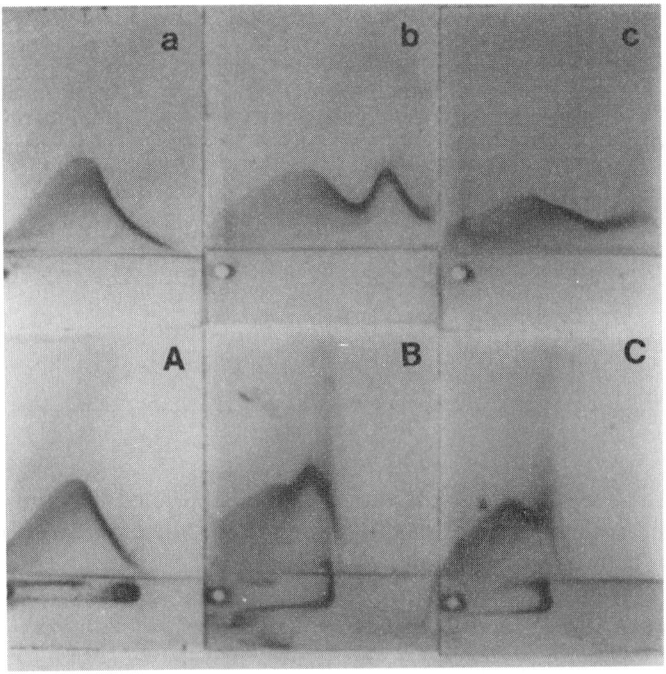

Fig. 21.1 Crossed immunoelectrophoresis of sera obtained from blood donor (a) and two patients with multiple myeloma (b,c), without (a,b,c) and with (A,B,C) ConA in the first dimension gel. A: R = 0.24; B: R(I) = 0.37, R(II) = 0.63; C: R(I) = 0.19, R(II) = 0.81.

peaks (Fig. 21.1b,c). The faster fractions, corresponding to myeloma IgG, were retarded by the interaction with Con A more than the slower fractions containing polyclonal IgG (Fig. 21.1B,C). Retardation coefficients for both examined samples of myeloma IgG are shown in the legend of Fig. 21.1.

A similar electrophoretic pattern was obtained by PSA–CAIE of normal sera, with slightly higher *R* values, ranging from 0.27 to 046. Retardation coefficients of some examined myeloma IgG, however, were several times higher in PSA–CAIE than in Con A–CAIE. For example, *R* values for the second peak of one myeloma IgG were 0.62 in PSA–CAIE and 0.17 in Con A–CAIE.

Affinity electrophoresis with PHA-E incorporated in the first-dimension gel gave generally lower *R* values, for myeloma samples ranging from 0.11 to 0.31, while application of WGA resulted in the highest retardation of myeloma IgG samples with *R* values between 0.90 and 1.42. The lectin PNA showed weak reactivity with all IgG examined, and in a few cases it was not reactive at all.

The results obtained for IgG examination by CAIE with the five lectins

Table 21.1 Concentration of IgG resulting in 50% inhibition of lectin binding to immobilized glycoproteins

	Monoclonal IgG (myeloma)			Polyclonal IgG (normal)
	1	2	3	
Lectins	Cp (mg/ml) $\times 10^{-3}$	Cp (mg/ml) $\times 10^{-3}$	Cp (mg/ml) $\times 10^{-3}$	Cp (mg/ml) $\times 10^{-1}$
Con A	2.1	4.3	1.1	1.2
PSA	2.2	3.7	8.6	1.3
PHA	16.0	4.0	22.0	1.4
WGA	7.8	3.9	15.0	1.3
PNA	16.0	7.8	3.9	4.9

applied were generally consistent with a high incidence of bisecting GlcNAc, bound to the trimannosyl core in IgG oligosaccharides, and with increased fucosylation in myeloma samples.

Competitive enzyme-lectin binding assay

In the applied competitive ELBA the lectin/IgG interaction was assessed by the IgG concentration necessary to achieve 50% inhibition of lectin binding to an immobilized glycoprotein. The results obtained by the examination of three myeloma samples and a pool of normal sera, are summarized in Table 21.1. All lectins used for this study had significantly higher affinity for the myeloma IgGs than for polyclonal IgG obtained from normal sera, and up to 100 times more polyclonal IgG was required for 50% inhibition of lectin binding, compared to monoclonal samples. Variation in lectin reactivity was also evident between myeloma IgGs. For example, Con A had the strongest affinity for Mo-IgG No3 (1.1×10^{-3} mg/ml necessary for 50% inhibition) while PSA, PHA and WGA had the least, suggesting that this IgG population had fewer bisecting GlcNAc residues, more exposed trimannosyl cores, and fewer Fuc residues than the other two examined Mo-IgGs.

IgE interaction with galectin-3

Solid phase system

The galectin-3 used in this study was isolated from rat livers and characterized by its specific properties. The affinity purified material (M_r 34 kDa) possessed agglutinating activity for trypsin-treated rabbit erythrocytes inhibitable by lactose. It also precipitated ^{125}I-labelled laminin in a dose-dependent manner, and precipitation was inhibited by the addition of lactose. Upon adsorption

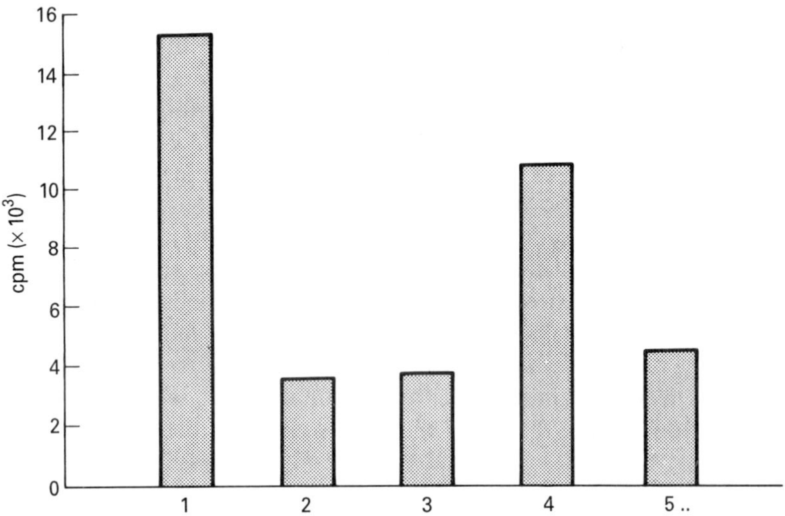

Fig. 21.2 Inhibition of galectin-3 interaction with ^{125}I-laminin in the solid phase assay. Inhibitors: (1) none; (2) laminin (2 μg/100 μl); (3) lactose (0.2 M); (4) human sera (1:10 000) containing 5 IU IgE/ml; (5) human sera (1:10 000) containing 8000 IU IgE/ml.

to polystyrene test tubes, the lectin retained the ability to react with ^{125}I-laminin. As shown in Fig. 21.2, this reaction was inhibited by the addition of an excess of unlabelled laminin or lactose. A pool of normal human sera diluted 10 000 times had a slight inhibitory effect, but sera with high IgE levels (equalized at 8000 IU/ml) possessed high inhibitory capacity towards the galectin-3/laminin interaction. This suggested examining IgE microheterogeneity by its interaction with an insolubilized endogenous lectin using the native IgE population, thus eliminating possible alterations of the glycoform ratios induced by the methods applied for IgE isolation from the examined sera. Owing to the limited amount of isolated galectin-3 available, it was possible to examine only five sera containing high IgE levels by the solid phase system and the variations found did not indicate microheterogeneity detectable by the applied method.

Binding assay with TG-elicited macrophages

Interaction of galectin-3 expressed on the surface of TG-elicited macrophages with polyclonal human IgE was examined using sera containing various IgE concentrations. The cell suspension was incubated with samples containing different IgE concentrations (30 min) and the IgE retained by the cells was then quantitated by the second incubation (30 min) with ^{125}I-labelled anti-IgE antibodies. The values obtained, shown as counts per minute in Fig. 21.3, indicated that IgE binding was a dose-dependent and saturable process. The samples used for this experiment were prepared by the dilution of sera containing high IgE concentrations, as explained in the legend. It is evident from the curve that, for the applied sera, IgE binding to macrophage receptors was not dependent on the source, but was related only to the IgE concentration. Addition of 0.2 M lactose solution to the macrophage suspension in vitro reduced IgE binding for all examined initial concentrations. A similar effect was obtained by the inhibition in vivo, when galactose solution was introduced intraperitoneally. In this experiment the group of mice treated with TG solution were intraperitoneally preinjected (3 h before TG injection) with 0.2 M D-galactose (1 mg/g body weight), and galactose solution was regularly administered at 6 h intervals for the subsequent 3 days. Macrophages were obtained from these animals using standard procedure. The results shown in Fig. 21.3 indicate that in vivo treatment of macrophages with galactose, reduced subsequent IgE binding to these cells in vitro.

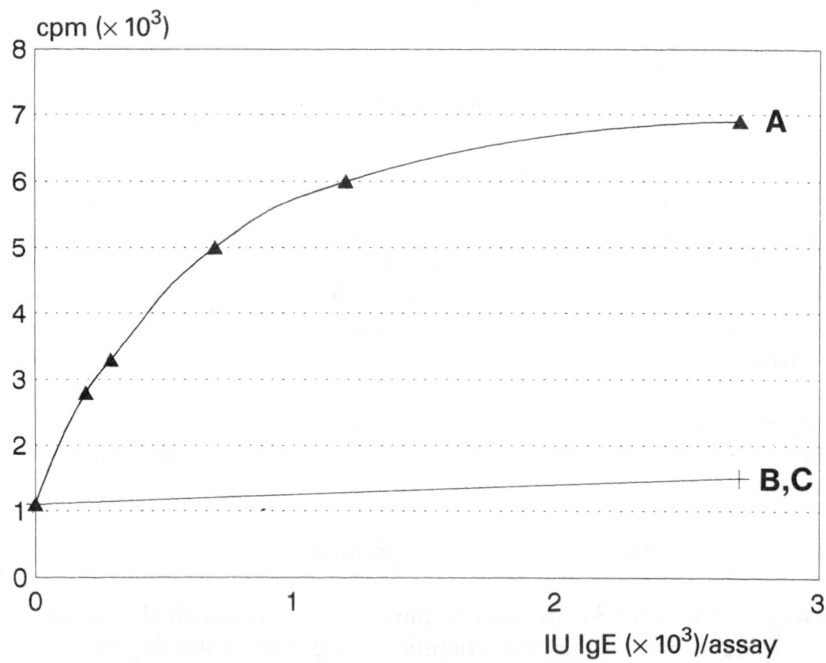

Fig. 21.3 Binding of human polyclonal IgE to mouse macrophage. Sera containing high IgE concentration were diluted and incubated with 10^6 cells, followed by incubation with ^{125}I-anti IgE (A). Inhibition in vitro with 0.2 M lactose (B). Inhibition in vivo with 0.2 M galactose (C).

DISCUSSION

A better understanding of the importance of immunoglobulin glycosylation for the performance of their functional activities (24) and the development of some autoimmune diseases (25) evoked the interest in the composition and changes of oligosaccharides bound to these proteins. The first methods employed for analysis of IgG and IgE glycosylation were lengthy and complicated chemical and physicochemical procedures (1,8,26). The possibility of determining some characteristics of the oligosaccharide chains and their alterations in diseases by using lectins of plant origin with known binding specificity was also tested soon after the first indications of immunoglobulin microheterogeneity (2,5,15). These simple and fast techniques were particularly successful in the characterization of abnormalities of IgG glycosylation connected with rheumatoid arthritis (RA) (27). Using lectin affinity methods it was shown that IgG from patients with RA possesses significantly fewer galactose residues in its sugar chains, and definite pathological consequences were attributed to this phenomenon (4). Lectin-based methods were also used to study glycosylation of myeloma IgG, and the results obtained with Con A and LCA indicated that some of the myeloma IgG proteins undergo unusual glycosylation processes (2). On the other hand, there is little information on the microheterogeneity of non-myelomatous IgE proteins. It was shown that IgE preparations obtained from allergic subjects reacted with several plant lectins, but without apparent variations in the reactivity of IgE samples from different individuals (14, our unpublished results). It was possible to detect the existence of IgE glycoforms only through the interaction with galectin-3, and variability was connected with the degree of sialylation (11).

Our results indicated that myeloma IgGs were generally more glycosylated than polyclonal IgG samples. In crossed affinity immunoelectrophoresis myeloma IgGs were more retarded by interaction with lectins incorporated in the first-dimension gel. When lectins were not added to the first gel, myeloma IgGs, owing to the higher content of sialic acid, usually migrated faster than polyclonal samples. Accordingly, about 100 times less monoclonal IgG was required in ELBA to achieve 50% inhibition of lectin binding to immobilized glycoprotein, compared to polyclonal IgG.

In CAIE the highest retardation effect was obtained with WGA, followed by PSA, Con A, PHA-E and finally PNA. The low reactivity of myeloma IgG with PNA was confirmed in ELBA, but the sequence of the other lectins was not the same. Although it is assumed that lectins incorporated into the gel do not move during electrophoresis at pH 8.6, it is possible that the electrophoretic mobility of different lectin-IgG complexes is not the same, which could have some influence on *R* values. ELBA would give more relevant data on the affinity of various lectins for IgGs; however, ELBA requires separation of IgG from the sera before examination, while CAIE could be performed with whole sera, which is a considerable advantage for the analysis of many samples.

Both methods showed significant variations in the glycosylation pattern of the examined myeloma IgGs. Differences are connected with the degree of fucosylation (PSA reactivity), with the presence of bisecting GlcNAc linked to the β-linked Man (PHA-E reactivity) and the exposure of a free mannosyl core (Con A reactivity). Glycosylation microheterogeneity was not related to the IgG subclasses or the type of light chain in the ten investigated samples. According to data in the literature (28) galactosylation of the Man (1–6) arm is preferred for IgG_1 and IgG_4, while IgG_2 and IgG_3 proteins exhibit a predominance of oligosaccharides having Gal on the Man (1–3) arm. However, such differences could not be detected with the applied lectins.

The reactivity of complex oligosaccharide chains of IgE with the applied plant lectins was similar to IgG. The work of Shibasaki *et al.* (14) indicated that IgE preparations obtained from allergic subjects were bound with high affinity to Con A, PSA and PHA-E, and with low affinity to WGA, and particularly PNA, among 12 lectins examined. However, in this study and in our recent trials, no variations were found in the reactivity of IgE from different individuals to the various plant lectins applied. Liu and Robertson (11) used galectin-3, as an endogenous ligand for IgE, for characterization of its heterogeneity. They found that galectin-3 recognized polyclonal IgE derived from four individuals with hyper-IgE syndrome or atopic dermatitis, while the proportion of binding ranged from over 60% to almost undetectable levels. It was concluded that galectin-3/IgE interaction is modulated by sialylation of IgE oligosaccharide chains and that the degree of sialylation is distributed in a distinct manner in different individuals. Following this approach, we attempted to determine IgE microheterogeneity by using its reactivity with galectin-3 insolubilized on polystyrene test tubes or exposed on the surface of elicited macrophages. In both systems IgE reacted with galectin-3 in a dose-dependent and lactose-inhibitable manner, but this reactivity did not show individual variations between the samples examined.

The IgE-binding capacity of galectin-3 points to the possible relevance of this lectin for IgE-mediated allergic reactions. Liu and coworkers, on the basis of their finding that IgE and IgE receptor (FcERI) on mast cells are the major glycoproteins recognized by galectin-3, and from the properties of the lectin itself, suggested that galectin-3 has a potential to modulate the function of mast cells (29). Two possible models were proposed:

- Galectin-3 mediates receptor aggregation and subsequent mast-cell activation by crosslinking of two or more FcERI, directly or through receptor bound IgE
- Galectin-3 augments receptor aggregation, induced by IgE immune complexes, by coupling two or more IgE receptor molecules.

The hypothesis that galectin-3 can affect the activation of mast cells was supported by the experimentally increased serotonin release induced by antigen, if RBL cells were pretreated with galectin-3 (30). Our finding that IgE binding by macrophages in vitro is inhibited by previous intraperitonal administration of galactose to TG-treated mice gave additional support to the opinion that the presence of active galectin-3 is essential for IgE binding to the surface of activated macrophages. It also suggests that lectin-mediated processes could be modulated in vivo by the addition of specific non-immunogenic oligosaccharides. The possible effects of such treatments on the functions of various lectins with similar sugar specificity are far beyond the scope of this work. Nevertheless, the idea that oligosaccharide treatment can present a new therapeutic approach in the attenuation of inflammation or in tumour spreading is appearing more and more frequently in the relevant literature.

ACKNOWLEDGEMENT

This study was supported by the Ministry of Science and Technology, Republic of Scrbia. The authors are grateful to the Central Clinic Chemical Laboratory of the Military Medical Academy for supplying samples from atopic patients.

REFERENCES

1. Baenziger, J. and S. Kornfeld. 1974. Structure of the carbohydrate units of IgA_1. *J. Biol. Chem.* **249**: 7260–9.
2. Kinoshita, N., M. Ohno, T. Nishiura *et al.* 1991. Glycosylation at the Fab portion of myeloma immunoglobulin G and increased fucosylated biantennary sugar chains: structural analysis by high-performance liquid chromatography and antibody–lectin enzyme immunoassay using lens culinaris agglutinin. *Cancer Res.* **51**: 5888–92.
3. Endo, T., A. Wright, S. L. Morrison and A. Kobata. 1995. Glycosylation of the variable region of immunoglobulin G – site specific maturation of the sugar chains. *Mol. Immunol.* **32**: 931–40.
4. Rademacher, T. W., R. B. Parekh, R. A. Dwek *et al.* 1988. The role of IgG glycoforms in the pathogenesis of rheumatoid arthritis. *Springer Semin. Immunopathol.* **10**: 231–49.
5. Harada, H., M. Kamei, Y. Tokumoto *et al.* 1987. Systematic fractionation of oligosaccharides of human immunoglobulin G by serial affinity chromatography on immobilized lectin columns. *Anal. Biochem.* **164**: 374–81.
6. Burton, D. R. 1985. Immunoglobulin G: functional sites. *Mol. Immunol.* **22**: 161–206.
7. Jefferis, R. 1993. The glycosylation of antibody molecules: functional significance. *Glycoconjugate J.* **10**: 357–61.

8. Fujii, S., T. Nishiura, A. Nishikawa *et al.* 1990. Structural heterogeneity of sugar chains in immunoglobulin G. *J. Biol. Chem.* **265**: 6009–18.
9. Mizuochi, T., T. Taniguchi, A. Shimizu and A. Kobata. 1982. Structural and numerical variations of the carbohydrate moiety of immunglobulin G. *J. Immunol.* **129**: 2016–20.
10. Baenziger, J. and S. Kornfeld, 1974. Structure of the carbohydrate units of IgE immunoglobulin. *J. Biol. Chem.* **249**: 1889–903.
11. Robertson, M. W. and F.-T. Liu. 1991. Heterogeneous IgE glycoforms characterized by differential recognition of an endogenous lectin (IgE-binding protein). *J. Immunol.* **147**: 3024–30.
12. Barondes, S. H., D. N. W. Cooper, M. A. Gitt and H. Leffer, 1994. Galectins: structure and function of a large family of animal lectins. *J. Biol. Chem.* **269**: 20 807–10.
13. Raz, A., G. Pazerini and P. Carmi. 1989. Identification of the metastasis-associated, galactoside-binding lectin as a chimeric gene product with homology to an IgE-binding protein. *Cancer Res.* **49**: 3489–94.
14. Shibasaki, M., R. Sumazaki, S. Isoyama and H. Takita. 1992. Interaction of lectins with human IgE: IgE-binding property and histamine-releasing activity of twelve plant lectins. *Int. Arch. Allergy Immunol.* **98**: 18–25.
15. Sumar, N., K. B. Bodman, T. W. Rademacher *et al.* 1990. Analysis of glycosylation changes in IgG using lectins. *J. Immunol. Meth.* **131**: 127–36.
16. Roff, C. F. and J. L. Wang. 1983. Endogenous lectins from cultured cells. isolation and characterization of carbohydrate-binding proteins from 3T3 fibroblasts. *J. Biol. Chem.* **258**: 10 657–63.
17. Agrawal, B. B. L. and I. J. Goldstein. 1972. Purification of carbohydrate-binding proteins. In: *Methods in Enzymology*, Vol. 28 (V. Ginsburg, ed.) Academic Press, New York, pp. 313–83.
18. Bog-Hansen, T. C. 1983. Affinity electrophoresis of glycoproteins. In: *Solid Phase Biochemistry: Analytical Synthetic Aspects* (W. H. Scouten, ed.) Wiley, New York, pp. 223–51.
19. Van der Schaal, J. A. M., T. J. J. Logman, C. L. Diaz and J. W. Kijne. 1984. An enzyme-linked lectin binding assay for quantitative determination of lectin receptors. *Anal. Biochem.* **140**: 48–55.
20. Timpl, R., H. Rohde, P. G. Robey *et al.* 1979. Laminin–a glycoprotein from basement membranes. *J. Biol. Chem.* **254**: 9933–7.
21. Hudson, L. and F. C. Hay. 1989. Radiolabelling of soluble proteins – Chloramin T method. In: *Practical Immunology* (3rd edn.) Blackwell Scientific Publications, Oxford, pp. 49–52.
22. Woo, H.-J., L. M. Shaw, J. M. Messier and A. M. Mercurio. 1990. The major non-integrin laminin binding protein of macrophages is identical to carbohydrate binding protein 35 (Mac-2). *J. Biol. Chem.* **265**: 7097–9.
23. Nowak, T. P., D. Koliber, E. L. Roel and S. H. Barondes. 1977. Developmentally regulated lectin from embryonic chick pectoral muscle. *J. Biol Chem.* **252**: 6026–30.
24. Jefferis, R., J. Lund and M. Goodall. 1995. Recognition sites on human IgG for Fcγ receptors: the role of glycosylation. *Immunol. Lett.* **44**: 111–17.
25. Parekh, R. B., R. A. Dwek, B. J. Sutton *et al.* 1985. Association of rheumatoid arthritis and primary osteoarthritis with changes in the glycosylation pattern of total serum IgG. *Nature* **316**: 452–7.
26. Takahashi, N., I. Ishii, H. Ishihara *et al.* 1987. Comparative structural study of the *N*-linked oligosaccharides of human normal and pathological immunoglobulin G. *Biochemistry* **26**: 1137–44.

27. Tsuchiya, N., T. Endo, M. Shiota *et al.* 1994. Distribution of glycosylation abnormality among serum IgG subclasses from patients with rheumatoid arthritis. *Clin. Immunol. Immunopathol.* **70**: 47–50.
28. Jefferis, R., J. Lund, H. Mizutani *et al.* 1990. A comparative study of the *N*-linked oligosaccharidc structures of human IgG subclass proteins. *Biochem. J.* **268**: 529–37.
29. Liu, F.-T. 1993. S-type mammalian lectins in allergic inflammation. *Immunol. Today* **14**: 486–90.
30. Frigeri, L. G. and F.-T. Liu. 1992. Surface expression of functional IgE binding protein, an endogenous lectin, on mast cells and macrophages. *J. Immunol.* **148**: 861–7.

22

Acute Phase Profile of Novel Plasma Protein sgp120 (PK–120)

Goran A. Nikolić, Milutin Mirić and Vojislav D. Miletić

The protein sgp 120 is a recently discovered plasma glycoprotein of 120 kDa relative molecular mass present in fresh plasma of healthy people at a concentration of 0.3 mg/ml (1,2). Because sgp120 was able to bind to a C4-Sepharose column and inhibit the early steps of the classical pathway of complement activation, it was classified as a complement regulatory protein (1). Degrading purified sgp120 during spontaneous activation of the contact system of coagulation or by plasma and tissue kallikrein generates multiple fragments in the range of 15 to 85 kDa (3,4, Basta, Miletic and Frank in preparation). High-molecular-weight kallikrein-generated fragments (HMWF, 65–85 kDa) show the N-terminal part of the amino acid sequence, whereas low-molecular-weight fragments (LMWF) are generated from the C-terminal half of the sgp120 molecule (Miletic, Basta and Frank in preparation). HMWF are recognized by monoclonal antibody E.1.9 prepared against purified sgp120, while LMWF can be recognised by goat polyclonal antiserum (Basta, Miletic and Frank in preparation). The sensitivity of sgp120 to kallikrein led Pu *et al.* to believe that sgp120 is a noval plasma kallikrein substrate, PK120 (4), but precise biological function of this protein is still not known.

The amino acid sequence of sgp120 (5, Hammer *et al.* in preparation) revealed a high sequence homology to the heavy chains of the abundant plasma protein, inter-α-trypsin inhibitor (IαI). Also, the mRNA for both sgp120 and IαI were found exclusively in the liver (5,6). IαI was discovered decades ago in plasma and serum samples. The relative molecular mass of IαI is 185–240 kDa (7), but related proteins (or protein fragments) of lower molecular mass have also been described (8). A limited degradation with hyaluronidase, *S. aureus* V8 proteinase, kallikrein, cathepsin G and neutrophil elastase and other molecular analyses show that IαI is composed

Immunoregulation in Health and Disease
ISBN 0–12–459460–3

of three polypeptide chains: two heavy chains (HC_1 and HC_2) connected to one light chain (HI–30, bikunin) by chondroitin sulfate links (8–10). The light chain of IαI contains the region for inhibitory activity against trypsin. Growth support activity for different cell lines was also ascribed to IαI (10–12). The amino acid sequence of IαI reveals 40% homology between HC_1 and HC_2 and no homology between the heavy and light chains (6,13,14).

Structural and functional similarities suport the growing evidence that IαI and some other protease inhibitors belong to the same protein family whose dominant biological function has yet to be discovered (7).

We investigated the relationship between sgp120 and IαI in acute phase response. In this chapter we present the evidence that sgp120 is an acute phase protein similar to complement components C3 and C4 and distinct from IαI.

MATERIALS AND METHODS

Blood samples were taken in plastic tubes containing EDTA (final concentration 10 mM) from 12 randomly selected patients awaiting cardiac surgery. Samples were taken at 2 h prior and every 2 h during the operation. Serial samples were taken every 2 h during the first postoperative day and daily up to 10 days. Two patients (No. 2 and No. 4) were later excluded from the study because massive transfusions were needed during surgery. Other patients received zero or 1–3 units of washed red cells during the first postoperative day. Cardiac surgery consisted of aortal or mitral valve exchanges (patients Nos. 1, 7, 10, 11), or arteriocoronary bypasses (patients Nos. 3, 4, 5, 6, 8, 9, 12). The duration of the operation was 3–5 h. Plasma samples were aliquoted and kept at −85°C until analysed.

Polyclonal anti-sgp120 antiserum was prepared by immunizing a goat with chromatographically purified sgp120 (2). The IgG fraction was isolated by caprylic acid–ammonium sulfate precipitation (15).

The concentrations of the following plasma proteins were determined in 185 patient plasma samples: CRP, α_1 antitrypsin, α_2 macroglobulin, haptoglobin, complement components C3 and C4, albumin, and sgp120. The concentrations were determined by laser nephelometry using equipment, standards and antisera of the Behring Institute, Marburg, Germany. The concentration of inter-α-trypsin inhibitor (IαI) was determined in 64 plasma samples from five patients (Nos. 1, 3, 5, 6 and 7). Both the sgp120 and IαI concentrations were determined by Laurells' rocket immunoasay (16) using polyclonal goat anti-sgp120 antiserum, and the IgG fraction of polyclonal sheep anti-IαI commercial antiserum (The Binding Site), respectively. Pooled plasma of 100 healthy adult blood donors served as an internal standard.

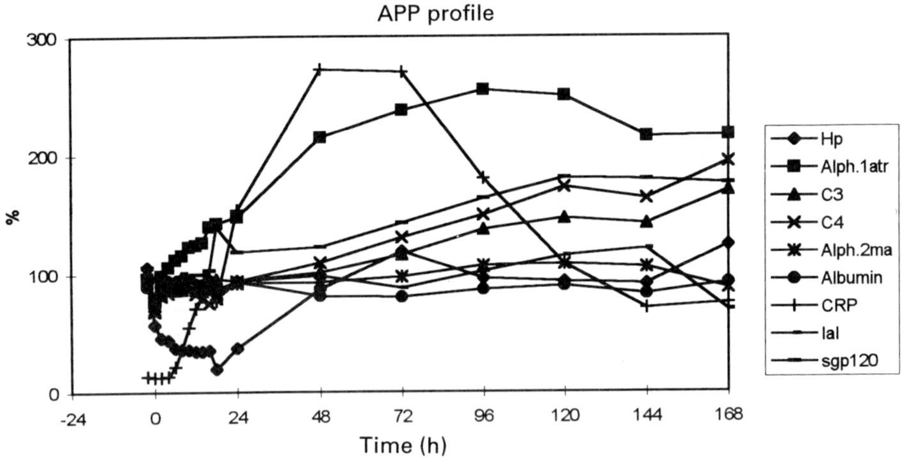

Fig. 22.1 Plasma concentrations of: haptoglobin, α_1 antitrypsin, C3, C4, α_2 macroglobulin, albumin, CRP, sgp120 and inter-α-trypsin inhibitor (IαI) in 10 (except IαI, 5) cardiac surgery patients during 10 postoperative days. Proteins serial labels are indicated in the legend. All concentrations are calculated as a percentage of standard plasma pool.

RESULTS

Plasma samples from 10 cardiac surgery patients were analysed during postoperative hospitalization in order to identify the AP behaviour of sgp120 and IαI compared to well-known AP reactants. All patients expressed typical AP responses after surgical trauma as shown by elevated concentrations of C-reactive protein, α_1 antitrypsin, C3 and C4 (Fig. 22.1).

The CRP concentration was below the detection limit (0.9 mg/l) in all but two (Nos. 7 and 10) preoperative samples and started to rise after 4 h (No. 11), 6 h (Nos. 8, 12), 8 h (Nos. 1, 3, 5, 7 and 9) or 14 h (Nos. 6 and 10). The peak concentration was achieved at 48 or 72 h after surgical trauma, followed by a slow decline during the next 3–4 days. Because the starting concentration could not be precisely determined by the method used in this study, the ratio beween the starting and maximal concentration cannot be determined, but Fig. 22.1 shows an extreme rise in CRP concentration.

The α_1 antitrypsin concentrations started to rise during or after the first postoperative day, reaching a peak after 3–5 days. The average maximal value was 2.893 times higher than the average starting concentration. Contrary to

Table 22.1 Statistical correlations among analysed proteins (Pearson's *r*)

sgp 120 vs:		C4 vs:		C3 vs:	
C3	0.7476	C3	0.8181	α1AT	0.7010
C4	0.7298	α1AT	0.6337	IαI	0.3786
α1AT	0.7220	Hp	0.3546	α2M	0.2703
IαI	0.5028	IαI	0.3463	Albumin	0.2751
CRP	0.2811	CRP	0.3078	Hp	0.2190
Hp	0.2690	α2M	0.2224		
α2M	0.1544	Albumin	0.1163		
Albumin	−0.0474				
a1AT vs:		**a2M vs:**		**Hp vs:**	
CRP	0.6640	IαI	0.2448	IαI	0.4277
IαI	0.4035	Albumin	0.2055	CRP	0.2768
α2M	0.2902	Hp	0.0606	Albumin	−0.1308
Hp	0.2958	CRP	−0.0274		
Albumin	−0.0328				
Albumin vs:					
CRP	−0.0984				
IαI	−0.0198				

the two previous acute phase proteins, the concentrations of C3 and C4 started to rise slowly during the second postoperative day with a continuous increase during all 10 days. The average maximal values for C3 and C4 were 1.618 and 2.053 times higher than their average starting concentrations, respectively.

The concentrations of α_2 macroglobulin, haptoglobin and albumin were practically unchanged (not shown here).

It is evident that sgp120 expresses an AP profile, and IαI shows no indication of an AP reaction. The sgp120 concentrations started to rise during the second postoperative day and continued to rise during all 10 days. The average maximal value was 2.364 times higher than the starting one. Statistical analysis (Table 22.1) showed the highest correlations between sgp120 and C3, C4, α_1 antitrypsin and IαI, and C3 and C4.

DISCUSSION

The recently discovered plasma protein sgp120 is present in all normal plasma samples at relatively high concentration (1,2). It was discovered during an attempt to purify complement component C2 by affinity chromatography on a C4-Sepharose column (1). Two different chromatographic procedures for sgp120 purification have since been described (2,4). Because sgp120 could bind to a C4-Sepharose column and inhibit the early steps in the complement classical pathway cascade, it was classified as a complement regulatory protein (1). Because of its exceptional sensitivity to degradation during contact system activation and digestion by purified kallikrein (1, 2, 3) it was later believed that sgp120 is a novel kallikrein substrate and it became known as PK-120 (4). Other than its sensitivity to kallikrein degradation, no other similarity, functional or structural, to other kallikrein substrates (high- and low-molecular-weight kininogens) has been described. Enormous efforts have produced no data indicating the possible physiological function of this abundant plasma protein. Even knowledge of the sgp120 primary structure and comparison to other well-known protein structures has produced no clues to the function(s) of sgp120 (5, Hammer *et al.* in preparation). The primary structure did show that sgp120 is a unique plasma protein having about 35% homology to the heavy chains of IαI, another abundant plasma protein with no precisely defined physiological function. Trypsin inhibitory activity and a role in the growth of some cell lines and extracellular matrix (11,12) are common functions of IαI and many of the low-molecular-weight enzyme inhibitors that belong to the superfamily of Kunitz-type inhibitors (7).

To investigate the relationship between sgp120 and IαI we determined sgp120 and IαI concentrations during the acute phase (AP) response. Since the AP response of sgp120 has not yet been determined, it is not known whether synthesis of sgp120 is controlled by inflammatory cytokines. It is known that HI30 (bikunin, IαI light chain) synthesis is up-regulated during the AP response but the heavy chains are not affected, suggesting that the synthesis of the heavy chains limits the AP response of IαI (7). Two related proteins having similarities in their primary structure may express similar antigenic epitopes and, as a result, can be recognized by specific antibodies in cross-reactions (17). The efficient purification of sgp120 by monoclonal antibody affinity chromatography (Miletic, Basta and Frank in preparation), without the copurification of IαI, indicate the absence of this particular epitope recognised by monoclonal antibody B1.9.E-2. Although IαI has anti-trypsin activity, this function may not be of great physiological importance because many other plasma inhibitors with a far higher inhibitory capacity toward this enzyme are present in the same biological fluids. Because of the absence of the HI-30 chain in sgp120, it is highly unlikely that sgp120 will express any trypsin inhibitory activity even though sgp120 expressed inhibitory activity against the early activation steps of the classical complement pathway (1).

To investigate the AP profile of sgp120 and IαI, for many reasons we have chosen patients who have undergone trauma during cardiac surgery. First, this type of surgical trauma is usually without an infectious component which may otherwise add new biochemical and immunological stimuli. Second, the operation is carefully planned and patients are well prepared. This is not normally the case in traumatic surgery. Third, the operations are serious and long-lasting, therefore inducing high acute phase response. The only drawback to this investigation is the possible influence of the large volume of donor blood circulating through the extracorporeal circulation and patient's body during operation. To minimize the influence of blood transfusions on our results, we carefully followed transfusion protocols during the postoperative period of the investigated patients. Two patients had complicated surgical procedures, heart attacks intraoperatively and massive transfusions during the postoperative period. Subsequently, these two patients were excluded from our final calculations. In all 10 analysed patients the acute phase response was highly evident according to the elevated concentrations of known acute phase proteins CRP, α_1 antitrypsin, C3 and C4. The concentrations of α_2 macroglobulin, haptoglobin and albumin remained almost unchanged. The acute phase profile presented in Fig. 22.1 and the correlation analysis presented in Table 22.1 show that sgp120 is an AP protein. The AP response of sgp120 is similar to complement components C3 and C4 and distinct from CRP, suggesting that the inflammatory cytokines IL-1β, IL-6, TNF and TGFβ1 may play a role in sgp120 synthesis induction (18–20). Observing elevated concentration levels and the time of response to the inflammatory stimuli, all acute phase proteins can be classified into three groups (19–22). The concentration in serum of group I AP proteins rises to less than twice the starting value 2–3 days after stimulation. Complement components C3 and C4 belong to this group. Group II proteins react 10–24 h after stimulation with a two- to fourfold increase in concentration. These proteins are represented by α_1 antitrypsin. Group III proteins react 6–10 h after initial stimulation and rise by a factor of over 1000 at the peak of the response. CRP is a dominant protein in this group. Because of its high correlation with C3, C4 and α_1 antitrypsin during the acute phase response, sgp120 may belong to either group I or group II AP proteins. The IαI concentration showed no change during an AP response, confirming previously published results (7). According to this investigation sgp120 and IαI are clearly distinct proteins whose synthesis is stimulated by different cytokines.

The homology in a primary structure (5, Hammer *et al.* in preparation) and the distinctions in AP response, presented in this paper, makes the relationship between sgp120 and IαI a very interesting puzzle. This discrepancy indicates either that common structural motifs (in this case homology in primary structure) are not critical for the prediction of common functions that sgp120 and IαI may have, or that the common and important physiological function of both proteins remains to be discovered and will confirm the predictions based on similar primary structures. Further investigations on transcriptional regulation of sgp120, organ and tissue colocalization of both sgp120 and IαI, and phylogenetic and ontogenetic studies of sgp120 are currently under way in our laboratories and will shed some light on this interesting phenomenon.

SUMMARY

The protein sgp120 is a recently discovered plasma glycoprotein. The biological function of this abundant protein is still unknown. The cDNA sequence of sgp120, however, is significantly homologous to another abundant plasma protein, inter-α-trypsin inhibitor (IαI). We investigated the sgp120 and IαI relationship in the acute phase response. The concentrations of sgp120, IαI and several well-known acute phase proteins such as CRP, albumin, α_1 antitrypsin, α_2 macroglobulin, C3, C4, haptoglobin were determined in serial plasma samples of 10 cardiac surgery patients. We show here that sgp120 is a novel acute phase protein similar in response time and magnitude to complement components.

Low correlations were observed between sgp120 and CRP, α_2-macroglobulin and haptoglobulin (0.2606, 0.2346, and 0.2581, respectively). The best correlation among the known acute phase reactants was found for C3 and C4 (0.8600), and α_1 antitrypsin and CRP (0.6720). These findings indicate that sgp120 is an acute phase reactant belonging to Kushners' group II and probably stimulated by the concerted action of IL-1, IL-6 and TNF as described for complement proteins. The concentration of IαI was stable without an acute phase response. Comparison of N-terminal sequences excluded any possibility that sgp120 may represent IαI heavy chain dimer. Therefore, sgp120 is a novel acute phase reactant distinct from IαI.

REFERENCES

1. Hammer, C. H., R. M. Jacobs and M. M. Frank. 1989. Isolation and characterization of a novel plasma protein which binds to activated C4 of the classical complement pathway. *J. Biol. Chem.* **264**: 2283–91.
2. Miletic, V. D. and M. M. Frank. 1994. Chromatographic isolation and determination of the concentration in human plasma of the novel plasma protein, sgp120. *Yug. Med. Biochem.* **13**: 95–102.
3. Langlois, P. F., Y. Pilatte, M. Basta *et al.* 1989. A newly identified plasma protein, sgp120, is cleaved after activation of the kinin-generating pathway. *Complement* **6**: 359 (Abstr).
4. Pu, X. P., A. Iwamoto, H. Nishimura and S. Nagasawa. 1994. Purification and characterisation of a novel substrate for plasma kallikrein (PK-120) in human plasma. *Biochim. Biophys. Acta* **1208**: 338–43.
5. Nishimura, H., I. Kakizaki, T. Muta *et al.* 1995. cDNA and deduced amino acid sequence of human PK-120, a plasma kallikrein-sensitive glycoprotein. *FEBS Lett.* **357**: 207–14.
6. Salier, J. P., M. Diarra-Mehrpour, R. Sesboue *et al.* 1987. Isolation and

characterization of cDNAs encoding the heavy chain of human inter-α-trypsin inhibitor (IαTI): Unambiguous evidence for multipeptide chain structure of IαTI. *Proc. Natl. Acad. Sci. USA* **84**: 8272–6.

7. Salier, J. P. 1990. Inter-α-trypsin inhibitor: emergence of a family within the Kunitz-type protease inhibitor superfamily. *Trends Biochem. Sci.* **15**: 435–9.
8. Enghild, J. J., I. B. Thogersen, S. V. Pizzo and G. Salvesen. 1989. Analysis of inter-α-trypsin inhibitor and a novel trypsin inhibitor, pre-α-trypsin inhibitor, from human plasma. *J. Biol. Chem.* **264**: 15 975–81.
9. Potempa, J., K. Kwon, R. Chawla and J. Travis. 1989. Inter-α-trypsin inhibitor. Inhibition spectrum of native and derived forms. *J. Biol. Chem.* **264**: 15 109–14.
10. Castillo, G. M. and D. M. Templeton. 1993. Subunit structure of bovine ESF (extracellular-matrix stabilizing factor(s)). A chondoritin sulfate proteoglycan with homology to human IαI (inter-α-trypsin inhibitors). *FEBS Lett.* **318**: 292–6.
11. McKeehan, W. L., Y. Sagakami, H. Hoshi and K. A. McKeehan. 1986. Two apparent human endothelial cell growth factors from human hepatoma cells are tumor-associated proteinase inhibitors. *J. Biol. Chem.* **261**: 5378–83.
12. Chen, L., S. J. T. Mao and W. J. Larsen. 1992. Identification of a factor in fetal bovine serum that stabilizes the cumulus extracellular matrix. A role for a member of the inter-α-trypsin inhibitor family. *J. Biol. Chem.* **267**: 12 380–6.
13. Gebhard, W., T. Schreitmuller, K. Hochstrasser and E. Wachter. 1988. Complementary DNA and derived amino acid sequence of the precursor of one of the three protein components of the inter-α-trypsin inhibitor complex. *FEBS Lett.* **229**: 63–7.
14. Gebhard, W., T. Schreotmuller, K. Hochstrasser and E. Wachter. 1989. Two out of three kinds of subunits of inter-α-trypsin inhibitor are structurally related. *Eur. J. Biochem.* **181**: 571–6.
15. Perosa, F., R. Carbone, S. Ferrone and F. Dammaco. 1990. Purification of human immunoglobulins by sequential precipitation with caprylic acid and ammonium sulphate. *J. Immunol. Meth.* **128**: 9–16.
16. Laurell, C. B. 1972. Electrophoretic and electro-immunochemical analysis of proteins. *Scand. J. Clin. Lab. Invest.* **29**: suppl. 124.
17. van Oss, C. J. 1994. Nature of specific ligand–receptor Bonds, in particular the antigen–antibody bond. In: *Immunochemistry* (C. J. van Oss and M. H. V. van Regenmortel, eds.) Marcel Dekker, New York, pp. 581–614.
18. Baumann, H., V. Onorato, J. Gauldie and G. P. Jahreis. 1987. Distinct sets of acute phase plasma proteins are stimulated by separate human hepatocyte-stimulating factors and monokines in rat hepatoma cells. *J. Biol. Chem.* **262**: 9756–68.
19. Whicher, J. T. and C. I. Westacott. 1992. The acute phase response. In: *Biochemistry of Inflammation* (C. T. Whicher and S. W. Evans, eds.) Kluwer, Dordrecht, pp. 243–71.
20. Rokita, H. and K. Szuba. 1991. Regulation of acute phase reaction by transforming growth factor β in cultured murine hepatocytes. *Acta Biochem. Polonica* **38**: 241–9.
21. Kushner, I. 1982. The phenomenon of acute phase response. *Ann. N.Y. Acad. Sci.* **389**, 39–48.
22. Kushner, I. and A. Mackiewicz. 1987. Acute phase proteins as disease markers. *Dis. Markers* **5**, 1–11.

23

Total Body Irradiation-induced Changes in Rat Serum IL-1, IL-6 and TNF Activities

Zvonko Magić, Zorka Kukić, Danilo Vojvodić, Nada Pejnović and Miodrag Čolić

The cytokines interleukin-1 (IL-1), interleukin-6 (IL-6) and tumor necrosis factor (TNF) are actively involved in the promotion and regulation of the acute phase response of an organism to different kinds of injury and infection. By performing their local and systemic effects they play a vital role in host defence mechanisms. Although high doses of IL-1 and TNF are toxic, they have been successful experimental radioprotective substances (1). Several of the recognized activities of IL-1, such as the production of colony stimulatory factors (CSFs), acute phase proteins (APPs) and IL-6, have been suggested to provide the basis for its radioprotective effect (1). Results of our previous studies have shown that high doses of ionizing radiation induced the increased synthesis of APPs (2) which was preceded by the increased expression of the appropriate genes in the liver. The APPs are essential for the re-establishment of homeostatic balance disturbed by the effect of different noxious agents. That is why some of these proteins, e.g. α_2-macroglobulin and ceruloplasmin, have been used as radioprotectors. The most important inducer of APP synthesis is IL-6. The first studies using IL-6 as a radioprotective substance were discouraging, although later investigations showed that IL-6 is an essential contributor to the natural resistance to lethal radiation (3). These findings also indicated that endogenous production and numerous in vivo interactions of these cytokines are important for the ability of lethally irradiated mice to increase their survival time. In the present study the effects of different radiation doses on the rat serum IL-1, IL-6 and TNF activities were determined. These cytokines belong to the two main groups of APP gene transcription inducers, i.e. the IL-1-type (IL-1α and β, TNFα and β) and IL-6-type (IL-6, IL-11, leukaemia inhibitory factor, oncostatin) cytokines. Their actions are, in turn, modulated by glucocorticoid hormones and growth factors. An aspect of their activities, such as those of IL-6 and

Immunoregulation in Health and Disease
ISBN 0–12–459460–3

dexamethasone on the expression of APPs genes in the hepatoma cell line (HTC) were also studied in this work.

MATERIALS AND METHODS

Experimental animals

Experiments were performed using male 8–10-week-old Albino Oxford (AO) strain rats. Rats were total body irradiated (Philips linear accelerator, 8 MeV) with 4 ($LD_{10/30}$), 6.7 ($LD_{50/30}$), 9 ($LD_{95-100/30}$) and 12 Gy ($LD_{100/30}$).

Serum cytokine level determinations

IL-1 activity was measured by incorporating tritiated thymidine into IL-1-sensitive D10S cells derived from the murine T-helper cell line D10.G4.1 (4).

Serum IL-6 activity was measured by a B9 bioassay (5).

TNF activity was determined by an L929 fibroblast cell lytic assay (6).

The specificity of the IL-1 and IL-6 assay was confirmed by using appropriate rabbit polyclonal anti-human IL-1 and IL-6 antibodies (Genzyme). For the TNF assay neutralizing anti-mouse TNFα antibody was used (Genzyme). Non-specific inhibition was excluded by using irrelevant rabbit immunoglobulin in identical protein concentrations.

Cell culture

The rat hepatoma tissue culture cell line (HTC-Morris hepatoma 7288C, Flow Laboratories) was cultivated to confluency for 3 days in the bicarbonate-buffered RPMI 1640 medium (Flow), 5% fetal calf serum (Flow), 2 mM glutamine (Serva) and 2% Gentamicin (ICN-Galenika) in a 5% carbon dioxide incubator at 37°C. The first group of cells (1×10^7 cells/ml) was 'pulsed' for 2 h at 37°C with constant shaking, either with 200 U/ml IL-6 (Genzyme), or with 1 μmol/l dexamethasone (Galenika). The cells were placed for 18 h in culture medium with 20-fold lesser concentrations of IL-6 or dexamethasone. In the second group HTC cells (0.5×10^6 cells/ml) were incubated for 20 h in the medium with 50 U/ml IL-6 or 1 μmol/l dexamethasone or both.

Isolation and analysis of RNAs

Total RNAs from HTC cells were isolated by the procedure based on the extraction with guanidine-HCl as described by Cox (7). After electrophoresis under denaturing conditions RNA was transferred onto Hybond nylon membranes (Amersham) and hybridized with nick-translated plasmid cDNA probes labelled with deoxycytidine 5′-[α-^{32}P]triphosphatetriethylammonium salt (Amersham) according to the manufacturer's instructions. After washing, the filters were exposed to Kodak X-OMAT AR films at −70°C for 3 days. Samples of 2, 5 and 10 μg of RNA isolated from four to six separate experiments were blotted onto nylon membranes, hybridized with the respective nick-translated cDNA probes, exposed to X-ray film and analysed by densitometry.

Plasmids

Plasmids carrying the cDNA inserts for rat α_1-acid glycoprotein (AGP) (pIRL 21), haptoglobin (Hp) (pIRL 25), cysteine inhibitor protease (CPI) (pIRL 28) and fibrinogen-α (Fb) (pIRL 14) mRNAs were kindly donated by Dr. Heinz Baumann (Roswell Park Memorial Institute, Buffalo, NY) and cDNA for rat albumin (Al) (pRSA 57) mRNA from Dr. T. D. Sargent of the California Institute of Technology, Pasadena, CA.

Statistical analysis

Statistical analyses were performed by a non-parametric Mann–Whitney *U* test.

RESULTS

In this work radiation doses ranging from a low lethal (4 Gy) to an absolutely lethal dose (12 Gy) were used to determine how they affect the activity of IL-1, IL-6 and TNF in rat serum during the first 7 days after total body irradiation. Doses of 4 and 12 Gy caused a significant increase of IL-1 activity 1 h after irradiation (1.9- and 1.6-fold, respectively), while for the 6.7 Gy dose the highest increase was found 3 h after irradiation (1.6-fold compared to the control values) (Fig. 23.1). Irradiation with 9 Gy did not cause a significant increase of IL-1 activity. After 6 h all of the examined doses caused a significant decrease in IL-1 activity, and values lower than controls were maintained until the end of the examination period (7 days). Similarly to IL-1, IL-6 increased activity that was observed at all doses was found in the first 3 h after irradiation (Fig. 23.1). At the first hour these values were 1.9-, 2.1- and 2.2-fold higher than the controls for 4, 9 and 12 Gy doses, respectively. A decrease in IL-6 activity with values that were similar to the controls was detected 6, 12 and 24 h after irradiation with all doses. A second peak of IL-6 activity (4.2-fold increase for the 12 Gy dose 3 days after irradiation), in a dose-dependent manner, was found 3–5 days after irradiation demonstrated a biphasic pattern of IL-6 activity in the serum of

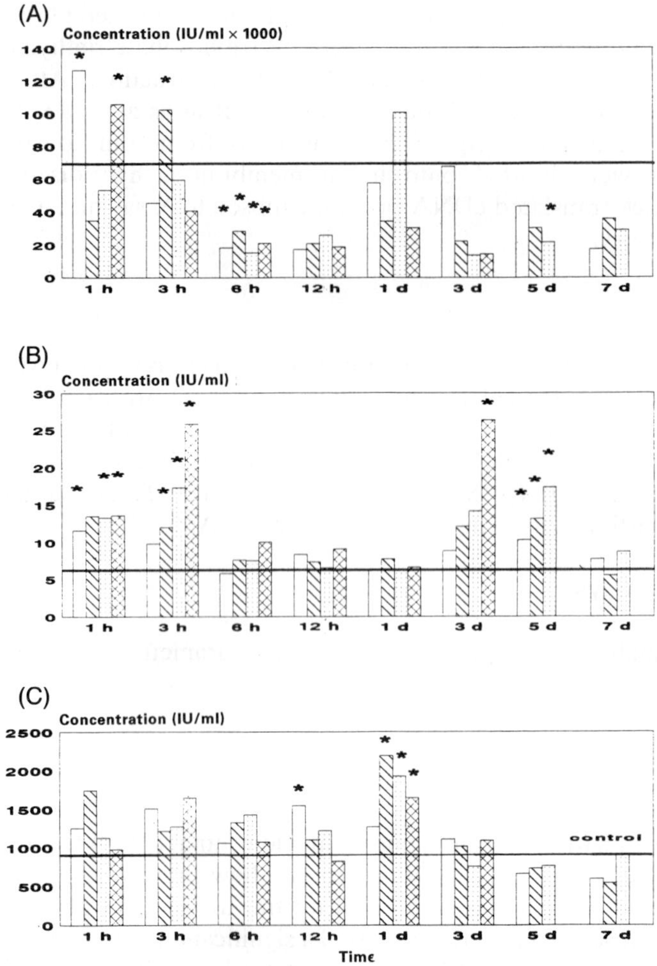

Fig. 23.1 Changes in (A) IL-1; (B) IL-6 and (C) TNF activity in the sera of rats after total body irradiation with 4, 6.7, 9 and 12 Gy. The sera were collected 1, 3, 6 and 12 h, and 1, 3, 5 and 7 days after irradiation. The activities of individual cytokines were tested by a specific bioassay with D10S, B9 and L929 cells for IL-1, IL-6 and TNF, respectively. Each experimental group consisted of at least five animals. The changes in cytokine activity were expressed as median values. The horizontal bar represents the control values. $*p < 0.05$. White bars, 4 Gy; hatched bars, 6.7 Gy; dotted bars, 9 Gy; cross-hatched bars 12 Gy.

irradiated rats. In contrast to these two cytokines, the maximal increase in TNF activity for the 4 Gy dose was found after 12 h (1.7-fold), and for higher doses after 24 h (2.5- and 2.2-fold for 9 and 12 Gy doses respectively) (Fig. 23.1). These values were higher than the controls at 1, 3 and 6 h after

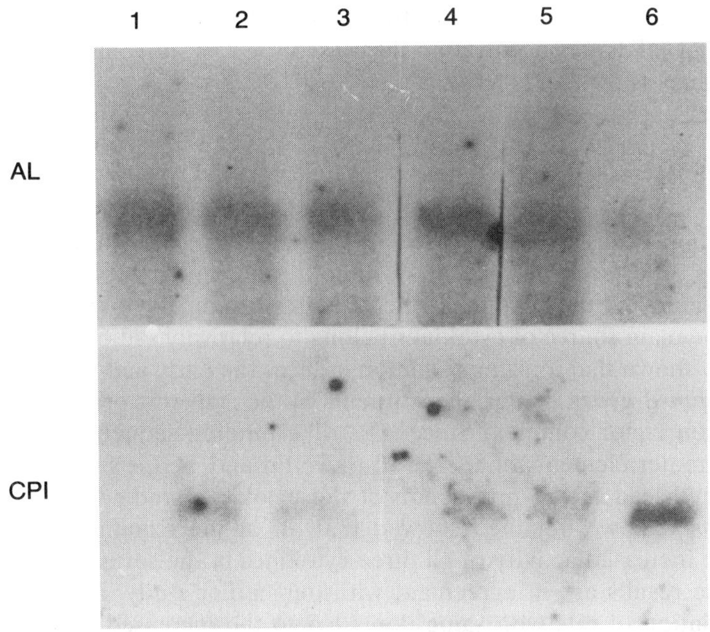

Fig. 23.2 Northern blot hybridization of total RNAs from the HTC cell line. 20 μg of RNAs were separated on a 1% agarose gel under denaturing conditions, transferred onto Hybond nylon membranes and hybridized with nick-translated onto plasmid AL and CPI cDNA probes that were labelled with [α^{32}P]-dCTP. X-ray films were exposed to the filters and the spots corresponding to Al and CPI mRNAs were quantified by densitometry. Line 1: control cells. Cells that were treated for 2 h with 1 μmol/l of dexamethasone (2) or with 200 U/ml of IL-6 (3). The second group of cells was treated 20 h with 1 μmol/l of dexamethasone (4), 50 U/ml of IL-6 (5), or with both (6).

irradiation, whereas after 3, 5 and 7 days they were lower or similar to the controls.

Further, we wanted to examine how IL-6 and dexamethasone alone or in combination affect the expression of AGP, Al, Hp, Fb and CPI genes in the HTC cell line. The 2 h treatment of cells with 200 U/ml of IL-6 or with 1 μmol/l of dexamethasone did not cause significant changes in the relative concentrations of mRNAs of the examined proteins, except for CPI whose concentration increased 2.1-fold after treatment with IL-6 (results not presented). Incubation of cells with 1 μmol/l of dexamethasone for 20 h induced a 2.0-fold increase in AGP mRNA concentration, whereas for the same incubation period 50 U/ml of IL-6 caused 1.6-, 2.1- and 2.3-fold increases in mRNA concentrations for AGP, Hp and CPI, respectively (results not shown). The most prominent changes in APP gene expression were found when the cells were treated with a combination of IL-6 and dexamethasone: the relative concentration of CPI mRNA increased 3.1-fold, while the Al mRNA concentration decreased for 25% in comparison to the control values (Fig. 23.2).

DISCUSSION

The radiation doses that were used in this study are life threatening with deleterious effects primarily on lymphoid and haematopoietic tissues. Although many of the cells from these tissues produce cytokines, the cells that are the main source of cytokines belong to relatively radioresistant cells. It was also shown that ionizing radiation induces the early activation of c-*fos*, c-*jun* and *jun*-B genes that are constituents of the activator protein-1 (AP-1) transcription factor complex. Since AP-1-like binding sequences are found in the promoter elements of IL-1α, IL-6, TNFα and TGFα genes (8), these signals could lead to the production of the cytokines studied in our work. The results that we obtained showed that all of the examined doses can induce the increased activity of all three cytokines in the serum of irradiated rats. These results are in agreement with our earlier study in which the in vivo irradiation of rats with same doses led to the increased production of IL-1 and IL-6 by peritoneal macrophages (9). Macrophages from irradiated rats (4 Gy) produced 10-fold more IL-1 in the first 3 h, whereas 6, 12 and 24 h after irradiation with all four doses these values were higher than in the controls. In the serum of irradiated rats 6 h after irradiation and at all of the subsequent times 2–3-fold lower values of IL-1 activity were found, indicating the presence of a naturally occurring IL-1 inhibitor. As it was shown (10) during endotoxaemia or sepsis, IL-1 specific inhibitory activities are probably caused by IL-1 receptor antagonist (IL-1RA). The radiation doses used in this study can lead to serious damage of the gastrointestinal system with consequent sepsis and endotoxaemia (11) and maybe with the possible production of IL-1RA. A more precise answer to this question could be given if besides IL-1 bioactivity, the concentration of IL-1 or its inhibitor were measured (ELISA; RIA). IL-1 induces its own production by autocrine or paracrine mechanisms, while TNFα seems to be the most important stimulator of IL-1 production. Although not as pronounced, the early increased activity of TNF might be adequate during the early IL-1 and IL-6 stimulation, whereas the peak of TNF activity that was found 24 h after irradiation is directed towards the induction of IL-6 activity found 3–5 days after irradiation. Since higher doses of IL-1 and TNF, in contrast to IL-6, have toxicological effects, efforts were made to establish the correlation between the severity of the injury/infection and the prognosis with the serum levels of these three cytokines (12). In these studies a correlation between the severity of the injury or infection and the serum levels of IL-6 was established (12). Our results are similar to these data in the way that the biphasic increase of IL-6 activity found 1–3 h and 3–5 days after irradiation was dose dependent. The importance of IL-6 and its interactions with IL-1 and TNF during the postirradiation period seems to be fundamental, not only because of their effects on neuroendocrine and immunological systems, but also because of their regulation of APP synthesis in the liver. In our previous study we found that total body irradiation caused a significant increase in the synthesis of some APPs (2). It is possible that these proteins, by their antiprotease, antioxidative, opsonic and immunomodulatory effects, down-regulate the inflammation produced by IL-1, IL-8 and TNF, as suggested by Dinarello (13). These functions of APPs are necessary for the host defence mechanisms against radiation. That is why we further wanted to determine how the major APP regulator protein, IL-6, and potent glucocorticoid-hormone analogue dexamethasone affect APP gene expression in the hepatoma cell line. The obtained results showed that the typical AP-response (3.1-fold increased concentration of CPI mRNA and 25% lower concentration of the 'negative' acute phase reactant Al mRNA) was provoked when IL-6 and dexamethasone were added to the cells together for the 20 h period (Fig. 23.2). A permissive effect of dexamethasone on APP gene transcription can be achieved by its stimulation of hepatoma cell lines to produce IL-6 or to synthesize IL-6 receptors (14). The lower induction of APP mRNAs when IL-6 was applied alone can be explained by their higher basal transcriptional level that was demonstrated by the production of 9 U/ml of IL-6 in the HTC cell line (15).

SUMMARY

The results presented in this study showed that radiation doses ranging from a low lethal dose to an absolutely lethal dose caused the early increase (1–3 h after irradiation) of the serum activity of IL-1 and IL-6, whereas the peak activity of TNF was found after 24 h. At 6 h and later, IL-1 activity in the sera of irradiated rats was significantly decreased. The second peak of IL-6 activity was found 3–5 days after irradiation. Also, it was shown that IL-6 and dexamethasone produce the typical pattern of acute phase protein gene expression in the hepatoma cell line when given in combination.

REFERENCES

1. Neta, R. and J. J. Oppenheim. 1991. Radioprotection with cytokines – learning from nature to cope with radiation damage. *Cancer Cells* **3**: 391–6.
2. Magić, Z., S. Matić-Ivanović, J. Savić and G. Poznanović. 1995. Ionizing radiation-induced expression of the genes associated with the acute response to injury in the rat. *Radiat. Res.* **143**: 187–93.
3. Neta, R., R. Perlstein, S. N. Vogel *et al.* 1992. Role of interleukin 6 (IL-6) in

protection from lethal irradiation and in endocrine responses to IL-1 and tumor necrosis factor. *J. Exp. Med.* **175**: 689–94.

4. Orcenole, F. S. and C. A. Dinarello, 1989. Characterization of subclone (D10S) of the D10.G4.1 helper T-cell line which proliferates to attomolar concentrations of interleukin-1 in the absence of mitogenes. *Cytokine* **1**: 14–22.
5. Shalaby, M. R., A. Waage, L. Aarden and T. Espevik. 1989. Endotoxin, tumor necrosis factor and interleukin 1 induce interleukin 6 production. *Clin. Immunol. Immunopathol.* **53**: 488–98.
6. Meager, A., H. Leung and J. Woolley. 1989. Assays for tumor necrosis factor and related cytokines. *J. Immunol. Meth.* **116**: 1–17.
7. Cox, A. R. 1986. The use of guanidinium chloride in the isolation of nucleic acids. In: *Methods In Enzymology* **123**: pp. 120–129. Academic Press, San Diego, CA.
8. Weichselbaum, R. R., D. E. Hallahan and V. Sukhatme. 1991. Biological consequences of gene regulation after ionizing radiation exposure. *J. Natl. Cancer. Inst.* **83**: 480–4.
9. Magić, Z., Z. Kukić, D. Vojvodić and N. Pejnović. 1994. Effect of in vivo irradiation on the production of IL-1 and IL-6 in rat peritoneal macrophages. *Vojnosanitet. Pregl.* **51** (Suppl.): 46–9.
10. Dayer, J. M. and D. Burger. 1994. Interleukin-1, tumor necrosis factor and their specific inhibitors. *Eur. Cytokine Netw.* **5**: 563–71.
11. Geraci, J. P., K. L. Jakson and M. S. Mariano. 1985. The intestinal radiation syndrome: sepsis and endotoxin. *Radiat. Res.* **101**: 442–550.
12. Svoboda, P., I. Kantorova and J. Ochmann. 1994. Dynamics of interleukin 1, 2, and 6 and tumor necrosis factor alpha in multiple trauma patients. *J. Trauma* **36**: 336–40.
13. Dinarello, C. A. 1992. Anti-cytokine strategies. *Eur. Cytokine Netw.* **3**: 7–17.
14. Snyers, L., L. DeWit and J. Content. 1990. Glucocorticoid up-regulation of high affinity interleukin 6 receptors on human epithelial cells. *Proc. Natl. Acad. Sci. USA* **87**: 2838–42.
15. Čolić, M., N. Pejnović, M. Kataranovski *et al.* 1991. Rat thymic epithelial cells in culture constitutively secrete IL-1 and IL-6. *Int. Immunol.* **3**: 1165–74.

Section 3

Hypersensitivity and autoimmunity

24

Two Sources of Programmed Flexibility in the Immune System: Variation in Structural and Regulatory Gene Segments

Avrion Mitchison, Brigitte Müller, Hannah Mitchison, Jerry Clarke and Angelika Daser

Genetic variation is of very great interest. Human civilization developed only when we learned how to domesticate plants and animals by manipulating genetic variation. The improvement of plant and animal strains by selection remains an important goal of agriculture. Horses and camels are bred with the utmost stringency for success in racing. And in humans, better understanding of the genetics of disease is leading to improvements in prevention, treatment and cure. Population genetics, the science behind these benefits, is moving forwards with explosive speed under the impact of molecular biology. That is what the human genome project is all about. Immunologists are beginning to recognize the importance of these developments: they realize that immunology will never be the same again.

Genetic variation in humans and other diploid organisms results mainly from the presence in the population of polymorphic genes. In contrast, rare mutations make only a small contribution. The polymorphisms are present for various reasons, chiefly balancing selection (i.e. a selective advantage for heterozygotes), and to a lesser extent migration and random drift. From the immunological standpoint random drift can be ignored, as it applies only to variation too slight to affect disease susceptibility, so we are left mainly with balancing selection (as will be discussed further).

A useful distinction, made possible by molecular genetics, is between variation in structural genes (i.e. in the coding regions of the genome, the

Immunoregulation in Health and Disease
ISBN 0–12–459460–3

exons) and variation in non-coding, regulatory regions. Regulatory regions are generally upstream of the corresponding structural genes but may include introns and downstream segments. In these regions are the promoter, often plus enhancer and silencer elements, plus splicing and spacer elements. Altogether these still make up only a minor fraction of total DNA, most of which is either nonsense or serves housekeeping functions. We shall use a terminology suggested to us by Jan Gimsa, of designating structural genes as *hardware* and their regulatory elements as *software*.

HARDWARE VARIATION

Within the immune system, polymorphism of structural segments is conspicuous only among genes encoding the antigen-handling proteins. The best known of these are the immunoglobulins, the T-cell receptors, and the class I and II MHC proteins. The TAP peptide transporters and the LMP proteasome components also handle antigens, and their structural gene-segments are also polymorphic although to a lesser extent. The relationship between structural polymorphism and antigen handling is particularly clear for the MHC molecules. These molecules are polymorphic only in the parts of their structure which bind antigenic peptides (1), and it is these parts which evolve most rapidly (2). Furthermore, when expression has been switched off by an alteration in the promoter region, these genes cease to evolve (3). Thus the evolution of these molecules nicely verifies Fisher's 'fundamental law' of natural selection, that the speed of evolutionary change is proportional to the amount of genetic variation. Less is known about the more recently discovered TAP and LMP polymorphisms. That of the TAP genes is clearly related to antigen-handling in the rat but not yet in man or mouse (4,5). Although searches have been carried out for association of TAP and LMP polymorphisms with most of the common human immunological diseases, no consistently positive evidence has been obtained, and none which rigorously excludes the effect of linkage disequilibrium with neighbouring class II MHC molecules. Perhaps a better place to look would be in infectious disease.

Polymorphism is of course not the only way in which these antigen-handling proteins acquire diversity within the body. All of them are encoded by gene clusters, which in the case of the MHC, TAP and LMC genes enable several proteins to be expressed in a single cell. The requirements of clonal selection prevent the immunoglobulin and TCR genes from doing so, but they have then adopted the unusual alternative of gene rearrangement accompanied by allelic exclusion. It has been argued from computer modelling that the number of MHC loci per cluster is determined by a balance between the need for diversity (tending to maximize the number) and the need to prevent overmuch negative selection (tending to minimize) (P. E. Seiden and F. Celada, quoted in 6).

It is worth looking briefly outside immunology. Antigen handling can be regarded as just one of the ways in which the body confronts the variable environment, in contrast to the constant *milieu interieur* in which the regulatory functions operate. How about other environmental inputs? The closest comparison is with smell, where the olfactory receptors (OR) ressemble to a remarkable extent the antigen receptors (7): like them, ORs have constant and variable domains, and are encoded in gene clusters (about 130 OR genes in humans, up to 1000 in rat). Although nothing is yet known about their polymorphism, extrapolation from the antigen receptors would lead one to expect that a high level will be found. Looking even further afield, the enormous allozyme variability of plants requires explanation. One might speculate that the lesser constancy of the plant *milieu interieur* encourages this form of polymorphism, although recent work on spruce indicates that migration and the mating system can be more important (8).

There is something fascinating about the breeding of race horses, for that is where the amateur geneticist can hope to make money. A good starting-point is some 300 years ago, when three Arab stallions, the Darley Arabian, the Godolphin Barb and the Byerley Turk (the latter being spoils of war when Buda was taken from the Turks in 1686) were imported into England to improve the speed of the indigenous breeds. In one form or another pedigrees and performance records have been kept in England ever since, where they provide a mine of information which is in constant use by breeders, owners, and the betting community (the 'punters'). They know that a fairly good predictor of 'form' (the likelihood that a horse will win) is the speed and stamina of its sire, dam, and dam's sire. The greatest race is the Derby. With very few exceptions, Derby winners are the most thorough of thoroughbreds.

ASSOCIATION OF CYTOKINE GENES WITH IMMUNOLOGICAL DISEASES IN HUMANS AND MOUSE

Current information concerning cytokine gene associations with human multifactorial immunological diseases in man is listed in Table 24.1. The studies there cited have been carried out on the diseases shown, by PCR typing of minor genetic polymorphisms in regulatory regions of the four genes shown. The TNFα gene is located within the MHC; the studies listed attempt to exclude associations resulting from linkage disequilibrium with MHC genes, but cannot rigorously succeed in doing so. Omitted from this table are reports from the older literature of an association between complement alleles and SLE (see e.g. 9), as well as those on association of the insulin gene with IDDM (10). Numerous reports of association with TAP genes have also been omitted, on the grounds that so many negative results were eventually reported that the few remaining positive ones must be regarded

Table 24.1 Cytokine gene polymorphisms associated with immunological diseases in humans

Disease	IL-1	IL-1R	IL-1RA	TNFα
Rheumatoid				
RA	No (15)		Yes (16)	Yes (15), No (17)
SLE			Yes (16)	
JRA	Yes (18)			
Endocrine				
IDDM		Yes (19)	Yes (19)	Yes 20, No (19)
Graves'			Yes (21)	
Addison's				Yes (22)
Dermal				
Alopecia areata			Yes (23,24)	
Dermatitis herpetiformis				No (25)
Lichen sclerosus			Yes (26)	
Psoriasis	Yes (27)			
Enteric				
Ulcerative colitis			Yes (23)	
Infectious				
Cerebral malaria				Yes (28)

as doubtful. So have reports of association with TCRβ alleles, on the grounds of possible confusion between polymorphism and V-gene usage. A promising single study on ICAM1 (11) should be mentioned, and attention is drawn to several recent reviews of the subject (12–14). Apart from these omissions, the table summarizes, to the best of our knowledge, the present literature on the association of these diseases with this group of markers. A collection of this sort is obviously open to bias. We do not know whether the polymorphic markers currently available for CD molecules (leukocyte surface glycoproteins) have not yet been tested for disease associations, or have been tested with negative results which have not been reported. The following polymorphisms are currently available for testing: CD18 (29–31), CD36 (32), CD37 (33), CD79 (34). Nor do we know why the third proinflammatory cytokine IL-6 does not figure on the list, although it does so in the mouse, see below. Failure to find an association does not imply that a gene is unimportant in the development of a disease: the gene may simply not be polymorphic in the population under study.

The main conclusion that can be drawn from this compilation is that polymorphisms of the two proinflammatory cytokines IL-1 and TNFα are repeatedly associated with immunological diseases; this applies also to the antagonist IL-1RA and probably also to the receptor IL-1R.

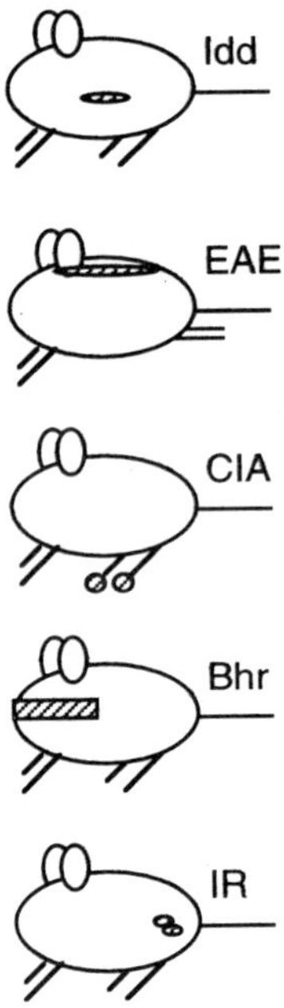

	IL-1	IL-7R	IL-2	IL-2R	TNFa	IL-6R	(IL-4)
Idd	Idd13				Idd1		
EAE		eae2				eae3	
CIA			n.n.				
Bhr	Bhr1			Bhr2	Bhr3		(?)
IR							(n.n.)

Fig. 24.1 Cytokines implicated in mouse disease models and in a mouse immune response. The principal sites affected are shown as hatched.

Information for the mouse is summarized in Fig. 24.1. The mouse genome has been scanned by means of microsatellite markers for loci determining susceptibility to the following diseases: insulin-dependent diabetes (Idd) (35), chronic experimental autoimmune encephalomyelitis (36), in a preliminary way for collagen-induced arthritis (CIA) (37), and airway hyperreactivity (Bhr) related to the asthma phenotype (38). Shown also is the outcome of genetic analysis of the cytokine response of mice to the well-defined single-epitope antigen allo-HPPD (39,40) The locus identified in the CIA study is designated n.n., as it has not yet been named. The IL-4 assignments are placed in brackets, to indicate that polymorphism has not been detected in this cytokine's gene; in the studies listed, the gene is likely to have been differentially activated by polymorphisms elsewhere in the genome.

This presentation of the data should be regarded with extreme caution, as in no case is the location known sufficiently accurately to identify any of these genes with certainty. The original publications emphasize this point, and make clear that larger numbers of mice and, ideally, congenic mouse strains will be required in order to do so. Even bearing this reservation in mind, the similarity in outcome of the mouse and human studies remains striking. Those in the mouse implicate the proinflammatory cytokines IL-1, and TNFα, together with a group of receptors for other cytokines which can loosely be regarded as proinflammatory. IL-4, probably the key anti-inflammatory cytokine, is also implicated indirectly. Taken together with the data from candidate human genes discussed above, the genetics tell us that the proinflammatory cytokines and their associated molecules may well be critically involved in susceptibility to immunological disease.

Reassuringly, we know that this conclusion will soon either be confirmed or rebutted by information emerging from the ongoing human genomic scans. The association of these cytokine polymorphisms with immunological diseases occurs so regularly as to suggest that they may well become a defining characteristic of these diseases: where an association is lacking, one begins to question whether the disease is truly immunological (multiple sclerosis will be a test case). The immunosuppressive drugs have had a similar history: cyclosporin A was introduced first as a treatment for immunological diseases, but a therapeutic response to it has become a defining feature of an immunological disease. It will be interesting to see how this response, and the response to the somewhat different drug thalidomide, will in the future line up disease by disease with the cytokine–gene associations.

SOFTWARE POLYMORPHISM IN THE MAJOR HISTOCOMPATIBILITY COMPLEX

Polymorphism in upstream regulatory regions of MHC genes is clearly important functionally. This form of polymorphism is conspicuous in class II MHC genes of both human and mouse (41). It has been suggested that it may provide differential expression of these molecules in diverse antigen-presenting cells, and may thus influence the balance of Th1 and Th2 cytokines (39,41). This is just one of the new ideas about MHC function, which supplement (but of course do not replace) the classical concept of determinant selection in the control of disease susceptibility; another possibility is that structurally polymorphic molecules may themselves donate different peptides to be presented by other MHC molecules (42).

CONCLUSION: THE SELECTIVE PRESSURE FOR CYTOKINE GENE POLYMORPHISM

What sustains these software polymorphisms in cytokine genes in humans and perhaps also in mouse? As with all forms of polymorphism, the null hypothesis is that they are unselected, reflecting only random drift in gene frequency or migration. The fact that disease associations are found with such regularity makes this unlikely. It is easy to imagine how having two promoters would confer flexibility on the immune response: for instance by allowing

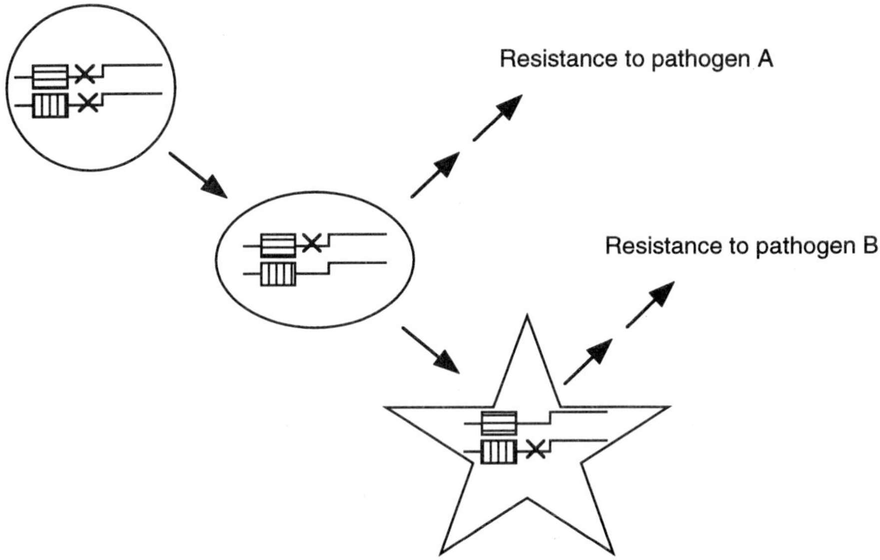

Fig. 24.2 How harbouring two cytokine genes differing in their software could provide valuable flexibility. Maternally and paternally derived genes are shown with both promoters initially switched off. As differentiation proceeds, one promoter switches on, causing cytokine production which produces resistance to pathogen A. At a later stage of differentiation the other promoter switches on, producing resistance to another pathogen, B.

a cytokine to have broader time-kinetics, or differential expression in response to a range of inducing signals (which might themselves be components of the cytokine network), or differential expression in different cells as shown in Fig. 24.2. The selective pressure probably has little to do with the immunological diseases considered here, if only because of their rarity and late time of onset. Flexibility of the sort proposed is surely more likely to have evolved in response to infection. Recent expression studies lend support to the flexibility hypothesis. Using a polymorphism in the 5′ region of the human TNFβ gene (and also affecting amino acid position 26 within the cytokine), a significantly higher response was found from one allele on days 2–4 after PHA-stimulation of peripheral blood mononuclear cells (43). In another study, a polymorphism in the IL-1 gene resulted in a quantitative difference in the response to LPS stimulation (44). It certainly makes sense that the greatest flexibility in expression would be found among these proinflammatory cytokines, since they are produced by the extraordinarily diverse cells of the monocyte/macrophage/microglia/dendritic cell lineage.

The argument advanced here strengthens the case for strategies of therapeutic intervention based on cytokines (45,46). By placing emphasis on the enormous diversity of the proteins engaged in antigen-handling, it weakens the case for antigen-based strategies, however attractive they may seem in principle. It will not be easy to discover the epitopes responsible for driving immunopathology, or to design effective antidotes. In contrast, the cytokines and their genes are available for therapeutic manoeuvres now.

Over the last 20 years immunologists have grown familiar with the distinction between features of the immune response concerned with specificity, and other features concerned with its appropriateness. It is one which is often proposed to provide a logical structure for the design of the immune system (47). The argument made here for a distinction between flexibility in antigen-handling and flexibility in expressing cytokines is saying much the same thing, only now dressed up in genetical clothing.

In the future it will be important to gain a better understanding of the molecular biology that governs the expression of cytokine and cytokine-receptor genes. Even more important will it be to understand the framework of cell biology into which their expression fits.

ACKNOWLEDGEMENTS

This work was supported by the Deutsche Forschungsgemeinschaft and the Senate Administration for Research and Education of the City of Berlin.

REFERENCES

1. Brown, J. H., T. S. Jardetzky, J. C. Gorga *et al.* 1993. Three-dimensional structure of the human class II histocompatibility antigen HLA-DR1. *Nature (Lond.)*. **364**:33–9.
2. Klein, J., Y. Satta, C. O'hUigin and N. Takahata. 1993. The molecular descent of the major histocompatibility complex. *Annu. Rev. Immunol.* **11**:269–95.
3. Begovich, A. B., T. H. Vu and P. P. Jones. 1990. Characterization of the molecular defects in the mouse E-beta f and E-beta q genes. Implications for the origin of MHC polymorphism. *J. Immunol.* **144**:1957–64.
4. Obst, R., E. A. Armandola, M. Nijenhuis *et al.* 1995. TAP polymorphism does not influence transport of peptide variants in mice and humans. *Eur. J. Immunol.* **25**:2170–6.
5. Schumacher, T. N., D. V. Kantesaria, D. V. Serreze *et al.* 1994. Transporters from H-2b, H-2d, H-2s, H-2k, and H-2g7 (NOD/Lt) haplotype translocate similar sets of peptides. *Proc. Natl. Acad. Sci. USA* **91**: 13004–8.
6. Mitchison, N. A. 1993. Will we survive? *Scientific American* **269**:136–44.
7. Ben-Arie, N., D. Lancet, C. Taylor *et al.* 1994. Olfactory receptor gene cluster on human chromosome 17: possible duplication of an ancestral receptor repertoire. *Hum. Mol. Genet.* **3**:229–35.
8. Isabel, N., J. Beaulieu and J. Bousquet. 1995. Complete congruence between gene diversity estimates derived from genotypic data at enzyme and random amplified polymorphic DNA loci in black spruce. *Proc. Natl. Acad. Sci. USA* **92**:6369–73.

9. Huang, D. F., K. A. Siminovitch, X. Y. Liu *et al.* 1995. Population and family studies of three disease-related polymorphic genes in systemic lupus erythematosus. *J. Clin. Invest.* **95**:1766–72.
10. Undlien, D. E., S. T. Bennett, J. A. Todd *et al.* 1995. Insulin gene region-encoded susceptibility to IDDM maps upstream of the insulin gene. *Diabetes* **44**:620–5.
11. Yang, H., D. K. Vora, S. R. Targan *et al.* 1995. Intercellular adhesion molecule 1 gene associations with immunologic subsets of inflammatory bowel disease. *Gastroenterology* **109**:440–8.
12. Duff, G. W. 1994. Interleukin-1 receptor antagonist and genetic susceptibility to inflammation. *J. Interferon Res.* **14**:305.
13. Rich, S. S. 1995. Positional cloning works! Identification of genes that cause IDDM. *Diabetes* **44**:139–40.
14. Ploski, R. and O. Forre. 1994. Non-HLA genes and susceptibility to juvenile chronic arthritis. *Clin. Exp. Rheumatol.* **12** S10:15–17.
15. Gomolka, M., H. Menninger, J. E. Saal *et al.* 1995. Immunoprinting: various genes are associated with increased risk to develop rheumatoid arthritis in different groups of adult patients. *J. Mol. Med.* **73**:19–29.
16. Danis, V. A., M. Millington, V. Hyland *et al.* 1995. Increased frequency of the uncommon allele of a tumour necrosis factor alpha gene polymorphism in rheumatoid arthritis and systemic lupus erythematosus. *Dis. Markers* **12**:127–33.
17. Wilson, A. G., N. de Vries, L. B. van de Putte and G. W. Duff. 1995. A tumour necrosis factor alpha polymorphism is not associated with rheumatoid arthritis. *Ann. Rheum. Dis.* **54**:601–3.
18. McDowell, T. L., J. A. Symons, R. Ploski *et al.* 1995. A genetic association between juvenile rheumatoid arthritis and a novel interleukin-1 alpha polymorphism. *Arthritis Rheum.* **38**:221–8.
19. Pociot, F., K. S. Ronningen, R. Bergholdt *et al.* 1994. Genetic susceptibility markers in Danish patients with type 1 (insulin-dependent) diabetes – evidence for polygenicity in man. Danish Study Group of Diabetes in Childhood. *Autoimmunity* **19**:169–78.
20. Davies, J. L., Y. Kawaguchi, S. T. Bennett *et al.* 1994. A genome-wide search for human type 1 diabetes susceptibility genes. *Nature* **371**:130–6.
21. Blakemore, A. I., P. F. Watson, A. P. Weetman and G. W. Duff. 1995. Association of Graves' disease with an allele of the interleukin-1 receptor antagonist gene. *J. Clin. Endocrinol. Metab.* **80**:111–15.
22. Partanen, J., P. Peterson, P. Westman *et al.* 1994. Major histocompatibility complex class II and III in Addison's disease. MHC alleles do not predict autoantibody specificity and 21-hydoxylase gene polymorphism has no independent role in disease susceptibility. *Hum. Immunol.* **41**:135–40.
23. Mansfield, J. C., H. Holden, J. K. Tarlow *et al.* 1994. Novel genetic association between ulcerative colitis and the anti-inflammatory cytokine interleukin-1 receptor antagonist. *Gastroenterology* **106**:637–42.
24. Cork, M. J., J. K. Tarlow, F. E. Clay *et al.* 1995. An allele of the interleukin-1 receptor antagonist as a genetic severity factor in alopecia areata. *J. Invest. Dermatol.* **104**:155–65.
25. Wilson, A. G., F. E. Clay, A. M. Crane *et al.* 1995. Comparative genetic association of human leukocyte antigen class II and tumor necrosis factor-alpha with dermatitis herpetiformis. *J. Invest. Dermatol.* **104**:856–8.
26. Clay, F. E., M. J. Cork, J. K. Tarlow *et al.* 1994. Interleukin 1 receptor antagonist gene polymorphism association with lichen sclerosus. *Hum. Genet.* **94**:407–10.

27. di Giovine, F. S., M. J. Cork, A. M. Crane *et al.* 1996. A specific interleukin-1 genotype associated with psoriasis and increased production of IL-1b. *J. Exp. Med.* submitted.
28. McGuire, W., A. V. Hill, C. E. Allsopp *et al.* 1994. Variation in the TNF-alpha promoter region associated with susceptibility to cerebral malaria. *Nature (Lond.)*. **371**:508–10.
29. Mastuura, S. and F. Kishi. 1994. Investigation of the polymorphic AvaII site by a PCR-based assay at the human CD18 gene locus. *Hum. Genet.* **93**:721.
30. Lopez, R. C., A. Nueda, B. Grospierre *et al.* 1993. Characterization of two new CD18 alleles causing severe leukocyte adhesion deficiency. *Eur. J. Immunol.* **23**:2792–8.
31. Law, S. K. and G. M. Taylor. 1991. Restriction fragment length polymorphism of the gene of the human leukocyte integrin beta-subunit (CD18). *Immunogenetics* **34**:341–5.
32. Lipsky, R. H., H. Ikeda and E. S. Medved. 1994. A dinucleotide repeat in the third intron of CD36. *Hum. Mol. Genet.* **3**:217.
33. Virtaneva, K. I., H. Nevanlinna and J. Schroder. 1993. BglII restriction fragment length polymorphism at the gene locus coding for the leukocyte surface antigen CD37. *Hum. Mol. Genet.* **2**:1336.
34. Hashimoto, S., N. Chiorazzi and P. K. Gregersen. 1994. The complete sequence of the human CD79b (Ig beta/B29) gene: identification of a conserved exon/intron organization, immunoglobulin-like regulatory regions, and allelic polymorphism. *Immunogenetics* **40**:145–9.
35. Wicker, L. S., J. A. Todd and L. B. Peterson. 1955. Genetic control of autoimmune diabetes in the NOD mouse. *Annu. Rev. Immunol.* **13**:179–200.
36. Sundvall, M., J. J. H. T. Yang, L. Jansson *et al.* 1995. Identification of murine loci associated with susceptibility to chronic experimental autoimmune encephalomyelitis. *Nature Genet.* **10**:313–17.
37. Bull, M. J., G. H. Nabozny, S. D. Kharc *et al.* 1994. Microsatellite analysis of chromosomes 1 and 3 on H-2q restricted murine collagen induced arthritis (CIA). *Arthritis Rheum.* **S9**:168.
38. De Sanctis, G. T., M. Merchant, D. R. Beier *et al.* 1995. Quantitative locus analysis of airway hyperresponsiveness in A/J and C57BL/6J mice. *Nature Genet.* **11**:150–4.
39. Brunner, M. C., S. Larsen, A. Sette, and N. A. Mitchison. 1995. Altered Th1/Th2 balance associated with the immunosuppressive/protective effect of the H-2Ab allele on the response to allo-HPPD. *Eur. J. Immunol.* **25**:3285–9.
40. Brunner, M. C. and N. A. Mitchison. 1996. Regulation by non-MHC genes of the allo-HPPD response. *Immunology* **88**:452–5.
41. Accolla, R. S., J. Guardiola, R. Lauster *et al.* 1996. Functional significance of polymorphism among MHC class II promoters. *Tissue Antigens* **48**.
42. Zanelli, E., M. A. Gonzalez-Gay and C. S. David. 1995. Could HLA-DRB1 be the protective locus in rheumatoid arthritis? *Immunol. Today* **16**:274–8.
43. Messer, G., U. Spengler, M. C. Jung *et al.* 1991. Polymorphic structure of the tumor necrosis factor (TNF) locus: an NcoI polymorphism in the first intron of the human TNF-beta gene correlates with a variant amino acid in position 26 and a reduced level of TNF-beta production. *J. Exp. Med.* **173**:209–19.
44. Pociot, F., J. Molvig, L. Wogensen *et al.* A TaqI polymorphism in the human interleukin-1 beta (IL-1 beta) gene correlates with IL-1 beta secretion in vitro. *Eur. J. Clin. Invest.* **22**:396–402.
45. Mitchison, N. A and J. Sieper. 1995. Immunological basis of oral tolerance. *Z. Rheumatol.* **54**:141–4.

46. Mitchison, N. A. 1995. Immunoregulation in T cell clusters. *The Immunologist* **3**:157.
47. Mitchison, N. A. Unique features of the immune system: their logical ordering and likely evolution. In: *Cell to Cell Interaction* (M. M. Burger, B. Sordat and R. M. Zinkernagel, eds.) S. Karger, Basel. pp. 201–14.

25

Down-regulation of Th1 Mediated Autoimmune Pathology

Miodrag L. Lukić, Lota Ejdus, Allen Shahin, Vera Pravica, Stanislava Stošić-Grujičić, Marija Mostarica Stojković, Sanja Kolarević, Eddy Liew, Zorica Ramić and Vladimir Badovinac

An immune response to autoantigen usually includes production of several types of cells and molecules which are either specific for the given antigen or production of which is specifically triggered by the autoantigenic stimulation. The analysis of the relevance of these different responses has led to the conclusion that in any given case a certain type of response is pathogenic while the other is irrelevant for the disease process but may be 'pathognomonic' in clinical situations. Thus, autoimmunity cannot be treated as being synonymous with the development of clinical disease. Destructive autoimmunity is associated with the development of clinical disease, whereas autoimmune responses that are non-destructive do not lead to disease. It appears that relative contribution of different functional subsets of $CD4^+$ T cells to the developing autoimmune responses determines whether the autoimmunity is expressed as either a destructive or a non-destructive process. It is therefore challenging to develop strategies which will alter the development of clinical autoimmune diseases by modulating the immune response. In order to achieve that it is necessary to completely understand the alteration of immunoregulatory balance which is responsible for disease induction and the molecular basis of the effector mechanisms leading to target cell destruction. In recent years, there is cumulative evidence that the relative contributions of T-helper type 1 (Th1) and T-helper type 2 (Th2) $CD4^+$ cells as landmarks of different effector pathways determine the destructive intensity of autoimmunity.

ORGAN-SPECIFIC AUTOIMMUNE DISEASES AND Th1 CELLS

Functions of Th1 and Th2 cells correlate well with production of their distinctive cytokines (reviewed in 1,2). Th1 cells, producing interleukin-2

Immunoregulation in Health and Disease
ISBN 0-12-459460-3

(IL-2) and interferon-γ (IFNγ), initiate cell-mediated inflammatory responses by activating cytotoxic T cells and inflammatory cells. Th2-derived cytokines (IL-4, IL-5) are required for optimal antibody production, particularly IgE responses, and enhance eosinophil production and functions. Th1-produced cytokine (IFNγ) and Th2-produced cytokine (IL-10) are mutually inhibitory for differentiation and effector functions of the reciprocal phenotype. This cross-regulation may partially explain the strong bias towards Th1 or Th2 response during different infections and autoimmune processes. However, Th1- and Th2-derived cytokine responses are not the only cytokine patterns possible. T cells expressing cytokines of both patterns have been called Th0 cells, while cells producing high amount of transforming growth factor-β (TGFβ) have been termed Th3 (3).

Although different patterns of cytokine production have been associated with different autoimmune diseases, the decision-making event in the initial phase of immune response leading to destructive or non-destructive autoimmunity is unknown. It may be argued that the inherent genetically determined pattern of cytokine production may be a decisive element in regulating induction of destructive or non-destructive autoimmunity and therefore determines susceptibility to a particular autoimmune disease (4–6).

It appears that organ-specific autoimmune diseases develop as a consequence of expansion of self-reactive Th1 cells specific for relevant organ-specific autoantigen(s). In recent literature, model diseases to study T-cell-mediated organ-specific autoimmunity had been myelin basic protein (MBP)-induced experimental allergic encephalomyelitis (EAE), collagen-induced arthritis and an insulin-dependent diabetes mellitus (IDDM). T cells in the lesions causing these diseases were found to produce IL-2 and IFNγ, but not IL-4 (7–9). It was therefore of interest to analyse the susceptibility to organ-specific autoimmune diseases in species where immune cells produce 'low' or 'high' quantity of Th1-type cytokines when triggered by the same stimuli (10). It might be assumed that the inherent capacity of the lymphoid cells to produce different quantities of Th1-type cytokines would correlate with susceptibility to organ-specific autoimmunity. This assumption appeared testable in two strains of rats (Albino Oxford (AO) and Dark August (DA)) which apparently differ in the level of IFNγ and IL-2 production (10). We have analysed Th1 cytokine production by T-cells and spleen cells after mitogenic and/or anti-CD3 antibody stimulation in these two strains (11,12). When lymph node cells derived from untreated animals were stimulated in vitro with T-cell mitogen, Con A, the level of IL-2 and IFNγ production was at least threefold higher in the culture supernatants derived from DA rats than in those obtained from AO rats. Immunization using either central nervous system tissue or MBP as an encephalitogen led to the induction of clinical and histological manifestations of EAE in DA rats, but induced only discrete subarachnoidal and perivascular infiltrates without clinical signs of disease in AO rats (13). We then tested the susceptibility of these two strains to developing a chemically induced autoimmune diabetes. To this end, we have used a model of diabetes induction with multiple subdiabetogenic doses of β-cell toxin-streptozotocin (STZ). Multiple low dose (MLD) of STZ induces diabetes in susceptible strains of mice (14,15). Two to three weeks following the treatment of five daily doses of 40 mg/kg body weight (b.w.), susceptible mice developed hyperglycemia accompanied by mononuclear cell infiltrates and consecutive β-cell destruction. We have attempted to induce the same disease in AO and DA rats (16). It was found that a single dose of 60–100 mg caused an outbreak of clinical diabetes in both strains, clearly as the direct effect of β-cell poisoning. However, five daily doses of 20 mg/kg b.w. did not have any effect on glycemia in IL-2 and IFNγ low producer AO rats, although it induced sustained hyperglycemia in DA rats. Histological and immunohistochemical analyses revealed only diffuse mononuclear infiltrates with characteristic early macrophage influx. In vivo treatment with anti-CD4 cytotoxic antibodies (W3/25 clone) demonstrated requirement for Th cells in the induction of the disease (16).

In order to demonstrate the genetic basis of susceptibility to cell-mediated autoimmunity and level of Th1 production, we have analysed the susceptibility to EAE and IL-2 production in $(DA \times AO)F_1$ hybrids and backcross generation rats (11). Taken together, results of several experiments have shown that autosomal dominant gene(s) control(s) both susceptibility to EAE and Th1 cytokine production. Both high production of IL-2 and susceptibility to EAE appear to be dominant traits. Finally, we have attempted to correlate susceptibility to autoimmune disease and IFNγ production in 7th backcross generation rats selected for susceptibility to EAE (12). The results were compatible with the notion that high IFNγ producers are more susceptible to EAE. Taken together, the results discussed strongly indicate that a genetically determined level of Th1 cytokine production after any stimulus contributes to susceptibility to organ-specific autoimmunity.

RT6$^+$ T DOWNREGULATORY CELLS

Diabetes-prone Bio-Breeding (BB) rats spontaneously develop insulin-dependent diabetes mellitus. All BB rat strains with high incidence of the disease suffer from a recessively inherited T-cell lymphopenia and failure to express CD45 RB and autoantigen RT6 on T-cells of lymph node and spleen (17). RT6 molecules are selectively expressed in subsets by CD4$^+$ and CD8$^+$ peripheral T-cells, but absent from B-cells and thymocytes (18). Groen *et al.* (19) have suggested that resting memory CD4$^+$ T-cells could be divided into CD45$^+$ RT6$^-$ and CD45$^-$ RT6$^+$. It was proposed that these two subsets can be regarded as Th1- and Th2-like resting memory populations.

We have analysed the quantitative participation of RT6$^+$ cells in the peripheral T-cell pool of Th1 autoimmune diseases-resistant AO and susceptible DA rats. To this end, peripheral lymphoid cells, nylon wool column non-adherent T cells, $CD4^+$ and $CD8^+$ T cells, isolated by a 'panning' technique (20) were incubated with anti-RT6, 6A5 monoclonal antibody followed by incubation with an $F(ab)_2$ fragment of fluorescein isothiocyanate-conjugated goat anti-rat IFNγ and analysed by flow cytometry. The results clearly indicated that $RT6^+$ cells were significantly more numerous in both major populations of peripheral T cells in AO rats. To test whether these findings were relevant for the strain-related differences in susceptibility to MLD-STZ-induced diabetes and EAE, we pretreated rats with five daily injections (1 ml intraperitoneally) of 6A5 hybridoma culture supernatants prior to the induction of these diseases. The treatment decreased the number of $RT6^+$ T cells for about 80% in both strains.

Lymphoid cells derived from AO rats produced significantly less IL-2 and IFNγ after stimulation with mitogen and depletion of $RT6^+$ cells enhanced the level of cytokines production (Table 25.1). These increases were fivefold in AO rats for both cytokines. However, in DA rats only IL-2 production was enhanced by anti-$RT6^+$ antibody. This treatment converted AO rats from resistant to diabetes to mildly diabetic and had a clear enhancing effect in DA rats. However, this treatment did not overcome the resistance of AO rats to the induction of clinical signs of EAE (Table 25.1). We then tested whether the proliferative response to MBP of the lymph node cells derived from immunized AO rats was affected by elimination of $RT6^+$ cells. The results indicated significant stimulation of antigen-driven proliferation. The fact that this stimulation was not sufficient to overcome the resistance to EAE induction, may have, at the moment, three possible explanations:

1. Although the production of IFNγ was enhanced by anti-RT6 antibody, the level reached after the treatment was three times lower than in normal DA rats. This may imply that the level of IFNγ required for the triggering of effector cells in CNS is higher than that required for the stimulation of effector cells in diabetes induction. In fact there is ample evidence that exogenous IFNγ may easily enhance diabetes in NOD mice (21) as well as MLD-STZ-induced diabetes (22).
2. An MBP-specific T cell line derived from (AO $\times$ DA) F_1 hybrids, was capable of inducing clinical EAE in F_1 hybrids and DA, but not in AO rats. *In vitro* restimulation with MBP presented by AO antigen presenting cells resulted in generation of an MBP-specific subline restricted by RT1u MHC products which induced clinical EAE in F_1 hybrids but not in the AO parental strain (23). Deletion of hosts' leukocytes using sublethal irradication and cytotoxic drugs did not abrogate the resistance of AO rats, which argues against involvement of hosts' lymphoid cells in EAE resistance. These findings suggested that the additional mechanisms operative at the level of the target tissue might be responsible for the differences in susceptibility to EAE. Indeed, our recent data (24) indicate

Table 25.1 The effects of depletion of $RT6^+$ cells on Th-1 cytokine production and induction of autoimmune diseases

Anti-RT6[a] mAbs	AO rats				DA rats			
	Th-1 cytokines[b]		Diabetes[c] Glycemia	EAE[d]	Th-1 cytokines[b]		Diabetes[c] Glycemia	EAE[d] Clinical
	IFN	IL-2			IFN-γ	IL-2		
−	18.46	11.57	8.50	0/5	315.19	34.36	12.97	3/3
+	97.30	56.6	13.96	0/5	302.13	97.54	18.97	3/3

[a]Rats were treated with five daily injections of anti-RT6.2 GA5 monoclonal antibody or control supernatant (1 ml) prior to induction of EAE or MLD-STZ.
[b]IFNγ and IL-2 were determined in supernatants of Con A (5 μ/ml) stimulated lymph node cell (5×10^5) culture (0.2 ml) derived from animals 24 h after the last injections of mAbs. Results are expressed as U/ml.
[c]Glycemia was determined 12 days (mean of six animals per group) after the last injection of STZ. Mean day 0 value for all animals tested was 7.65 mmol/l.
[d]Animals immunized with 100 μg MBP-CFA were observed daily from clinical signs of EAE. Results are given as ratio of diseased/immunized animals.

that such a difference exists at the level of accessory cells. We assumed that the capacity of accessory cells to produce proinflammatory cytokines and/or nitric oxide (NO) may be related to the differences in susceptibility to EAE. Therefore we analysed the production of tumor necrosis factor-α (TNFα) and NO by IFNγ activated macrophages derived from AO and DA rats. It was found that the differences in the level of TNFα production as evaluated by bioassay (L929 cells) and ELISA of cytokine content in 24 and 48 h culture supernatant are significantly higher ($p < 0.001$) in susceptible DA rats while NO production, as determined by generation of nitrate, was slightly but not significantly higher in the cell cultures derived from disease-resistant AO rats. Thus, the resistance to EAE may be due to the incapacity of accessory cells to produce sufficient amount of TNFα in response to IFNγ stimulation.

3. Finally, the difference in production of down-regulatory cytokine transforming TGFβ may also play a role (as discussed below). It is possible to assume that enhanced disease-inducing capacity of the lymphocytes depleted RT6$^+$ cells was not sufficient to overcome down-regulation by TGFβ produced by non-lymphoid cells in CNS. Indeed, it has been increasingly appreciated that cytokines play an important role in inflammatory reactions of the CNS but the source of cytokines for each inflammatory event is not always known (25). For example, active TGFβ has shown to be made by endothelial cells in vitro when they are cocultured with pericytes (26).

INTERLEUKIN-1 INHIBITORS

Endogenous glucocorticoid hormones play an important role in the normal regulation of the immune system and act as physiological immunosuppressants involved in the control of immune and inflammatory hyperreactivity (27). Although glucocorticoids have a direct effect on T-cell cytokine production (especially IL-2) (28), it is also documented that they suppress monokine production, IL-1 in particular (29,30). Additionally, we have shown that accessory cells pretreated with glucocorticoid in vivo or in vitro produce, in absence of IL-1, an inhibitor of IL-1 activity (31). It is not established whether this inhibitor represents the released IL-1 receptors (32,33) or is identical to the IL-1 receptor antagonist (34).

We have attempted to modulate the induction of Th1 mediated autoimmunity by these inhibitors of IL-1. When CBA mice were injected with either IL-1 inhibitor derived from macrophage cultures or human recombinant IL-1 receptor antagonist (IL-1RA) during the induction of MLD-STZ diabetes, they remained normoglycemic for at least 18 weeks after the induction of the disease (Lukic, Stosic and Dinarello, submitted). There is evidence in vitro that proinflammatory cytokines such as IL-1 and TNF

Table 25.2 Effect of IL-1 inhibitor on the development of insulitis islet cell damage and glycemia[a]

Animal number	Treatment[b]	Cellular infiltration	Islet cell damage		Glycemia (mmol/l)
			Vacuolization	Pyknosis	
1	STZ + Control	+	+	+	14.8
2	STZ + Control	++	++	+	11.9
3	STZ + Control	++	++	+	13.5
4	STZ + INH	+	+	−	6.7
5	STZ + INH	+	+	−	5.5
6	STZ + INH	+	+	−	6.6

[a]The results represent functional and morphological data on day 48 after induction of MLD-STZ. The histological data are based on a minimum of 50 islets per pancreas.
[b]Beginning with the third day of STZ injections, mice were injected intraperitoneally with 1 ml of either dialyzed cell-free supernatant containing the glucocorticoid induced rat IL-1 inhibitor. Control mice received 10 daily injections of 1 ml of rat peritoneal cell culture supernatant to which hydrocortisone was added prior to dialysis.

directly, via specific receptors, affect β cells in the islet of Langerhans and that IL-1RA can protect these cells from the deleterious effects of recombinant IL-1β (35). At the first glance, it seems that our results suggest that the same mechanisms might be operative in vivo. Similarly, when young diabetes-prone BB rats were treated with 2 mg/kg per day of IL-RA from day 30 to day 90 of age, none of them had developed diabetes, whereas 32% of the vehicle-injected rats did (36). At day 150, however, the incidence of diabetes was similar in both groups. The fact that much briefer treatment of animals with IL-1 inhibitor or IL-1RA may more profoundly affect the induction of MLD-STZ-induced diabetes (Table 26.2) may be due to the differences in the availability of relevant autoantigen(s) in spontaneous and induced-disease models.

It is tempting to speculate that the in vitro protective effect of IL-1RA in immune mediated diabetes is due to its direct binding to the IL-1 receptor on β cells. However, Bodovinac *et al.* (in preparation) found that pretreatment with IL-1RA down-regulates induction of EAE in susceptible DA rats. Thus it appears that alteration of inflammatory process and/or expansion of autoreactive cells may also be targeted in the prevention of Th1-mediated autoimmunity by the inhibitors of IL-1 activity.

TRANSFORMING GROWTH FACTOR-β AND Th2-DERIVED CYTOKINES

Active cellular suppression has not been unequivocally demonstrated as a mechanism for peripheral tolerance because of difficulties in cloning and in demonstrating that cloned T-cells can activity-regulate the responses of other antigen-specific disease-producing cells in vivo. Most recently, Ke and Kapp (37) revived the classical suppressor cells showing that orally administered ovalbumin activated spleen suppressor T cells transferred unresponsiveness to naive syngeneic recipients. These suppressor cells were $CD4^-$ $CD8^+$ T cells phenotypically distinguished from cytotoxic cells by reactivity with monoclonal antibody that recognizes activated suppressor T cells (38). The fact that in repeated experiments resistance to EAE in AO rats could be partially overcome by the procedures which preferentially affect suppressor cells suggests that the level of active suppression may play a role in genetically determined differences in susceptibility to autoimmunity (39,40).

Oral administration of 'low antigen dose' is a classical method of inducing autoantigen-specific immune tolerance through active suppression. T-cell clones isolated from the mesenteric lymph nodes of mice tolerized to MBP were $CD4^+$ and were structurally identical to Th1 encephalitogenic $CD4^+$ clones in T-cell receptor usage, major histocompatibility complex restriction and epitope recognition. However, they produced mainly TGFβ with various amounts of IL-4 and IL-10 (3). Thus, mucosally derived $CD4^+$ cells producing mainly TGFβ may be considered another T helper subset, Th3, with both mucosal T-helper function and down-regulatory properties for Th1 cells. The immunosuppressive and anti-inflammatory properties of TGFβ have been exploited in the amelioration of EAE (41,42) and collagen-induced arthritis (43,44). However, there is no evidence whether TGFβ may down-regulate experimental T-cell mediated diabetogenesis. Therefore, we attempted to comparatively study the effects of TGFβ on the development of EAE and MLD-STZ-induced diabetes in disease-susceptible DA rats. We have tried to manipulate the susceptibility to EAE and diabetes by oral administration of human TGFβ expressed in attenuated AMoA-*Salmonella typhimurium* (22). Rats given orally 10^{10} TGFβ-producing *S. typhimurium* developed EAE with later onset and significantly milder than the animals receiving control microorganisms (Table 25.3).

However, the same treatment in repeated experiments was completely ineffective in altering the development of MLD-STZ-induced diabetes in mice or rats (Table 25.3). It is not completely established how TGFβ exerts a protective effect in EAE. Santambrogio *et al.* (45) have found that TGFβ treatment in EAE does not influence the appearance of sensitized cells in peripheral blood and lymph nodes, but does prevent accumulation of T cells in brain and spinal cord. We have found significantly lower numbers of $CD4^+$ T cells in the draining lymph nodes of MBP-CFA immunized rats treated with TGFβ-positive *S. typhimurium* (unpublished) but it is not clear if it reflects the suppressed expansion of encephalitogenic cells. The ability of TGFβ to modulate migration through the blood–brain barrier composed of endothelial cells and astrocytes appeared to lead to reduction of lymphocyte infiltration into CNS (25). It seems that similar TGFβ-controlled mechanisms

Table 25.3 Effect of TGF-β on induction of Th-1 mediated autoimmune diseases

TGF-β[a]	MLD-STZ diabetes (glycemia)[b]		EAE clinical score[c]	
	BALB/c mice	DA rats	AO rats	DA rats
–	11.5	11.6	0	2.7
+	15.8	12.1	0	0.5

[a]Animals were given orally 10^{10} TGFβ producing attenuated AMoA-*Salmonella typhimurium* or control *S. typhimurium* on day −2, 0, 2, 6 and 10 in relation to encephalitogenic challenge or first day of STZ treatment.
[b]MLD-STZ diabetes was induced by four daily injections of 40 mg/kg body weight (mice) or 20 mg/kg body weight (rats) of STZ. Glycemia was evaluated weekly during 8 weeks. Maximum values (mml/l) were given.
[c]EAE was induced by foot-pad injection of 100 μg MBP in CFA and rats observed daily for the presence of clinical signs (10, 40). Peak clinical disease was seen by day 14 in both groups (4–6 animals per group).

are not operative in the influx of macrophages and T cells into the islet after low-dose STZ treatment.

Th1 mediated autoimmunity may be suppressed by targeting autoantigen to the antigen presenting cell which preferentially stimulates Th2-type cells (46). Saoudi *et al.* (47) have demonstrated that if rats protected from EAE were treated with MBP covalently linked to anti-rat immunoglobulin D, lymph node cells from these pretreated animals, although proliferating in vitro to MBP, produced less IFNγ but generated markedly increased level of messenger RNA for IL-4 and IL-13. Additionally, pretreatment greatly reduced the level of leukocyte infiltration into the central nervous system. This finding seems to confirm a previous report indicating that IFNγ plays an essential role in the recruitment of lymphocytes into delayed-type hypersensitivity lesions (48). The data also implicate that alteration of the balance between IFNγ producing and IL-4 producing cells may influence the susceptibility to EAE and MLD-STZ-induced diabetes.

It had been reported that repeated injections of mercuric chloride may lead in susceptible strains to an autoimmune disease characterized by the production of various autoantibodies, a striking enhancement of serum IgE level with concomitant increase of MHC class II molecule expression on B cells. These findings indicated that mercuric chloride treatment induces a Th2 mediated systemic autoimmunity (49). This treatment apparently down-regulates Th1 mediated organ-specific autoimmunity (49). Indeed, subtoxic doses of mercuric chloride prevented induction of experimental autoimmune uveoretinitis in Lewis rats (49) and down-regulated the induction of MLD-STZ-induced diabetes in DA rats (to be published). It is of interest to note that the effect in diabetes was achievable even if the treatment started 12 days after the STZ treatment, suggesting that the enhancement of Th2-

type cytokines may reduce the mononuclear cell infiltration in the islet as previously shown in EAE.

INHIBITORS OF NITRIC OXIDE SYNTHASE

Nitric oxide is important in many biological functions. We (50) and others (51–53) have argued that a free radical synthesized from L-arginine by nitric oxide synthase mediates the destruction of target tissues in some autoimmune pathology such as IDDM and glomerulonephritis and arthritis. The role of nitric oxide in islet cell damage was first shown in an MLD-STZ-induced model of diabetes (50) and recently extended to spontaneously diabetic BB rats (54,55). Administration of N^6-monomethyl-L-arginine (NMMA) an inhibitor of nitric oxide synthase ameliorated MLD-STZ-induced diabetes (50,51) in mice and significantly reduced the incidence of IDDM in diabetes-prone BB rats (54,55). Inhibitors of nitric oxide synthase have been shown to protect against both cytokine-induced inhibition of insulin secretion (56) and cytotoxicity of cytokines and activated macrophages on pancreatic islet β cells in vitro (57,58). However, the source of production of nitric oxide during diabetes development was not readily identified in any of the above studies. The activated macrophages infiltrating the islets are likely to be an important source of nitric oxide in vivo. Macrophages have been implicated as playing an essential role in the autoimmune destruction of pancreatic islet cells (59). Thus, it was of interest to test whether macrophages derived from rats susceptible and resistant to induction of MLD-STZ diabetes differ in their inherent capacity to produce nitric oxide. As indicated earlier, no significant difference was observed (24) although DA macrophages did produce significantly more TNFα. We assume that macrophage-derived proinflammatory cytokines induce nitric oxide-dependent apoptotic cell death triggered by nitric oxide in pancreatic β cells. Indeed such a mechanism appears to be operative in isolated rat pancreatic cells exposed to IL-1 (60). Finally, failure to completely suppress development of diabetes in BB rats and MLD-STZ treated mice by the inhibitor of nitric oxide synthase may indicate that development of diabetes involves both nitric oxide-sensitive and nitric oxide-insensitive phases as proposed for the NOD mouse (61). The generation of inducible nitric oxide synthase knock-out mice (62) offers an opportunity to dissect out possible nitric oxide-dependent and nitric oxide-independent pathways in the induction of Th1 mediated immunopathology (our work in progress).

CONCLUSION

The evidence obtained, mainly in experiments analysing the molecular and cellular basis of the differences in susceptibility to EAE and experimental autoimmune diabetes, argues that the destructive autoimmune process may be modified at the level of the target tissue. The balance of cytokines and other mediators (e.g. nitric oxide) released locally by T cells, macrophages and resident tissue cells seems to determine the outcome of autoimmunity. The local balance of cytokines and other mediators, rather than autoreactivity per se, determines the interplay between autoimmune and inflammatory mechanisms and severity of the disease.

The realization that alterations in Th1/Th2 balance can be achieved by various means and that the production of proinflammatory cytokines and nitric oxide may be effectively blocked, opens the way for new therapeutic strategies.

ACKNOWLEDGEMENT

The studies discussed were supported by RSF (Belgrade) and FMHS (Al Ain) grants. The secretarial help of Mr. M. V. Raghavan and Mrs. G. Dawood is gratefully acknowledged.

REFERENCES

1. Mosmann, T. R. and S. Sad. 1996. The expanding universe of T-cell subsets: Th1, Th2 and more. *Immunol. Today* **17**:138–76.
2. Swain, S. L., L. M. Bradley, M. Croft *et al.* 1991. Helper T-cell subsets: phenotype, function and the role of lymphokines in regulating their development. *Immunol. Rev.* **123**:115–28.
3. Chen, Y., V. K. Kuchzoo, J. Inobe *et al.* 1994. Regulatory T-cell clones induced by oral tolerance: Suppression of autoimmune encephalomyelitis. *Science* **265**:1237–40.
4. Lukic, M. L., V. Pravica, S. Stosic and A. Shahin. 1995. Cytokine network determines susceptibility to low dose streptozotocin-induced diabetes. *Int. J. Diabetes* **3**:156–7.
5. Charlton, B. and K. J. Lafferty. 1995. The Th1/Th2 balance in autoimmunity. *Curr. Opin. Immunol.* **7**:793–8.
6. Liblau, R. S., S. M. Singer and H. O. McDevitt. 1995. Th1 and Th2 $CD4^+$ T-cells in the pathogenesis of organ-specific autoimmune diseases. *Immunol. Today* **16**:34–8.
7. Renno, T., R. Zeine, J. M. Girard *et al.* 1994. Selective enrichment of Th1 $CD45RB^{low}$ $CD4^+$ T-cells in autoimmune infiltrates in experimental allergic encephalomyelitis. *Int. Immunol.* **6**:347–54.
8. Renno, T., M. Krakowski, C. Piccirillo *et al.* 1995. TNF-alpha expression by resident microglia and infiltrating leukocytes in the central nervous system of mice with experimental allergic encephalomyelitis. Regulation by Th1 cytokines. *J. Immunol.* **154**:944–53.
9. Kolb, H., V. Kolb-Bachofen and B. O. Roep. 1995. Autoimmune versus inflammatory type 1 diabetes: a controversy? *Immunol Today* **16**:170–2.

10. Vukmanovic, S., M. Mostarica Stojkovic and M. L. Lukic. 1989. Experimental autoimmune encephalomyelitis in 'low' and 'high' Interleukin 2 producer rats. I. Cellular basis of induction. *Cell. Immunol.* **121**:237–46.
11. Lukic, M. L., M. Mostarica Stojkovic, M. Kostic *et al.* 1987. Cellular and genetic basis of the strain differences in IL2 production in rats. *Transpl. Proc.* **19**:3137–9.
12. Arsov, I., V. Pravica, L. Ejdus *et al.* 1995 Selection for the susceptibility to experimental allergic encephalomyelitis also selects for high IFN-γ production. *Transplan. Proc.* **27**:1537–8.
13. Vukmanovic, S., M. Mostarica Stojkovic, I. Calud *et al.* 1990. Analysis of T cell subsets after induction of experimental autoimmune encephalomyelitis in susceptible and resistant strains of rats. *J. Neuroimmunol.* **27**:63–9.
14. Like, A. A. and A. A. Rossini. 1976. Streptozotocin induced pancreatic insulitis: new model of diabetes. *Science* **193**:415–17.
15. Elias, D., H. Prigozin, N. Polak *et al.* 1994. Autoimmune diabetes induced by B-cell toxin STZ. Immunity to the 60 Kda heat shock protein and insulin. *Diabetes* **43**:992–8.
16. Lukic, M. L., R. Al-Sharif, M. Mostarica *et al.* 1991. Immunological Basis of the strain differences in susceptibility to low-dose streptozotocin-induced diabetes in rats. In: *Lymphatic Tissues and In Vivo Immune Responses* (Imhof *et al.*, eds.) Marcel Dekker, New York, pp. 643–7.
17. Greiner, D. Y., J. P. Mordes, E. S. Handler *et al.* 1987. Depletion of RT6.1$^+$ lymphocytes induces diabetes in resistant BB/W rats. *J. Exp. Med.* **166**:461–9.
18. Fangmann, J., R. Schwinzer, H. J. Hedrick *et al.* 1991. Diabetes prone BB rats express the RT6 alloantigen on intestinal intra-epithelial lymphocytes. *Eur. J. Immunol.* **21**:2011–15.
19. Groen, H., F. A. Klatter, A. S. Van Peterson *et al.* 1993. Composition of rat CD4$^+$ resting memory T-cell pool is influenced by major histocompatibility complex. *Transplant Proc.* **25**:2782–3.
20. Wisocky, L. J. and V. L. Sato. 1978. 'Planning' for lymphocytes: a method for cell selection. *Proc. Natl. Acad. Sci. USA* **75**:2844–8.
21. Campbell, I. L., T. W. H. Kay, L. Oxbrow and L. C. Harrison. 1991. Essential role for interferon gamma and interleukin 6 in autoimmune insulin-dependent diabetes in NOD/Wehi Mice. *J. Clin. Investig.* **87**:739–42.
22. Shahin, A., T. A. M. Mahmoud and M. L. Lukic. 1995. Transforming growth factor β and Inteferon gamma modulate the development of Th-1 mediated autoimmunity in susceptible and resistant strains of rats. *Transpl. Proc.* **27**:1535–6.
23. Mostarica-Stojkovic, M., S. Vukmanovic, Z. Ramic and M. L. Lukic. 1992. Evidence for target tissue regulation of the resistance to experimental allergic encephalomyelitis in AO rats. *J. Neuroimmunol.* **41**:95–106.
24. Lukic, M. L., A. Shahin, K. Broadbent and S. Stephen. 1996. Tumor necrosis factor alpha but not nitric oxide production by macrophages correlates with susceptibility to T-cell mediated interferon gamma dependent autoimmunity. *FACEB J.* (in press).
25. Fabry, Z., D. J. Topham, D. Fee *et al.* 1995. TGF-β2 decreases migration of lymphocytes in vitro and homing of cells into the central nervous system in vivo. *J. Immunol.* **155**:325–32.
26. Antonelli-Orlidge, A., K. B. Saunders, S. R. Smith and P. A. D'Amore. 1989. An activated form of transforming growth factor β is produced by cocultures of endothelial cells and pericytes. *Proc. Natl. Acad. Sci. USA* **86**:4544–7.
27. Arya, S. K., F. Wong-Staal and R. C. Gallo. 1984 Dexamethasone-mediated

inhibition of human T-cell growth factor and gamma-interferon messenger RNA. *J. Immunol.* **133**:273–6.
28. Boumpas, D. T., E. D. Anastassiou, S. A. Older *et al.* 1991. Dexamethasone inhibits human interleukin 2 but not interleukin 2 receptor gene expression in vitro at the level of nuclear transcription. *J. Clin. Invest.* **87**:1739–47.
29. Stosic-Grujicić, S. and M. M. Simić. 1982. Modulation of Interleukin 1 production by activated macrophages: in vitro action of hydrocortisone, colchicine and cytochalasin B. *Cell. Immunol.* **69**:235–42.
30. Lew, W., J. J. Oppenheim and K. Matsushima. 1988. Analysis of the suppression of IL-1 alpha and IL-1 beta production in human peripheral blood mononuclear adherent cells by a glucocorticoid hormone. *J. Immunol.* **140**:1895–902.
31. Stosić-Grujicić, S. and M. L. Lukic. 1992. Glucocorticoid-induced keratinocyte-derived interleukin-1 receptor antagonist(s). *Immunology* **75**: 293–8.
32. Giri, J. G., J. Wells, S. K. Dower *et al.* 1994. Elevated levels of shed type II IL-1 receptor in sepsis. *J. Immunol.* **153**:5802–13.
33. Sims, J. E., J. G. Giri and S. K. Dower. 1994. The two interleukin-1 receptors play different roles in IL-1 activities. *Clin. Immunol. Immunopathol.* **72**:9–14.
34. Dinarello, C. A. and R. C. Thompson. 1996. Blocking IL-1: Effects of IL-1 receptor antagonist in vitro and in vivo. *Immunol Today* **12**:404–10.
35. Mandrup-Poulsen, T., U. Zumsteg, J. Reimers *et al.* 1993. Involvement of interleukin-1 and interleukin-1 antagonist in pancreatic β-cell destruction in insulin-dependent diabetes mellitus. *Cytokine* **5**:185–91.
36. Dayer-Métroz, M. D., D. Duhamel, W. Rufer *et al.* 1992. IL-1 receptor antagonist delays spontaneous autoimmune diabetes in BB rats. *Eur. J. Clin. Invest.* **22**:A50.
37. Ke, Y. and F. A. Kapp. 1996. Oral antigen inhibits priming of $CD8^+$ CTL, $CD4^+$ T cells, and antibody responses while activating $CD8^+$ suppressor T cells. *J. Immunol.* **156**:916–21.
38. Kapp, J. A., C. W. Pierce, D. R. Webb *et al.* 1995. Characterization of the epitope recognized by a monoclonal antibody that reacts differentially with murine suppressor T cells. *Int. Immunol.* **7**:1319–26.
39. Mostarica Stojkovic, M., M. Petrovic and M. L. Lukic. 1982. Cellular and genetic basis of the relative resistance to the induction of experimental allergic encephalomyelitis in Albino Oxford rats. *Adv. Exp. Med. Biol.* **149**:699–702.
40. Mostarica Stojkovic, M., M. Petrovic and M. L. Lukic. 1982. Resistance to the induction of EAE in AO rats: its prevention by the pretreatment with cyclophosphamide or low dose of irradiation. *Clin. Exp. Immunol.* **50**:311–17.
41. Racke, M. E., S. Dhib-Jalbut, B. Cannella *et al.* 1991. Prevention and treatment of chronic relapsing experimental allergic encephalomyelitis by transforming growth factor-β1. *J. Immunol.* **146**:3012–16.
42. Racke, M. K., S. Sriram, J. Carlino *et al.* 1993. Long-term treatment of chronic relapsing experimental allergic encephalomyelitis by transforming growth factor-β2. *J. Neuroimmunol.* **46**:175–84.
43. Kuruvilla, A. R., R. Shah, G. M. Hochwald *et al.* 1991. Protective effect of transforming growth factor β1 on experimental autoimmune diseases in mice. *Proc. Natl. Acad. Sci. USA* **88**:2918–21.
44. Brandes, M. E., J. B. Allen, Y. Ogawa and S. M. Wahl. 1991. Transforming growth factor β1 suppresses acute and chronic arthritis in experimental animals. *J. Clin. Invest.* **87**:1108–13.
45. Santambrogio, L., G. M. Hochwald, B. Sazena. 1993. Studies on the mechanisms by which transforming growth factor-β (TGF-β) protects against allergic encephalomyelitis. *J. Immunol.* **151**:1116–21.

46. Eynon, E. E. and D. C. Parker. 1993. Parameters of tolerance induction by antigen targeted to B lymphocytes. *J. Immunol.* **151**:2958–64.
47. Saoudi, A., S. Simmonds, I. Huitinga and D. Mason. 1995. Prevention of experimental allergic encephalomyelitis in rats by targeting autoantigen to B cells: Evidence that the protective mechanism depends on changes in the cytokine response and migratory properties of the autoantigen-specific T cells. *J. Exp. Med.* **182**:335–44.
48. Issekutz, T. B., J. M. Stoltz and P. Van der Meide. 1988. Lymphocyte recruitment in delayed-typed hypersensitivity. The role of IFNγ. *J. Immunol.* **140**:2989–93.
49. Saoudi, A., J. Kuhn, K. Huygen *et al.* 1993. TH2 activated cells prevent experimental autoimmune uveoretinitis, a TH1-dependent autoimmune disease. *Eur. J. Immunol.* **23**:3096–103.
50. Lukic, M. L., S. Stosic-Grujicic, N. Ostojic *et al.* 1991. Inhibition of nitric oxide generation affects the induction of diabetes by streptozotocin in mice. *Biochem. Biophys. Res. Commun.* **178**:913–20.
51. Kolb, H., U. Kiesel, K. D. Kroncke and W. Kolb-Bachofen. 1991. Suppression of low dose streptozotocin induced diabetes in mice by administration of a nitric oxide synthase inhibitor. *Life Sci.* **49**:P1213–P1217.
52. Corbett, J. A. and M. L. McDaniel. 1994. Reversibility of interleukin-1β-induced islet destruction and dysfunction by the inhibition of nitric oxide synthase. *Biochem. J.* **299**:719–24.
53. Weinberg, J. B., D. I. Granger, D. S. Piselsky *et al.* 1994. The role of nitric oxide in the pathogenesis of spontaneous murine autoimmune disease: Increased nitric oxide production and nitric oxide synthase expression in MRL-1ps/1pr mice, and reduction of spontaneous glomerulonephritis and arthritis by orally administered N^G-monomethyl-L-arginine. *J. Exp. Med.* **179**:651–60.
54. Lindsay, R., W. Smith, S. P. Rossiter *et al.* 1995. N^W-Nitro-L-arginine methyl ester reduces the incidence of IDDM in BB/E rats. *Diabetes* **44**: 365–8.
55. Wu, G. 1995. Nitric oxide synthesis and the effect of aminoguanidine and N^G-monomethyl-L-arginine on the onset of diabetes in the spontaneously diabetic BB rat. *Diabetes* **44**:360–4.
56. Welsh, N. and S. Sandler. 1993. Interleukin-1β induces nitric oxide production and inhibits the activity of aconitase without decreasing glucose oxidation rates in isolated mouse pancreatic islets. *Biochem. Biophys. Res. Commun.* **182**:333–40.
57. Kronche, K. D., V. Kolb-Bachofen, B. Berschick *et al.* 1991. Activated macrophages kill pancreatic syngeneic islet cells via arginine-dependent nitric oxide generation. *Biochem. Biophys. Res. Commun.* **175**:752–8.
58. Fehsel, K., A. Jalowy, S. Qi *et al.* 1993. Islet cell DNA is a target of inflammatory attack by nitric oxide. *Diabetes* **42**:496–500.
59. Amano, K. and J. W. Yoon. 1990. Studies on autoimmunity for initiation of β-cell destruction. V. Decrease of macrophage-dependent T-lymphocytes and natural killer cytotoxicity in silica-treated BB rats. *Diabetes* **39**:590–6.
60. Kaneto, H., J. Fujii, H. G. Seo *et al.* 1995. Apoptotic cell death triggered by nitric oxide in pancreatic β-cells. *Diabetes* **44**: 733–8.
61. Corbett, J. A., A. Mikhael, J. Shimizu *et al.* 1993. Nitric oxide production in islets from non-obese diabetic mice: aminoguanidine-sensitive and resistant stages in the immunological diabetic process. *Proc. Natl. Acad. Sci. USA* **90**:8992–5.
62. Wel, X. Q., I. G. Charles, A. Smith *et al.* 1995. Altered immune responses in mice lacking inducible nitric oxide synthase. *Nature* **375**:408–10.

26

Immunotherapy of Atopic Allergic Diseases

Bogdan Petrunov

Elimination of allergens from the external and internal environment of the body as well as immunotherapy is nowadays the most commonly used means for specific treatment of allergic patients. The possible drug treatments, including corticosteroids, are not very efficient in decreasing or reducing the allergic symptoms. This could explain the enormous and long-lasting interest in specific immunotherapy. It must be remembered that drug treatment cannot essentially change the spontaneous and long-lasting course of the disease. This is why intensive research has been carried out for the last 10–15 years on specific immunotherapy hyposensitization in controlled and non-controlled trials (1–10). To decrease the risks of side-effects and to obtain better clinical results, many experiments have been made on treatment methods. From 1911 when Freeman and Cook (3) first applied allergenic pollen extracts for treatment of pollen-allergic rhinitis, until now, specific hyposensitization has been the subject of many controversial opinions. Different results have been obtained but there is no doubt that 'specific immunotherapy is a cornerstone in the complex treatment of the allergic diseases. No better treatment could contemporary allergology offer to patients suffering from atopic hypersensitivity', as Professor Shapin (former president of the International Association of Allergology and Clinical Immunology) has stated. The European Academy of Allergology and Clinical Immunology is also greatly interested in specific immunotherapy of allergic diseases. The Academy periodically evaluates the development of the problem, regularly publishing official documents on this essential aetiopathogenic treatment method (3,11). Allergens for specific diagnosis and immunotherapy have been produced in Bulgaria for 30 years. In this country specific immunotherapy is the most commonly used method for treatment of respiratory allergy, and the clinical results are very promising, comparable to those reported by the leading scientists in the field of allergology.

Immunoregulation in Health and Disease
ISBN 0-12-459460-3

MECHANISMS OF SPECIFIC IMMUNOTHERAPY (HYPOSENSITIZATION)

The aim of hyposensitization is to achieve a change (modulation) of the immune system which is favourable for patients. As a result, different pathological abnormalities in the immune response (genetically determined or acquired) must be corrected. Allergic diseases are evoked by many different immunological mechanisms. Specific immunotherapy, directed to the specific allergen, provides different possibilities for influence. They could be summarized as follows:

- Production of specific 'blocking' (IgG1 or IgG4) antibodies, having 1000 times higher affinity to the proper allergen compared with the IgE antibodies (reaginic antibodies). Thus the blocking antibodies prevent binding of IgE to the specific allergen.
- Increasing the suppressed functional capacity of the CD8 T lymphocytes (T-suppressor lymphocytes), which suppress the IgE antibody synthesis.
- Influence on the IgE DRB and DQB genes of the HLA system, encoding for IgE antibody synthesis.
- Suppressing the expression of the Fc receptors for IgE antibodies on the surface of the T and B lymphocytes.
- Induction of specific switching of Th2 lymphocyte differentiation into Th1. As a result the secretion of IL-3, IL-4 and IL-5 (stimulating IgE synthesis) is depressed and the secretion of IL-2 and interferon-γ (suppressing the synthesis of IgE antibodies) is stimulated.
- Decreasing the activity of the mast cells as a result of blocking IL3 secretion, followed by suppression of mediators (histamine, PAF, ECF, etc.) release.
- Suppressing the activity of eosinophilic leukocytes, decreasing the secretion of IL-5. As a result the inflammatory reaction is diminished.
- Amelioration of non-specific bronchial hyperactivity by decreasing the release of mediators.
- Stimulation of the histamine-binding activity of the serum.
- Stimulation of the synthesis of protecting secretory IgA antibodies.
- Stimulation of the non-specific mechanisms of the immune defence (phagocytosis, production of interferon, lysozyme and alveolar surfactants) by bacterial allergens containing lipopolysaccharide (endotoxin).

INDICATIONS FOR SPECIFIC IMMUNOTHERAPY (HYPOSENSITIZATION)

One of the basic factors for successful specific immunotherapy is to define exactly the indications for its implementation. Thus the following circumstances should be taken into consideration. Their consecutive evaluation and application would guarantee higher clinical effectiveness of this method of treatment.

Conditions for application of immunotherapy (hyposensitization)

- Convincing data for the onset and the clinical course of the disease (case history, skin tests, serological factors).
- Availability for immunotherapy of high-quality, effective and standardized allergenic extracts lacking side-effects.
- Possibility that the immunotherapy be carried out for at least 5 years.

Reasons for carrying out immunotherapy/hyposensitization

- Decreasing the symptoms of the disease.
- Decreasing the need of drug therapy.
- Decreasing the risk of disease progressing – prophylactic effect of immunotherapy.
- Establishment of better quality of life for the patients (BQL).

It is important to point out the pronounced prophylactic effect of specific immunotherapy/hyposensitization, which is its major advantage over all other well-known methods for treatment of allergic diseases. There are convincing data on this in the literature. Mosbech (12) examined patients with allergic rhinitis (pollen allergy) over 8 years and found that those who had been subjected to specific hyposensitization developed asthma only half as often. Rackemann and Edwards (13) observed 688 asthmatic children for a period of more than 20 years and found that in their maturity only 25% of children treated by specific immunotherapy develop bronchial asthma. In the group of children treated with drugs, 75% became asthmatic. Malling (14), as a result of the observation on approximately 400 patients with bronchial asthma over 10 years, concluded that the specific immunotherapy significantly decreased the risk of lethal outcome in these patients. Bousquet (15), based on his investigations over 5000 patients with allergic rhinitis over 5 years, confirmed that the risk of developing bronchial asthma is 5% in the group receiving complete specific immunotherapy, 12% in the group treated with corticosteroids, antihistamine drugs and xanthins and 23% in the control group (patients treated with placebo).

SIDE-EFFECTS DURING SPECIFIC IMMUNOTHERAPY (HYPOSENSITIZATION)

In the course of the immunotherapy, local or systemic side-effects may be observed. The physician should be aware of them since successful immunotherapy depends on them. The value of the side-effects should be neither underestimated nor overestimated, since they are not very frequent. Overestimation of side-effects could restrict the application of highly effective specific immunotherapy and deprive the patient of a surely positive outcome of the disease. In support of this opinion, some of the most important investigations of the frequency of the serious side-effects (anaphylactic shock-like reactions) appearing during the specific immunotherapy may be cited:

- Walls (16) observed 20 000 patients treated by specific hyposensitization, receiving 150 000 injections. He found that only 0.01% of the patients developed anaphylactic shock.
- Lockey (17) found that in the USA during the period 1945–1987, 46 cases of anaphylactic shock were registered among patients subjected to specific immunotherapy.
- A similar investigation was carried out in the Centre for Drug Side-effects Control in England during 1991 (18). It was found that for the period 1980–1990 only 11 patients had developed anaphylactic shock as a result of immunotherapy.
- The famous English allergologist Frankland (19) reported one single case of anaphylactic shock during his practice, administering 750 000 shots of different allergens.

A major principle in the specific hyposensitization is the *individual* approach for each patient during the treatment. The achievement of excellent clinical results and avoidance of the side-effects depend to a great extent on the individual approach to immunotherapy. The treatment must comply with the immunological reactivity of each patient and the specificity of the proper allergen.

ALLERGEN EXTRACTS FOR SPECIFIC IMMUNOTHERAPY (HYPOSENSITIZATION)

The quality of the allergen extract used for specific hyposensitization is another major factor that determines the success of the treatment. Three basic conditions should be borne in mind:

- the choice and the quality of the initial raw material
- the method of extraction of the allergen
- isolation and purification of the allergen and its standardization and characterization.

Taking account of these basic conditions makes it possible to produce allergens with identical chemical and immunological properties as well as standard biological activity in each batch, which guarantees high-quality immunotherapy.

Allergenic preparations

- *Liquid extracts* have been widely used for many years.
- *Depo-extracts* have limited application since it is impossible for the side-effects to be controlled and corrected.
- *Lyophilized extracts*: their major disadvantage is that during the process of lyophilization there is a possibility of uncontrolled changes in the allergen molecule.
- *Mixtures of allergenic extracts* are not recommended for use, since mixing allergens of different origin and different chemical and immunological properties could lead to unwanted interference between them, leading to change or loss of allergenic activity.
- *Modified allergens* (*allergoids, tolerogens*) are at present the most promising preparations for specific immunotherapy with little or no allergenic activity, but with retained immunogenicity.
- *Liposome extracts* comprise extracts of allergens included in liposomes. This allows their better effect in the body. They are still under investigation, but it seems likely they will have great success in the future.

ALTERNATIVE SPECIFIC IMMUNOTHERAPY (HYPOSENSITIZATION)

Although specific immunotherapy by the subcutaneous administration of the allergen, as discussed above, is the most widely known, some alternative possibilities for immunotherapy exist. They have very limited application, being used by a few specialists only, in some particular cases, and they cannot replace classical methods. Specific hyposensitization has great advantages over the alternative methods in effectiveness and harmlessness, standardization of the preparations, and method of administration.

The alternative routes of application for immunotherapy are:

- oral immunotherapy
- sublingual immunotherapy
- local intranasal immunotherapy
- local bronchial immunotherapy
- quick (rush) immunotherapy.

FUTURE TRENDS FOR SPECIFIC IMMUNOTHERAPY (IMMUNOMODULATION)

The rapid development of immunology during the past 10–15 years, as well as of molecular biology, genetics, biochemistry and biotechnology, has given a great impetus to our understanding of the mechanisms of body allergization.

Opportunities have arisen for better diagnosis, treatment, prophylaxis and especially improvement of specific immunotherapy. These are in different theoretical and practical stages of realization, depending on the level of our knowledge in the field of applied and clinical allergology. In general, they could be summarized as follows:

- Infusion of allergen-specific T-suppressor lymphocytes.
- Simultaneous application of cyclosporin and the allergen. As a result the function of T-helper lymphocytes is suppressed, followed by diminished IgE synthesis.
- Administration of immune complexes, consisting of allergen and allergen-specific IgG. The aim is to obtain immunological tolerance against the allergen.
- Elimination of those B-lymphocyte clones which produce IgE, by irradiation.
- Infusion of radiolabelled allergens which damage the IgE antibodies fixed on the cells.
- Treatment with a variety of monoclonal antibodies, directed to some mediators of the allergic reactions, to IgE and IgG4 antibodies or to Fc receptors for these antibodies on the surface on the mast cells and basophilic leukocytes.
- Therapy with enzyme-treated allergens that have partially or totally lost the epitopes for B lymphocytes but have retained their T lymphocyte epitopes.
- Administration of synthetic or monovalent peptides isolated from the allergens, which mimic the amino acid sequence of the Fc fragment of IgE heavy chain and prevent its binding with the Fc receptor on the surface of mast cells and basophilic leukocytes.
- Application of antiidiotypic IgE antibodies.
- Administration of synthetic and recombinant allergens. As a result of intensive investigations in this field, several synthetic and recombinant allergens are already available. They could be used for diagnostic purposes (skin tests, RAST), but unfortunately they have too low immunogenicity and clinical effectiveness to be used for specific immunotherapy.

CLINICAL AND IMMUNOLOGICAL STUDY ON THE EFFECTIVENESS OF POLLEN ALLERGOID IN SPECIFIC HYPOSENSITIZATION

With a view to improving the effectiveness of specific hyposensitization, during the last 10–15 years there has been intensive work on the creation, study and clinical use of chemically modified allergens or allergoids, on which great hopes have been placed (20–25). The allergoids, with strongly reduced or completely eliminated allergenic properties but preserved immunogenicity, stimulate the formation of the sensitizing IgE antibodies much less than their initial allergens. They lead to the synthesis by an organism's immune system mainly of 'blocking' IgG antibodies, which is known to be one of the basic mechanisms explaining the effect of the specific immunotherapy. With the introduction of allergoids into clinical practice two very important effects have been achieved:

- The risk of unpleasant side reactions in the course of treatment has significantly decreased, because of the lower allergenic activity of the preparation.
- There is a possibility of introducing higher doses of allergen (allergoid) in the patient and thus obtaining better clinical results.

Bearing all this in mind, and on the basis of our long-standing experimental experience of allergoid preparation (26–28), we have applied our group's pollen allergoid in clinical practice and estimated its effectiveness.

We have studied and treated 53 patients suffering from pollen allergy (allergic rhinitis and conjunctivitis) with proved sensitization to the grass pollen allergens from which the group of pollen allergoids was prepared. For the purposes of specific hyposensitization we used group grass pollen allergoid, obtained by us using Marsh's modified method (29) on the basis of treatment of the initial allergens with formaline. The group pollen allergoid (Pald) contains allergens from the pollen of the following six which are grass species basic for our country: *Dactylis glomerata*, *Festuca* species, *Lolium perenne*, *Secale cereale*, *Phleum pratense*, *Arrhenaterum elatius*. The hyposensitization was carried out by the well-known classical schedule with gradually increasing concentration and quantities of the allergoid, starting with 10 PNU and going up to 12 500 PNU in quantities of 0.1 up to 0.8 ml subcutaneously. The symptoms were scored objectively and subjectively during the 3 years period treatment. The total IgE, IgE specific to two of the grass pollens (*D. glomerata* B6 and *Ph. pratense* B10) of the group grass pollen allergoid, and specific IgG (blocking antibodies) to group pollen allergens and pollen allergoid obtained from it were determined before and after 1, 2 and 3 years of immunotherapy.

Clinical results from the application of the pollen allergoid in the three groups of patients treated by hyposensitization during 1, 2 and 3 years respectively are presented in Table 26.1. In 83% of the treated patients excellent or very good effects were observed, and if the number with a good result is added to them we see that in 90.5% of all patients favourable clinical results were achieved. Only 5 patients (9.5%) showed no effect of the immunotherapy.

Of the 53 treated patients with pollinosis, 42 were studied immunologically. These results, in relation to the duration of the treatment, are shown in Fig. 26.1. A statistically significant decrease in the level of the total IgE ($p < 0.05$) and significant increase in the specific 'blocking' antibodies to the pollen allergen and allergoid ($p < 0.01$) in the three groups of patients was

Table 26.1 Clinical results from specific hyposensibilization carried out with group pollen allergoid

Term of treatment	Treated patients	Clinical results from specific hyposensibilization							
		Excellent		Very good		Good		Without effect	
		number	%	number	%	number	%	number	%
1 year	24	9	37.5	9	37.5	3	12.5	3	12.5
2 years	17	7	41.2	7	41.2	1	5.8	2	11.8
3 years	12	10	83.3	2	16.7	–	–	–	–
Total	53	26	49.0	18	34.0	4	7.5	5	9.5

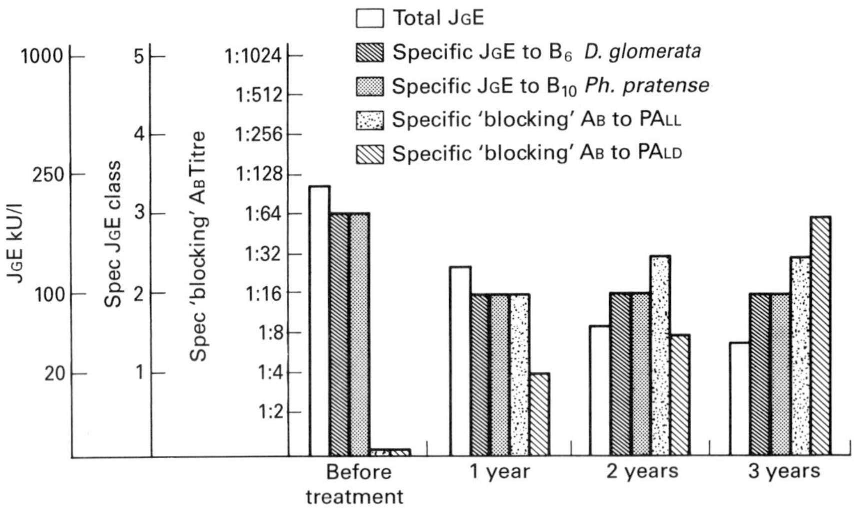

Fig. 26.1 Level of total IgE, specific IgE to the allergens of *D. glomerate* (B6) and *Ph. pratense* (B10) pollens and specific 'blocking' antibodies against PALL and PALd in patients before and after specific hyposensibilization with group pollen allergoid (PALd), carried on for 1, 2 and 3 years, respectively. The results are expressed as median values of the units and classes (ELISA, PRIST, RAST) and titres (passive hemagglutination).

established after treatment. Patients treated by hyposensitization for 3 years presented a statistically significant decrease of the specific IgE to two of the pollen allergens included in the allergoid. It was established that patients who had excellent or very good clinical results had a statistically significant decrease of the total IgE ($p<0.05$) in comparison with their level before treatment (Fig. 26.2). The same result was established for the level of the specific IgE in the patients with excellent clinical results from immunotherapy with pollen allergoid (Fig. 26.3). The results of the titre of the 'blocking' antibodies versus the pollen allergen and the allergoid obtained from it respectively in relation to the clinical result of immunotherapy are shown in Figs. 26.4 and 26.5. It is evident that practically in all patients there is a significant increase in the titre of these antibodies in comparison with their level before treatment ($p<0.01$) when an excellent or very good result was obtained from the hyposensitization treatment.

Bearing in mind the results obtained, we can conclude that the pollen allergoid possessed good therapeutic effectiveness. Increasing the duration of treatment (1, 2 or 3 years) improves the clinical results. These encouraging results have the even greater value in that, in the course of treatment, there were single, weak local reactions observed in patients and in only four (7.7%)

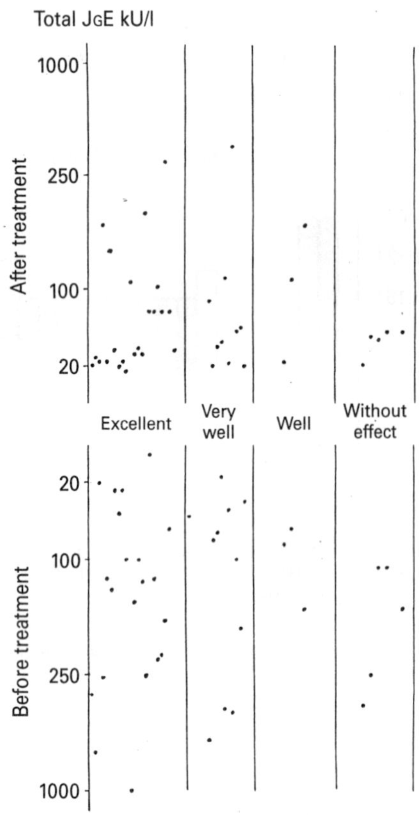

Fig. 26.2 The level of total IgE antibodies, expressed as kU/L (ELISA, PRIST) in 42 patients investigated, treated with group pollen allergoid (PALd), before and after immunotherapy, depending on clinical result.

of them were we compelled to discontinue the increase of the allergoid dose, because of reinforcement of disease symptoms. On the other hand, the significantly decreased activity of the allergoid permitted its introduction to the patients in much higher doses (10 000–12 000 PNU) than the raw allergens without danger of side-effects, which is one explanation for the good clinical result of the immunotherapy. It is obvious that the therapeutic effectiveness of the pollen allergoid could be explained with sufficiently preserved specific immunogenicity and the formation of high titres of 'blocking' antibodies. At the same time there is a clear tendency for the total and specific IgE to decrease in most of the patients treated with pollen allergoid.

All this is in favour of the wide introduction of allergoids into clinical practice, which is confirmed by the publication in recent years of papers in many countries (1,2,4,27,30,31) presenting allergoids as

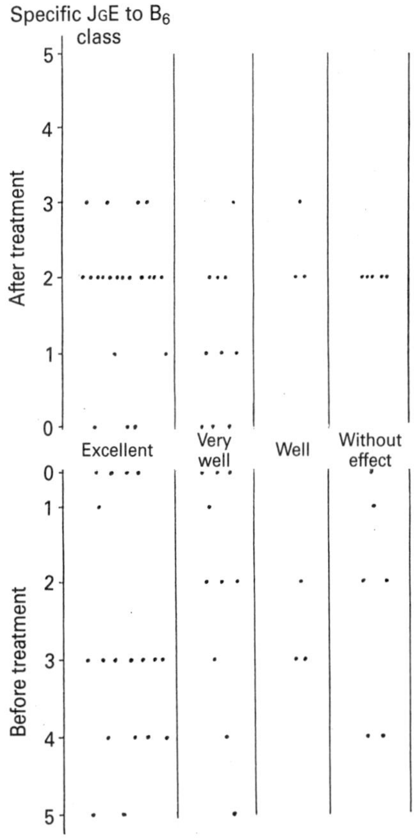

Fig. 26.3 Level of specific IgE antibodies to the allergen of *D. glomerate* pollen (B6) in classes (ELISA, RAST) in investigated 42 patients, treated with group pollen allergoid (PALd), before and after immunotherapy, depending on clinical result.

appropriate biological preparations for the purposes of the specific hyposensitization/immunotherapy of atopic allergy.

CONCLUSION

Finally I would like to cite the conclusion of the recent Programme of the European Academy of Allergology and Clinical Immunology concerning the problems of the specific immunotherapy/hyposensitization, published in 1993. It expresses the opinion of prominent allergologists in a very concise way:

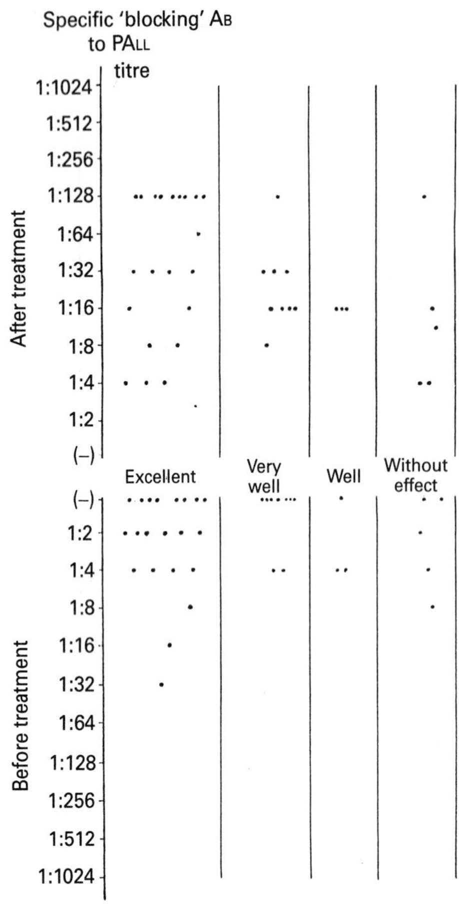

Fig. 26.4 Level of specific 'blocking' antibodies to the group pollen allergen (PALL) in titres (passive haemagglutination) in investigated 42 patients, treated with group pollen allergoid (PALD), before and after immunotherapy, depending on clinical results.

A significant clinical efficacy of immunotherapy has been documented in a number of controlled studies. The capacity of drug treatment is limited to the elimination or decrease of symptoms, and no studies have been able to show that pharmacological treatment of allergic diseases, not even corticosteroids, modifies the spontaneous, long-term course of the disease. We recommend that immunotherapy forms an integrated part of the treatment of allergic disorders, thus reducing the disease severity, improving the quality of life of allergics, and diminishing the risk and cost of pharmacotherapy. The logical approach in the treatment of allergic diseases must be to impede the natural course of the disease. Not only the direct clinical benefit, but

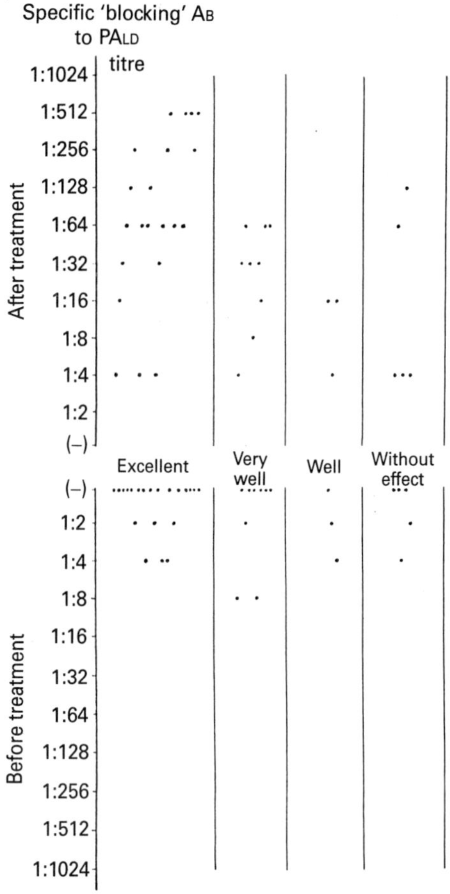

Fig. 26.5 Level of specific 'blocking' antibodies to the group pollen allergoid (PALD) in titres (passive haemagglutination) in investigated 42 patients, treated with group pollen allergoid (PALD), before and after immunotherapy, depending on clinical results.

also the possible preventive aspects of immunotherapy should be considered.

REFERENCES

1. Bousquet, J. and F. B. Michel. 1989. Specific immunotherapy, past, present and future. *Proceedings, XIV Congress of the EAACI*, Berlin (West), 193–7.
2. Bousquet, J., A. Hejjaoui and F. B. Michel. 1990. Specific immunotherapy in asthma. *J. Allergy Clin. Immunol.* **86**:292–305.
3. Malling, H. J. and B. Weeke. 1993. Position paper: Immunotherapy. *Allergy* **48**, Suppl. 14:9–35.

4. Malling, H. J. 1995. The future of immunotherapy. *Proceedings XVI European Congress of Allergology and Clinical Immunology. Madrid*, 693–700.
5. Nelson, H., J. Oppenheimer and G. Vatsia. 1993. A double-blind placebo-controlled evaluation of sublingual immunotherapy with standardized cat extract. *J. Allergy Clin. Immunol.* **93**:229–36.
6. Norman, P. 1981. Immunotherapy. *Prog. Allergy* **32**:318–355.
7. Norman, P. and T. Van Metre. 1990. The safety of allergenic immunotherapy. *J. Allergy Clin. Immunol.* **85**:522–5.
8. Rebhun, L., L. Thouin, F. Russel and D. Rebhun. 1981. Extracorporal hyposensitization. *Ann. Allergy* **46**:140–2.
9. Rebien, W., E. Puttonen and H. Maasch. 1982. Clinical and immunological response to oral and subcutaneous immunotherapy with grass pollen extract. *Eur. J. Pediatr.* **138**:341–4.
10. Terde, N. and R. Urbanek. 1989. Combination of parenteral and oral immunotherapy in grass pollen-allergic children. *Allergy* **44**:272–80.
11. Thompson, R. 1989. The current status of allergen immunotherapy. Report of WHO/IUIS working group. *Allergy* **44**:369–79.
12. Mosbech, H. and O. Østerballe. 1988. Does the effect of immunotherapy last after termination of treatment. *Allergy* **43**:523–9.
13. Rackemann, F. and M. Edwards. 1972. Asthma in children. 1972. **246**:815–63.
14. Malling, H. J. 1990. New ideas in allergen-specific immunotherapy. *Am. J. Rhinol.* **4**:155–8.
15. Bousquet, J. and F. B. Michel. 1994. Specific immunotherapy in asthma: Is it effective. *J. Allergy Clin. Immunol.* **194**:1–11.
16. Walls, A. 1992. Liposome for allergy immunotherapy. *Clin. Exp. Allergy* **22**:1–12.
17. Lockey, R. F., L. M. Benedict and P. C. Turkeltaub. 1987. Fatalities from immunotherapy and skin testing. *J. Allergy Clin. Immunol.* **79**:660–7.
18. Committee on Safety of Medicine. 1986. CSM update: desensitizing vaccines. *Br. Med. J.* **293**:948.
19. Frankland, A. W. 1980. Anaphylactic reactions to desensitisation. *Br. Med. J.* **281**:1429.
20. Bousquet, J., M. Frank, R. Soussana *et al.* 1987. Comparison of parameters assessing the efficacy of immunotherapy with allergoid in grass pollinosis. *Int. Arch. Allergy Appl. Immunol.* **77**:542–5.
21. Bousquet, J., A. Hejjaoui, W. Skassa-Brociek *et al.* 1987. Double blind placebo controlled immunotherapy with mixed grass pollen allergoid. *J. Allergy Clin. Immunol.* **80**:591–8.
22. Grammer, L. and M. Shaughnessy. 1984. Persistence of efficacy after a brief course of polymerized rageed allergens. *J. Allergy Clin. Immunol.* **73**:484–9.
23. Marsh, D., J. Alexander and P. Norman. 1982. Bosting of patients with high and low doses of allergoid. *J. Allergy Clin. Immunol.* **69**:99–105.
24. Sehon, A. and W. Lee. 1979. Suppression of IgE antibodies with modified allergens. *J. Allergy Clin. Immunol.* **64**:242–50.
25. Warner, J. 1978. Controlled trial of hyposensitization to *D. pteronyssinus* in children with asthma. *Lancet* **11**:912–16.
26. Petrunov, B. 1980. Preparation and immunological characteristics of allergoids from house dust and grass pollen. *Days of Bulgarian Science and Technology in Canada. Montreal.*
27. Petrunov, B., V. Yomtova and E. Stanoeva. 1988. A study on chemically modified pollen allergen (allergoid). *Problems of Infectious and Parasitic Diseases, Sofia*, 90–8.

28. Petrunov, B., E. Stanoeva, D. Baltadjieva and D. Konstantinova. 1994. Clinical effectiveness of immunotherapy with grass pollen allergoid. *Acta Medica Bulgarica. Sofia.* **XVI**:56–67.
29. Marsh, D., P. Norman, M. Roebber and L. Lichtenstein. 1981. Studies of allergoids from naturally occurring allergens. *J. Allergy Clin. Immunol.* **68**:449–55.
30. Dreborg, S. and A. Frew, eds. 1993. Allergen standardization and skin tests. Position paper. *Allergy* **48** Suppl. 14:49–54.
31. Weise, F., C. Haase and E. Frank. 1989. Statistical implications of side effects and other parameters registered during pollen-specific hyposensitization with depot allergoid. *XIV Congress of the EAACI, Berlin (West).*

27

Altered Functions of Peripheral Blood Mononuclear Cells and Granulocytes in Patients with Active Psoriasis

Danilo Vojvodić, Nada Pejnović, Djordjije Karadaglić, Zorka Kukić and Aleksandar Dujić

Psoriasis is defined as an inflammatory immune-mediated skin disease. Its hallmarks are epidermal hyperproliferation and altered differentiation with local inflammatory infiltrate composed mainly of neutrophils and T lymphocytes (1). The central role in psoriatic lesions belongs to the $CD4^+$ T lymphocyte, whose soluble products activate antigen-presenting cells, polymorphonuclear leukocytes and keratinocytes (2). $CD4^+$ T lymphocytes extracted from psoriatic plaque and propagated in vitro produce Th1-type cytokines, namely IFNγ and IL-2 (3), which induce increased expression of class II MHC and adhesion molecules on keratinocytes and production of another wave of inflammatory cytokines, leading to further keratinocyte proliferation and increased migration of T lymphocytes and neutrophils into skin lesions (2).

Reports concerning IL-8 found locally in psoriatic skin lesions (4) further indicate a possible important role for polymorphonuclear cells in regulation of psoriatic plaque genesis by producing significant levels of IL-1β, TNFα, IL6, IL-1 receptor antagonist (IL-1RA) and especially IL-8 (5). Moreover, recent data stress the importance of T lymphocytes in regulating neutrophil functions and vice versa (6,7).

However, recent findings suggest that altered peripheral blood cell functions in psoriaric patients could contribute to the ongoing local inflammatory response (8–10). A number of studies point out systemically altered immunoreactivity in patients with psoriasis, such as elevated plasma IL-6 levels (9), activation of neutrophils (10) by soluble factors of unstimulated

Immunoregulation in Health and Disease
ISBN 0–12–459460–3

monocytes and increased adhesiveness of psoriatic PB mononuclear cells to endothelial cells (8).

In order to obtain further insight into the functions of peripheral blood cells in patients with psoriasis we investigated the mitogen and phorbol ester-induced proliferative lymphocyte response, as well as neutrophil activation, adhesion and TNF production.

MATERIAL AND METHODS

Isolation of cells

Cells were isolated from venous blood of 16 patients (13 men, 3 women) with severe and active generalized forms of psoriasis, hospitalized at the Clinic for Dermatovenerology, MMA, Belgrade, without any systemic therapy. Six healthy volunteers were included as controls.

Peripheral blood cells were isolated by centrifugation on a Lymhoprep density gradient (Nycomed, Norway). The mononuclear cells were washed and resuspended in RPMI (ICN Pharmaceuticals, USA) supplemented with 5% fetal calf serum (FCS ICN Pharmaceuticals, USA). Polymorphonuclear cells were recovered from the pellet, and after haemolysis of erythrocytes with isotonic ammonium chloride, cells were washed and reconstituted in RPMI 5% FCS. The purity of these cell populations was more than 95% as estimated by May–Gruenwald–Giemsa staining.

Proliferation assay

Peripheral blood mononuclear cells were seeded in 96-well flat-bottom microtitre plates at 3×10^6 ml in complete medium (RPMI 1640 containing 10% FCS, 2 mM L-glutamine and 100 mg/ml garamycin). After stimulation with mitogens (phytohaemaglutinin-PHA, Sigma, St. Louis, MO, 20 and 40 μg/ml), phorbol myristate acetate-PMA (Sigma, St. Louis, MO, 50 ng/ml), or with calcium ionophore (Sigma, St. Louis, MO, 0.25 μg/ml) cells were cultivated for 72 h at 37°C in 5% carbon dioxide and pulsed with 0.5 μCi/ml of 3H TdR (5 Ci/mM, Amersham) for the last 18 h of culture.

NBT reduction assay

Polymorphonuclear cells were resuspended at 5×10^5/well of 96-well flat-bottom microtitre plates. The various concentration of PMA and LPS were added with NBT dye (NBT, Sigma, St. Louis, MO, 10 μl/well at a concentration of 5 mg/ml) at the beginning of culture, cells incubated for 30 min and colour dissolved with SDS-HCl. The absorbance of dissolved colour was determinated using a microplate spectrophotometer (Berhing ELISA processor II, Behringwerke AG Diagnostica) at 570 nm.

Adhesion assay

Polymorphonuclear cells resuspended at a concentration of 5×10^6/ml were seeded 100 μl cell suspension/well, in 96-well plates. After adding the various concentration of PMA and LPS, cells were incubated for 30 min in 5% carbon dioxide at 37°C and non-adherent cells washed out. Adherent cells were stained with 0.1% methylene blue, and absorbance of dissolved colour (0.1N HCl) determined using a microplate spectrophotometer (Berhing ELISA processor II, Behringwerke AG Diagnostica) at 650 nm.

TNF production

PMNs were resuspended at a concentration of 5×10^6/ml in RPMI 5% FCS, stimulated with PMA and LPS and incubated for 24 h. After centrifugation the supernatants were collected and stored at −20°C until use.

The TNF activity was detected using an L-929 mouse fibroblast cell line. Cells were seeded at 2.5×10^4 cells per well and left overnight to adhere. One hour before different dilutions of test samples or recombinant mouse TNFα were added, actinomicin D (Sigma, St. Louis, MO) was added at a final concentration of 0.2 mg/l. After overnight incubation at 37°C in 5% carbon dioxide, the non-adherent cells were discarded, and the viable cells that were left were determined by staining with methylene blue, The optical density of dye that was solubilized by 0.1 N hydrochloric acid was determinated using a microplate spectrophotometer (Berhing ELISA processor II, Behringwerke AG Diagnostica) at 650 nm. The specificity of TNF-induced cytotoxicity was confirmed by neutralizing anti-mouse TNFα antibody.

Statistical analysis

Statistical analyses were made using the Mann–Whitney test.

RESULTS AND DISCUSSION

Peripheral blood lymphocyte proliferation

The level of spontaneous lymphocyte proliferation did not differ between psoriatic patients and healthy controls. PHA (40 μg/ml)-induced lymphocyte proliferation showed a significantly lower level ($p < 0.05$) in patients with psoriasis compared to healthy controls, which was even more pronounced in response to 20 μg/ml PHA ($p < 0.001$) (Fig. 27.1, top).

Extremely low proliferative response was detected in comparison with the controls when MNC from psoriatic patients were stimulated with PMA alone or with addition of calcium ionophore ($p < 0.01$) (Fig. 27.1, bottom).

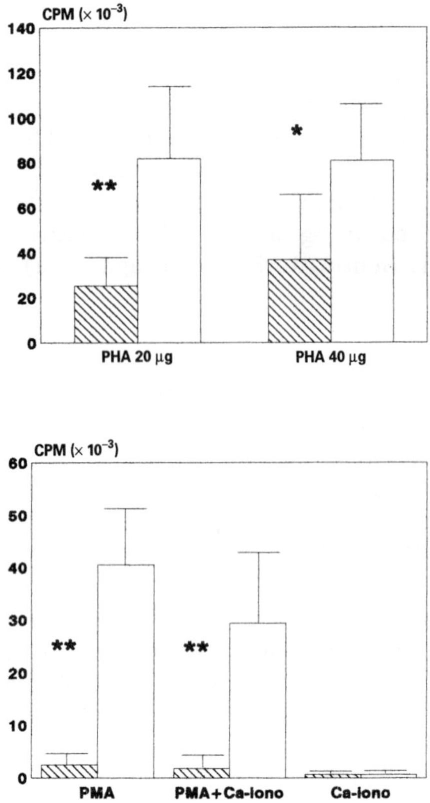

Fig. 27.1 PB lymphocyte proliferative response. Top: Stimulation with PHA. Bottom: Stimulation with PMA, PMA and calcium ionophore and ionophore alone. Data are presented as mean ± SD of proliferative responses of studied groups. $*p<0.05$, $**p<0.01$ between groups (Mann–Whitney test). Shaded bars, patients; white bars, control group.

Various factors found to be present in skin lesions or in the circulation of patients with psoriasis could inhibit the lymphocyte proliferative response. Phytohaemagglutinin-activated human blood lymphocytes release 15-HETE (15-mono hydroxyeicosatetraenoic acid) and LTB4 (5,12 diHETE or leukotriene B_4), which are potent inhibitors of lymphocyte proliferation (11).

High concentrations of both of these metabolites have been found in acute psoriatic skin lesions (12), along with a high concentration of neuropeptide VIP (13) which is also known as an inhibitor of mitogen-induced proliferative response (14).

On the other hand, two reports stress that PB MNC in psoriatic patients are activated by as yet unknown stimuli. This was demonstrated by enhanced psoriatic MNC adhesiveness to endothelium (8) and increased levels of IL-6 (9) produced by PB monocytes. It could be speculated that IL-6 produced by monocytes could induce release of TGFβ which is known as a potent inhibitor of lymphocyte proliferation (15) and could also lead to more general cytokine imbalance such as inhibiting IL-1 and TNF production which could seriously impair the activation of lymphocytes (16).

Addition of PMA and calcium ionophore as direct activators of cytoplasmic biochemical processes in lymphocytes resulted in very low proliferative response, as with PHA, a membrane-acting stimulator which requires normal antigen presenting cell functions. PMA-induced low proliferative response could not be explained by altered PKC activity, since it was shown that patients with psoriasis have normal PKC activity (either in membrane or in cytosol) in peripheral blood lymphocytes (17). The obtained results warrant further investigation employing pure lymphocytes to delineate the cell population responsible for impaired proliferative response.

Peripheral blood polymorphonuclear cells (PMN) activation

Neutrophils from patients with psoriasis showed significantly lower spontaneous ($p<0.05$) and LPS induced NBT reduction ($p<0.05$), but when triggered by PMA reduction level was significantly higher compared to healthy controls ($p<0.05$) (Fig. 27.2, top). PMN from psoriatic patients were less adherent to polystyrene substrates, either without simulation or after addition of PMA or LPS ($p<0.01$) (Fig. 27.2, middle). There are limited data about peripheral blood neutrophil functions in psoriasis. The significant difference in neutrophil NBT reduction level is possibly due to primed state of psoriatic PMN (18), since no spontaneous increase in oxidase activity, but subsequent stimulation with suboptimal PMA (10 ng/ml) provoked a response that was far more intensive than in healthy controls.

Possible priming factors for granulocytes are TNF and GM-CSF shown to be produced from unstimulated monocytes from patients with active psoriasis (10). Decreased granulocyte adhesion to plastic was also described for PB PMN from patients with rheumatoid arthritis, another systemic inflammatory disease, and it was additionally shown that all the adhesion molecules relevant for neutrophil adhesive functions (CD11a,b/CD18) were expressed significantly less (19).

TNF production by peripheral blood polymorphonuclear cells

Spontaneous neutrophil TNF production did not differ between psoriatic patients and healthy controls, except that 4 out of 16 patients with psoriasis had extremely high levels. PMA induced similar amounts of TNF in both groups, in contrast to LPS stimulation which evoked significantly higher

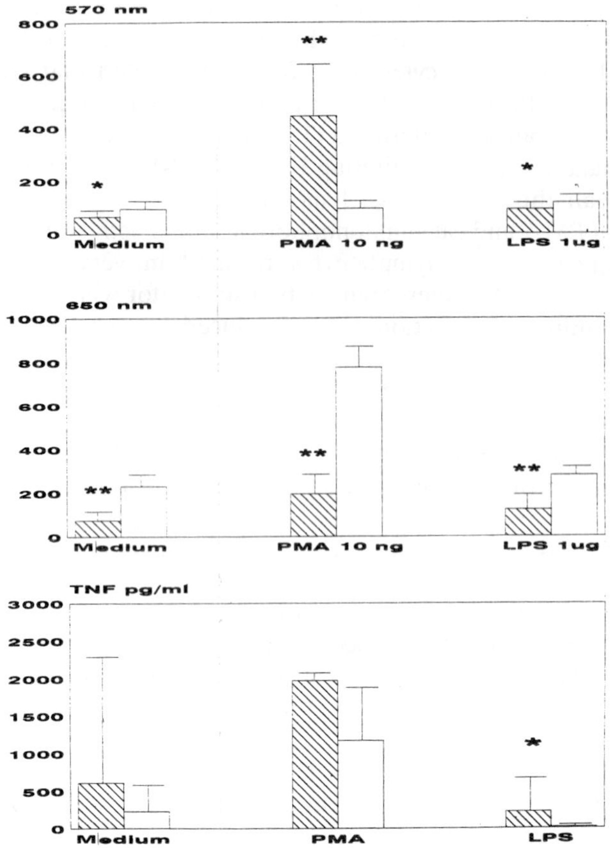

Fig. 27.2 Assessment of peripheral blood polymorphonuclear cells functions. Top: Activation of PB PMN (NBT test). Data are presented as the mean ± SD of NBT reduction from a representative experiment. Centre: PB PMN adhesion to polystyrene substrates. Data are presented as the mean ± SD of adhesion from a representative experiment. Bottom: PB PMN TFN production. Data are presented as the mean ± SD cytokine activity from a representative experiment. *$p<0.05$. **$p<0.01$ between groups (Mann–Whitney test). Shaded bars, patients; white bars, control group.

TNF production in psoriatic patients' granulocytes ($p<0.01$) (Fig. 27.2, bottom).

Investigations of the beneficial effects of cyclosporin A (CsA) in the treatment of psoriasis (2), showed that CsA inhibits TNF and GM-CSF production by peripheral blood monocytes, and revealed the importance of TNF in psoriasis. It was already shown that unstimulated peripheral blood monocytes from patients with active psoriasis produce factors such as TNFα and GM-CSF (10). Our results imply that spontaneous TNF production was not significant (except for a few patients), but was higher only when granulocytes were stimulated with LPS, which suggests their higher capacity for TNF production. Therefore, along with the aforementioned results the higher stimulated TNF production implies a steady state of neutrophils in patients with psoriasis which could possibly contribute to the ongoing inflammatory process.

CONCLUSION

The results of our study demonstrated impaired peripheral blood lymphocyte proliferative response and altered functions of PB neutrophils in patients with active psoriasis. Further investigation should indicate whether these systemic phenomena are causes or merely consequences in the pathogenesis of psoriasis.

REFERENCES

1. Gunter, M., L. Kemeny, B. Homey and T. Ruzicka. 1996. FK 506 in the treatment of inflammatory skin disease: promises and perspectives. *Immunology Today* **17**:106–7.
2. Wong, R. L., C. M. Winslow and C. D. Cooper. 1993. The mechanisms of action of cyclosporin A in the treatment of psoriasis. *Immunology Today* **14**:69–74.
3. Schlaak, J. F., M. Buslay, W. Jochum *et al.* 1995. T cells involved in psoriasis belong to the Th1 subset. *J. Investigative Dermatol.* **102**:145–9.
4. Anttila, Heli S. I., S. Reitamo, P. Erkko *et al.* 1992. Interleukin-8 immunoreactivity in the skin of healthy subjects and patients with palmoplantar pustulosis and psoriasis. *J. Investigative Dermatol.* **98**:96–101.
5. Lloyd, A. R. and J. J. Openheim. 1992. Polys lament: the neglected role of the polymorphonuclear neutrophil in the afferent limb of the immune response. *Immunol. Today* **13**:169–72.
6. Prior, C., P. J. Townsend, D. A. Hughes and P. L. Haslam. 1992. Induction of lymphocyte proliferation by antigen-pulsed human neutrophils. *Clin. Exper. Immunol.* **87**:485–92.
7. Zhang, J. H., A. Ferrante, A. P. Arrigo and J. M. Dayer. 1992. Neutrophil stimulation and priming by direct contact with activated human T lymphocytes. *J. Immunol.* **148**:177–81.
8. LeRoy, F., L. A. Brown, M. W. Greaves *et al.* 1991. Blood mononuclear cells from patients with psoriasis exhibit an enhanced adherence to cultured vascular endothelium. *J. Investigative Dermatol.* **97**:511–16.
9. Neuner, P., A. Urbanski, F. Trautinger *et al.* 1991. Increased IL6 production by monocytes and keratinocytes in patients with psoriasis. *J. Investigative Dermatol.* **97**:27–33.
10. Pigatto, P. D., L. B. Pigatto, A. Bigardi *et al.* 1990. Factors secreted by untreated psoriatic monocytes enhance neutrophil function. *J. Investigative Dermatol.* **94**:373–6.
11. Hadden, J. W. 1988. Transmembrane signals in the activation of T lymphocytes by mitogenic antigens. *Immunol. Today* **9**:235–9.

12. Pleszczynski, M. P. 1992. Arachidonic acid and the leukotrieens. In: *Encyclopedia of Immunology* (I. M. Roit and P. J. Delves, eds.) Academic Press, London, pp. 155–8.
13. Anand, P., D. R. Springall, M. A. Blank *et al.* 1991. Neuropeptides in skin disease: increased VIP in eczema and psoriasis but not axillary hyperhydrosis. *Br. J. Dermatol.* **124**:547–9.
14. Sirinek, L. P. and M. S. O'Dorisio. 1991. Modulation of immune function by intestinal neuropeptides. *Acta Oncol.* **30**:509–17.
15. Zhou, D., A. M. Minster and R. A. Winchurch. 1992. Inhibitory effects of interleukin 6 on immunity: possible role in burn patients. *Arch. Surg.* **127**:65–9.
16. Aderka, D., J. Le and J. Vilcek. 1989. IL6 inhibits lipopolisaharide-induced tumor necrosis factor production in cultured human monocytes, and U937 cells in mice. *J. Immunol.* **143**:3515–23.
17. Raynaud, F. and D. Evian-Brion. 1991. Protein kinase C activity in normal and psoriatic cells: cultures of fibroblasts and lymphocytes. *Br. J. Dermatol.* **124**:542–6.
18. Hallet, M. B. and D. Lloyds. 1995. Neutrophil priming: the cellular signals that say amber but not green. *Immunol. Today* **16**:264–8.
19. Jones, J., I. Laffafian, A. M. Cooper *et al.* 1994. Expression of complement regulatory molecules and other surface markers and neutrophils from synovial fluid and blood of patients with rheumatoid arthritis. *Br. J. Dermatol.* **33**:707–12.

28

$CD4^+$ T Lymphocyte Subsets Influence Duration of Clinical Remission in Recent-onset Insulin-dependent Diabetes Mellitus

Nebojša M. Lalić, Miodrag L. Lukić, Duško Kosec, Miroslava Zamaklar, Katarina Lalić, Aleksandra Jotić and Predrag Đorđević

Previous studies have suggested that changes in the $CD4^+$ T lymphocytes might modulate the clinical course of the disease in recent-onset insulin-dependent diabetes mellitus (IDDM) patients (1–4). Simultaneously, it has been postulated that $CD4^+$ T cells represent a heterogeneous subpopulation of T lymphocytes in humans and it has been demonstrated that the presence of the isoforms of the cell surface antigen CD45, determined by four different types of N-terminal exon products (CD45RA, CD45RB, CD45RC and 'no-exon' or CD45R0 isoforms), was found to be suitable for characterization of different $CD4^+$ T-cell subsets with specific monoclonal antibodies (5). Thus, it has been shown that $CD4^+CD45RA^+$ T cells represent 'virgin' or immunologically naive cells whereas $CD4^+CD45R0^+$ T cells are found to be 'primed' or memory cells which acquire their CD45R0 marker upon antigenic stimulation (6). In addition, the $CD4^+CD45R0^+$T cells are found to promote other lymphocyte responses (T helper–inducer lymphocytes) whereas $CD4^+CD45RA^+$ T cells are suggested to suppress other responses of T lymphocytes (T suppressor–inducer lymphocytes) (7). The role of CD45R0 and CD45RA subsets of $CD4^+$ T lymphocytes in the pathogenesis of IDDM and especially in relations to the clinical course of the disease has

Immunoregulation in Health and Disease
ISBN 0-12-459460-3

not been extensively studied. In this study, we have demonstrated that duration of clinical remission (CR) in recent-onset IDDM patients is strongly related to the level of the $CD45R0^+$ subset of $CD4^+$ T cells in the peripheral blood.

PATIENTS AND METHODS

In the study we included 25 recent-onset IDDM patients (<6 months after diagnosis) showing a complete remission (CR) (a non-insulin-requiring state of normoglycemia lasting >30 days) within the first year of the disease. The patients were divided into two groups according to the duration of remission: a long-term remission (>6 mo) (group A, $n = 12$) and a short-term remission (<6 mo) (group B, $n = 13$). Also, 10 healthy control age-matched subjects were included in the study (group C) (Table 28.1). Informed consent was obtained from each subject before inclusion in the study.

The follow-up analysis of lymphocyte subsets in the peripheral blood was done in each subject of groups A and B in (a) insulin-requiring state (IRS) and (b) state of CR, while in group C a single measurement was done. Human mononuclear lymphocytes were separated by Ficoll-Hypaque density centrifugation (Pharmacia) from the heparinized fresh blood taken from the subjects in fasting euglycemic conditions, and the lymphocyte subsets were determined by immunofluorescence using specific monoclonal antibodies (8). $CD3^+$, $CD4^+$ and $CD8^+$ lymphocyte subsets were detected by one-colour staining using fluorescein isothiocyanate (FITC)-conjugated antibodies (Anti-Leu 4, Anti-Leu 3a and Anti-Leu 2a, respectively, Becton Dickinson). $CD45R0^+$ and $CD45RA^+$ subsets of $CD4^+$ cells were detected by using a

Table 28.1 Long-term vs. short-term clinical remission in recent-onset IDDM: characteristics of patients and controls

Characteristics	Group A	Group B	Group C
Number of subjects	12	13	10
Age (yr)	23.4 ± 0.5	24.2 ± 0.8	22.7 ± 0.9
Duration of diabetes before inclusion (mo)	3.4 ± 0.8	2.9 ± 0.9	–
Duration of clinical remission (mo)	3.1 ± 0.9	8.9 ± 0.8	–
Total leucocyte number ($\times 10^3$/ml)	6.2 ± 0.4	5.8 ± 0.3	5.4 ± 0.5
Fasting blood glucose (mmol/l)	5.9 ± 0.6	5.4 ± 0.7	4.1 ± 0.8

Group A: long-term remission (>6 mo); Group B: short-term remission (<6 mo); Group C: healthy controls.

two-colour staining with FITC-conjugated Anti-Leu 3a for $CD4^+$ lymphocytes and phycoerythrin-conjugated UCHL-1 (kindly provided by Dr. Peter Beverly, Imperial Cancer Research Fund, London) and Anti-Leu 18 (Becton Dickinson) antibodies for $CD45R0^+$ and $CD45RA^+$ subsets respectively. Specific immunofluorescence was detected by flow cytometry.

The significance of the differences was determined by one-way variance analysis.

RESULTS

The analysis of the percentage of $CD3^+$, $CD4^+$ and $CD8^+$ T lymphocytes in the peripheral blood did not show significant differences among the long-term remission IDDM patients (group A), the short-term remission IDDM patients (group B), and the healthy control subjects (group C), in either IRS or CR. Also, within groups A and B, we could not detect significant differences between IRS and CR (Table 28.2).

When we analysed the percentage of $CD4^+CD45R0^+$ T lymphocytes, we found that in both patient groups (A and B) it was higher than in the healthy controls (group C), both in IRS and in CR. Also, within groups A and B, it was higher in IRS than in CR. Moreover, in the state of CR, the percentage of $CD4^+CD45R0^+$ T cells was significantly lower in the long-term remission (group A) compared to the short-term remission IDDM patients (group B) (Table 28.3).

The percentage of $CD4^+CD45RA^+$ lymphocytes was lower in IRS in both patients groups (A and B) compared to the controls (group C). However, in the state of CR, it increased in both patient groups and there was no difference among groups A, B and C (Table 28.4).

Table 28.2 Long-term vs. short-term clinical remission in recent-onset IDDM: percentage of $CD3^+$, $CD4^+$ and $CD8^+$ lymphocytes in the peripheral blood

Patients	Clinical phase of disease	Lymphocyte subsets		
		$CD3^+$	$CD4^+$	$CD8^+$
Long-term remission (Group A)	IRS	80.2 ± 2.0[a]	44.2 ± 1.5	25.1 ± 2.4
	CR	77.2 ± 2.9	42.9 ± 1.7	24.1 ± 2.5
Short-term remission (Group B)	IRS	78.4 ± 2.3	43.7 ± 1.2	25.7 ± 2.6
	CR	75.7 ± 3.3	42.0 ± 1.9	24.5 ± 2.8
Controls (Group C)	–	73.5 ± 4.6	45.9 ± 2.9	26.1 ± 2.7

[a]Percentage of total number of lymphocytes in the peripheral blood determined by immunofluorescence and flow cytometry; the results are expressed as mean ± SE.

Table 28.3 Long-term vs. short-term clinical remission in recent-onset IDDM: percentage of $CD4^+$, $CD45R0^+$ lymphocytes in the peripheral blood

Patients	Clinical phase of disease	Lymphocyte subsets	
		$CD4^+CD45R0^+$	$CD4^+CD45R0^-$
Long-term remission (Group A)	IRS	32.3 ± 2.2[a]	11.9 ± 1.4
	CR	28.4 ± 2.0	14.5 ± 1.7
Short-term remission (Group B)	IRS	35.2 ± 2.1	8.5 ± 0.9
	CR	32.7 ± 2.0	9.3 ± 0.9
Controls (Group C)	–	24.3 ± 1.3	21.6 ± 1.8

[a]Percentage of total number of lymphocytes in the peripheral blood determined by immunofluorescence and flow cytometry; the results are expressed as mean ± SE.
IRS: Group A vs. Group C and Group B vs. Group C, $p < 0.05$.
CR: Group A vs. Group C and Group B vs. Group C, $p < 0.05$; Group A vs. Group B, $p < 0.05$.

Table 28.4 Long-term vs. short-term clinical remission in recent-onset IDDM: percentage of $CD4^+$, $CD45RA^+$ lymphocytes in the peripheral blood

Patients	Clinical phase of disease	Lymphocyte subsets	
		$CD4^+CD45RA^+$	$CD4^+CD45RA^-$
Long-term remission (Group A)	IRS	22.8 ± 1.9[a]	21.7 ± 1.6
	CR	25.8 ± 1.9	18.1 ± 1.3
Short-term remission (Group B)	IRS	23.2 ± 2.1	21.0 ± 1.9
	CR	24.9 ± 2.1	17.4 ± 1.3
Controls (Group C)	–	25.5 ± 1.9	20.1 ± 1.8

[a]Percentage of total number of lymphocytes in the peripheral blood determined by immunofluorescence and flow cytometry; the results are expressed as mean ± SE.
IRS: Group A vs. Group C and Group B vs. Group C, $p < 0.05$.
CR: Group A vs. Group C and Group B vs. Group C, $p = \text{NS}$; Group A vs. Group B, $p = \text{NS}$.

DISCUSSION

Our results have shown that, although there was no difference in total number of $CD4^+$ cells, a longer duration of CR in recent-onset IDDM patients was associated with increased percentage of $CD4^+CD45R0^+$ T lymphocytes. In contrast, in the CR the percentage of $CD4^+CD45RA^+$ T cells increased compared to the IRS and reached levels similar to those in healthy controls, but it did not differ in relation to the duration of the CR.

The lack of the change in total number of CD4$^+$ and CD8$^+$ T lymphocytes is in agreement with the findings of the majority of the studies of the peripheral blood T-cell phenotypes in recent-onset IDDM patients (2–4).

In this study, we found that an increased percentage of CD4$^+$CD45R0$^+$ T cells was found in all recent-onset IDDM patients compared to the healthy controls, both in IRS and in CR irrespective of its duration, which is consistent with the recent findings of over-representation of the CD45R0 molecule on CD4$^+$ T lymphocytes of diabetic children (9). The presence of excess of the primed CD4$^+$CD45RO$^+$ T cells and the decrease in naive CD4$^+$CD45RA$^+$ T cells in the recent-onset IDDM patients could be a result of an activated immune response to the antigens involved in the pathogenesis of IDDM (6). The increased percentage of CD4$^+$CD45R0$^+$ T lymphocytes which was found in this study is in agreement with the data revealing an expansion of this CD4$^+$ T-cell subset at onset of other different autoimmune diseases, e.g. multiple sclerosis (10) and systemic lupus erythematosus (11).

The predominance of CD4$^+$CD45R0$^+$ over CD4$^+$CD45RA$^+$ in the recent-onset IDDM patients might be an inherited trait associated with the pathogenesis of the disease in these patients, as suggested by the fact that the same type of imbalance between the CD4$^+$ T-cell subsets has been found in the first degree relatives of diabetic children, especially in those at high risk for the development of IDDM expressed as islet cell antibody positivity (9). In this sense, our results imply that the subjects with an inherited increase in the number of memory cells among CD4$^+$ T lymphocytes or the predominance of T helper–inducer lymphocytes would be prone to develop IDDM.

Although the increased levels of CD4$^+$CD45R0$^+$ T lymphocytes has been shown to be a universal characteristic of recent-onset IDDM patients, irrespective of the clinical phase of the disease, in our study we have found that higher levels of CD4$^+$CD45R0$^+$ T cells in the state of CR correlate with shorter duration of remission. This might be a consequence of the higher intensity of the immune response more frequently activated by the beta cell autoantigens (6). Alternatively, our results might reveal a predominance of T helper–inducer lymphocytes which is inherited in the patients predisposed to a shorter duration of CR (7). Thus, our results imply that higher number of CD4$^+$CD45R0$^+$ T cells might represent a suitable marker for a short-term remission, while lower CD4$^+$CD45R0$^+$ T-cell number would characterize a long-term duration of the CR. Finally, the association of short-term duration of remission with a higher percentage of CD4$^+$CD45R0$^+$ T lymphocytes is a complementary finding suggesting that increased presence of the CD4$^+$CD45R0$^+$ subset of CD4$^+$ T cells might play a major role in the activation of the recurrent autoimmune destruction of beta cells underlying the onset of IDDM.

In our study we found that the percentage of CD4$^+$CD45RA$^+$ T lymphocytes has increased in the CR compared to IRS, reaching levels similar to those in healthy controls. These findings might imply that the increases in the number of T suppressor–inducer lymphocytes in the peripheral blood, which were found in the state of CR, represent a mechanism of re-establishing homeostasis in the immune system during CR (3,7). However, the fact that there was no difference in the number of $CD4^+CD45RA^+$ T cells between patients with short-term and long-term remission, whereas they differed significantly in the number of $CD4^+CD45R0^+$ T lymphocytes, suggests that $CD4^+CD45RA^+$ T cells do not influence the duration of the CR in the recent-onset IDDM patients.

CONCLUSION

In recent-onset IDDM, the patients with short-term remission exhibited higher levels of $CD45R0^+$ T cells in the peripheral blood compared to those with long-term remission. The results imply that duration of remission might be regulated by the balance of immunoregulatory $CD4^+$ T cell subsets.

REFERENCES

1. Rossini, A. A., G. L. Greiner, H. P. Friedman and J. P. Mordes. 1993. Immunopathogenesis of diabetes mellitus. *Diabetes Rev.* **1**:43–75.
2. Al-Kassab, A. S. and S. Raziuddin. 1990. Immune activation and T cell subset abnormalities in circulation of patients with recently diagnosed type I diabetes mellitus. *Clin. Exp. Immunol.* **81**:267–71.
3. Faustman, D., G. S. Eisenbarth and J. Breitmeyer. 1990. Analysis of T lymphocyte subsets in all stages of diabetes. *J. Autoimmunity* **3**(Suppl):111–16.
4. Ilonen, J., H. M. Surcel and M. Kaar. 1991. Abnormalities within CD4 and CD8 T lymphocyte subsets in type I (insulin-dependent) diabetes. *Clin. Exp. Immunol.* **85**:278–81.
5. Fowell, D., A. J. McKnight, F. Powrie *et al.* 1991. Subsets of $CD4^+$ T cells and their roles in the induction and prevention of autoimmunity. *Immunol. Rev.* **123**:37–64.
6. Peakman, M., A. G. S. Buggins, K. H. Nicolaides *et al.* 1992. Analysis of lymphocyte subpopulations in cord blood from early gestation fetuses. *Clin. Exp. Immunol.* **90**:345–50.
7. Beverly, P. V. C. 1990. Is T cell memory maintained by crossreactive stimulation? *Immunol. Today* **11**:203–5.
8. Parks, D. R., L. L. Lanier and L. A. Herzenberg. 1985. Flow cytometry and fluorescence activated cell sorting (FACS). In: *Handbook of Experimental Immunology* (D. M. Weir, ed.) C. V. Mosby, St. Louis, pp. 107–17.
9. Peakman, M., T. Warnock, A. Vats *et al.* 1994. Lymphocyte subset abnormalities, autoantibodies and their relationship with HLADR types in children with Type 1 (insulin-dependent) diabetes and their first degree relatives. *Diabetologia* **37**:155–65.

10. Morimoto, C., D. A. Hafler, H. L. Weiner *et al.* 1987. Selective loss of suppressor-inducer T cell subset in progressive multiple sclerosis: analysis with anti-2H4 monoclonal antibody. *N. Engl. J. Med.* **316**:67–73.
11. Morimoto, C., E. Reinherz, J. Distaso *et al.* 1984. Relationship between systemic lupus erythematosus T cell subsets, anti-T cell antibodies and T cell function. *J. Clin. Invest.* **73**:669–70.

29

Increased Levels of TGFβ1 in Cerebrospinal Fluid of Multiple Sclerosis Patients

Jelena Drulović, Marija Mostarica Stojković, Zvonimir Lević, Nebojša Stojsavljević, Vera Pravica, Dragoslav Sokić and Šarlota Mesaroš

Multiple sclerosis (MS) is a chronic inflammatory demyelinating disease of the central nervous system (CNS). Although the aetiology is not known, it is widely accepted that immune system abnormalities are crucial in the development of MS lesions. In recent years, a growing body of data has suggested a central role for a dysregulated cytokine network in MS (1–4). Cytokines mediate a wide range of activities and often have pleiotropic effects. It has been postulated that some cytokines may be deleterious, and may affect the initiation and perpetuation of immune pathology in MS, whereas others may have a protective role inducing a regression of disease.

Transforming growth factor-β (TGFβ) is one of the putative down-regulating cytokines in MS. This cytokine has a beneficial effect in an experimental animal model of MS, experimental allergic encephalomyelitis (EAE) (5,6). Treatment of rats or mice with TGFβ counteracts EAE (5), while in vivo blocking with antibody against TGFβ exacerbates the disease (6). Furthermore, it has been demonstrated that the expression of TGFβ mRNA is increased in peripheral blood (PB) mononuclear cells (MNC) from MS patients with slight disability (7) or stable disease (8). In longitudinal study, TGFβ mRNA expression in PB MNC declined prior to a relapse and returned to baseline values 4–8 weeks after the relapse of MS (9). Consistent with this finding, proteolipid protein (PLP)-stimulated T-cell clones from PB of MS patients failed to secrete TGFβ during acute attacks, whereas the cytokine secretion was restored during remission (10).

Little is known of the pattern of TGFβ production within the CNS in MS. We assayed TGFβ1 in the cerebrospinal fluid (CSF) of patients with MS and investigated whether its presence correlated with clinical disease activity.

Immunoregulation in Health and Disease
ISBN 0–12–459460–3

PATIENTS AND METHODS

We studied CSF samples from 32 patients (23 female and 9 male) with definite MS (11). The mean age was 35 years (range 17–48 years). The duration of the disease varied between 3 months and 19 years (mean 4 years). Disease severity was scored on Kurtzke's Expanded Disability Status Scale (EDSS) (12). The EDSS score varied from 3.5 to 8.0 (mean 4.0). Patients were classified as having either active or inactive MS. The active form of the disease was further subdivided into acute relapse and chronic progressive disease. Thirteen patients were in acute relapse, and 7 patients had chronic progressive MS. Twelve patients with inactive MS had been clinically stable for at least 3 months at the time of CSF analysis. None had received steroids or other immunosuppressive drugs in the previous 3 months.

Control samples were obtained from 11 patients undergoing lumbar puncture during the investigation of other non-inflammatory neurological disorders (NIND), namely: migraine (2), tension headache (2), epilepsy (2), normal pressure hydrocephalus (1), pseudotumour cerebri (1), brain tumour (1), cervical spondylotic myelopathy (1) and lumbar radiculopathy (1).

CSF samples were obtained by non-traumatic lumbar puncture and cells were immediately removed by centrifugation. Samples were stored at −70°C until use.

TGFβ1 measurements in CSF samples were carried out in blind fashion with an ELISA kit (Quantikine, R&D systems, Minneapolis, MN, USA) according to the manufacturer's instructions. The detection limit for TGFβ1 was 5 pg/ml.

For statistical analysis, Fisher's exact test, a two-tailed Mann–Whitney test and the Spearman rank correlation coefficient were used. All values were expressed as mean ± standard error of the mean (SE).

RESULTS

TGFβ1 was detected in 23 of 32 patients (72%) with MS and in 2 of 11 (18%) control patients ($p = 0.004$, Fisher's exact test) (Table 29.1). Control patients with detectable TGFβ1 had diagnoses of cervical spondylotic myelopathy and brain tumour. The incidence of detectable TGFβ1 was similar in active and inactive MS patients (70% and 75% of patients, respectively).

CSF TGFβ1 concentrations in MS patients (836.0 ± 191.8 ng/ml, mean ± SE) were significantly higher than in controls (112.6 ± 35.5 ng/ml) ($p = 0.001$), whereas the concentrations failed to differentiate between patients with active MS and those with inactive disease ($p = 0.72$) (Table 29.1).

There was no correlation between the CSF concentrations of TGFβ1 and disease duration or clinical severity as assessed by EDSS.

Table 29.1 TGF β1 concentrations in CSF of MS patients and controls (ng/ml)

	Proportion of patients with detectable CSF TGF β1	Mean	SE	Min.	Max.
MS					
Active	14/20 (0.70)	862.3*	257.8	0.4	2274.6
Inactive	9/12 (0.75)	786.7**	287.4	0.9	2274.6
Total	23/32 (0.72)	836.0***	191.8	0.4	2274.6
Controls	2/11 (0.18)	112.6	35.5	77.0	148.1

*active MS vs. controls, $p = 0.0007$.
**inactive MS vs. controls, $p = 0.033$.
***total MS vs. controls, $p = 0.001$.

DISCUSSION

Our present report shows that the levels of TGFβ1 in the CSF of patients with MS were significantly increased compared with NIND controls. We detected TGFβ1 in the CSF of 23 (72%) MS patients and 2 (18%) patients with NIND who had diagnoses of brain tumour and cervical spondylotic myelopathy. We have previously shown that there is no difference in TGFβ1 levels between MS patients and controls, but only a few specimens were available for this analysis (13). This is, as far as we know, the only report on TGFβ1 in CSF. However, it has recently been found that CSF from MS patients contain high numbers of TGFβ mRNA-expressing MNC after stimulation with myelin basic protein (MBP) and PLP (14).

We were not able to find any correlation between CSF TGFβ1 levels in MS patients and the clinical parameters of disability, disease duration or clinical disease activity. MS patients with active disease had higher CSF concentrations of TGFβ1 than those with inactive MS, but this difference did not reach the level of statistical significance. This is in agreement with a recently published report on the detailed immunohistochemical analysis of early postmortem CNS tissue from 18 cases of MS, which indicates that the expression of TGFβ1 is relatively uniformly high in acute and chronic MS lesions (3). The level of TGFβ1 expression was higher in acute MS lesions than in chronic active and chronic silent lesions, but the difference was not statistically significant. In all types of MS lesions, TGFβ1 was associated with endothelial cells and the extracellular matrix around blood vessels. Accordingly, it was suggested that TGFβ1 could have a regulatory role at the blood–brain barrier.

TGFβ1 and its homologues TGFβ2 and TGFβ3 are pleiotropic cytokines with predominant immunosuppressive activities (15). It has been shown that TGFβ:

- inhibits the activation and proliferation of MBP-specific T lymphocytes (5,16)
- strongly suppresses MBP- and PLP-induced mRNA expression of certain pro-inflammatory cytokines, in particular interferon-γ (IFNγ) and tumor necrosis factor-α (TNFα) in blood MNC of MS patients (17)
- suppresses astrocyte autoantigen presentation and antagonizes hyper-induction of MHC class II antigen by IFNγ and TFNα (18).

In contrast to these effects, which have been proposed to be beneficial in MS, it seems that TGFβ may also exert proinflammatory activities within the CNS. Thus, for example, Hurwitz *et al.* have demonstrated that TGFβ1 up-regulates a monocyte chemoattractant protein (MCP)-1 expression by astrocytes (19). MCP-1 is a member of the chemokine family which could induce a progression of the CNS inflammatory disease by stimulation and recruitment of monocytes to sites of inflammatory lesions.

Our study supports the notion that the role of TGFβ1 in MS is more complex than initially thought. This should be taken into consideration in a discussion of TGFβ1 as a putative therapeutic agent in MS.

CONCLUSION

Recently conducted studies have implicated the potential role of TGFβ1 in MS. We have examined TGFβ1 levels in the CSF of MS patients and investigated whether their presence correlated with clinical disease activity. The concentrations of TGFβ1 were measured in CSF samples from MS patients and non-inflammatory neurological controls. CSF TGFβ1 concentrations were significantly higher in the MS group than in controls. No significant difference in CSF TGFβ1 levels was found between MS patients with active disease and those with inactive MS. These findings document the in situ involvement of TGFβ1 in the pathogenesis of MS.

REFERENCES

1. Selmaj, K., C. S. Raine, B. Cannella and C. F. Brosnan. 1991. Identification of lymphotoxin and tumor necrosis factor in multiple sclerosis lesions. *J. Clin. Invest.* **87**:949–54.
2. Woodroofe, M. N. and M. L. Cuzner. 1993. Cytokine mRNA expression in inflammatory multiple sclerosis lesions: detection by non-radioactive in situ hybridization. *Cytokine* **5**:583–8.
3. Cannella, B. and C. S. Raine. 1995. The adhesion molecule and cytokine profile of multiple sclerosis lesions. *Ann. Neurol.* **37**:424–35.
4. Windhagen, A., J. Newcombe, F. Dangond *et al.* 1995. Expression of co-stimulatory molecules B7-1 (CD80), B7-2 (CD86), and interleukin-12 cytokine in multiple sclerosis. *J. Exp. Med.* **182**:1985–96.
5. Racke, M. K., S. Dhib-Jalbut, B. Cannella *et al.* 1991. Prevention and treatment of chronic relapsing experimental allergic encephalomyelitis by transforming growth factor-β1. *J. Immunol.* **146**:3012–17.
6. Racke, M. K., B. Cannella, P. Albert *et al.* 1992. Evidence of endogenous regulatory function of transforming growth factor-β1 in experimental allergic encephalomyelitis. *Int. Immunol.* **5**:615–20.
7. Link, J., M. Soderstrom, T. Olsson *et al.* 1994. Increased transforming growth factor-β, interleukin-4, and interferon-γ in multiple sclerosis. *Ann. Neurol.* **36**:379–86.
8. Rieckmann, P., M. Albrecht, B. Kitze *et al.* 1994. Cytokine mRNA levels in mononuclear blood cells from patients with multiple sclerosis. *Neurology* **44**:1523–6.
9. Rieckmann, P., M. Albrecht, B. Kitze *et al.* 1995. Tumor necrosis factor-α messenger RNA expression in patients with relapsing-remitting multiple sclerosis is associated with disease activity. *Ann. Neurol.* **37**:82–8.
10. Correale, J., W. Gilmore, M. McMillan *et al.* 1995. Patterns of cytokine secretion by autoreactive proteolipid protein-specific T cell clones during the course of multiple sclerosis. *J. Immunol.* **154**:2959–68.

11. Poser, C. M., D. W. Paty, L. Scheinberg *et al.* 1983. New diagnostic criteria for multiple sclerosis: guidelines for research protocols. *Ann. Neurol.* **13**:227–31.
12. Kurtzke, J. F. 1983. Rating neurologic impairment in multiple sclerosis: an expanded disability status scale (EDSS). *Neurology* **33**:1444–52.
13. Drulović, J., M. Mostarica-Stojković, N. Stojsavljević *et al.* 1995. Measurement of IL-12, TNF-α and TGF-β in sera and CSF of MS patients. *J. Neuroimmunol.* (suppl. 1):33.
14. Link, J., S. Fredrikson, M. Soderstrom *et al.* 1994. Organ-specific autoantigens induce transforming growth factor-β mRNA expression in mononuclear cells in multiple sclerosis and myasthenia gravis. *Ann. Neurol.* **35**:197–203.
15. Fontana, A., D. B. Constam, K. Frei *et al.* 1992. Modulation of immune response by transforming growth factor β. *Int. Arch. Allergy Immunol.* **99**:1–7.
16. Schluesener, H. J. and O. Lider. 1989. Transforming growth factor β1 and β2: Cytokines with identical immunosuppressive effects and a potential role in the regulation of autoimmune T-cell function. *J. Neuroimmunol.* **24**:249–58.
17. Link, J., B. He, V. Navikas *et al.* 1995. Transforming growth factor-β1 suppresses autoantigen-induced expression of pro-inflammatory cytokines but not of interleukin-10 in multiple sclerosis and myasthenia gravis. *J. Neuroimmunol.* **58**:21–35.
18. Schluesener, H. J. 1990. Transforming growth factors type β1 and β2 suppress rat astrocyte autoantigen presentation and antagonize hyperinduction of class II major histocompatibility complex antigen expression by interferon-γ and tumor necrosis factor-α. *J. Neuroimmunol.* **27**:41–7.
19. Hurwitz, A. A., W. D. Lyman and J. W. Berman. 1995. Tumor necrosis factor α and transforming growth factor β upregulate astrocyte expression of monocyte chemoattractant protein-1. *J. Neuroimmunol.* **57**:193–8.

30

Specificity and Cross-reactivity of the 01 IgM Mouse Monoclonal Antibody

Slobodan Apostolski, Terence McAlarney and Norman Latov

01 is a monoclonal antibody obtained from a fusion of mouse myeloma P3-NS1/1-Ag4-1 with spleen cells from BALB/c mice immunized with white matter from bovine corpus callosum (1). It belongs to the IgM immunoglobulin subclass and recognizes antigens on the surface of developing oligodendrocytes. It has been shown that 01 antibody has multiple specificities, reacting with galactocerebroside (GalC), monogalactosyl-diglyceride, lactosylceramide, and psychosine (2). In our previous work we found that 01 antibody inhibits HIV-1 gp120 envelope glycoprotein binding to human neuroblastoma cells (NB) and rat dorsal root ganglion (DRG) neurons (3). Since antibodies directed against carbohydrate determinants are known to cross-react with other glycolipids and glycoproteins that express similar oligosaccharides (4), we investigated the binding of 01 antibody to a panel of neuronal glycolipids, and to glycoproteins extracted from human NB cells, rat DRG and oligodendroglial (ODG) cells, as well as to human NB, rat DRG and ODG cells in culture in order to examine their specificities and cross-reactivities.

MATERIALS AND METHODS

Detection of 01 antibody binding by enzyme-linked immunosorbent assay (ELISA)

The mouse hybridoma cells producing the monoclonal 01 antibody were grown in culture, and the supernatants containing the antibodies used directly for the experiments. The lipids (Sigma Immunochemicals) included sulfatide (GalS), galactocerebroside (GalC), GM1-ganglioside (GM1), ceramides type

Immunoregulation in Health and Disease
ISBN 0-12-459460-3

IV, GM2-ganglioside, asialo-GM1 ganglioside (AGM1), psychosine, cholesterol, cholesterol-3-sulfate, monogalactosyl digliceride (MG), lysosulfatide, and GD1b-ganglioside (GD1b). Anti-glycolipid antibodies were measured by ELISA according to a method described by Sadiq *et al.* (5). Absorbance was measured at 450 nm with a BioRad ELISA reader and the absorbance in BSA-coated control wells was subtracted from that in antigen-coated wells. In other controls, the 01 antibody was omitted from the reaction in the microwells. All determinations were done in triplicate and results were the average of triplicate determinations. The adherence of GalS and GM1 to the wells was confirmed by ELISA using antibodies specific to each of the glycolipid antigens.

Antibody binding to neuronal cells by immunofluorescence

The human NB cell line LAN-5 (6) was grown in Dulbecco's modified Eagle's medium containing 15% fetal bovine serum, 1% penicillin-streptomycin, 2 mM glutamine, and 1 mM sodium pyruvate. DRG neurons were isolated from day-15 embryonic rats (Sprague-Dawley), prior to appearance of Schwann cells (3). For immunofluorescence microscopy, the LAN-5 cells and DRG neurons were grown on poly-D-lysine and laminin-treated coverslips in six-well plates. ODG cells were isolated from neonatal rat pup cerebral cortices, and the cell suspension was plated on to coverslips treated with poly-D-lysine hydrobromide in 16 nm 24-well plates and maintained in a modified nitrogen chemically defined medium (7). Cells grown on coverslips were washed twice in PBS for 10 min and then immunostained unfixed. They were first exposed to 50% normal goat serum (NGS) for 10 min, incubated with 01 antibody at a dilution of 1 : 2 in medium at 4°C for 2 h, washed twice in PBS containing 1% NGS for 10 min, and then incubated with FITC- or Texas red-conjugated anti-mouse IgM antibodies (Accurate Chemical Sci.) for 30 min. After final washing in 1% NGS in PBS for 10 min, the cells were fixed in 4% paraformaldehyde, mounted with gel medium containing 2% DABCO (Sigma), and viewed with a Zeiss fluorescence microscope. The human monoclonal IgM from the patient with monoclonal gammopathy of undetermined significance served as a control antibody. In addition, cells fixed in 4% paraformaldehyde were treated with 0.05% trypsin, or with chloroform : methanol (C:M) (1:1) for 20 min at room temperature, prior to immunostaining with 01 antibody.

Antibody binding to SDS-protein extracts of the neuronal cells by Western blot

To determine whether 01 antibody also binds to proteins, it was tested for binding to SDS–protein extracts of the LAN-5 human NB cell line, rat DRG and rat ODG cells. Cells were delipidated with C:M (1:1, v:v) and solubilized for 10 min at 65°C in 2% SDS containing enzyme inhibitor cocktail (0.7/μM pepstatin, 1.1 μM leupeptin, 50 μg/ml trypsin inhibitor, 2 mM EDTA, 0.23 mM PMSF and 3 mM benzamidine). The solubilized proteins were then separated on a 7% SDS–PAGE gel and transferred to nitrocellulose sheets. The sheets were then saturated in 8% BSA in 0.9% NACl, 10 mM Trizma base, pH 7.4 for 1 h at room temperature, and washed 5 times with washing solution (PBS with 1% BSA, 0.05% Tween-20, 10 mM Trizma base, pH 7.4). They were then incubated with the 01 antibody at a dilution of 1:10 in washing solution or with control solution overnight at 4°C, the sheet washed 5 times, and the bound 01 antibody detected using affinity-purified peroxidase-conjugated goat antibodies to mouse IgM at a concentration of 1:1000 in washing solution for 2 h at 4°C. Reaction products were developed with 0.1% 3,3′-diaminobenzidine tetrahydrochloride, 0.1% imidazole, 0.01% hydrogen peroxide (DAB). The 01 antibody was omitted from control nitrocellulose blots. To confirm that 01 antibody was binding to glycoproteins rather than to glycolipids, the protein extract was subjected to proteolytic digestion with pronase prior to separation by SDS–PAGE. To confirm that 01 antibody reacted with an oligosaccharide determinant of the reactive glycoproteins, the cell proteins on nitrocellulose blots were deglycosylated by periodate oxidation and examined for binding to the 01 antibody.

RESULTS

In the ELISA system, the 01 IgM monoclonal antibody bound to GalC, GM1, AGM1, GD1b, monogalactosyl diglceride, and psychosine (Fig. 30.1). Immunofluorescence showed that the 01 antibody bound not only to rat ODG cells, but also to the surface of unfixed human NB and rat DRG cells (Fig. 30.2). As control, the NB, DRG, and ODG cells were not immunostained by the human monoclonal IgM from the patient with monoclonal gammopathy of undetermined significance (not shown). The pretreatment of the neuronal cells with trypsin slightly reduced the intensity of the 01 binding from +3 to +2, mostly as a consequence of reduction of cytoplasmic but not membrane staining. The pretreatment with C:M, which removes glycolipids, did not eliminate the 01 binding, indicating an existence of additional protein antigens recognized by 01 antibody.

In Western blot studies of DRG, NB, and ODG SDS–protein extracts, the 01 antibody bound to several glycoprotein bands in the DRG and NB cells (46 kDa, 120 kDa, 200 kDa), and to a single protein band (200 kDa) in the ODG cells (Fig. 30.3), indicating that the 01 antibody also bound to proteins. Pretreatment of the protein extracts with pronase or exposure of the proteins on nitrocellulose strips to 5 mM periodate abolished the 01 antibody binding.

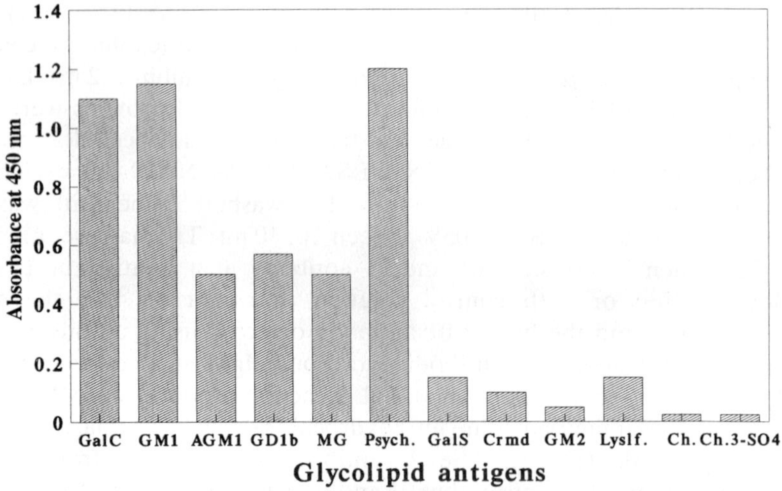

Fig. 30.1 Binding of mouse monoclonal IgM 01 antibody by ELISA. The lipids included galactocerebroside (GalC), GM1-ganglioside (GM1), Asialo-GM1 ganglioside (AGM1), GD1b-ganglioside (GD1b), monogalactosyl diglyceride (MG), psychosine (psych.), sulfatide (GalS), ceramides type IV (Crmd), GM2-ganglioside (GM2), lysosulfatide (Lyslf), cholesterol (Ch.), and cholesterol-3-sulfate (Ch.3-SO4). The 01 antibody binds to GalC, GM1, psychosine, GD1b, MG, and AGM1.

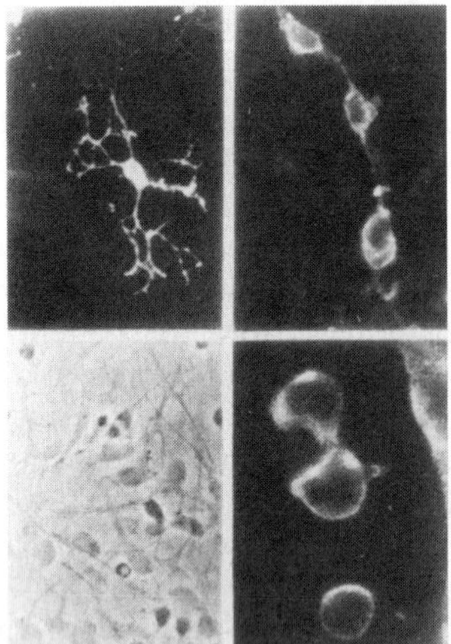

Fig. 30.2 The mouse monoclonal IgM 01 antibody binds to rat oligodendroglia (ODG), rat dorsal root ganglion (DRG), and human neuroblastoma (NB) cells. The 01 antibody binds to rat ODG. The same microscopic field viewed with rhodamine optics (top left) or with phase-contrast optics (bottom left) (×500). The 01 antibody binds to the surface of unfixed rat DRG (top right), and human NB cells (bottom right) (×640).

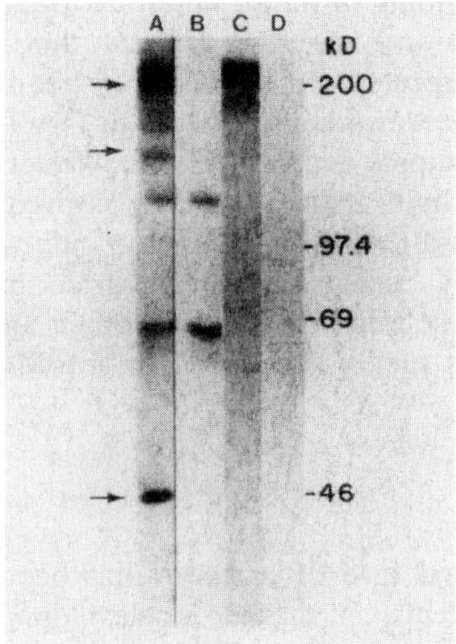

Fig. 30.3 Binding of mouse monoclonal IgM 01 antibody to protein extracts of rat dorsal root ganglion (DRG) neuron and oligodendrocytes (ODG) by Western blot. A, The 01 recognizes three protein bands in the protein extracts of DRG neurons. B, As control, the biotinylated anti-mouse IgM antibody binds to two protein bands, but not to the other 01 reactive proteins. C, The 01 antibody binds to a single protein band in ODG. D, As control for C, biotinylated antibody to mouse IgM shows no binding.

DISCUSSION

The mouse monoclonal IgM 01 antibody has been used as specific antigenic marker for oligodendroglia in the CNS and for Schwann cells in peripheral nerve (1, 8–10). It has been designated as an anti-GalC antibody and as a specific marker for galactocerebroside-positive developing neuronal cells. Bansal *et al.* (2) showed the specificity of the 01 antibody not only for GalC but also for the monogalactosyl-diglyceride and psychosine, and for an unidentified species in rat brain extracts. The cross-reactivity of the anti-GalC antibodies with gangliosides and galactosyl diglycerides has been previously reported, and there was only an assumption that they might react with glycoproteins carrying the same hapten group (11). However, as shown in these studies, the 01 anti-GalC antibody definitely reacts with several other glycolipids and glycoproteins in the nervous system in addition to GalC. In ELISA studies, the cross-reactivity appears to be restricted as the antibody recognizes glycolipids with terminal β_1-linked galactosyl group, particularly GM1, AGM1, monogalactosyl diglyceride, and psychosine. This interaction is stereospecific since other glycolipids with the same terminal galactosyl linkage are not recognized by the 01 antibody. In immunofluorescence, in addition to specific binding of the 01 antibody to ODG cells, it binds to the surface of human NB and rat DRG cells, so that its use as a cell-specific marker should be interpreted with caution. Neither pretreatment with trypsin nor with C:M prevented binding of the 01 to DRG cells, indicating that 01 reacts with both glycolipids and proteins. In Western blot, the results show that the antibody reactivity is due to binding to glycoprotein oligosaccharides which might also contain terminal β_1-linked galactosyl groups. It is likely that the 01 antibody recognizes carbohydrate determinants shared by glycoproteins and glycolipids similarly to other antibodies that recognize carbohydrate epitopes such as anti-GM1 or anti-MAG antibodies (4,12).

CONCLUSION

The mouse monoclonal IgM 01 antibody has been used as an anti-GalC antibody and as a specific cell marker for developing oligodendrocytes. We examined the binding of the 01 antibody to a panel of purified glycolipids by ELISA, and to neuronal cells by immunofluorescence and by western blot. The 01 antibody bound strongly to GalC, GM1 ganglioside, monogalactosyl diglyceride, asialo-GM1, GD1b and psychosine. By immunofluorescence, in addition to binding to ODG cells, the 01 antibody bound to the surface of non-fixed human NB and rat DRG cells. In Western blot, the 01 bound to several glycoprotein bands in human NB and rat DRG cells, and to a single high molecular weight in rat ODG cells. These results demonstrate that the use of 01 as an 'anti-GalC' must be interpreted with caution, because it cross-reacts with oligosaccharide determinants of other glycolipids and glycoproteins in the nervous system.

REFERENCES

1. Sommer, I. and M. Schachner. 1981. Monoclonal antibodies (01 to 04) to oligodendrocyte cell surfaces: An immunocytological study in the central nervous system. *Dev. Biol.* **83**:311–27.
2. Bansal, R., A. E. Warrington, A. L. Gard *et al.* 1989. Multiple and novel specificities of monoclonal antibodies 01, 04, and R-mAb used in the analysis of oligodendrocyte development. *J. Neurosci. Res.* **24**:548–57.
3. Apostolski, S., T. McAlarney, A. Quattrini *et al.* 1993. The gp120 glycoprotein of human immunodeficiency virus type 1 binds to sensory ganglion neurons. *Ann. Neurol.* **34**:855–63.
4. Latov, N. 1990. Antibodies to glucoconjugates in neurologic disease. *Clin. Aspects Autoimmun.* **4**:18–29.
5. Sadiq, S. A., F. P. Thomas, K. Kilidireas *et al.* 1990. The spectrum of neurologic disease associated with anti-GM1 antibodies. *Neurology* **40**:1067–72.
6. Srinivasan, J., A. P. Hays, F. P. Thomas *et al.* 1990. Autoantigens in human neuroblastoma cells. *J. Neurochem.* **26**:43–50.

7. Levison, S. W. and K. D. McCarthy. 1991. Astroglia in culture. In: *Culturing Nerve Cells* (G. Banker and K. Groslin, eds.) MIT Press, Cambridge, MA, pp. 309–36.
8. Raff, M. C., R. Mirsky, K. L. Fields *et al.* 1978. Galactocerebroside: A specific cell surface antigenic marker for oligodendrocytes in culture. *Nature* **274**:813–16.
9. Mirsky, R., J. Winter, E. R. Abney *et al.* 1980. Myelin-specific proteins and galactolipids in rat Schwann cells and oligodendrocytes in culture. *J. Cell Biol.* **84**:483–94.
10. Schachner, M. 1982. Cell type-specific surface antigens in the mammalian nervous system. *J. Neurochem.* **39**:1–8.
11. Latovitzki, N. and D. H. Silberberg. 1975. Ceramide glycosyltransferases in cultured rat cerebellum: Changes with age, with demyelination, and with inhibition of myelination by 5-bromo-2′-deoxyuridine or experimental allergic encephalomyelitis serum. *J. Neurochem.* **24**:1017–22.
12. Latov, N., A. P. Hays and W. H. Sherman. 1988. Peripheral neuropathy and anti-MAG antibodies. *CRC Crit. Rev. Neurobiol.* **3**:301–32.

31

Humoral Immune Response to Oxidized Low-density Lipoprotein in Patients with Coronary Artery Disease

Stanimir Kyurkchiev, Ivan Kehayov, Assen Gudev and Chudomir Nachev

Atherosclerosis is generally accepted to be a multifactorial disease which leads to severe complications in the heart, brain or peripheral vessels. Immunoinflammatory phenomena which are triggered either by the oxidation of low-density lipoprotein (1) or by response to injury (2) are thought to be the basic mechanisms in the pathogenesis of atherosclerosis.

Oxidative modification of low-density lipoprotein (LDL) which has been shown to take place in vivo (3) leads to the generation of novel epitopes on the molecule (4). In that way the oxidized LDL (oxi-LDL) can be recognized as a 'foreign' antigen and can induce a variety of immune reactions in patients with atherosclerosis. Salonen *et al.* (5) reported that autoantibodies against oxi-LDL could be detected in patients with carotid atherosclerosis and their titres could be an independent predictor of the progression of the disease. On the other hand, it has been demonstrated that cell-mediated immunity is involved in the pathogenesis of atherosclerosis since T cells isolated from atherosclerostic plaques recognize oxi-LDL in a specific manner (6).

In this paper data are presented that autoantibodies against oxi-LDL can be detected in a cohort of patients with coronary artery disease (CAD) using a sensitive immunoenzyme assay. It should be mentioned that LDL oxidized in vitro by treatment with peroxidase was used as a specific antigen in the immunoenzyme assay. Peripheral blood leukocytes from a CAD patient with a high titre of anti-oxi-LDL autoantibodies were used for construction of a heterohybridoma secreting human monoclonal antibodies against oxi-LDL.

Immunoregulation in Health and Disease
ISBN 0-12-459460-3

MATERIALS AND METHODS

Selection of patients

Blood serum samples were collected by vein puncture of 51 patients with angiographically proven CAD and 51 age-matched controls.

Isolation and oxidation in vitro of LDL

Native low-density lipoprotein (nLDL) was isolated by potassium bromide gradient (density 1.020–1.050 g/cm^3) ultracentrifugation at 25 000 rev/min from fresh human blood plasma collected in the presence of 1 mg/ml EDTA in order to prevent the spontaneous oxidation of LDL. After extensive dialysis against phosphate-buffered saline (PBS), pH 7.4 containing 1 mg/ml EDTA, nLDL was aliquoted and stored at 4°C for no longer than 6 weeks. Protein content of the isolated LDL was determined by the method of Lowry *et al.* (7).

Samples of nLDL were oxidized by treatment with peroxidase as followed: 25 IU peroxidase (type XII, Sigma, USA) and 6 μl hydrogen peroxide were added to 500 μg nLDL in 4.4 ml PBS and the mixture was incubated at 37°C for 16–18 h. The mixture was passed through a Sephadex G-25 column (Pharmacia LKB Biotech., Sweden) to separate the free peroxidase, and the purified oxi-LDL was collected.

Production of heterohybridomas

Peripheral blood leucocytes (PBL) were isolated from patients with CAD by gradient centrifugation on Ficoll-Paque. The cells were incubated in vitro in the presence of oxi-LDL and polyclonal activators such as pokeweed mitogen (PWM, Sigma, USA) for 5 days and fused with mouse myeloma cells. Supernatants from wells with growing hybridomas were screened for the presence of human IgG by a sandwich ELISA. Clones secreting human IgG were cloned by the method of limiting dilutions and stored in liquid nitrogen. The specificity of each monoclonal antibody was determined by testing it against a number of purified human proteins and saline extracts from human organs or samples from atheromas collected after death.

Immunoenzyme assay (ELISA)

Polyvinylchloride microtitre 96-well plates were coated with 50 ng/ml nLDL or oxi-LDL by incubation overnight at 4°C and washed with PBS containing Tween 20 (T-PBS). Unoccupied binding sites were blocked with an excess of protein (2% bovine serum albumin, BSA) for 1 h at room temperature (RT) and sera (diluted 1/100) from CAD patients or controls were applied to each well and incubated for 2 h at RT. After extensive washing with T-PBS, anti-human IgG serum conjugated with peroxidase (Sigma, USA) was added and the mixture incubated for 1 h at RT. Subsequently the enzyme reaction was developed with 0.4 mg/ml *ortho*-phenylendiamine and 0.05% hydrogen peroxide for 5 min in the dark. The colour reaction was stopped by adding 10% sulfuric acid and the OD values at 492 nm were read using a microELISA reader (Dynatech, Switzerland). In some experiments a variant of the immunoenzyme assay was used and that was absorption ELISA. The only difference in the procedure was that patients' sera were preabsorbed with oxi-LDL or nLDL.

A sandwich ELISA was used to detect IgG secretion from growing hybrids cultured in vitro as previously described (8).

RESULTS

LDL was purified from patient's blood plasma by density gradient centrifugation ($d = 1.020$) and oxidized by treatment with peroxidase. Both nLDL and oxi-LDL were used for development of an immunoassay (ELISA) for detection of autoantibodies against oxidized LDL in patients with coronary artery disease. To demonstrate the specific character of this immunoassay, serial dilutions of positively reacting human serum were tested against a fixed amount of oxi-LDL coated on PVC wells. Under such experimental conditions the dose-dependent curve clearly showed the specific binding of antibodies to the antigen (Fig. 31.1). This kind of dose-dependent curve was obtained when individual sera from CAD patients were tested repeatedly.

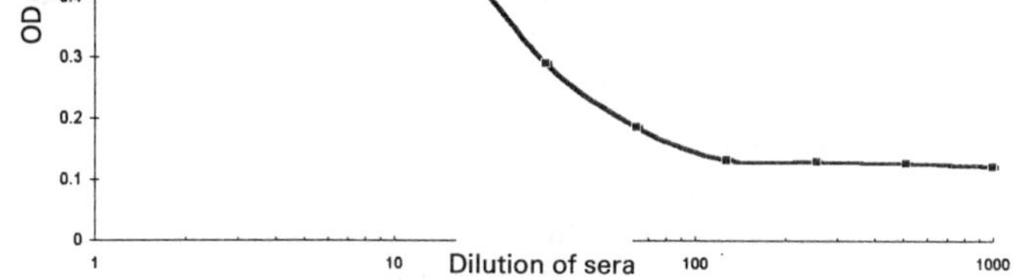

Fig. 31.1 Dose-dependent curve outlined by testing serial dilutions of an anti-oxi-LDL positive serum against fixed amount of oxi-LDL (5 μg/ml) coated on PVC wells.

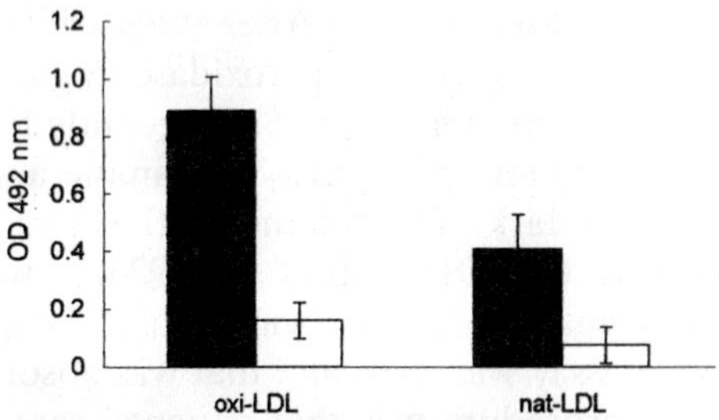

Fig. 31.2 Reactions of sera from: (a) patients with coronary artery disease (CAD) and (b) healthy donors against oxi-LDL and nLDL coated wells by ELISA.

Table 31.1 Effectiveness of fusion experiments to produce hybridomas secreting human immunoglobulins

Patients	Disease	Hybs IgG+
NMD	IDDM	4
IvCo	CAD	0
JoSim	Polyend	4
MiSto	IDDM	2
NiSim	Polyend	0
IvNi	CAD	4
VaMi	CAD	2
Vel	CAD	0

IDDM, insulin dependent diabetes mellitus; Polyend, poly-endocrynological syndrome; CAD, coronary artery disease.

Contrary to that, sera from age-matched control donors gave low-background OD values which were not changed with serial dilution of the serum. At dilutions of 1/100 positive reactions were recorded with sera from CAD patients. The mean OD 492 nm values in these patients were found to be 0.886 ± 0.124 with oxi-LDL and 0.407 ± 0.076 when tested against native LDL, while in the control groups mean OD values in ELISA were 0.159 and 0.075 ± 0.064 respectively (Fig. 31.2).

PBL from eight patients with CAD or insulin-dependent diabetes mellitus (IDDM) were used in independent fusion experiments to produce heterohybridomas secreting monoclonal antibodies against oxi-LDL. In these experiments a total of 16 hybridomas secreting human IgG were selected, cloned by limiting dilutions and stored in liquid nitrogen (Table 31.1). Further assessment of the specificity of each monoclonal antibody demonstrated that the heterohybridoma designated as IvNi 2D2 secreted an IgG antibody which

Table 31.2. Specificity of human monoclonal antibodies secreted by hybridomas constructed with lymphocytes from CAD patients

Hybridomas	IgG	oxiLDL	nLDL	MDA-lys[a]	SA[b]
IvNI 1C10[c]	(+)	(−)	(−)	(−)	(−)
IvNi 2D2	(+)	(+) (?)	(+)	(−)	(−)
IvNi 2G5	(+)	(−)	NT	NT	(−)
IvNi 2G7	(+)	(−)	NT	NT	(−)
MiSto 2B3	(+)	(−)	NT	NT	(−)
MiSto 1H11	(+)	(−)	NT	NT	(−)
VaMi 1H6	(+)	(−)	NT	NT	(−)
VaMi 2G6	(+)	(−)	NT	NT	(−)

[a]Malondialdehyde lysine.
[b]Human serum albumin.
[c]Code number.
NT, not tested.

reacted with oxi-LDL in ELISA. Somewhat controversial results were obtained when IvNi 2D2 was tested against samples of LDL individually isolated and oxidized in vitro. In some cases the antibody reacted positively with both oxi-LDL and nLDL isolated from one patient, whereas it reacted only with oxi-LDL but not with the nLDL from other patients. No reactions against a number of other proteins could be detected (Table 31.2). The specific reaction of IvNi 2D2 was confirmed by testing serial dilutions of the antibody against a constant amount of the oxi-LDL and under those experimental conditions a dose-dependent curve was obtained. When Mab IvNi 2D2 was tested against saline extracts from human organs it was found that the antibody did not react with the water-soluble proteins of these organs.

DISCUSSION

High titres of autoantibodies of IgG specific to LDL oxidized in vitro are detected in sera from patients with CAD, which substantiates the data reported by Salonen *et al.* (5). However, it is not clear whether changes in the titres of the anti-oxi-LDL autoantibodies can be reliable predictors of atherosclerosis progression. In our experiments LDL was oxidized with peroxidase treatment which was much closer to the mode of LDL oxidation in vivo than treatment with copper. It can be speculated that the in vitro treatment of LDL with peroxidase causes the expression of neoepitopes which are recognized as 'foreign' and consequently can induce the secretion of autoantibodies. The biological role of the anti-oxi-LDL autoantibodies is rather controversial. It can be speculated that such autoantibodies are involved in the pathogenesis of vascular damage or that they might have some protective effect. A major restriction for detailed studies of the biological role of anti-oxi-LDL antibodies is the rather heterogeneous populations of IgG molecules which can be isolated from human serum. A possible approach to overcome such restrictions is the production of human hybridomas secreting homogeneous IgG reacting against oxi-LDL. In these studies a human monoclonal antibody reacting in a specific manner with oxi-LDL has been produced after fusion of lymphocytes from a CAD patient with mouse myeloma cells. This antibody may be used as a specific probe for studies on the biological role of autoantibodies in atherosclerosis.

CONCLUSION

Recently, substantial evidence has been collected that the humoral immune response is involved in the pathogenesis of atherosclerosis. LDL modified by oxidation is rendered immunogenic and autoantibodies are generated against the neoepitopes. The real significance of these antibodies is not yet fully understood, owing to the lack of well-defined specific anti-oxi-LDL human antibodies. Construction of human hybridomas secreting monoclonal antibodies against oxi-LDL, is quite a promising approach to studying the pathogenetic role of the humoral immune response in atherosclerosis.

REFERENCES

1. Witztum, J. L. 1994. The oxidation hypothesis of atherosclerosis. *Lancet* **344**:793–5.
2. Ross, R. 1993. The pathogenesis of atherosclerosis: a perspective for the 1990s. *Nature* **362**:801–9.
3. Palinski, W., M. E. Rosenfeld, S. Yla-Herttuala *et al.* 1989. Low-density lipoprotein undergoes oxidative modification in vivo. *Proc. Natl. Acad. Sci. USA* **86**:1372–6.
4. Palinski, W., S. Yla-Herttuala, M. E. Rosenfeld *et al.* 1990. Antisera and monoclonal antibodies specific for epitopes generated during oxidative modification of low-density lipoprotein. *Arteriosclerosis* **10**:325–35.
5. Salonen, J. T., S. Yla-Herttula, R. Yamamato *et al.* 1992. Autoantibody against oxidized LDL and progression of carotid atherosclerosis. *Lancet* **339**:883–7.
6. Stemme, S., B. Faber, J. Holm *et al.* 1995. T lymphocytes from human atherosclerotic plaques recognize oxidized low density lipoprotein. *Proc. Natl. Acad. Sci. USA* **92**:3893–7.
7. Lowry, O. H., N. J. Rosenbrough, A. L. Farr and R. J. Randall. 1951. Protein measurement with the Folin phenol reagent. *J. Biol. Chem.* **193**:165–75.
8. Kyurkchiev, S., M. Shigeta, K. Koyama and S. Isojima. 1986. A human-mouse hybridoma producing monoclonal antibody against human sperm-coating antigen. *Immunology* **57**:489–92.

32

Biopsy-proven Dilated Heart Muscle Disease Treated with Immunomodulators: 2-year Follow-up

Milutin Mirić, Jovan D. Vasiljević, Srđjan Brkić, Milovan Bojić, Zoran Popović, Mirjana Vukičević and Aleksandar Dujić

Enteroviruses and other viruses have recently been documented in cardiac tissues of patients with idiopathic myocarditis (MC) and idiopathic dilated cardiomyopathy (IDC) (1–3). It is possible that cardiotropic viruses not only cause a symptomatic or asymptomatic initial infection but also persist in the myocardium of some patients (4–6). A deficiency of host defences might contribute to the development of persistent infections. Presuming the viruses to be the causative agent in idiopathic MC and some patients with IDC, therapeutic use of interferon-alpha (IFNα) or its inducers seems to be appropriate. This rationale was the basis for the clinical trial we conducted, in which IFNα or thymic hormones were administered to patients with dilated heart muscle disease. We chose IFNα because it is highly diffusible and easily reaches distant organs after subcutaneous injection, and thymic hormones because they induce a rise of the endogenous IFN level and stimulate NK and T cell activities (7).

METHODS

Thirty-eight patients with biopsy-proven diagnosis of idiopathic MC or idiopathic dilated cardiomyopathy and left ventricular ejection fraction (LVEF) at angiography below 45%, formed the study group. Initial evaluation included clinical symptoms, immunological tests, chest

Immunoregulation in Health and Disease
ISBN 0–12–459460–3

radiographs, electrocardiogram, two-dimensional echocardiographic examination, right- and left-heart haemodynamic studies and right-ventricular endomyocardial biopsy. Three or four myocardial tissue samples were taken and studied by light microscopy to establish the histological diagnosis, according to Dallas's criteria (8).

All patients were thoroughly evaluated for their immunological status. Blood was taken for measurement of virus neutralizing antibody titres, humoral and cellular studies. Humoral studies included:

- a search for circulating antibodies against cardiac muscle, skeletal muscle, smooth muscle and parietal cells as well as those against components of the nuclei and the mitochondria (9)
- quantitation of the sera for IgM, IgG, IgA, IgD and IgE (10)
- a detection of circulating immune complexes (11).

Among cellular studies, phenotyping of peripheral blood mononuclear cells and NK cell assay (^{51}Cr release assay) (12) were performed to define the patient's lymphocyte subpopulations and non-specific cell-killing ability. For phenotyping of peripheral blood mononuclear cells we used monoclonal antibodies (OKT3, OKT4, OKT8 and Leu-7) (13). Total ($CD3^+$) T lymphocytes were expressed as a percentage of the total lymphocytes, and $CD4^+$ and $CD8^+$ T lymphocytes as a percentage of total T cells. Immunological studies were repeated weekly and monthly during the first 6-month follow-up.

The study design was a prospective, randomized, open-label comparison of conventional therapy versus conventional therapy plus immunomodulation with IFNα or thymic hormones. After approval by the Institution Review Board and after consent forms were signed, the patients were randomly assigned to three treatment limbs:

- group 1, 12 patients, received conventional therapy for congestive heart failure
- group 2, 13 patients, received conventional therapy as well as IFNα therapy
- group 3, 13 patients, received conventional therapy as well as thymic hormone therapy.

Treatment lasted for 3 months. During the next 3 months all patients received conventional therapy alone.

Purified leucocytic IFNα (Torlak, Beograd) was given at 3 million U/m^2 of body surface area subcutaneously 3 times a week.

Thymus-TFX Thymomodulin (Thymoorgan GmbH, Pharmazie, Vienenburg) was administered at 10 mg subcutaneously three times a week. Thymus-TFX Thymomodulin is a biologically active extract of the thymus gland of calves consisting of a polypeptide family of 4–6 kDa.

At 6-month, 1-year and 2-year follow-up we performed clinical evaluation, echocardiographic studies, chest radiographs and Holter monitoring. At 1 year, repeated right-ventricular endomyocardial biopsy was done if the initial diagnosis was MC. At 2 years radionuclide ventriculography at rest and during exercise was performed.

Peripheral blood platelet counts, serum transaminases and bilirubin were repeatedly monitored during the study.

Measurements were recorded as mean ± SEM values. Statistical analysis was performed using analysis of variance for repeated measures (Newman–Keuls multiple comparisons), and analysis of variance modified *t*-test (Bonferroni) as appropriate. Results were considered significant if p was less than 0.05.

RESULTS

Thirty-eight patients were included in the study, 15 females and 23 males. Four patients had histological diagnosis of active and 11 patients of borderline MC. Their average age at presentation was 29.3 years. Twenty-three patients had a histological diagnosis of IDC and average age at presentation of 31.7 years.

According to the criteria established by the New York Heart Association, 2 patients were in functional clinical class II, 26 patients were in class III and 10 in class IV.

There was no significant baseline medical difference among the three treatment groups. Left ventricular function assessed by angiography at the beginning of the study was similar (LVEF was 22.7 ± 1.2% in patients treated with IFNα, 22 ± 1.4% in patients treated with thymomodulin and 23.9 ± 1.1% in conventionally treated patients).

In 33 patients the relative number of $CD3^+$ and $CD4^+$ cells was low at presentation (56.7 ± 2.4%, and 38.7 ± 1.3% respectively). NK cells were absent or significantly decreased in all patients, while NK cell activity was low in 35 patients.

The relative number of $CD4^+$ cells increased significantly only in IFNα-treated patients after 4 weeks of treatment and reached 45.2 ± 1% at 6-month follow-up ($p < 0.0001$). IFNα-treated patients showed a reduction in the frequency of $CD8^+$ cells after 2 weeks of therapy (from 29.9 ± 0.9% to 21.7 ± 1.2%), while frequency of $CD8^+$ cells remained constant in other patient groups ($p < 0.0001$). Statistically significant increase in the $CD4^+/CD8^+$ ratio was found in the IFNα group after the second week of treatment ($p < 0.0001$).

The relative number of NK cells increased significantly after 2 weeks of treatment in the IFNα group and returned to baseline level after 1 month (Fig. 32.1). Instead of a sharp, short-lasting increase in NK cell number, progressive, long-lasting increase was found in the Thymomodulin group.

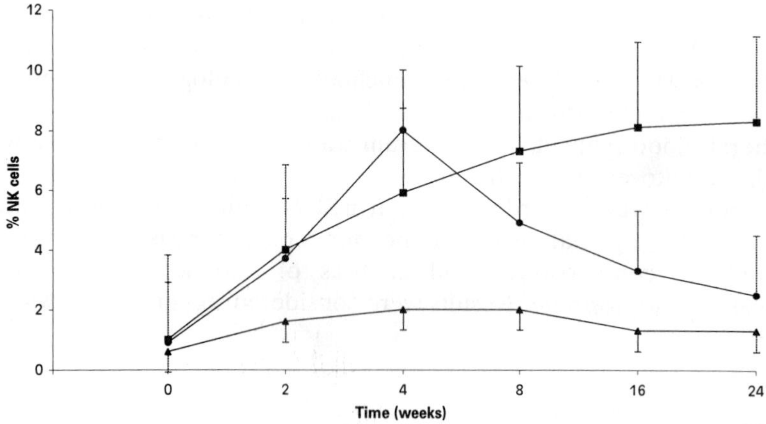

Fig. 32.1 NK cells in 38 patients with dilated heart muscle disease during therapy. IFN = IFNα (circles), TH = thymomodulin (squares), Conv. = conventional therapy alone (triangles). $p < 0.0001$ (ANOVA for repeated measures, Newman–Keuls multiple comparisons, error bars = SEM).

The relative number of NK cells remained constantly low in conventionally treated patients. A significant increase in NK cell activity was observed in IFNα and Thymomodulin-treated patients starting at 2 weeks and lasting for months (from $30.6 \pm 1.4\%$ to $48.5 \pm 1.9\%$ in the IFNα group, and from $28.6 \pm 1.2\%$ to $44.7 \pm 1.6\%$ in the Thymomodulin group). We did not find a change in NK cell activity in conventionally treated patients ($p < 0.0001$). Increase in relative number of NK cells and NK cell activity was followed by a significant decrease in neutralizing antibody viral titres in patients treated with immunomodulators. In patients treated conventionally, viral titres did not change significantly during 6-month follow-up, correlating well with the unchanged activity of NK cells.

In 10 IFNα-treated and 11 Thymomodulin-treated patients, resting LVEF assessed by echocardiography improved at 6 months and showed further improvement at 2-year follow-up (Fig. 32.2). Resting LVEF improved in eight conventionally treated patients. This improvement was significantly lower than in patients treated with immunomodulators ($p < 0.05$).

Repeated biopsies were done at 1 year. Five patients treated with IFNα with initial diagnosis of MC (2 active and 3 borderline), had resolved MC at 1 year. Out of five patients treated with Thymomodulin (1 active and 4 borderline MC), one had resolving MC and four had resolved MC at 1 year. In the conventionally treated group, one patient with active MC initially had resolving MC at 1 year, two with borderline MC initially had resolved MC at 1 year, and two with borderline MC initially had a histological diagnosis of dilated cardiomyopathy at 1 year.

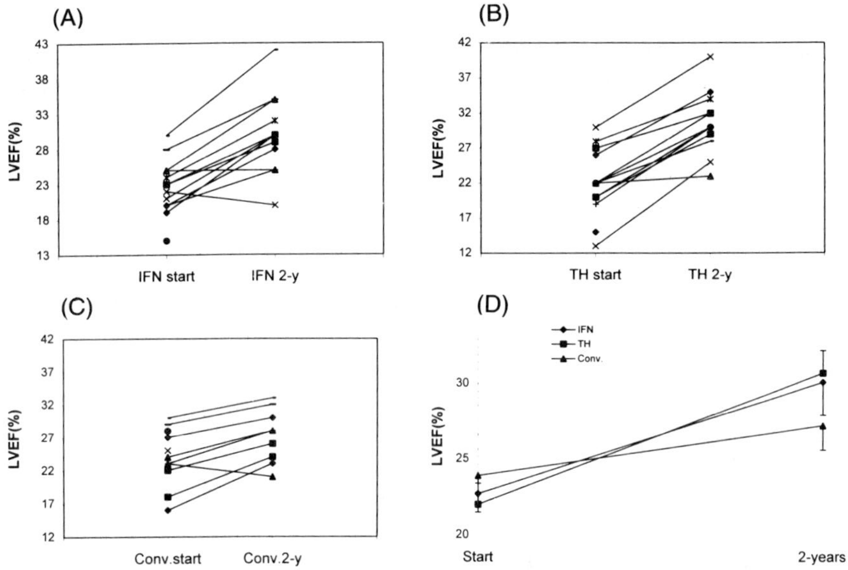

Fig. 32.2 Left ventricular ejection fraction (LVEF) in 38 patients with dilated heart muscle disease under therapy. (A) patients treated with IFNα and conventional therapy; (B) patients treated with thymomodulin and conventional therapy; (C) patients treated with conventional therapy alone; (D) mean values ± SEM. $p < 0.0001$ (ANOVA for repeated measures, Newman–Keuls multiple comparisons). Key as for Fig. 32.1.

Nine patients treated with IFNα and six treated with Thymomodulin improved their functional class at 1 year. At 2-year follow-up these patients maintained their improvement. Five conventionally treated patients improved their functional class at 1 year, and one of them worsened again at 2-year follow-up.

One IFNα-treated patient with biopsy-proven IDC died 5 months after presentation. It was a sudden death outside hospital. One Thymomodulin-treated patient died at 9 months with embolic cerebrovascular accident. Three patients died during 2-year follow-up in the conventionally treated group – one sudden death and two end-stage cardiac failures.

DISCUSSION

Dilated heart muscle disease can be idiopathic (IDC), or secondary to other causes, such as viral MC or viral perimyocarditis (14). Criteria for IDC in our study were cardiomegaly in angiocardiography, reduced ejection fraction (<45%), exclusion of coronary artery disease, valvular heart disease, hypertension and other forms of secondary heart muscle diseases, and histopathological findings of hypertrophy and branching of myocytes, with diffuse or focal fibrosis. Criteria for idiopathic MC were biopsy-determined inflammation of the myocardium with infiltrate, focal necrosis and interstitial edema with or without fibrosis.

Although there are multiple causes of dilated cardiomyopathy and the aetiology is frequently difficult to determine, it is becoming increasingly apparent that following an acute or subacute episode of MC due to a virus infection, the virus might persist in the cardiac tissues causing a dilated cardiomyopathy (6,15).

Presuming that heart in idiopathic MC and IDC may represent a site of low-grade persistent infection, protracted intermediate or lower doses of IFNα could be considered as a treatment schedule (16).

Thymic hormones have been shown to enhance host defense mechanisms important against virus spreading, such as cytotoxic T cell activity, NK cell activity and IFN production (7). They also exhibit immunoreconstructive effects in vivo enhancing the expression of IL-2 receptors when this expression is suboptimal and had been triggered by the competent signals (17). Besides induction of T-cell maturation and differentiation markers, thymic hormones might also affect the activity of mature lymphocytes (18).

LVEF improved in 21 of 26 patients (81%) after IFNα or Thymomodulin administration and in lesser extent in eight of 12 conventionally treated patients (66%, $p < 0.01$) at 6-month follow-up. At 2-year follow-up, 19 of 26 patients treated with immunomodulators (73%) and four of 12 conventionally treated patients (25%) improved their functional class.

As observed by Mason *et al.* (19), increased NK cell activity is associated with a more effective inflammatory response and less severe initial forms of MC. NK cell response is mainly responsible for elimination of virus in early phase of the disease, but could also be important for elimination of virus in late phase of the disease in cases of persistent viral infection. Our findings are in agreement not only with suggestions of Mason *et al.* (19) that a strong spontaneous immune response could be a benefit rather than an initiating factor of MC, but also that a stimulation of immune response by immunomodulators could be of benefit even in IDC.

CONCLUSION

Patients with a left ventricular ejection fraction <30% have a poor prognosis; many such patients are on a progressive downhill course and likely to die within a few years. We believe that the improvement in cardiac function that occurred during 2-year follow-up in patients with idiopathic MC or IDC treated with IFNα or Thymomodulin may result from the immunoenhancing effects achieved in patients with possible chronic myocardial viral infection.

The results reported here even suggest that combining of IFNα and Thymomodulin could induce better improvement than either drug alone, due to earlier IFN-achieved and more sustained Thymomodulin-accomplished immunological effects.

REFERENCES

1. Kandolf, R., P. Kirschner, D. Ameis *et al.* 1988. Enteroviral heart disease: diagnosis by in situ hybridization. In: *New Concepts in Viral Heart Disease* (H. P. Schultheiss, ed.) Springer-Verlag, Berlin, pp. 337–48.
2. Kandolf, R., D. Ameis, P. Kirschner *et al.* 1987. In situ detection of enteroviral genomes in myocardial cells by nucleic acid hybridization: an approach to the diagnosis of viral heart disease. *Proc. Natl. Acad. Sci. USA* **84**:6272–6.
3. Archard, L., C. Freeke, P. Richardson *et al.* 1988. Persistence of enterovirus RNA in dilated cardiomyopathy: a progression from MC. In: *New Concepts in Viral Disease* (H. P. Schultheiss, ed.) Springer-Verlag, Berlin, pp. 349–62.
4. Bowles, N. E., P. J. Richardson, E. G. J. Olsen and L. C. Archard. 1986. Detection of Coxsackie-B-virus-specific RBA sequences in myocardial biopsy samples from patients with MC and dilated cardiomyopathy. *Lancet* **I**:1120–3.
5. Weiss, L. M., X. F. Liu, K. L. Chang and M. E. Billingham. 1992. Detection of enteroviral RNA in idiopathic dilated cardiomyopathy and other human cardiac tissues. *J. Clin. Invest.* **90**:156–9.
6. Klingel, K., C. Hohenadl, A. Canu *et al.* 1992. Ongoing enterovirus-induced MC is associated with persistent heart muscle infection: quantitative analysis of virus replication, tissue damage, and inflammation. *Proc. Natl. Acad. Sci. USA* **89**:314–18.
7. Aiuti, F., G. Russo, M. Carbonari *et al.* 1985. A rational approach for the use of thymic hormones in viral infection and primary immunodeficiencies. In: *Peptide Hormones as Mediators in Immunology and Oncology* (R. D. Hesch, ed.) Serono Symposia Vol. 19. Raven Press, New York, pp. 185–9.
8. Aretz, H. T., M. E. Billingham, W. D. Edwards *et al.* 1987. Myocarditis: a histological definition and classification. *Am. J. Cardiovasc. Pathol.* **1**:3–13.
9. Woodruff, J. F. 1980. Viral myocarditis: a review. *Am. J. Pathol.* **101**:427–9.
10. Maisch, B., R. Trostel-Soeder, E. Stechemesser *et al.* 1982. Diagnostic relevance of humoral and cell-mediated immune reactions in patients with acute viral MC. *Clin. Exp. Immunol.* **48**:533–4.
11. Disis, M. L., T. L. McDonald, J. L. Colombo *et al.* 1986. Circulating immune complexes in cystic fibrosis and their correlation to clinical parameters. *Pediatr. Res.* **20**:385–90.
12. Kay, H. D., R. Fagnani and G. D. Bonnard. 1979. Cytotoxicity against the K562 erythroleukemia cell line by human NK (NK) cells which do not bear free Fc receptors for IgG. *Int. J. Cancer* **21**:141–50.
13. Hirsch, R. L. and K. P. Johnson. 1986. The effects of long-term administration of recombinant Alpha-2 Interferon on lymphocyte subsets, proliferation, and suppressor cell function in multiple sclerosis. *J. Interferon Res.* **6**:171–7.
14. Maisch, B., M. Herzum and U. Schoenian. 1993. Pathogenesis of disease: humans. In: *Viral Infections of the Heart* (J. E. Banatvala, ed.) Edward Arnold, London, pp. 138–75.
15. Huber, S. A. 1992. Viral myocarditis: a tale of two diseases. *Lab. Invest.* **66**:1–3.

16. Evans, T. and D. Secher. 1984. Kinetics of internalization and degradation of surface-bound interferon in human lymphoblastoid cells. *EMBO J.* **3**:2975–8.
17. Sztein, M., S. A. Serrate and A. L. Goldstein. 1986. Modulation of interleukin 2 receptor expression on normal human lymphocytes by thymic hormones. *Proc. Natl. Acad. Sci. USA* **83**:6107–11.
18. Talmadge, J. E., K. A. Uithoven, B. F. Lenz and M. Chrigos. 1984. Immunomodulation and therapeutic characterization of thymosin fraction five. *Cancer. Immunol. Immunother*. **18**:185–9.
19. Mason, J. W., J. B. O'Connell, A. Herskowitz *et al.* 1995. A clinical trial of immunosuppressive therapy for myocarditis. *N. Engl. J. Med.* **333**:269–75.

33

IL-1, TNF and IL-6 Release by Wound- inflammatory Cells During the Healing Process in Two Strains of Rats

Tatjana Banović, Nada Pejnović, Milena Kataranovski and Aleksandar Dujić

The wound-healing process involves a well-coordinated cascade of cellular and molecular events designed to enable restoration of the injured tissue (1). The initial haemostasis is followed by inflammatory and proliferative phases, ending with a remodelling stage that overlaps in time (2). The inflammatory stage in particular is characterized by intense participation of blood-borne cells which, in a time-dependent manner, and through specific adhesive interactions, infiltrate the injured tissue and cooperate to promote tissue remodelling. The early inflammatory phase of wound repair is initiated by the infiltration of polymorphonuclear granulocytes, whereas in the later events macrophages, T lymphocytes and their soluble products play a major role (3). It is believed that cytokine balance is essential for the control of the various cellular interactions within a healing wound. Interleukin 1 (IL-1), tumor necrosis factor (TNF) and interleukin 6 (IL-6)) secreted at the site of injury could influence both the early and later events of the healing process (4). Secreted by various cell types that infiltrate the injured tissue, these cytokines can affect cell adhesion, movement, proliferation and synthesis of extracellular matrix proteins (4,5). A few recent studies showed significant levels of IL-1, TNF and IL-6 within the normal healing wound (5). This study was undertaken to investigate the cellular responses during the course of wound healing in two different inbred rat strains: Albino Oxford (AO) and Dark August (DA), which exhibit genetically determined differences in the

Immunoregulation in Health and Disease
ISBN 0–12–459460–3

production of IL-2 (6), IFNγ (7) and TNF (8). Several studies indicate that AO rats are 'low' and DA strain 'high' producers Th1-derived cytokines (7,8,9). To our knowledge this is the first study undertaken to investigate wound-healing course, cellular response and cytokine production in repair processes in those two rat strains. To that end, a wound-healing model in animals was used that permitted investigation of time-dependent cellular changes within the healing wound. We measured the rate of wound closure of full-thickness wounds, the type of wound-infiltrating cells and the time course of IL-1, IL-6 and TNF production by wound-derived cells using a sponge-matrix model.

MATERIALS AND METHODS

Animals

Female Albino Oxford (AO) and Dark August (DA) rats (age range 12–16 weeks) bred at the Farm for Experimental Animals, Military Medical Academy, Belgrade, Yugoslavia, were used in all experiments.

Reagents and cytokines

Recombinant human IL-6, ultrapure human IL-1, recombinant mouse TNFα, polyclonal rabbit anti-human IL-1 antibody, and anti-mouse TNFα antibody were obtained from the manufacturer (Genzyme, Cambridge, MA).

Assessment of wound healing

Two round full-thickness wounds were prepared dorsally in both strains with a sharp, round metal blade, diameter 1 cm. Wound diameters were measured during 7 days of the healing process and wound area calculated.

Sponge matrix model

Sterile polyvinyl sponges ($2 \times 1 \times 0.5$ cm) were implanted subcutaneously (10,11) and at various time points excised and squeezed to collect the fluid in the wound. The sponge-derived cells were then seeded (1×10^6 cells/ml) for 20 h in RPMI medium with 5% fetal calf serum (ICN Pharmaceuticals, Costa Mesa, CA). A differential cell count was performed after staining the sponge cellular infiltrate with the May–Grunwald–Giemsa method at various time points.

D10 (N4) M bioassay for IL-1

IL-1 activity was measured by using the IL-1 sensitive D10 (N4) M cell line (12). D10 (N4) M cells were seeded at a concentration of 1×10^4 cells/well, and the supernatants of cells of the wound were added. After 72 h each culture well received MTT solution, and plates were incubated for additional 4 h. The optical density of formazan solubilized by SDS-HCl was measured with a microplate spectrophotometer (Behring ELISA Processor, Behringwerke AG Diagnostica, Marburg, Germany) at 570 nm. The specificity of IL-1-induced proliferation was confirmed by neutralizing rabbit polyclonal anti-human IL-1 antibody (cross-reactive with rat IL-1).

B9 bioassay for IL-6

IL-6 activity was measured by using the IL-6 dependent murine hybridoma cell line B9 (13). The B9 cells were seeded at 5×10^3 cells per culture and test performed as described for IL-1. The specificity of IL-6-induced proliferation was confirmed by neutralizing polyclonal anti-human IL-6 antibody (cross-reactive with rat IL-6).

L929 bioassay for TNF

The TNF activity was detected by using the L-929 mouse fibroblast cell line (14). Cells were seeded at 2.5×10^4 cells per well and after overnight culture actinomycin D (Sigma, St. Louis, MO) was added (0.2 mg/l) 1 h before test samples. After overnight incubation the non-adherent cells were removed and the viable cells stained with methylene blue. The optical density of dye that was solubilized by 0.1 N HCl was determined with microplate spectrophotometer (Behring ELISA Processor, Behringwerke AG Diagnostica) at 650 nm. The specificity of TNF-induced cytotoxicity was confirmed by neutralizing anti-mouse TNFα antibody (cross-reactive with rat TNF).

Statistical methods

Statistical significance was calculated by using a Mann–Whitney *U* test and Student *t* test.

RESULTS

Rate of wound closure

Healing wound area decreased during 7 days in both strains of rats. In the DA strain it significantly decreased over all time points after wounding. In

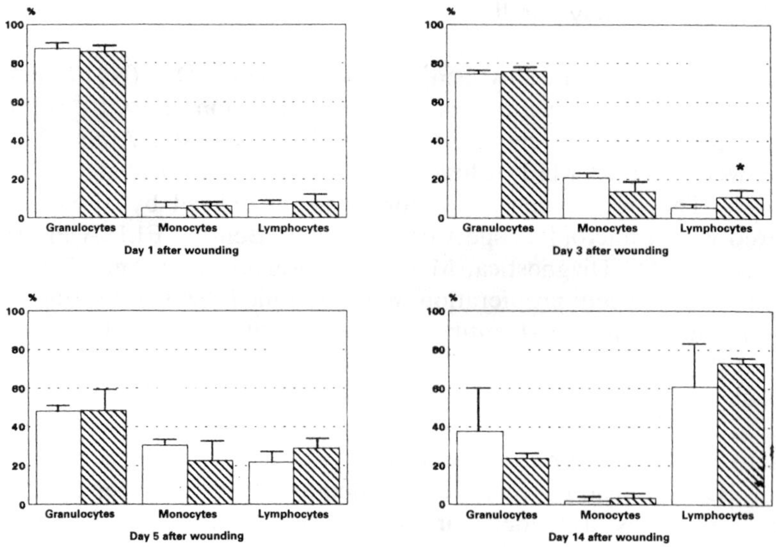

Fig. 33.1 The type of inflammatory cells that migrated to sponges. Data are presented as the mean ± SD of the percentage of cells from a representative experiment. $*p<0.05$ between groups (Student's *t* test). Shaded bars, DA rats; white bars, AO rats.

AO rats it decreased significantly from day 1 to 3 and from day 5 to 7 after wounding. Compared to the AO strain, DA rats showed significantly smaller wound area on days 1 (487.23 vs. 658.87 mm^2, $p<0.05$) and 7 (47.80 vs. 120.74 mm^2, $p<0.05$) after injury.

Type of inflammatory cells

Granulocytes predominated on days 1 and 3 in wounds in both strains. Mononuclear cells with a predominance of macrophages constituted the majority of the infiltrated cells on day 5 in both strains, and with a predominance of lymphocytes on day 10 after injury in DA strain (data not shown). Lymphocytes were the predominant cell type on day 14 after wounding in both strains (Fig. 33.1). In DA rats compared to the AO strain a significantly higher percentage of wound infiltrating lymphocytes was observed on days 3 (10.67% vs. 5.33%) and 7 (34.75% vs. 19.50%, $p<0.05$).

IL-1, IL-6 and TNF in supernatants of wound-derived cells

In the early inflammatory phase the time course of IL-1 production was similar in both strains. It was significant on day 3, decreased on day 5 and then again increased reaching peak levels on day 14 in DA, and on day 10 in AO strain with a trend towards decrease in the 14-day supernatants. There

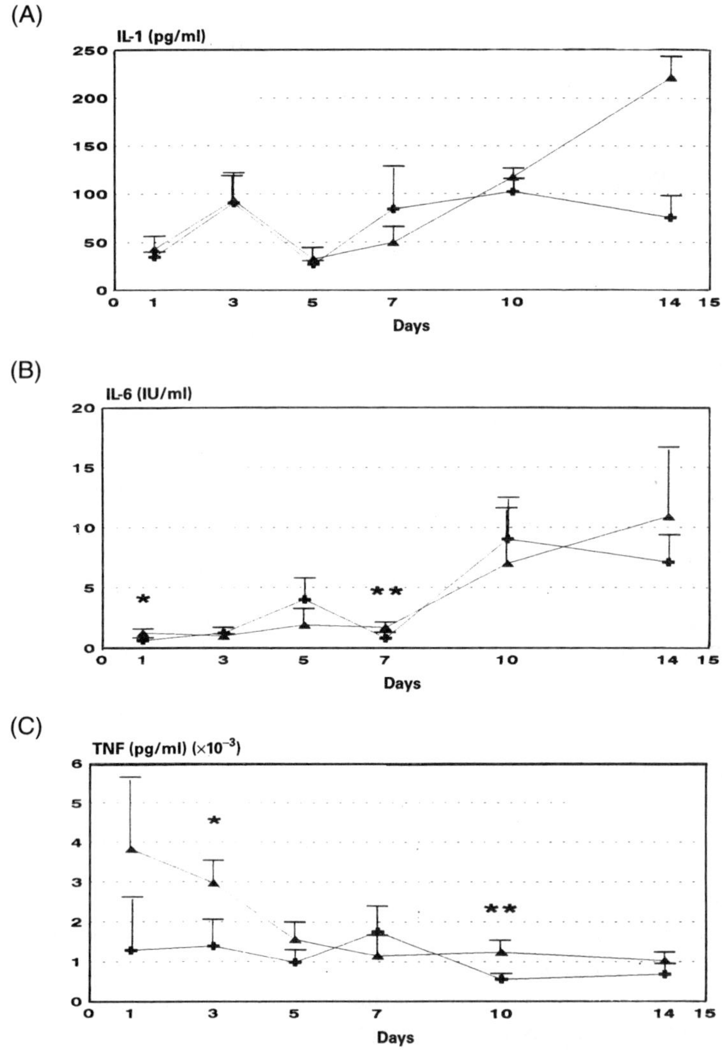

Fig. 33.2 Cytokine activity in the supernatants of sponge-derived inflammatory cells. A, IL-1; B, IL-6; C, TNF. Data are presented as the mean ± SD cytokine activity from a representative experiment. $*p<0.05$, $**p<0.001$ between groups (Mann–Whitney *U* test). Crosses, AO rats; triangles, DA rats.

were no significant differences in IL-1 production between strains at each time point (Fig. 33.2A). Similarly, IL-6 production increased on day 5, decreased on day 7 and then gradually increased over time with the highest levels detected on days 10 and 14 (in AO and DA respectively). Significantly higher activities in supernatants of wound cells from DA rats were observed on days 1 and 7 postwounding (Fig. 33.2B). In contrast, TNF production in DA rats was significant in the first 3 days and then gradually decreased over all time points. In the AO strain, however, peak TNF activity was not seen until day 7 and then decreased on day 10 after injury. On days 3 and 10 after wounding, significantly higher activities were observed in supernatants of wound cells from DA rats (Fig. 33.2C).

DISCUSSION

Our study demonstrates that DA and AO rats differ in their healing capabilities: DA rats showed an accelerated wound-healing course which was accompanied with different pattern of wound cellular infiltration and significantly higher levels of IL-6 and TNF in supernatants of wound-derived cells compared to AO strain. It is apparent that complex regulatory network involving various inflammatory cells that accumulate within the wound and their soluble products could influence the normal healing process (4). The role of lymphocytes in wound healing is still poorly defined and it seems that its participation is restricted to T lymphocytes (1) which, acting with macrophages, can send discrete molecular signals to stimulate fibroblast chemotaxis, proliferation and collagen production (15). We can hypothesize that the accelerated wound-healing course exhibited in DA rats by the significantly smaller wound area on days 1 and 7 after wounding could be influenced by the significantly more intensive accumulation of lymphocytes within the healing wound observed on days 3 and 7 after wounding compared to AO rats. This could be supported by recent reports suggesting that increased infiltration of T lymphocytes within a wound often results in extended scar formation and fibrosis (16) and that accumulation of active T lymphocytes (17,18) at the site of injury may result in increased adhesiveness, proliferation and fibronectin production of connective tissue fibroblasts (19). This study shows that accelerated wound closure in DA rats is accompanied by higher levels of IL-6 and TNF in wound-derived cell supernatants observed in this rat strain. This is in agreement with the recent data which showed that a prolonged presence of IL-6 increased collagen synthesis in liver tissues (20). However, there are studies which show that TNF down-regulated collagen synthesis (21) and suggest that reduced production of TNF corresponds with an improvement of the healing process (22). On the other hand, several in vitro studies showed that TNF can have both positive and negative effects on fibroblasts and endothelial cell growth (1). It was therefore suggested that tissue level and exact time of production of this cytokine may dictate its in vivo effects (3). The levels of IL-1 production by wound-inflammatory cells in AO and DA rats did not differ significantly in our study. This result should be interpreted with care because of the possibility of the production of IL-1 inhibitor (23) or IL-1 receptor antagonist

(24) by wound-infiltrating cells. Previous studies have shown that DA and AO strain exhibit genetically inherited differences in the level of IL-2 (25), IFNγ (7) and TNF (8) production, as well as in the capacity to mount T-cell-dependent immune response to several foreign antigens (26). We can therefore speculate that the accelerated wound-healing course seen in DA rats could be also due to the altered production of some other cytokines, especially of the Th1 profile which was not investigated in this study. Our data represent constitutive IL-1, IL-6 and TNF production of sponge-derived wound-inflammatory cells. This study did not point out the specific cellular sources of the elevated IL-6 and TNF since the total wound infiltrate consisted of sponge-derived polymorphonuclear granulocytes, macrophages and lymphocytes that were seeded for the cytokine production. Despite the fact that mononuclear cells make substantially greater quantities of cytokines than polymorphonuclear cells on a single-cell basis, granulocytes constitute the majority of infiltrating cells in the inflamed and injured tissue (24) and may thus represent an important source of IL-1, IL-6 and TNF (27) in the tissue during the early healing phase. It is therefore possible that differences at the level of the functions of granulocytes and their interactions with other cell types involved in wound healing could be responsible for the observed difference in the healing capacities of DA and AO rats.

CONCLUSION

DA rats were shown to have a faster closure rate of full-thickness wounds compared to the AO strain. A higher proportion of infiltrating lymphocytes and higher IL-6 and TNF activities in wound-cell supernatants could be one of the mechanisms which underline the accelerated wound-healing course seen in DA rats.

REFERENCES

1. Barbul, A. 1990. Immune aspects of wound repair. *Clin. Plast. Surg.* **17**: 433–41.
2. Ortonne, J. P. and J. Clevy. 1994. Physiology of cutaneous cicatrization. *Rev. Prat.* **44**:1733–7.
3. Di Pietro, L. A. 1995. Wound healing: the role of the macrophage and other immune cells. *Shock* **4**:233–40.
4. Ford, H. R., R. A. Hoffman, E. J. Wing *et al.* 1989. Characterization of wound cytokines in the sponge matrix model. *Arch. Surg.* **124**:1422–8.
5. Pejnovic, N., D. Lilic, G. Zunic *et al.* 1995. Aberrant levels of cytokines within the healing wound after burn injury. *Arch. Surg.* **130**:999–1006.
6. Mostarica-Stojkovic, M., L. Ejdus-Konstantinovic, M. Kostic and M. L. Lukic. 1985. Resistance to the induction of T cell mediated autoimmunity correlates with lower IL2 production. *Adv. Exp. Med. Biol.* **186**:713–20.

7. Arsov, I., V. Pravica, V. Badovinac *et al.* 1995. Selection for the susceptibility to experimental allergic encephalomyelitis also selects for high IFN gamma production. *Transpl. Proc.* **27**:1537–8.
8. Stosic-Gruicic, S., M. L. Lukic, A. Shanin *et al.* 1995. Relationship between Th1 and Th2 associated cytokines and susceptibility to multiple low dose of streptozotocin induced diabetes in rats. *Autoimmunity* **21**:44.
9. Lukic, M. L., M. Mostarica-Stojkovic, M. Kostic *et al.* 1987. Cellular and genetic basis of the strain differences in IL2 production in rats. *Transplant Proc.* **19**:3137–9.
10. Schilling, A. J., W. Joel and H. M. Shurley. 1959. Wound healing: a comparative study of the histochemical changes in granulation tissue contained in stainless steel wire mesh and polyvinyl sponge cylinders. *Surgery* **46**:702–10.
11. Middleton, M. M. and P. A. Campbell. 1989. Functions of purified neutrophils isolated from gelatin sponges. *J. Leukoc. Biol.* **46**:461–6.
12. Hopkins, S. J. and M. Humphrey. 1989. Simple, sensitive and specific bioassay of interleukin 1. *J. Immun. Meth.* **120**:271–6.
13. Shalaby, M. R., A. Waage, L. Arden and T. Espevik. 1989. Endotoxin, tumor necrosis factor-alpha and Interleukin 1 induce Interleukin 6 production in vivo. *Clin. Immunol. Immunopathol.* **53**:488–9.
14. Meager, A., H. Leung and J. Wooley. 1989. Assays for tumor necrosis factor and related cytokines. *J. Immunol. Meth.* **116**:1–17.
15. Postlethwaite, A. E., G. N. Smith, C. L. Mainard *et al.* 1984. Lymphocyte modulation of fibroblast function in vitro. Stimulation and inhibition of collagen production by different effector molecules. *J. Immunol.* **132**:2470–7.
16. Agelli, M. and S. M. Wahl. 1986. Cytokines and fibrosis. *Clin. Exp. Rheumatol.* **4**:379–82.
17. Fishel, R. S., A. Barbul, W. E. Beschorner *et al.* 1986. Lymphocyte participation in wound healing. *Ann. Surg.* **206**:25–9.
18. Peterson, J. M., A. Barbul, R. J. Brelin *et al.* 1987. Significance of T-lymphocytes in wound healing. *Surgery* **102**:300–5.
19. Wojciak, B. and J. F. Crossan. 1993. The accumulation of inflammatory cells in synovial sheat and epitenon during adhesion formation in healing rat flexor tendons. *Clin. Exp. Immunol.* **93**:108–14.
20. Choi, I., H. S. Kang, Y. Yang and K. H. Pyun. 1994. IL6 induced hepatic inflammation and collagen synthesis in vivo. *Clin. Exp. Immunol.* **95**:530–5.
21. Regan, M. C., S. G. Kirk, M. Hurson *et al.* 1993. Tumor necrosis factor-a inhibits in vivo collagen synthesis. *Surgery* **113**:173–7.
22. Bettinger, D. A., J. V. Pellicane, W. C. Tarry *et al.* 1994. The role of inflammatory cytokines in wound healing: accelerated healing in endotoxin-resistant mice. *J. Trauma* **36**:810–13.
23. Tiku, K., M. L. Tiku, S. Liu and L. Skoskey. 1986. Normal human neutrophils are a source of a specific interleukin 1 inhibitor. *J. Immunol.* **136**:3686–92.
24. Cassaleta, M. 1995. The production of cytokines by polymorphonuclear neutrophils. *Immunol. Today* **16**:21–6.
25. Vukmanovic, S., M. Mostarica-Stojkovic, I. Zalud *et al.* 1990. Analysis of T cell subset after induction of experimental autoimmune encephalomyelitis in susceptible and resistant strains of rats. *J. Neuroimmunol.* **27**:63–9.
26. Kostic, M., M. Mostarica-Stojkovic, L. Ejdus-Konstantinovic *et al.* 1986. Genetic determinants of the strain differences in interleukin 2 (IL-2) production in inbred strains of rats. *Period. Biol.* **88**:310–11.
27. Cassatella, M. A. 1995. The production of cytokines by polymorphonuclear neutrophils. *Immunol. Today* **16**:21–6.

Section 4

Host reactivity to graft, tumour and infection

34

Cytotoxic Mechanisms of Natural Killer Cells

Nikola L. Vujanović, Shigeki Nagashima,
Ronald B. Herberman and Theresa L. Whiteside

To protect the host from pathogens or transformed cells, under the pressure of evolutionary selection, highly efficient and powerful immune mechanisms have developed, including cell-mediated cytotoxicity. Among several types of immune cells capable of cytotoxic activity, the best characterized and most extensively evaluated for anti-viral and anti-tumour cytotoxic functions are antigen-specific cytotoxic T lymphocytes (CTLs) (1) and non-specific natural killer (NK) cells (2). These effector cells can be activated and expanded in vivo as well as in vitro. On activation, they develop more powerful cytotoxic and other effector functions (3–5). In recent clinical studies in cancer patients with advanced metastatic disease, immunotherapy based on transfer of activated effector cells, such as tumour-infiltrating lymphocytes (TILs) (6) or highly purified NK cells (7,8), was found associated with clinical responses in a subset of these patients. The anti-tumour therapeutic effect has been related to cytotoxic activity of transferred effector cells. Thus, studies of cytotoxic mechanisms mediated by immune effector cells are of major importance not only for a better understanding of the relationships between the immune system and pathogens or malignant cells but also for development of novel strategies for anti-viral and anti-cancer therapy.

NK cells are a phenotypically and functionally distinct lymphocyte population (2,7,8). They can be defined functionally as 'professional' cytotoxic effector cells of the immune system with the ability to kill virus-infected or tumour cells spontaneously (without previous stimulation). Because of those properties, NK cells have been long considered to be the first line of immune defence and are anticipated to act as the major constitutive (non-adaptive) effectors of immunosurveillance against virus and cancer (2,7,8). More direct support for this hypothesis comes from recent studies that have begun to define several multigene families of cell surface-bound receptors and ligands, as well as secretory cytotoxic molecules, which are selectively engaged in NK cell-mediated killing. Two different cytotoxic pathways, which selectively induce death of abnormal

Immunoregulation in Health and Disease
ISBN 0-12-459460-3

cells, are apparently utilized by NK cells: secretory/necrotic and non-secretory/apoptotic killing. These pathways are mediated via ligand/receptor-initiating signal transduction in either effector or target cells, respectively. Here, we review evidence for the presence of these two cytotoxic pathways in NK cells.

SECRETORY/NECROTIC PATHWAY OF KILLING

Receptors

The secretory/necrotic pathway model of killing is based on the hypothesis that NK cells, interacting with susceptible targets, are triggered via specific receptors to actively release cytolytic granules and molecules capable of damaging the target cell membrane (9). Studies have recently been commenced to determine the nature of these receptors on NK cells and corresponding ligands on NK-sensitive targets (10,11). Initially, it was demonstrated that NK cells can kill target cells expressing allogeneic major histocompatibility complex (MHC) molecules as well as those completely lacking the MHC antigens. These observations suggested that NK cells might play an important role in elimination of cells with changed or lost expression of the MHC class I molecules. A concept has been introduced that NK cells can discriminate between normal self and abnormal self. In the last few years, two different types of receptors have been recognized on the surface of NK cells:

- triggering receptors, able to recognize specific oligosaccharide ligands present on target cells
- inhibitory receptors, which recognize self MHC class I molecules (10,11, Fig. 34.1A).

Triggering receptors

A considerable body of evidence indicates that NK cells can be activated and mediate lysis of NK-sensitive targets through ligation of a variety of receptors, including CD2, CD16, CD69, NK-TR1, 2B4, p38 and NKR-P1 (10). Based on these findings, it has been proposed that no one unique NK cell-specific receptor is responsible for triggering the cytolytic response. However, recent studies have seriously challenged this notion and have indicated that NK cells might utilize a particular receptor to recognize and directly lyse NK-susceptible targets. Thus, NKR-P1 receptors, 60–80 kDa transmembrane homodimers of disulfide-linked glycoproteins, belonging to the C-type animal lectin superfamily (10,12), can recognize sulfated oligosaccharide sequences of cell membrane ligands, such as heparan and chondroitin sulfate

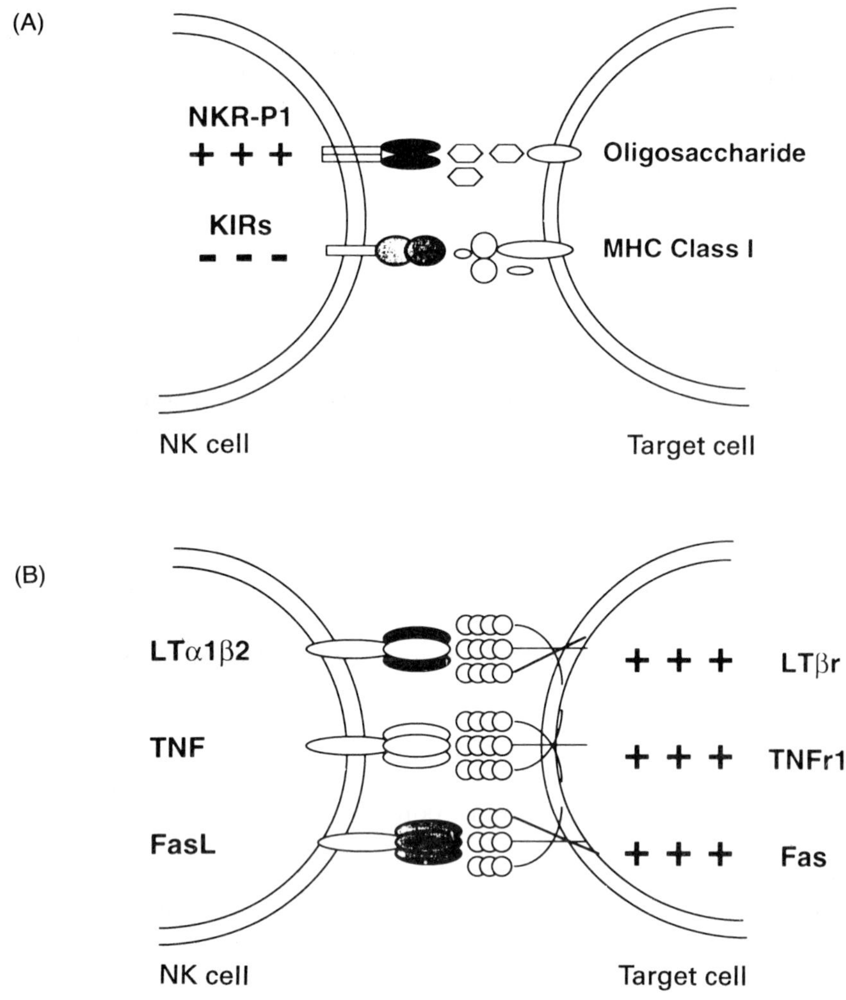

Fig. 34.1 Receptors and ligands involved in secretory/necrotic (A) and non-secretory/apoptotic (B) killing of tumour cells by NK cells.

proteoglycans, expressed on the membrane of NK-cell-susceptible targets (13,14). These ligands in soluble form showed the ability to inhibit binding of soluble NKR-P1 to and killing of YAC-1 targets by rat NK cells. In addition, NK-resistant P815 targets exposed to liposomes containing the NKR-P1 ligands became sensitive to NK cell-mediated lysis and able to trigger NK cells for cytolytic activity against these targets (13). Interactions of NKR-P1 on NK cells and oligosaccharide ligands on NK susceptible targets appeared to be able to induce calcium ion influx and signalling of the protein tyrosine kinase (PTK)-dependent, phosphatidyl-inositol 3-kinase (PI-3)-independent pathway in the effector cells, leading to their cytolytic granule release and killing of targets (13,14). Three mouse NKR-P1 genes, five rat and one human homologue have been discovered so far (10). Several laboratories are now attempting to determine whether NK cells can express and utilize various NKR-P1 isoforms to recognize different oligosaccharide ligands and to kill different tumour targets.

Inhibitory receptors

The ability of NK cells to selectively kill NK-sensitive tumour cells and to spare normal cells appears to be determined by a distinct family of NK-cell surface receptors and corresponding ligands expressed on target cells. Several of these receptors have been recently discovered both in humans and rodents and defined to belong to the Ig and C-type animal lectin superfamilies, respectively (11,15). Both types of receptors recognize polymorphic MHC class I molecules, which signals inhibition of killing of target cells expressing appropriate alleles. These receptors were called killer-cell inhibitory receptors (KIRs). Human KIRs (11) are encoded by genes located on chromosome 19 at 19q13.4. They contain Ig-like loops in the extracellular domains. According to the number of these loops, two different KIRs have been defined: 58 kDa (p58) with two Ig-like loops and 70 kDa (p70) with three Ig-like loops. Up to now, 13 members of the human KIR family differing in extracellular, transmembrane and intracytoplasmic domains have been discovered. The KIRs have immunoreceptor tyrosine-based activation motifs (ITAMs) in the intracytoplasmic domains. Two different human KIRs characterized by two Ig loops, defined by mAbs GL183 and EB6, recognize two groups of HLA-C alleles. A human KIR with three Ig loops, defined by mAb DX9 (NKB1), recognizes HLA-Bw4. In contrast, mouse KIRs (11,15) are represented by Ly-49 differentiation antigens. Seven murine KIRs that have been defined are type II membrane proteins and are coded by related genes on chromosome 6 and preferentially expressed by NK cells. Ly-49 genes do not rearrange, but alternatively splice, resulting in allelic polymorphism. Murine KIRs are expressed as disulfide-bonded homodimers on subsets of NK cells. The subsets of NK cells expressing different Ly-49s (A, C and G.2) largely overlap, indicating that individual NK cells express more than one Ly-49 gene. Ly-49s recognize MHC class I molecules, interacting with a sulfated polysaccharide, fucoidin, present on the α_1 and α_2 domains of H-2 (15). Signalling pathways through KIRs have not been defined. However, recent studies suggest that when a complete inhibition of cytolysis by MHC recognition is achieved, target cell recognition fails to generate tyrosine phosphorylation of phospholipase C (PLC)-γ-derived second messengers in NK cells (14).

Cytolytic granules

NK cells contain characteristic azurophilic granules in cytoplasm (2,9). This morphologic characteristic of NK cells has been long thought to be related to their cytolytic function. The cytoplasmic granules are 0.3–1.0 μm in size and are found in cytotoxic NK cells (1,16). Ultrastructural analysis using transmission electron microscopy (TEM) showed that the granules have two compartments: a dense core domain and a multivesicular cortical domain (1,16). The former contains secretory molecules, such as the cytotoxic proteins perforin and granzymes, chondroitin sulfate proteoglycans with a presumed storage function and the calcium-binding protein calreticulin with calcium-sequestering activity. In contrast, the multivesicular domain contains lysosomal proteins, including acid phosphatase, α-glucosidase, cathepsin D, and LGP120. The multivesicular region demonstrates additional properties in common with lysosomes, including acidic pH, the presence of the 270-kDa mannose-6 phosphate receptor (Man6-P, a marker of early endocytic compartments) and endocytic uptake of exogenous cationized ferritin. Thus, the cytoplasmic granules represent unique dual-functional organelles, which combine both secretory and prelysosomal compartments/functions (1,16). Based on their characteristics, composition, and distribution during lysis mediated by NK cells, the cytoplasmic two-compartment granules are thought to be essential for cytotoxic function of NK cells. Cytolytic molecules found in the two-compartment cytoplasmic granules, such as perforin and granzymes, are considered to be the most important effector molecules mediating secretory/necrotic killing.

Perforin

Biochemical analysis of purified cytoplasmic granules on Percoll gradients from CRNK-16 rat LGL leukaemia cells showed that they contain the 66–70 kDa calcium-dependent lytic glycoprotein, perforin, composed of 534 amino acids (17). Perforin is partially homologous to the terminal components of the membrane attack complex (MAC) of complement (C6–C9) (17). Perforin, like complement, is able to bind, insert and polymerize into the target-cell membrane. During this process, perforin monomers can form 5–20 nm cell membrane pores. Recent studies have substantially added to our understanding of the perforin function. Non-cytolytic rat basophilic leukaemia cells transfected with perforin cDNA acquired cytolytic activity against erythrocytes coated with specific IgE antibodies (17–20). Thus, perforin alone could lyse at least some target cells, i.e. erythrocytes. In a complementary study, inhibition of perforin expression in cytolytic lymphocytes by perforin antisense oligonucleotides produced a significant, but not complete, inhibition of cytolytic activity of these cells against nucleated targets. This observation confirmed the importance of perforin in cytotoxic activity but also indicated that perforin is not solely responsible for target cell lysis. Definitive evidence for the role of perforin in NK-cell killing has been obtained from the studies with perforin-deficient (P^0) mice (21). Cytolytic activity of NK cells from these mice was found to be drastically reduced and they were unable to clear in vivo lymphocytic choriomeningitis virus. However, growth of syngeneic fibrosarcoma cells was not different in P^0 than in normal mice up to day 10 after tumour cell inoculation. These findings argue against the role of secretory cytolytic activity mediated by NK cells in antitumour activity in vivo. It is, therefore, possible that NK cells mediate antitumour functions by an alternative mechanism not involving perforin.

Granzymes

Granzymes are serine proteinases capable of cleaving a variety of substrates (22). Initially, it was found that granzyme A can degrade several extracellular matrix (ECM) proteins, while granzyme B can prevent adhesion of adherent tumour cell lines to extracellular matrix (ECM) proteins. Thus, it was postulated that granzymes play a role in lymphocyte extravasation and migration (22). Granzyme A was then shown to cleave and activate the thrombin receptor at the Leu-Asp-Pro-Arg/Ser site. The enzymatic activities of granzymes have been further defined by hydrolysis of synthetic substrates, such as Boc-Lys-SBzl specific for tryptase (granzyme A), Asp-ase (granzyme B), chymase and Met-ase (22). The significance of granzymes in NK cytotoxicity has been indicated by the findings that a variety of proteinase inhibitors, particularly specific inhibitors of granzyme B Asp-ase activity, e.g. isocoumarin or tripeptide chloromethylketone, inhibits NK activity as well as cytolysis mediated by cytoplasmic granules purified from NK cells (1,18–20,22). It appears that proteolytic activity of granzymes inside target cells is necessary for their cytotoxic function, as loading of target cells with aprotinin blocks granzyme-mediated killing (22). However, granzymes by themselves are not cytolytic. Only cotreatment of target cells with sub-lytic concentrations of purified perforin or digitonin and granzyme A or granzyme B, but not with granzymes alone, induces DNA fragmentation (17,22). In addition, rat basophilic leukaemic cells transfected with perforin and both granzyme A and granzyme B cDNA could both lyse and induce DNA fragmentation in nucleated target cells (17,22). In contrast, these effector cells transfected with either cDNA alone induced only insignificant changes in target cells.

Cytotoxic cells from granzyme B-deficient mice mediate lysis with reduced efficiency and are unable to induce rapid DNA fragmentation in target cells (23). However, this defect could be corrected by longer incubation, indicating that other cytotoxic proteins in effector cells might also be involved (23). Thus, it is currently believed that perforin is necessary to provide access for granzymes to their substrates in target cells (17,22). DNA damage induced by granzyme B does not require de novo protein synthesis in target cells, indicating that they contain the molecules pre-made for a cytotoxic event. However, the nature of these molecules is unknown (22). More recent studies demonstrate that these granule proteinases can activate an endonuclease and degrade target cell DNA into the oligosome-sized fragments. This effect may be indirect, because, like the cysteine protease interleukin-1β converting enzyme (ICE) , which is homologous with the product of the *Caenorhabditis elegans* cell-death gene, *ced-3*, granzyme A is able to cleave the 31 kDa inactive IL-1β precursor after asparatic acids and to generate the 17 kD proinflammatory cytokine IL-1β (24). In addition, granzyme B has a similar aspase activity to ICE (22). These data indicate that granzymes might induce apoptosis in target cells by activating certain common intracellular pathways of programmed cell death (PCD).

Current model of lysis of NK-cell susceptible targets

A mechanistic model of NK cell-mediated lysis of susceptible targets was independently proposed by Henkart and Podack more than 10 years ago (1,18–20). Combining all the supporting evidence that has accumulated since then, the model could be summarized as follows (1,18–20): NK cells are presumed to play an active role in killing NK-sensitive targets. Interaction of NK cells with susceptible targets activates a regulated calcium-dependent secretory mechanism in these effector cells. This secretory mechanism starts with magnesium-dependent, but calcium- and temperature-independent rapid binding of effector cells to appropriate target cells via CAMs (i.e. LFA-1 on NK cells and ICAM-1 on target cells). The second stage of NK cytotoxicity involves calcium- and temperature-dependent recognition of target cells by the putative NK receptors, resulting in triggering of the cytolytic machinery in NK cells. The triggering event results in a characteristic intracytoplasmic movement and reorientation of the Golgi apparatus, microtubule-organizing centre and cytoplasmic granules towards the target. It is followed by calcium-dependent granule exocytosis into an extracellular space located in the contact zone between the NK cell and target cell membranes. Degranulation of NK cells is followed by the release of cytotoxic molecules, perforin and granzymes, from exocytosed granules and formation of pores in the target cell membrane by perforin insertion and polymerization. The cytolytic process progresses with influx of calcium and sodium ions, efflux of potassium ions and penetration of granzymes through the cell membrane pores formed by polymerized perforin. As a consequence of an osmotic imbalance, entry of water and swelling of mitochondria and cytoplasm in target cells, cellular necrosis occurs, with rupture of the cell membrane and leaking out of the cytoplasmic content. Usually, a low level of DNA fragmentation and other symptoms of apoptosis follow necrosis in target cells, apparently as a consequence of granzyme activity.

This cytotoxic mechanism, largely defined in 4 h ^{51}Cr-release assays, has been considered as the major pathway of target cell killing by NK cells (2,9). However, only rare transformed cultured cell lines, such as K562 myeloid leukaemia, in humans, or YAC-1 T-cell lymphoma, in rodents, can be efficiently lysed by freshly isolated non-activated NK cells (2). In contrast, a large majority of normal or transformed cells is apparently resistant to NK-cell lysis (2).

NON-SECRETORY/APOPTOTIC PATHWAY OF KILLING

In vivo studies have indicated that NK cells might play an important role in antitumour defence, particularly in the control of metastasis development (7,8). However, a long-standing unexplained paradox has been the finding of rapid in vivo elimination of tumour cells derived from lines defined as NK-resistant in in vitro ^{51}Cr-release assays, which measure necrotic cell death (7,8). A possible explanation for the contrasting ubiquitous in vivo antitumour effects and limited in vitro cytotoxicity of NK cells is that the classical NK assay reflects perforin-mediated lysis, but fails to detect an alternative pathway of tumour cell killing apparently operative in vivo. Thus, it is likely that NK cells utilize, in addition to the secretory cytolytic pathway, an alternative cytotoxic mechanism. For example, membrane-bound cytotoxic ligands expressed on NK cells might be able to trigger apoptotic cell death in tumour cells by engagement of corresponding receptors on these targets.

The tumour necrosis factor (TNF) family of ligands

Recent studies have identified a large family of related, biologically important, functionally pleiotropic, cell membrane-bound and secreted cytokines, the TNF family of ligands (25,26). One of the most prominent characteristics of these molecules is their capability of inducing apoptotic cell death. Eleven different family members have been identified so far, as listed in Table 34.1. Among them, TNF and LTα were shown to be coded by three genes, each containing three introns and four exons, located in a cytokine locus in the middle of the MHC complex. Most of the TNF family ligands are 26–40 kDa type II membrane-anchored proteins with the intracellular N-terminus, a single transmembrane domain, and the extracellular C-terminus with a homologous 150 amino acid receptor binding residue (25,26). LTα is an exception. It does not have the intracytoplasmic and transmembrane domains and is directly secreted, forming soluble homotrimers (25,26). However, LTα is also found as a membrane-anchored form incorporated into a heterotrimeric complex with a second subunit, the transmembrane protein LTβ, in a 1:2 stoichiometric ratio (LTα1β2) (25,26). This indicates that members of the TNF family of ligands have not only homotypic but also heterotypic binding properties and, thus, the

Table 34.1 The TNF family of ligands and their receptors

Ligands	Receptors
TNFα (tm p26, s p17)	TNFR1 (p60, CD120a)^{dd*}
LTα (TNFβ, s p21–25)	TNFR2 (p80, CD120b)*
LTβ (tm p33), LTα1β2 (tm p87–90)	LT–βR (p50–55, TNFRrp)^{dd*}
FasL (tm p40, s p27)	Fas (p48, APO–1, CD95)^{dd*}
CD27L (tm p50)	CD27 (p55)
CD30L (tm p40)	CD30 (p120)*
CD40L (tm p39, s p18)	CD40 (p50)^{dd*}
OX40L (tm p30)	OX40 (p50)
4-1BBL (tm p35)	4-1BB (p50)*
NGF	NGFR (p75, p140)^{dd}
TRAIL (tm p40, s p28)	?*

TRAIL, TNF-related apoptosis-inducing ligand; tm, transmembrane form; s, soluble form; ^{dd}, presence of an intracytoplasmic death domain; *, receptor which can signal apoptosis.

potential to make not only homo-oligomers but also hetero-oligomers and multiply the number of their structural and functional varieties. The 17 kDa extracellular portion of the transmembrane (26 kDa) form of TNFα can be released in a soluble (secreted) form by proteolytic cleavage mediated via the matrix metalloproteinases. It forms homotrimers and folds into a β-pleated sheet sandwich. Similarly, the 40 kDa transmembrane FasL can be cleaved by the matrix metalloproteinases, generating 27 kDa soluble fragments of the extracellular portion (27). Furthermore, the secreted form of TNFα has been found in cell-free body fluids under a variety of pathophysiological circumstances, including septic shock, autoimmune diseases, graft-versus-host reaction or cancer development (25,26). These data indicate that the TNF family ligands may be expressed not only as membrane-bound but also as secreted forms, depending on the functional status of immune cells and, thus, be able to act both in a direct cell–cell contact and at a distance, respectively. Soluble TNF and LTα homotrimers were shown to have a particularly high homology at the external portions of the protomer interfaces. Crystallographic analysis demonstrated that these particular regions of the ligand trimers are the specific acceptor sites for receptors and that one LTα homotrimer can bind three TNFR1 (26). These findings indicate the possible mode of interaction between the TNF family ligands and their corresponding receptors.

The TNF family of receptors

A complementary family of molecules to the TNF family of ligands, the TNF family of receptors, has been defined in parallel (25,26). Ten members, all representing type I transmembrane proteins, have been discovered (25,26,

Table 34.1). Two soluble members have been also found, i.e. T2 and A53R poxvirus gene products (soluble TNFR). With the exception of TNFα and LTα, each of the TNF family ligands has a single specific receptor. TNFα and LTα have two common receptors, TNFR1 and TNFR2, and thus show functional redundancy. All members of the TNF receptor family have characteristic extracellular cysteine-rich pseudorepeats, which share significant intersubunit sequence homology. Soluble forms of these receptors are released by proteolysis. An exception is soluble 4-1BB, which is generated by alternative splicing. The TNF family receptors have cytoplasmic domains which are generally short (46–221 residues) and without sequence homology. However, TNFR1 and Fas have an intracytoplasmic motif spanning 65 amino acids of 29% residue homology, named the death domain (26,28). A similar motif was recently found in the C-terminus of NGFRp75, CD40 and LTβR (26,28–30). The death domain has some similarity to a motif of the protein reaper in *Drosophila*, specifically expressed in cells induced to die by apoptosis. Fas also contains a negative regulatory domain, a 15 amino acid 'salvation' domain at the C-terminus, not present on TNFR1. This Fas domain is able to associate with the protein–tyrosine phosphatase identified in basophils (PTP-BAS) and thus to block apoptotic function of the receptor (26). Because of that, cells expressing PTP-BAS are resistant to FasL-mediated killing, while those without it are sensitive.

Intracytoplasmic regions of the TNF family receptors differ in size and structure, and, in spite of the absence of catalytic domains, they are able to mediate a variety of signalling pathways by binding to and engagement of particular cell signalling mediators. Thus, homotypic clustering was shown not only of Fas, TNFR1, LTβR and CD40, which have the intracytoplasmic death domain, but also of TNFR2, CD30, 4-IBB, or of a putative TRAIL receptor that can signal apoptotic cell death in sensitive targets (26,29–31). This signalling through TNFR1 and Fas was found to be accompanied by the receptor ligation-recruitment/activation of three intracytoplasmic molecules, i.e. 34 kDa TRADD (by TNFR1), 23 kDa FADD (by Fas), and 71 kDa RIP (by both receptors) (28). TRADD and FADD N-terminus lack a defined protein motif, while RIP contains a kinase domain. However, all three cytoplasmic molecules have in the C-terminus a domain with a considerable homology to the receptor death motif, and showed the ability to associate through these domains with the receptors (26). TRADD (TNFα)- and FADD (FasL)-mediated (induced) apoptosis was found to be inhibited by crmA (a poxvirus gene product of the serpin family), which encodes a specific inhibitor of ICE, and by the specific tetrapeptide ICE inhibitors (32). Thus, ICE might play an important role in apoptosis induced by these ligands. In addition, Bcl-2, baculovirus p35 protein and p53 are also able to down-regulate TNFα- or FasL-induced apoptosis (26). These data indicate that apotosis mediated through the TNF family of receptors might utilize certain intracellular pathways common for PCD. In addition, the TNF family receptors can couple ligand binding to induction of tyrosine and serine/threonine phosphorylation, and sphingomyelinase activation (33–35). The latter was shown to lead to generation of ceramides, potent intracellular mediators of a variety of biological responses, including cell differentiation (via NF-kB), cell-cycle arrest (via c-myc) and apoptosis (via phospholipase D, PLD) (36). These findings illustrate the complexity and still incomplete understanding of signal transduction and its regulation leading to apoptosis induced by the TNF family ligands.

Biological role of the TNF family ligands

Expression of the TNF family of ligands and their receptors appears to be tissue (cell) type dependent and cell differentiation (development)/activation dependent (25,26). Whereas the ligands are almost exclusively expressed by cells of the immune system, the receptors have a much wider distribution, and are expressed with certain variability not only by the immune cells but also by a variety of cells in different tissues and at different stages of differentiation (25,26). Thus, cellular response to the TNF family ligands might depend not only on the type of interacting ligands and receptors but also on the type of target tissues (cells) and their differentiation/activation stage. Consequently, the TNF family of ligands are involved in a variety of physiological and pathophysiological processes, including cell differentiation and tissue development, anti-viral and anti-tumour defence, self-tolerance, costimulation in immune responses, immunoregulation and inflammatory responses (25,26,37). These cytokines also have an important ability to induce apoptotic death in tumour cells (25,26,28–31,37). Thus, certain members of the TNF family of ligands might have a significant role in the immunosurveillance of newly appearing malignant cells as well as in anti-tumour defense. As NK cells have been considered as the major constitutive effectors of these immune functions, it is possible that they express and utilize the TNF family of cytotoxic ligands.

Expression of the TNF family of ligands by NK cells and corresponding receptors by tumour cells

It has been shown that activated NK cells express membrane-bound and/or secrete several of the TNF family of ligands, including TNFα, LTα, LT$\alpha 1\beta 2$ and FasL, and are capable of inducing lysis of TNFα-sensitive and some Fas$^+$ targets in prolonged cytotoxicity assays (1,38–40). In contrast to the induced expression, constitutive expression of these cytotoxic ligands on NK cells has not been established. Recent studies have indicated that non-activated mouse NK cells express functional membrane-bound FasL and can kill Fas$^+$ thymocytes from normal mice and Fas transfectants upon a prolonged coincubation (41,42). More recently, we have performed extensive studies examining constitutive expression of the TNF family of ligands on human NK cells and corresponding receptors on tumour cells (8,43–45). We demonstrated by RT-PCR and flow cytometry that freshly isolated, highly purified (≥95% $CD3^-CD56^+$), non-activated human peripheral blood NK cells constitutively express the TNFα, LT$\alpha\beta$ and FasL mRNAs and cell surface proteins. The levels of expression of the ligands by NK cells from different donors showed substantial variations. On the other hand, various solid tissue-derived tumour cell lines showed simultaneous expression of the several corresponding cell surface receptors, including TNFR1, TNFR2, LTβR and Fas. However, the levels of expression of different receptors varied in different tumour cell lines. In contrast to solid tissue-derived tumour cell lines, leukaemia cell lines showed expression of one or none of these receptors. These findings demonstrated that NK cells and solid tissue-derived tumour cells express complementary sets of cell surface bound ligands and receptors, respectively, that can potentially interact and mediate apoptotic death in targets.

NK-cell membrane-mediated apoptotic cell death

To relate the above-described findings to a particular cytotoxic function of NK cells, we next examined whether freshly isolated, non-activated, highly purified human peripheral blood NK cells can directly induce not only the well-known necrotic death but also apoptotic death in tumour cells, and whether they can do so in the absence of secretory function (46). To this end, we simultaneously used several cytotoxicity assays selective for either necrotic (4 h ^{51}Cr release assay and TEM) or apoptotic (1 h [^{3}H]-thymidine release or terminal deoxynucleotidyl transferase (TdT)-mediated dUTP nick end labelling (TUNEL) assays, and TEM) cell death. NK cells used as effector cells were either untreated or pre-treated with calcium chelators (EDTA and EGTA) or mild fixation (10 min exposure to 1% paraformaldehyde), to eliminate their secretory activities. These treatments were shown to completely abrogate NK-cell BLT-esterase release induced by PMA (secretion of granzyme A), lysis of sheep red blood cells in the presence of specific antibodies (secretion of perforin), IL-2-induced secretion of TNFα and IFNγ, and necrotic killing of K562 (granule release and secretion of both perforin and granzymes). A large variety of normal cell types (7) and transformed cell lines (28) of either haematopoietic or solid tissue origin, either NK sensitive or NK resistant, were used as target cells. We showed that, whereas untreated NK cells were able to induce necrosis (i.e. cell swelling, rupture of cell membrane, and ^{51}Cr release) only in K562 leukaemia cell targets, both untreated NK cells and NK cells treated with calcium chelators or fixed with paraformaldehyde were fully capable of inducing a rapid and significant apoptosis (i.e. cell shrinking, chromatin condensation, and DNA fragmentation detected by dUTP binding and [^{3}H]-thymidine release) in all 25 solid tissue-derived tumour cell lines tested in this study. The apoptotic pathway of killing mediated by NK cells was effective against a variety of tumour cell targets, including gliomas, melanomas, squamous cell carcinomas of the head and neck, breast carcinomas, lung squamous cell carcinomas, lung small cell carcinomas as well as gastric, colon, renal cell and ovarian carcinomas (46). However, this pathway was ineffective against leukaemia cell lines, including K562, and normal cells of haematopoietic origin (46). NK cells showed an inconsistent and low level of this type of killing against normal solid tissue-derived targets. In addition, fixed NK cells showed similar apoptotic killing ability as untreated NK cells. The ability of fixed (i.e. not alive) NK cells to effectively induce apoptosis in tumour cell targets suggests that, in this type of killing, an active involvement (i.e. receptor signalling, motility and secretion) of NK cells does not take place, and, thus, an active participation of target cells via their receptor-induced suicidal mechanisms is likely. In our further analyses a positive correlation between the susceptibility of target cells to this type of NK-cell killing and expression of the TNF family receptors on these targets could be established. Therefore, it is possible that the apoptotic mechanism of killing might be mediated by the interactions between membrane-bound cytotoxic ligands on NK cells and corresponding receptors on targets.

Role of the membrane-bound TNF family of ligands in apoptotic killing by NK cells

To directly test the possibility that NK cells induce apoptosis in tumour cells by utilizing the membrane-bound TNF family ligands, we employed a variety of neutralizing antibodies and receptor–Fc constructs with the specificity for the TNF family of ligands and their receptors (8,43–45). As discussed above, we observed that coincubation of solid tissue-derived tumour cell lines with NK cells inducted rapid DNA fragmentation, as measured in 1 h [^{3}H]-thymidine release assays. Using three different solid tissue-derived human tumour cell lines (i.e. BT-20 breast carcinoma, LS-174 colon carcinoma and OVCAR-3 ovarian carcinoma) as targets, the NK cell-induced DNA fragmentation was shown to be inhibited significantly and to a similar extent by the pretreatment of effector cells either with anti-TNFα or anti-LTα neutralizing antibodies, or with TNFR–Fc or LTβR–Fc constructs. Similar effects were obtained by the preincubation of target cells with either anti-TNFR1, anti-TNFR2 or anti-Fas blocking antibodies. In addition, the levels of this inhibition varied depending on the levels and multiplicity of the TNF family receptors expressed on tumour cell targets. Furthermore, while coincubation of tumour cells with either recombinant TNFα, LTα or FasL was without appreciative cytotoxic effect, the combined treatment with either TNFα plus FasL or LTα plus FasL induced a rapid DNA fragmentation. These data showed that rapid non-secretory/apoptotic killing of tumour cells by NK cells is signalled by simultaneous ligation of the several TNF family receptors expressed on targets by the corresponding cytotoxic ligands expressed on the effector cells (Fig. 34.1B). It seems that at least two different simultaneous signals coming from NK cell membrane are a minimal requirement for the rapid induction of apoptosis in tumour cells.

SUMMARY

NK cells are 'professional' cytotoxic effector cells of the immune system which have spontaneous ability to selectively kill virus-infected and tumour cells without damaging normal cells. Recent studies have shown that cytotoxic functions of NK cells are mediated and regulated by several different multigene families of cell membrane receptors and ligands (Fig. 34.1). Engagement of appropriate receptors on effector or target cells by corresponding ligands on target or effector cells, respectively, can induce signal transduction in either of the participants, leading to activation of two different antitumour cytotoxic pathways: i.e. secretory/necrotic and non-secretory/apoptotic. The type and range of target cells susceptible to these killing mechanisms mediated by NK cells appear to be different. Whereas the classic secretory/necrotic killing mechanism can induce cell death in only a few leukaemia cell lines, the non-secretory/apoptotic pathway can kill a large variety of solid tissue-derived tumour cell targets. The novel pathway is mediated by the TNF family ligands and is highly promiscuous. It may, therefore, be potentially important in immune surveillance, antimetastatic/antitumour functions and immunoregulation.

ACKNOWLEDGEMENTS

This research was supported in part by American Cancer Society grants IM-713 (NLV) and IM-696 (TLW), NIH grant RO1-CA63513 (TLW) and the Pathology, Education and Research Foundation, Pittsburgh, PA.

REFERENCES

1. Berke, G. 1994. The binding and lysis of target cells by cytotoxic lymphocytes: Molecular and cellular aspects. *Annu. Rev. Immunol.* **12**:735–73.
2. Trinchieri, G. 1989. Biology of natural killer cells. *Adv. Immunol.* **47**:187–376.
3. Rosenberg, S. A. and M. T. Lotze. 1986. Cancer immunotherapy using interleukin-2 and interleukin-2-activated lymphocytes. *Annu. Rev. Immunol.* **4**:681–709.
4. Yannelli, J. R., C. Hyatt, S. McConnell *et al.* 1996. Growth of tumor-infiltrating

lymphocytes from human solid cancers: summary of a 5-year experience. *Int. J. Cancer* **65**:413–21.
5. Vujanovic, N. L., R. B. Herberman, A. A. Maghazachi and J. C. Hiserodt. 1988. Lymphokine-activated killer cells in rats. III. A simple method for the purification of large granular lymphocytes and their rapid expansion and conversion into lymphokine-activated killer cells. *J. Exp. Med.* **67**:15–29.
6. Rosenberg, S. A., J. R. Yanelly, J. C. Yang *et al.* 1994. Treatment of patients with metastatic melanoma with autologous tumor infiltrating lymphocytes and interleukin 2. *J. Natl. Cancer. Inst.* **86**:1159–66.
7. Whiteside, T. L. and R. B. Herberman. 1995. The role of natural killer cells in immune surveillance of cancer. *Curr. Opin. Immunol.* **7**:704–10.
8. Vujanovic, N. L., P. Basse, R. B. Herberman and T. L. Whiteside. 1996. Antitumor functions of natural killer cells and control of metastases. METHODS: A Comparison to Methods in Enzymology **9**:394–408.
9. Henkart, P. 1986. Mechanism of NK-cell mediated cytotoxicity. In: *Cancer Immunology: Innovative Approaches to Therapy* (R. B. Herberman, ed.) Martinus Nijhoff Publishers, Boston, pp. 123–50.
10. Chambers, W. H. and C. S. Brissette-Storkus. 1995. Hanging in the balance: natural killer cell recognition of target cells. *Chem. Biol.* **2**:429–35.
11. Lanier, L. L. and J. H. Phillips. 1996. Inhibitory MHC class I receptors on NK and T cells. *Immunol. Today* **17**:86–91.
12. Bezouska, K., G. Vlahas, O. Horvath. 1994. Rat natural killer cell antigen, NKR-P1, related to C-type animal lectins is a carbohydrate-binding protein. *J. Biol. Chem.* **269**:16 945–52.
13. Bezuska, K., C.-T. Yuen, J. O'Brien *et al.* 1994. Oligosaccharide ligands for NKR-PL protein activate NK cells and cytotoxicity. *Nature* **372**:150–7.
14. Liebson, P. J. 1995. Viewpoint: Signal transduction during natural killer cell activation. *Nat. Immun.* **14**:117–22.
15. Yokoyama, W. M. and W. E. Seaman. 1993. The Ly-49 and NKR-P1 gene families encoding lectin-like receptors on natural killer cells. The NK gene complex. *Annu. Rev. Immunol.* **11**:613–35.
16. Burkhardt, J. K., S. Hester, C. K. Lapham and Y. Argon. 1990. The lytic granules of natural killer cells are dual-function organelles combining secretory and pre-lysosomal compartments. *J. Cell. Biol.* **111**:2327–40.
17. Liu, C.-C., C. M. Walsh and J. D.-E. Young, 1995. Perforin: structure and function. *Immunol. Today* **16**:192–201.
18. Henkart, P. A. 1994. Lymphocyte-mediated cytotoxicity: Two pathways and multiple effector molecules. *Immunity* **1**:343–6.
19. Podack, E. R. 1995. Functional significance of two cytolytic pathways of cytotoxic T lymphocytes. *J. Leuk. Biol.* **57**:548–52.
20. Berke, G. 1995. The CTL's kiss of death. *Cell* **81**:9–12.
21. Welsh, C. M., M. Matloubian, C.-C. Liu *et al.* 1994. Immune function in mice lacking the perforin gene. *Proc. Natl. Acad. Sci. USA* **91**:10 854–8.
22. Smith, M. J. and J. A. Trapani. 1995. Granzymes: exogenous proteinases that induce target cell apoptosis. *Immunol. Today* **16**:202–6.
23. Heusel, J. W., R. L. Wesseischmidt, S. Shresta *et al.* 1994. Cytotoxic lymphocytes require granzyme B for the rapid induction of DNA fragmentation and apoptosis in allogeneic target cells. *Cell* **76**:977–87.
24. Irmler, M., S. Hertig, H. R. MacDonald *et al.* 1995. Granzyme A is an interleukin 1β-converting enzyme. *J. Exp. Med.* **181**:1017–22.
25. Beutler, B. and C. van Huffel. 1994. Unraveling function in the TNF ligand and receptor families. *Science* **264**:667–8.

26. Smith, C. A., T. Farrah and R. G. Goodwin. 1994. The TNF receptor superfamily of cellular and viral proteins: activation, costimulation, and death. *Cell* **76**:959–69.
27. Kayagaki, N., A. Kawasaki, T. Ebata *et al.* 1995. Metalloproteinase-mediated release of human Fas ligand. *J. Exp. Med.* **182**:1777–83.
28. Cleveland, J. L. and J. N. Ihle. 1995. Contenders in Fas/TNF death signaling. *Cell* **81**:479–82.
29. Hess, S. and H. Engelmann. 1996. A novel function of CD40: Induction of cell death in transformed cells. *J. Exp. Med.* **183**:159–67.
30. Browning, J. L., K. Miatkowski, I. Sizing *et al.* 1996. Signaling through the lymphotoxin-β receptor induces the death of some adenocarcinoma tumor lines. *J. Exp. Med.* (in press).
31. Wiley, S. R., K. Schooley, P. J. Smolak. 1995. Identification and characterization of a new member of the TNF family that induces apoptosis. *Immunity* **3**:673–82.
32. Tewari, M. and V. M. Dixit. 1995. Fas- and tumor necrosis factor-induced apoptosis is inhibited by the poxovirus crmA gene product. *J. Biol. Chem.* **270**:3255–60.
33. Tian, Q., J.-L. Taupin, S. Elledge *et al.* 1995. Fas-activated serin/threonine kinase (FAST) phosphorylates TIA-1 during fas-mediated apoptosis. *J. Exp. Med.* **182**:865–74.
34. Kim, M.-Y., C. Linardic, L. Obeid and Y. Hannun. 1991. Identification of sphingomyelin turnover as an effector mechanism for the action of tumor necrosis factor α and γ-interferon. Specific role in cell differentiation. *J. Biol. Chem.* **266**:484–9.
35. Cifone, M. G., R. De Maria, P. Roncaioli *et al.* 1993. Apoptotic signalling through CD95 (Fas/Apo-1) activates an acidic sphingomyelinase. *J. Exp. Med.* **177**:1547–52.
36. Pushkareva, M., L. M. Obeid and Y. A. Hannun. 1995. Ceramide: an endogenous regulator of apoptosis and growth suppression. *Immunol. Today* **16**:294–7.
37. Lynch, D. H., F. Ramsdell and M. R. Alderson. 1995. FasL in the homeostatic regulation of immune responses. *Immunol. Today* **16**:569–73.
38. Ware, C. F., P. D. Crowe, M. H. Grayson *et al.* 1992. Expression of surface lymphotoxin and TNF on activated T, B and NK cells. *J. Immunol.* **149**:3881–8.
39. Vitolo, D., N. L. Vujanovic, H. Rabinowich *et al.* 1993. Rapid IL-2-induced adherence of human natural killer cells. Expression of mRNA for cytokines and IL-2 receptors in adherent NK cells. *J. Immunol.* **151**:1926–37.
40. Miyake, M., A. Horiuchi, K. Kimura *et al.* 1992. Correlation between killing activity towards the murine L929 cell line and expression of membrane-associated lymphotoxin-related molecule of human lymphokine-activated killer cells. *Eur. J. Immunol.* **22**:2174–52.
41. Montel, A. H., M. R. Bochan, J. A. Hobbs *et al.* 1995. Fas involvement in cytotoxicity mediated by human NK cells. *Cell. Immun.* **166**:236–46.
42. Arase, H., N. Arase and T. Saito. 1995. Fas-mediated cytotoxicity by freshly isolated natural killer cells. *J. Exp. Med.* **181**:1235–8.
43. Vujanovic, N. L., S. Nagashima, R. B. Herberman and T. L. Whiteside. 1995. A novel mechanism of direct killing utilized by human resting NK cells against malignant cells. *FASEB J.* A1022.
44. Vujanovic, N. L., S. Nagashima, R. B. Herberman and T. L. Whiteside. 1995. Apoptotic killing of tumor cells by human resting natural killer cells. *Abstract*

Book of the 9th International Congress of Immunology, San Francisco, California, p. 777.

45. Vujanovic, N. L., S. Nagashima, Y. Kashii *et al*. 1996. Constitutive expression of the TNF family ligands by human natural killer cells and their utilization in apoptotoic killing. Manuscript in preparation.
46. Vujanovic, N. L., S. Nagashima, R. B. Herberman and T. L. Whiteside. 1996. Non-secretory apoptotic killing by human natural killer cells. *J. Immunol.* **157**:1117–26.

35

MHC and Other Antigens at the Feto-maternal Interface

Marighoula Varla-Leftherioti

THE IMPORTANCE OF STUDYING FETAL ANTIGENIC EXPRESSION

The paradox of the survival of the semiallogeneic fetus in the uterus is a problem, and its answer would not only be of interest for understanding physiological and pathological pregnancies, but could also result in new approaches to infertility, to immunosuppression in transplantation and to tumour immunotherapy. Studies on fetal antigenic expression contribute to obtaining such an answer, and have attracted the interest of scientists since early in this century. The initial approaches started in the 1920s, when it was suggested that the embryo has no definite physiological characteristics individual enough to be recognized by the mother. For many years afterwards, there was little activity in this field apart from studies that tended to refute the above hypothesis by furnishing evidence of the effective antigenecity of embryonic and fetal tissues. In the 1950s, transplant immunologists focused on this central immunological enigma and a series of possible explanations for the embryo's survival appeared (antigenic immaturity of fetal tissues, immunological incompetence of the mother, immunologically privileged nature of the uterus, presence of an anatomical barrier inhibiting either the afferent or the efferent arm of the maternal immune response) (1,2). After 1980, proposed mechanisms for the survival of the fetus became more precise:

- the immunological barrier was localized at the feto-maternal interface (failure to express or masking of paternal alloantigens)
- inhibition of maternal alloreactivity was attributed to decidual factors under hormonal control
- the detection of immunosuppressive cells, antibodies and other specific and non-specific factors of fetal or maternal origin started (3–9).

In all classic studies the maternal immune mechanisms were considered

Immunoregulation in Health and Disease
ISBN 0-12-459460-3

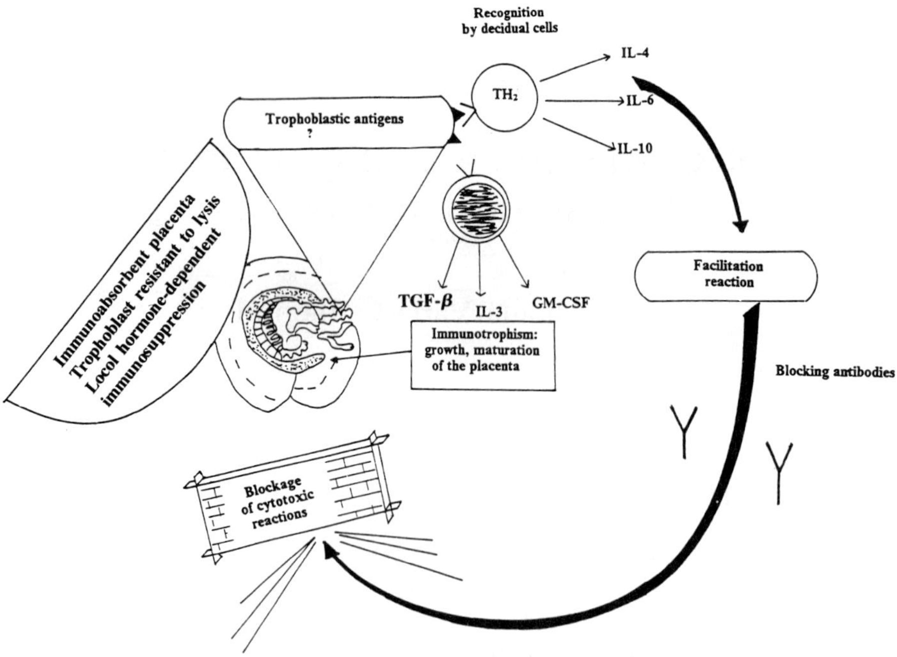

Fig. 35.1. Possible mechanisms for fetal survival.

as potentially harmful for the fetus, but progress in knowledge of the immunocompetent cells and tissue growth factors led scientists to investigate the hypothesis that the maternal immune response is favourable for the embryo's growth and survival (10). Data for establishing this hypothesis had come from both experimental (11,12) and clinical studies and mainly from cases of recurrent spontaneous abortions, where it was shown that, when women were immunized with their partner's lymphocytes, they had successful pregnancies (13,14). The explanation was that their immune response was stimulated by paternal alloantigens expressed on lymphocytes, which are also found on fetal tissues but, for some reason, they do not provide enough stimulus for the enhancing maternal response (15–17).

Today, it is accepted that, for a successful pregnancy, fetal antigens must be recognized by local (at the fetal–maternal interface) maternal cells of the Th2 type, which secrete anti-inflammatory cytokines, such as IL-4 and IL-10, and the classical cellular 'rejection response' is diverted to an enhancing, humoral 'facilitating response' (18,19). Produced antibodies block harmful reactions, while other local maternal cells secrete other cytokines (IL-3, GM-CSF, TGFβ), which promote growth and maturation of the placenta (20,21) (Fig. 35.1).

So, the survival of the fetus is dependent on fetal–maternal interactions

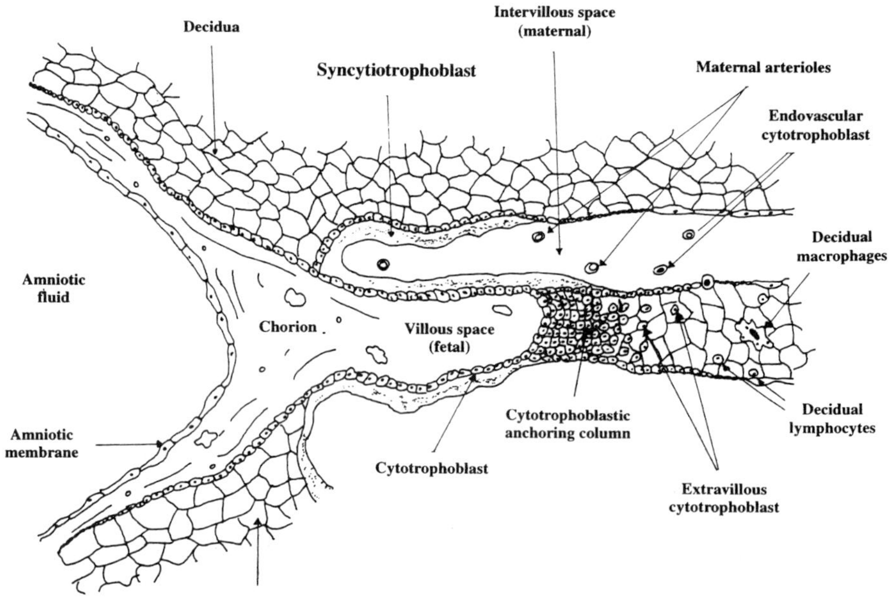

Fig. 35.2. Decidual–trophoblastic interface.

and it is obviously important to know the nature of the antigens which are recognized by the mother in the feto-maternal interface, as this recognition initiates the enhancing response.

FETO-MATERNAL INTERFACE

Throughout most of pregnancy, there is a complicated type of maternal–fetal contact in the placenta, which is formed by fetal (amnion and chorion) and maternal tissues (decidua) (22) (Fig. 35.2). The last layer of the placental fetal tissues, which is in contact with the maternal decidua, is trophoblast. So, the embryo and its extraembryonic envelope allow the maternal cells to encounter just one type of tissue: the trophoblast (materno-trophoblastic interface or decidual–trophoblastic interface). The trophoblast also lines fetal placental villi and forms a direct interface with maternal blood. Chorionic villi are covered by two layers: the outer layer, which faces the maternal component, is the syncytiotrophoblast, a non-mitotic covering, which consists of individual cells but matures into an acellular syncytium. This layer also lines the intervillous blood spaces. Beneath the syncytiotrophoblast is the cytotrophoblast, which is more metabolically active and pushes the syncytiotrophoblast, helping to join the villi to the maternal tissue.

Some cytotrophoblast cells push through the syncytiotrophoblast to make cytotrophoblast columns that help to join the villi to the maternal tissue, being in direct tissue contact with the maternal uterine decidual tissue. Also, some cytotrophoblastic cells migrate into the myometrium (extravillous cytotrophoblast) or invade the spiral arteries of the uterus (endovascular trophoblast) (23,24).

To study maternal immunological recognition of the fetus, we have to know antigenic expression of the trophoblast in its contact to maternal tissues, that is syncytiotrophoblast and extravillous cytotrophoblast.

TROPHOBLAST ANTIGENIC EXPRESSION

Whether the trophoblast–decidual interface contains parental transplantation antigens or other antigens that could initiate an alloimmune response has been the most important point in investigating the immunological paradox of pregnancy. A series of studies has shown expression of molecules of different antigenic systems on trophoblastic tissues, including MHC antigens, antigens of the erythrocyte blood groups, complement regulatory proteins, Fc receptors, isoenzymes, adhesion molecules, etc. (25,26). These antigens are presented here, with emphasis on those of them that fulfil the criteria for allorecognition and initiation of an alloimmune response, that is the ones that are polymorphic and present on trophoblastic tissues in direct contact with maternal tissue.

Antigens of the major histocompatibility complex (MHC)

Initial studies examining the reactivity of HLA antisera with human extraembryonic cells have not shown reactivity with either cytotrophoblast or syncytioptrophoblast (27,28). The use of monoclonal HLA antibodies has revealed no reaction for class II antigens, while class I binding concerned cytotrophoblast, which was found positive with some but not all monoclonals (mAb w6/32$^+$, mAb 61D2$^-$ (29–31). Next, by Southern blot and in situ hybridization techniques, HLA class I mRNA was detected in isolated cytotrophoblastic but not in syncytiotrophoblastic cells (32). The conclusion from all these studies was that trophoblastic cells regulate HLA class I expression differently from other types of cells, and it was accepted that MHC are not expressed on syncytiotrophoblast although they are expressed on cytotrophoblast. However, it was not clear if the message in cytotrophoblast arises from classical or non-classical HLA genes.

Our knowledge concerning the exact nature of cytotrophoblast HLA antigens is recent, following the discovery that MHC class I region has more genes than those responsible for the known, A, B, C products (33). Three non-classical class I loci were identified: HLA-E, HLA-F and HLA-G. Genes

E, F and G have very high homologies with classical HLA class I genes but they are truncated and they have a restricted tissue distribution and very low polymorphism. HLA-E and HLA-G molecules are present on the cell surface, while HLA-F appears rather as a cytoplasmic protein (34). They are all present on some choriocarcinomas; HLA-E and HLA-F are more confined to lymphoid cells and the distribution of HLA-G is more limited to tissues of fetal and/or embryonic origin (35,36).

HLA-E appears to have the widest distribution among those non-classical HLA genes. HLA-E mRNA is present in many tissues and has also been detected in human placenta villous cytotrophoblast and in vitro differentiated syncytiotrophoblast isolated from term placenta (37–39). HLA-E mRNA was clearly identified only in small round cells present in first-trimester decidua and term membranes (40). However, no cell surface expression of HLA-E has been demonstrated on trophoblast cells. For the cytoplasmic HLA-F, things are more complicated and, although HLA-F transcripts in human placenta have been shown by an RNase protection technique, our knowledge is very limited (37).

HLA-G appears to have a more limited distribution than HLA-E, but it is nevertheless the most important because its distribution is mainly to trophoblastic tissues. Other than trophoblast, various other embryonic and adult tissues have been found to transcribe HLA-G (ex fetal liver, heart, lung and kidney, adult keratinocytes, eye, peripheral blood leukocytes, spleen, thymus, liver, kidney, skin, prostate, testicle, ovary, small intestine, colon) (34,41,42). It is of interest that HLA-G is expressed in the anterior eye, which is recognized as an immune privileged site like placenta. This observation supports the hypothesis that HLA-G is involved in inducing immune tolerance.

The HLA-G gene is composed of eight exons, encoding a signal peptide, extracellular, transmembrane and cytoplasmic domains. HLA-G sequences are highly conserved in humans but not among different species into the same extent as the classical antigens. HLA-G differs from classical class I because a large part of the cytoplasmic domain (24 of the 30 amino acids) is not translated. Owing to this lack of translation, HLA-G cytoplasmic tail has lost a serine in position 336, a potential site of phosphorylation. Six different HLA-G transcriptional isoforms have been described. Four of them encode membrane-bound products: HLA-G1, which is the full-length isoform with three external domains, HLA-G2 with splicing out of exon 3 (the $\alpha 2$ domain is missing), HLA-G3 with splicing out of exons 3 and 4 (the $\alpha 2$ and $\alpha 3$ domains are missing) and HLA-G4 with splicing out of exon 4 (the $\alpha 3$ domain is missing). Two other transcripts contain part of intron 4: G1s, which encodes the soluble form of G1, and G2s or G6, which encodes a soluble product of G2 lacking the $\alpha 2$ domain (33,43).

The presence of the different HLA-G transcriptional isoforms has been shown in the first-trimester and term villous and extravillous cytotrophoblast cells, placental villous mesenchymal cells in first trimester, as well as in term amnion cells. In contrast, very low or no levels of specific HLA-G messages were detected in the syncytiotrophoblast (34,39,40,43). HLA-G transcripts are present in quite significant amounts in the extravillous membranes of first-trimester placenta, while the opposite relationship occurs at term (40). This seems to be important because, conversely, class I classical MHC genes are only slightly expressed in the first-trimester placenta and their activity increases up to the stage of the term placenta (37).

By use of polyclonal and monoclonal HLA-G antibodies that have recently been described, HLA-G was detected on several transfectants and cell lines (44,45). McMaster *et al.*, using monoclonal antibodies, showed that on first- and second-trimester placental tissue sections, HLA-G was expressed only on extravillous cytotrophoblast cells that derive from anchoring villi and invade the uterus and blood vessels (45). Third-trimester placental tissue sections exhibited the same pattern but cytotrophoblast within the uterine wall stained less brightly. Although HLA-G transcripts were also found in other human tissues, extravillous cytrotrophoblast cells from first-trimester placenta appear to be the only cell type in which HLA-G is translated and expressed on the cell surface. This strongly suggests the involvement of a highly cell type- and stage-specific post-transcriptional regulation. Very little is known about molecular regulatory mechanisms that control expression of HLA-G in the human placenta. According to the cell type and time of gestation, HLA-G expression may be regulated at the levels of transcription, translation and/or transport to the cell membrane. Positive constitutive transcriptional regulatory mechanisms are operating in extravillous cytotrophoblast cells. In villous cytotrophoblast, HLA-G is transcribed and translated but not expressed and many post-transcriptional regulatory mechanisms are involved. In syncytiotrophoblast, HLA-G transcripts are not translated and thus transcriptional repressor mechanisms are likely to occur (46).

The role of non-classical MHC antigens in pregnancy is an open question as there are somewhat conflicting theories on their function. They are found at rather low levels at the cell surface and they have very limited (or absent) polymorphism which does not allow them to present a large set of peptides. Most of the discussions and speculations concern HLA-G gene and its isoforms. Its differential expression in extraembryonic tissues, dependent on the stage of pregnancy and different from that of classical HLA class I genes, implies that it plays an important role at the feto-maternal interface, thus influencing the outcome of pregnancy. If it has to be considered as an alloantigen recognized on fetal tissues by the mother in order for her to develop an immune response, polymorphism must exist for its alloimmunogenicity. Such a polymorphism seems to exist, since, although HLA-G was at first thought to be monomorphic, recent studies started to show different HLA-G alleles, being in linkage disequilibrium with HLA-A, and to suggest that nearly all individuals are heterozygous for them (47–49). Sequence variations concern α1- and α2-domains and polymorphism is, thus, located in the peptide binding region (50).

The possible (proposed) roles of HLA-G during pregnancy are:

- It has been demonstrated that the CD8 α/α homodimer can recognize and bind to HLA-G expressed by a lymphoblastoid cell line (LCL.221) transfectant (51). Perhaps, then, HLA-G can serve as a recognition element by suppressor cells which are $CD8^+$ and thus prevent rejection of the fetus.
- Although contradictory data have been obtained, it is hypothesized that HLA-G can reduce lytic activity by IL-2-activated NK (52–54). The same can exist for T cells bearing $\gamma\delta$ receptors (present in decidua), which have been found to bind to G (55).
- HLA-G may stimulate the decidual lymphocytes to produce either positive or negative acting cytokines that mediate either growth and activation or suppression of other cells in the microenvironment of the placenta. It is possible that aberrations in the HLA-G gene may affect placental growth, and missense mutations in the α2-domain were found in neonates with idiopathic intrauterine growth (50).
- HLA-G may mediate placenta-localized immune responses that protect the fetus from infection. Recent evidence that both the membrane-bound and soluble forms of HLA-G have a motif for binding endogenous peptides (56) makes it possible that they can present viral peptides to TCR and lysis of infected trophoblast cells may prevent spread of the infection in the placenta.
- Soluble HLA-G α chain may suppress maternal cytotoxic T cells by binding directly to TCR and inhibiting its interaction with MHC/peptide complex on a target cell (52).

Complement-regulatory proteins

In initial studies, McIntyre *et al.* immunized rabbits with human trophoblast and antisera were developed which recognized antigens on the trophoblast that differed between individuals and which could be fitted into several groups (57,58). The same antisera reacted also with lymphocytes from the parents who gave rise to the placenta, in particular, with the father. This led to the concept of a paternally derived trophoblast-lymphocyte cross-reactive antigen (TLX) and also to the hypothesis that an immune response by the mother may facilitate successful pregnancy through a variety of mechanisms including immunosuppression and blocking of recognition of trophoblast by potentially aggressive maternal lymphocytes (59). It was thought that TLX might be minor histocompatibility antigens and immunization with them results in protection of the blastocysts. It was also suggested that TLX may be in linkage with MHC in such a way that incompatibilities will stimulate production of blocking antibodies and suppressor cells (28).

In 1986, a monoclonal antibody, H316, was obtained, recognizing structures on human trophoblasts, peripheral blood lymphocytes and some tumour cells including choriocarcinomas (60). It was thought that it was directed to TLX antigens. However, H316 was not alloreactive and did not block MLRs. These results agree with the concept that anti-TLX are not anti-MHC. They hypothesize that all pregnancies generate anti-TLX antibodies which are blocked by anti-idiotypic antibodies (61). More recently, immunochemical analysis of the binding of this monoclonal antibody showed that H316 recognizes CD46, a complement-regulatory protein also called membrane cofactor protein (MCP) or Huly-m5 (62). CD46 is present on a number of cells including trophoblast, sperm and leukocytes (63,64) and is one of the several types of proteins that serve to prevent spontaneous lysis of cells by complement. Although the relationship between TLX and CD46-MCP is not fully understood, it is proposed that the binding of C3b to CD46 induces a conformational change exposing an antigenic TLX epitope (65,66).

CD46 is not the only complement regulatory protein found on trophoblast. Decay-accelerating factor (DAF, CD55) and membrane attack complex-inhibiting factor (CD59) are also found on trophoblast and may protect it from complement lysis. Trophoblast expresses these complement inhibitors exclusively to sites of direct contact with maternal blood tissues at the feto-maternal interface (67). So, they may function specifically to inhibit amplification convertases formed at this site either directly or indirectly as a result of maternal complement activation (direct by the alloantigens, indirect after a response to infections). Thus, they may have an important role in protecting semi-allogeneic human conceptus from maternal C-mediated attack (68). This protective function seems to be the only mechanism which is clear among all other mechanisms underlying the relationship between mother and the fetus and shows that the embryo contributes directly to its own survival in the pregnant uterus. Another important point is that the above complement-regulatory proteins are expressed throughout the female genital tract and may protect the transversing sperm and implanting blastocyst from complement-mediated damage (69). As cells deficient in these regulatory molecules may be more susceptible to lysis by antibody plus complement, if there were deficient embryos, they would possibly die very early, never surviving to be detected as a pregnancy (26).

Although the contribution of the complement regulatory proteins in the protection of the embryo by the inhibition of complement activation is clear, their role in initiating an alloimmune response is difficult to justify. Polymorphism, which is not required for them to function as complement inhibitors, but which is needed for alloantigenicity, does not exist in all of them. CD46 appears to be the only one exhibiting a degree of polymorphism. RFLP analysis of the CD46 gene has shown polymorphic bands, which occur significantly less frequently in women having recurrent spontaneous abortion who also show increased sharing of TLX antigens with their partners (70,57). Thus, TLX may fulfil the criteria as a potential of alloantigenic system, stimulating the mother for an immune response, where enhancing factors are developed in the same time that possibly harmful anti-TLX antibodies are blocked by anti-idiotypic antibodies.

Other antigens expressed on trophoblast

Erythrocyte blood group antigens

Antigens of the ABO blood group system are not expressed by human trophoblast. On extravillous trophoblast in normal and molar pregnancies and in choricarcinoma tumour cells, the sialyl-Le^X antigen has been found, which, after neuraminidase treatment, becomes the Le^X itself (71). A possible role of this carbohydrate antigen could be the protection of trophoblast from NK lysis.

Rh-D factor is present on plasma membrane and cytoplasm of the villous trophoblasts (72). However, since Rh sensitization is known to occur at delivery, it seems that the presence of Rh alloantigens on the trophoblast is not sufficient for an immune response.

Placental-specific alkaline phosphatase

A placental isoenzyme of alkaline phosphatase (PLAP) is found on syncytiotrophoblast but not on most other cytotrophoblast cells. It is polymorphic but maternal immunity to this antigen has never been shown. Besides, it appears after the first trimester and thus it makes it unlikely to initiate the maternal immune response (73,74).

Fc receptors for IgG

Fc receptors are present in the placenta but their importance is questionable since Fc receptor blocking antibodies are not found in all normal pregnancies (75). Their role presumably relates to the transplacental passage of maternal IgG.

Adhesion molecules and cytokine receptors

Several adhesion molecules and cytokine receptors are expressed on trophoblast cells and they are probably involved in interactions between the trophoblast and the local environment.

Trophoblastic adhesion molecules undergo a dramatic alteration during normal cytotrophoblast differentiation along the invasive pathway in vivo (76). A delicate balance of adhesive interactions normally permits cytotrophoblast invasion. Migrating-invasive trophoblast cells bear integrins such $\alpha5/\beta1$ which binds fibronectin (stimulation of trophoblast migration) and lack integrins such as $\alpha3/\beta1$ which binds laminin (inhibition of trophoblast migration) (77). Some other adhesion molecules are not expressed on trophoblastic cells and their absence is also important: intercellular adhesion molecule-1 (ICAM-1) is not expressed on endovascular cytotrophoblast normally, but it appears in abnormal pregnancies, as happens with DR antigens (78).

Receptors for cytokines produced by decidual cells (CSF-1, TGFβ) and possibly responsible for changing the differentiation stage of trophoblast, are also present on trophoblastic cells and may be important in regulating placental growth (26).

The R80K protein

R80K is a highly polymorphic protein alloantigen present on the microvesicles prepared from human term placental syncytiotrophoblast, to which the mother produces an immune response (79). The antigen is also expressed by the father's lymphocytes and immunization of a woman lacking the antibody with her partner's lymphocytes generates it. R80K is very immunogenic and covered with antibody in successful pregnancies, since IgG was found to bind it on the syncytiotrophoblast of all term placentas studied (80). Consequently, it is a possible candidate for being the recognition antigen on the trophoblast, but so far we do not know whether it is present on first-trimester trophoblast.

CONCLUSIONS

We now have a better knowledge of the antigens expressed on trophoblast. However, no final answer has yet been given as to which of the antigen(s) expressed in the feto-maternal interface initiates the facilitating pregnancy response. New evidence on this antigenic expression is found every day, and it remains to prove how it assures fetal survival.

REFERENCES

1. Medawar, P. B. 1953. Some immunological and endocrinological problems raised by the evolution of viviparity in vertebrates. *Symp. Soc. Exp. Biol.* **7**: 320–38.
2. Simmons, R. L. and P. S. Russel. 1962. The antigenicity of mouse trophoblast. *Ann. NY Acad. Sci.* **99**:717–32.

3. Beer, A. E. and R. E. Billingham. 1980. Mechanisms of non-rejection of fetal–placental allografts. *Folia Biol.* **26**:225–43.
4. Lala, P. K., S. Chatterjee-Hasrouni, M. Kearns *et al.* 1983. Immunobiology of the feto-maternal interface. *Immunol. Rev.* **75**:87–116.
5. Bell, S. C. and D. Billington. 1983. Anti-fetal allo-antibody in the pregnant female. *Immun. Rev.* **75:**5–30.
6. Daya, S., D. A. Clark, C. Devlin and J. Jarrell. 1985. Preliminary characterization of two types of suppressor cells in the human uterus. *Fertil. Steril.* **44**:778–85.
7. Sargent, I. L. and C. W. G. Redman. 1985. Maternal cell-mediated immunity to the fetus in human pregnancy. *J. Reprod. Immunol.* **7**:95–104.
8. Antczak, D. F. 1989. Maternal antibody responses in pregnancy. *Curr. Opin. Immunol.* **1**:1135–40.
9. Bulmer, J. N. 1989. Decidual cellular responses. *Curr. Opin. Immunol.* **1**:1141–7.
10. Wegman, T. 1984. Foetal protection against abortion: Is it immunosuppression or immunostimulation? *Ann. Immunol. (Inst. Pasteur)* **135**:309–12.
11. Chaouat, G., J.-P. Kolb, N. Kiger *et al.* 1985. Immunologic consequences of vaccination against abortion in mice. *J. Immunol.* **134**:1594–8.
12. Athanassakis, I., C. Bleackley, V. Paetkau *et al.* 1987. The immunostimulatory role of T cells and T cell-derived lymphokines on murine fetally-derived placental cells. *J. Immunol.* **138**:37–44.
13. Taylor, C. and W. P. Faulk. 1981. Prevention of recurrent abortion with leukocyte transfusions. *Lancet* **2**:68–70.
14. Beer, A. E., J. F. Quebberman, J. W. I. Ayers and R. F. Haines. 1981. Major histocompatibility complex antigens, maternal and paternal immune responses and chronic habitual abortion in humans. *Am. J. Obstet. Gynecol.* **141**:987–99.
15. Faulk, W. P. and J. A. McIntyre. 1981. Trophoblast survival. *Transplantation* **31**:1–5.
16. Mowbray, J. F. 1988. Success and failures of immunisation for recurrent spontaneous abortion. In: *Early Pregnancy Loss. Mechanisms and Treatment* (R. W. Beard and F. Saarp, eds.) Peacock Press, Ashton-under-Lyne, pp. 325–31.
17. Carp, H. J. A., V. Toder, S. Mashiach *et al.* 1990. Recurrent miscarriage: A review of current concepts, immune mechanisms and results of treatment. *Obstet. Gynecol. Surv.* **45**:657–69.
18. Wegmann, T. G., H. Lin, L. Guilbert and T. R. Mosmann. 1993. Bidirectional cytokine interactions in the maternal–fetal relationship: is successful pregnancy a TH2 phenomenon? *Immunol. Today* **14**:353–6.
19. Voisin, G. A. and R. Raghuparthy. 1995. Immunodeviation of the immune response during pregnancy. In: *Immunology of Human Reproduction* (M. Kurpisz and N. Fernandez, eds.) BIOS Scientific Publishers, Oxford, pp. 335–49.
20. Wegmann, T. G. 1987. Placental immunotrophism: Maternal T cells enhance placental growth and function. *Am. J. Reprod. Immunol.* **15**:67–9.
21. Wegmann, T. G., I. Athanassakis, L. Guilbert *et al.* 1989. The role of M-CSF and GM-CSF in fostering placental growth, fetal growth, and fetal survival. *Transpl. Proc.* **21**:566–8.
22. Boyd, J. D. and W. J. Hamilton. 1970. *The Human Placenta.* Heffers, Cambridge, England.
23. Pijneborg, R., J. M. Bland, W. B. Robertson and I. Brosens. 1983. Uteroplacental arterial changes related to interstitial trophoblast migration in early human pregnancy. *Placenta* **4**:397–414.
24. Loke, Y. W. and B. H. Butterworth. 1987. Heterogeneity of human trophoblast

populations. In: *Immunoregulation and Fetal Survival* (T. G. Wegmann and T. J. Gill, eds.) Oxford University Press, New York, pp. 197–209.

25. Claman, H. M. 1993. Matero-fetal relationships. Immunological aspects. In: *The Immunology of Human Reproduction* (H. M. Claman, ed.) Humana Press, Totowa, NJ, pp. 51–79.
26. Clark, D. A. 1995. Immunobiological characterization of the trophoblast–decidual interface in human pregnancy. In: *Immunology of Human Reproduction* (M. Kurpisz and N. Fernandez, eds.), BIOS Scientific Publishers, Oxford, pp. 301–11.
27. Faulk, W. P. and A. Temple. 1976. Distribution of β2-microglobulin and HLA in chorionic villi of human placentae. *Nature* **262**:799–802.
28. Faulk, W. P. and J. A. McIntyre. 1983. Immunological studies of human trophoblast: Markers, subsets and functions. *Immunol. Rev.* **75**:140–75.
29. Sunderland, C. A., W. G. Redman and G. M. Stirrat. 1981. HLA-A,B,C antigens are expressed on nonvillous trophoblasts of the early human placenta. *J. Immunol.* **127**:2614–15.
30. Redman, C. W. G., A. J. McMichael, G. M. Stirrat *et al.* 1984. Class I major histocompatibility complex antigens on human extravillous trophoblast. *Immunology* **52:**457–68.
31. Hsi, B. L., C. J. Yeh and W. P. Faulk. 1984. Class I antigens of the major histocompatibility complex on cytotrophoblast of human chorion laeve. *Immunology* **52**:621–9.
32. Hunt, J. S., J. L. Fishback, G. K. Andrews and G. W. Wood. 1988. Expression of class I HLA genes by trophoblast cells. *J. Immunol.* **140**:1293–9.
33. Geragthy, D. E., B. H. Koller and H. T. Orr. 1987. A human major histocompatibility complex class I gene that encodes a protein with a shortened cytoplasmic segment. *Proc. Natl. Acad. Sci. USA* **84**:9145–9.
34. Le Bouteiller, P. 1994. HLA class I chromosomal region, genes and products: facts and questions. *CRC Crit. Rev. Immunol.* **14**:89–129.
35. Ellis, S. A., M. S. Palmer and A. J. McMichael. 1990. Human trophoblast and choriocarcinoma cell line BeWo express a truncated HLA class 1 molecule. *J. Immunol.* **144**:731–5.
36. Kovats, S., E. L. Main, C. Librach *et al.* 1990. A class 1 antigen, HLA-G, expressed in human trophoblasts. *Science* **248**:220–3.
37. Wei, X. and H. T. Orr. 1990. Differential expression of HLA-E, HLA-F and HLA-G transcripts in human tissue. *Hum. Immunol.* **29**:131–42.
38. Ulbrecht, M., T. Honka, T. S. Person *et al.* 1992. The HLA-E gene encodes two differentially regulated transcripts and a cell surface protein. *J. Immunol.* **149**:2945–53.
39. Guillaudeux, T., A. M. Rodriguez, M. Girr *et al.* 1995. Methylation status and transcriptional expression of the MHC class I loci in human trophoblast cells from term placenta. *J. Immunol* **154**:3283–9.
40. Yelavarthi, K. K., J. L. Fishback, and J. S. Hunt. 1991. Analysis of HLA-G mRNA in human placental and extraplacental membrane cells by in situ hybridization. *J. Immunol.* **146**:2847–54.
41. Omno, M., T. Guillaudeux, L. Amiot *et al.* 1994. The HLA-G gene is expressed at a low mRNA level in different human cells and tissues. *Hum. Immunol.* **41**:79–86.
42. Kurpisz, M., N. Fernandez and D. Fiszer. 1995. The expression of MHC genes in reproductive organs and their role in reproduction. In: *Immunology of Human Reproduction* (M. Kurpisz and N. Fernandez, eds.) BIOS Scientific Publishers, Oxford, pp. 163–84.

43. Ishitani, A. and D. E. Geraghty. 1992. Alternative splicing of HLA-G transcripts yields proteins with primary structures resembling both class I and class II antigens. *Proc. Natl. Acad. Sci. USA* **89**:3947–51.
44. Chumbley, G., A. King, K. Gardner *et al.* 1994. Generation of an antibody to HLA-G in trangenic mice and demonstration of the tissue reactivity of this antibody. *J. Reprod. Immunol.* **27**:173–86.
45. McMaster, M. T., C. L. Librach, Y. Zhou *et al.* 1995. Human placental HLA-G expression is restricted to differentiated cytotrophoblasts. *J. Immunol.* **154**:3771–8.
46. Le Bouteiller, P. 1995. Molecular regulatory mechanisms that might control HLA class I gene expression in human trophoblast cells. In: *Immunology of Human Reproduction* (M. Kurpisz and N. Fernandez, eds.) BIOS Scientific Publishers, Oxford, pp. 205–15.
47. Alizadeh, M., C. Legras, G. Semana *et al.* 1993. Evidence for a polymorphism of HLA-G gene. *Hum. Immunol.* **38**:206–12.
48. Van der Ven, K. and C. Ober. 1994. HLA-G polymorphisms in African Americans. *J. Immunol.* **153**:5628–33.
49. Morales, P., A. Corell, J. Martinez-Laso. 1993. Three new HLA-G alleles and their linkage disequilibria with HLA-A. *Immunogenetics* **38**:323–31.
50. Van der Ven, K. and C. Ober. 1994. Evidence for polymorphism in the $\alpha 2$ domain of the human leukocyte antigen (HLA)-G gene. *Am. J. Reprod. Immunol.* **31**:220–1.
51. Sanders, S. K., P. A. Giblin and P. Kavathas. 1991. Cell–cell adhesion mediated by CD8 and human histocompatibility leukocyte antigen G, a nonclassical major histocompatibility complex class I molecule on cytotrophoblasts. *J. Exp. Med.* **174**:737–40.
52. King, A. and Y. W. Loke. 1991. On the nature and function of human uterine granular lymphocytes. *Immunol. Today* **12**:432–5.
53. Kovats, S., C. Librach, P. Sisch *et al.* 1991. Expression and possible function of the HLA-G~ chain in human cytotrophoblast. In: *Cellular and Molecular Biology of the Materno-Fetal Relationship* (G. Chaouat and J. Mowbray, eds.) Colloque INSERM/John Libbey Eurotext, Paris, pp. 21–9.
54. Chumbley, G., A. King, K. Robertson *et al.* 1994. Resistance of HLA-G and HLA-A2 transfectants to lysis by decidual cells. *Cell. Immunol.* **155**:312–22.
55. Heyborn, K., Y. X. Fu, A. Nelson *et al.* 1994. Recognition of trophoblast by $\gamma\delta$ T cells. *J. Immunol.* **153**:2918–26.
56. Lee, N., A. Malacko, A. Ishitani *et al.* 1995. The membrane bound and soluble forms of HLA-G bind identical sets of endogenous peptides but differs with respect to glycosylation and TAP association. *9th International Congress of Immunology, San Francisco*, Abstract 1414.
57. McIntyre, J. A. and W. P. Faulk. 1982. Allotypic trophoblast-lymphocyte cross-reactive (TLX) cell surface antigens. *Hum. Immunol.* **4**:27–35.
58. McIntyre, J. A., W. P. Faulk, S. J. Verhulst and J. A. Colliver. 1983. Human trophoblast-lymphocyte cross-reactive (TLX) antigens define a new alloantigen system. *Science* **222**:1135–7.
59. Goto, S., K. Takakuwa, K. Kanazawa and A. Takeuchi. 1989. MLR-blocking antibodies are directed against alloantigens expressed on cytotrophoblasts. *Am. J. Reprod. Immunol.* **21**:50–3.
60. Stern, P. L., N. Beresford, S. Thompson *et al.* 1986. Characterization of the human trophoblast-leukocyte antigenic molecules defined by a monoclonal antibody. *J. Immunol.* **137**:1604–9.
61. McIntyre, J. A. 1988. In search of trophoblast-lymphocyte cross-reactive (TLX)

antigens. *Am. J. Reprod. Immunol. Microbiol.* **17**:100–10.
62. Purcell, D. F. J., I. F. C. McKenzie, D. M. Lublin *et al.* 1990. The human cell surface glycoproteins HuLY-m5, membrane cofactor protein (MCP) of the complement system and trophoblast-leukocyte common (TLX) antigen are CD46. *Immunology* **70**:155–61.
63. Bulmer, J. N. and P. M. Johnson. 1985. Antigen expression by trophoblast populations in the human placenta and their possible immunological relevance. *Placenta* **6**:127–40.
64. Anderson, D. J., J. S. Michaelson and P. M. Johnson. 1989. Trophoblast/leukocyte-common antigen is expressed by human testicular germ cells and appears on the surface of acrosome-reacted sperm. *Biol. Reprod.* **41**:285–9.
65. Vanderpuye, O. A., C. A. Laberrere, C. J. Thaler *et al.* 1991. Syncytiotrophoblast brush border proteins recognized by monoclonal antibody TRA-2-10 and rabbit anti-TLX sera. *Placenta* **12**:199–215.
66. Golberg, J. S., M. K. Haynes, F. S. Cowchock *et al.* 1995. Alloantibody responses to antigens recognized by rabbit antitrophoblast antisera in trophoblast and mononuclear cell (MNC) membranes by primary aborting women before and after paternal leukocyte immunization. *Am. J. Reprod. Immunol.* **33**:21–30.
67. Holmes, C. H., K. L. Simpson, S. D. Wainwright *et al.* 1990. Preferential expression of the complement regulatory protein decay accelerating factor at the fetomaternal interface during human pregnancy. *J. Immunol.* **144**:3099–105.
68. Tedesco, F., G. Narchi, O. Radillo *et al.* 1993. Susceptibility of human trophoblast to killing by human complement and the role of the complement regulatory proteins. *J. Immunol.* **151**:1562–70.
69. Jensen, T. S., L. Bjorge, A.-L. Wollen and M. Ulstein. 1995. Identification of the complement regulatory proteins CD46, CD55, and CD59 in human fallopian tube, endometrium and cervical mucosa and secretion. *Am. J. Reprod. Immunol.* **34**:1–9.
70. Risk, J. M., B. F. Flanagan and P. M. Johnson. 1991. Polymorphism of the human CD46 gene in normal individuals and in recurrent spontaneous abortion. *Hum. Immunol.* **30**:162–7.
71. King, A. and Y. W. Loke. 1988. Differential expression of blood-group-related carbohydrate antigens by trophoblast subpopulations. *Placenta* **9**:513–22.
72. Goto, S., H. Nishi and Y. Tomoda. 1980. Blood group Rh-D factor in human trophoblast determined by immunofluorescent method. *Am J. Obstet. Gynecol.* **137**:707–12.
73. Johnson, P. M., J. M. Risk and J. N. Bulmer. 1987. Antigen expression at human maternofetal interfaces. In: *Immunoregulation and Fetal Survival* (T. G. Wegmann and T. J. Gill III, eds.) Oxford University Press, New York, pp. 181–6.
74. Thaler, C. J. and J. A. McIntyre. 1990. Fetal wastage and non-recognition in human pregnancy. *J. Reprod. Immunol.* **1**:79–102.
75. Sedmak, D. D., D. H. Davis, U. Singh *et al.* 1991. Expression of IgG Fc receptor antigens in placenta and on endothelial cells in humans. An immunohistochemical study. *Am. J. Pathol.* **138**: 175–81.
76. Damsky, C. H., M. L. Fitzgerald and S. J. Fisher. 1992. Distribution patterns of extracellular matrix components and adhesion receptors are intricately modulated during first trimester cytotrophoblast differentiation along the invasive pathway in vivo. *J. Clin. Invest.* **89**:210–22
77. Burrows, T. D., A. King and Y. W. Loke. 1993. Expression of intergrins by human trophoblast and differential adhesion to laminin or fibronectin. *Hum. Reprod.* **8**:475–84.

78. Laberrere, C. A. and W. P. Faulk. 1995. Intercellular adhesion molecule-1 (ICAM-1) and HLA-DR antigens are expressed on endovascular cytotrophoblasts in abnormal pregnancies. *Am. J. Reprod. Immunol.* **33**:47–53.
79. Jalali, G. R., J. L. Underwood and J. F. Mowbray. 1989. IgG on normal human placenta is bound to both antigen and Fc receptors. *Transplant. Proc.* **81**:572–4.
80. Jalali, G. R., A. Rezai, J. L. Underwood *et al.* 1995. An 80-kDa syncytiotrophoblast alloantigen bound to maternal alloantibody in term placenta. *Am. J. Reprod. Immunol.* **33**:213–20.

36

Conserved Bacterial Proteins: Implications for the Pathogenesis of Reactive Arthritis

Sanja Ugrinović, Andreas Mertz, Roland Lauster and Joachim Sieper

Reactive arthritis (ReA) is a common human inflammatory disease affecting mainly peripheral joints, and occurs following genitourinary infection (*Chlamydia trachomatis*) or enteral infection (*Yersinia*, *Salmonella*, *Shigella*, *Campylobacter* spp.) (1). All these bacteria are obligate (*C. trachomatis*) or facultative intracellular bacteria. Scrutiny of ReA population reveals that 60–70% of the patients are HLA-B27 positive, compared with 7% of healthy people (2). Despite extensive research, the interaction of environmental and genetical factors in the pathogenesis of ReA is still unknown, and there is currently no cure for this disorder.

The fact that ReA is triggered by several, biologically different, bacteria raises the question of a common antigen shared among these microbes. In most cases of ReA, the triggering bacterium can be identified by means of antigen-specific proliferative response of synovial fluid (SF) T cells (3,4). Bacteria contain some 1000 proteins, all of which represent potential antigens for T cells. The existence of T cells recognizing conserved bacterial proteins has been proposed as one explanation of why in some patients with ReA there appears to be recognition of more than one bacterium (5). The identification of immunodominant proteins and peptides is of great importance both for better understanding of the disease, and for developing new forms of immunotherapy. Among the immunodominant proteins of *Yersinia* and *Chlamydia* are highly conserved ribosomal protein L2 (30 kDa), L23 (13 kDa), the 19 kDa subunit of the urease (5), and the 60 kDa heat-shock protein (Gro El homologue) of *Yersinia*; conserved the 18 kDa histone-like protein and the 57 kDa heat-shock protein (Gro EL homologue) of *Chlamydia* (6).

Intracellular pathogens residing in vacuoles are normally presented via

Immunoregulation in Health and Disease
ISBN 0-12-459460-3

MHC class II Ag presentation. However, the ReA triggering bacteria, *Salmonella* (7,8), *Yersinia* (9), and *Chlamydia* (10,11) can also induce a $CD8^+$ T-cell response. In the context of the HLA-B27 association, therefore, the question arises as to whether or not an arthritogenic bacterial peptide presented by HLA-B27 to $CD8^+$ T cells drives the pathogenesis. Furthermore, recognition of $CD8^+$ T cells is mostly confined to a few proteins and often to only one epitope on each bacterium. This makes it more likely that $CD8^+$ T cells would recognize a common epitope shared by different bacteria. To date, it has been shown (9) that it is possible to raise $CD8^+$, HLA-B27 restricted clones for *Yersinia*. The same authors (12) described clones which recognize 19 kDa-derived HLA-B27 nonapeptide in patients with early ReA. Another group (13) reported about a line from a *Salmonella*-induced ReA patient recognizing a *C. trachomatis* 75 kDa-derived HLA-B27 nonapeptide. These findings imply that $CD8^+$ T cells from ReA patients are able to recognize bacterial peptides in the context of HLA-B27, but whether or not it is a common epitope is still not clear.

Here we describe recognition of conserved bacterial proteins by SF T cells of *Chlamydia* and *Yersinia*-induced ReA patients, both on the level of $CD4^+$ and $CD8^+$ T cells.

MATERIALS AND METHODS

Patients

Patients with ReA were selected according to the clinical picture, i.e. an asymmetrical or monoarthritis predominantly in the lower limbs, a clear history of recent urethritis or gastroenteritis, and specific proliferation of SF T cells to *Chlamydia* or *Yersinia* antigens (SI > 5) (4).

Cell separation and proliferation assays

Mononuclear cells (MNC) were separated as previously described (4) from peripheral blood and synovial fluid by density gradient centrifugation (Ficoll-Paque, Pharmacia Biotech AB, Sweden) and resuspended in tissue culture medium comprising RPMI 1640 (GIBCO, UK) with 10% human serum pool, 100 U/ml penicillin, 100 μg/ml streptomycin and 2 mM glutamine (Biochrome KG, Germany). Cells were plated into 96-well plates at 10^5 cells/well and stimulated in triplicates with following antigens: tissue culture medium alone (background proliferation); pokeweed mitogen (1 μg/ml, Sigma, UK); heat-inactivated *C. trachomatis* serotype L2/434 (5 μg/ml, kindly provided by Dr. Groh, Department of Microbiology, Jena); heat-inactivated *Yersinia enterocolitica* O:3 (5 μg/ml, kindly provided by Dr. Mielke, Department of Microbiology, UKBF, Berlin), recombinant forms of *Yersinia*-

derived proteins: 19 kDa, 13 kDa, 30 kDa, *Chlamydia*-derived 57 kDa and 18 kDa proteins, and where indicated the native form of 19 kDa protein (17). The cells were cultured for 6 days at 37°C in 5% carbon dioxide and ^{3}H-thymidine (7.4 kBq/well, Amersham, UK) incorporation was measured as previously described (4).

Recombinant protein gene expression and protein purification

The complete open reading-frames of *Chlamydia* 57 kDa and 18 kDa and *Yersinia* 19 kDa, 13 kDa, 30 kDa and 60 kDa proteins were amplified by PCR using the following primers:

57 kDa: 1. GATCCCATGGTCGCTAAAAAC
2. GATCAGATCTATAGTCCATTCCTGC
18 kDa: 1. CATGCCATGGCGCTAAAAGATACG
2. GATCGGATCCTTTTTTTGTTGAGCGAG
19 kDa: 1. CATGCCATGGGCAGCACAAAGACAA
2. GACTAGATCTTTTAGACGATTTGAAGCCAC
13 kDa: 1. CATGCCATGGCAATTCGTGAAGAACGTCGTC
2. GATCAGATCTCTCTGCGCCGCCGATG
30 kDa: 1. CATGCCATGGCAATTGTTAAATG
2. GATCAGATCTTTTTTTACTACGGCGAC

Amplification conditions were: 94°C, 5 min; 94°C, 1.5 min; 72°C, 2 min; 35 cycles.

The amplification fragments were isolated from agarose gel with a Jet Sorb Kit (Genome, Germany), digested with Nco I and Bgl II endonucleases (Boerhringer Mannheim, Germany) and ligated into Nco I and Bgl II digested vector pQE 60 (Qiagen, Germany).

Positive clones were selected after transformation of electrocompetent *E. coli* strain M15 (pREp 4) (Qiagen, Germany). Expression of the cloned genes was induced by addition of 1 mM IPTG (isopropyl-β-D-thiogalactopyranosid). Cells were harvested in a French press after 2 h and the fusion protein was separated from crude extract on an Ni–NTA–Resin column according to the manufacturer's instructions (Qiagen, Germany).

CTL assays

10^6 target cells (macrophages infected with bacteria or Epstein–Barr transformed B cells pulsed with peptides) were labelled with 100 μCi of ^{51}Cr (Amersham, Germany) for 1–1.5 h. Cells were washed twice with RPMI 1640 resuspended at 5×10^3 cells/100 μl and added to the serial dilutions of CTL in round-bottomed 96 well-plates (Nunc, UK). In cases in which peptides were added as antigens, these were also present during CTL assay at a final concentration of 10 μM. Spontaneous release was determined in wells with target cells but without CTL. Maximum release was determined by adding 1.5% Triton X100 (Sigma, UK) to wells containing targets but no CTL. After 4 h incubation at 37°C supernatant from each well was assayed for ^{51}Cr release in a gamma counter. Percentage of specific lysis was determined as follows:

$$\textit{percentage of specific lysis} = \frac{\textit{experimental release} - \textit{spontaneous release}}{\textit{maximum release} - \textit{spontaneous release}} \times 100$$

Spontaneous release was less than 20% of maximal release by detergent in all experiments.

Stimulation and propagation of *Yersinia*-specific CTL lines

After separation, SF MNC were placed in 24-well tissue culture plates (Costar, USA) (1×10^6 cells/ml) and incubated for 1.5–2 h at 37°C. Non-adherent cells were removed and adherent macrophages (Mϕ) were infected with live *Yersinia enterocolitica* (kindly provided by Dr. Mielke, Department of Microbiology, UKBF, Berlin) at a ratio of 1:10 in a medium without antibiotics, centrifuged for 10 min at 3000 rev/min and incubated at 37°C for 1 h. After incubation, infected Mϕ were washed three times with prewarmed medium to remove free bacteria. Cultures containing infected Mϕ (2×10^5/ml) and T cells (8–9 $\times 10^5$/ml) were established in a 24-well tissue culture plate and 100 U/ml rIL2 (Eurocetus GmbH, Germany) was added on day 3. After 7 days, cells were harvested, washed, and restimulated with autologous infected Mϕ and rIL-2. Weekly stimulations were conducted for 3 weeks, at which time CTL assays were performed.

Transformation of B cells

Peripheral blood (PB) MNC from all investigated patients were resuspended in a medium containing RPMI 1640, 10% FCS (GIBCO, UK), glutamine, penicillin/streptomycin, and sodium pyruvate (Sigma) and plated in 24-well Costar tissue culture plate (2×10^6 cells). 1 ml supernatant (kindly provided by Dr. Notter, Department of Haematology, UKBF, Berlin) of Epstein–Barr virus-producing cell line B95-8 was added. Cyclosporine A (600 ng/ml) was added weekly to the culture and after at least 10 days small colonies of transformed lymphoblastoid cells could be seen. These were grown and used as described. B cell lines were periodically checked for mycoplasma infection (Mycoplasma Detection Kit, Enzyme Immunoassay, Boehringer Mannheim, Germany).

Preparation of target cells

Monocytes/macrophages were isolated from peripheral blood and infected with *Yersinia enterocolitica* as described above, except the cells were incubated overnight, after removing free bacteria.

Epstein–Barr virus cell lines matched for HLA-B27, but mismatched for all other HLA class I molecules, were pulsed with relevant peptides at a concentration of 50 μM and incubated overnight.

Synthetic peptides

Nonapeptides from proteins of interest were chosen according to the HLA-B27 binding motif and synthesized on a robot system developed for multiple peptide syntesis (MyltiSynTech, Bochum, Germany). The peptides were tested in a standard HLA-assembly assay as described elsewhere (5).

RESULTS

SF CD4^{+} T cells response to conserved proteins in *Yersinia*-induced ReA patients

We described earlier (5) that three major protein fractions, i.e. membrane pellet, cytoplasmatic protein fraction and ribosomal pellet, of *Yersinia* have different capacities to stimulate SF T cells from patients with *Yersinia*-triggered ReA. The strongest proliferation was seen in response to the ribosomal pellet, from which two main proteins could be extracted – L23 (13 kDa) and β-urease subunit (19 kDa).

Both proteins from the ribosomal fraction elicited the strong proliferative response in 10 tested patients with *Yersinia*-induced ReA (Fig. 36.1). In contrast, the majority of ribosomal pellet proteins judged to be anionic or neutral proteins (ANP) elicited only moderate or weak proliferative response.

The 57 kDa heat shock protein elicits a proliferative response in *Chlamydia*-induced ReA patients

In order to define the relevant antigens in patients with *C. trachomatis*-induced ReA, recombinant forms of *Yersinia*-derived conserved proteins (19 kDa, 13 kDa, 30 kDa) and *Chlamydia*-derived conserved proteins

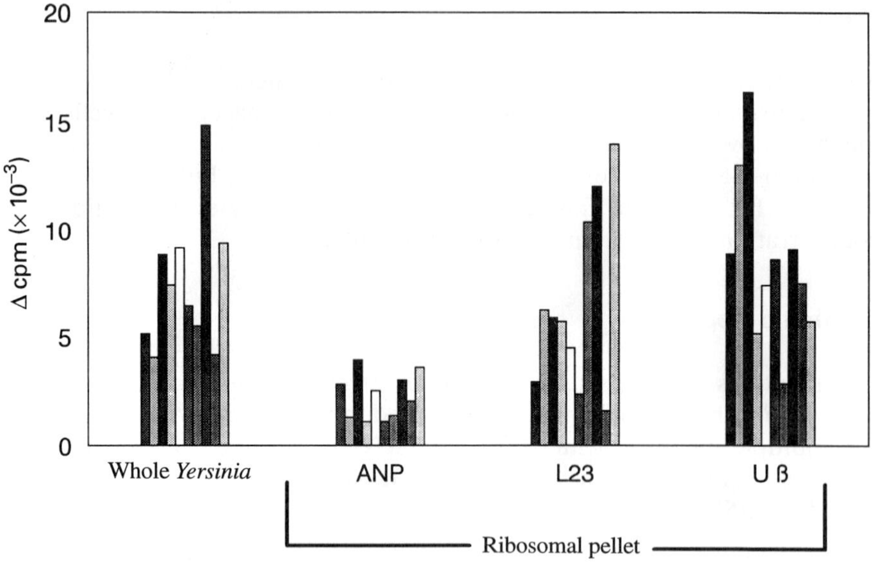

Fig. 36.1 Proliferative response of synovial fluid mononuclear cells of all 10 reactive arthritis patients to whole *Yersinia* and purified ribosomal pellet proteins and protein fractions. The highest proliferation is seen in response to the urease β-subunit (Uβ) and to a slightly less degree in response to ribosomal protein L23. The fraction of anionic and neutral proteins (ANP) induced only weak proliferation.

(57 kDa and 18 kDa were used to stimulate proliferative response of SF T cells from *C. trachomatis*-triggered arthritis patients (Fig. 36.2).

In all cases, only the 57 kDa protein was able to induce a proliferative response.

Yersinia can induce a specific cytotoxic response in both HLA-B27-positive and HLA-B27-negative ReA patients

Five patients with *Yersinia*-induced arthritis (one HLA-B27 negative, five HLA-B27 positive) were chosen for evaluating the question whether it is possible to generate SF *Yersinia*-specific CTL. After 1 week of stimulation with live *Yersinia* no cytotoxicity was observed (date not shown). The specific cytotoxicity could be obtained only after 3 weeks of repetitive stimulation by Mϕ infected with live *Yersinia* (Fig. 36.3). This cytotoxicity was due to infection of targets with *Yersinia*, since non-infected Mϕ did not induce any cytotoxicity. Moreover, when Mϕ were preincubated with heat-inactivated *Yersinia*, no cytotoxicity was induced (Fig. 36.4). The cytotoxicity could be suppressed in the presence of anti-class I antibody by 50%, as shown in Fig. 36.4.

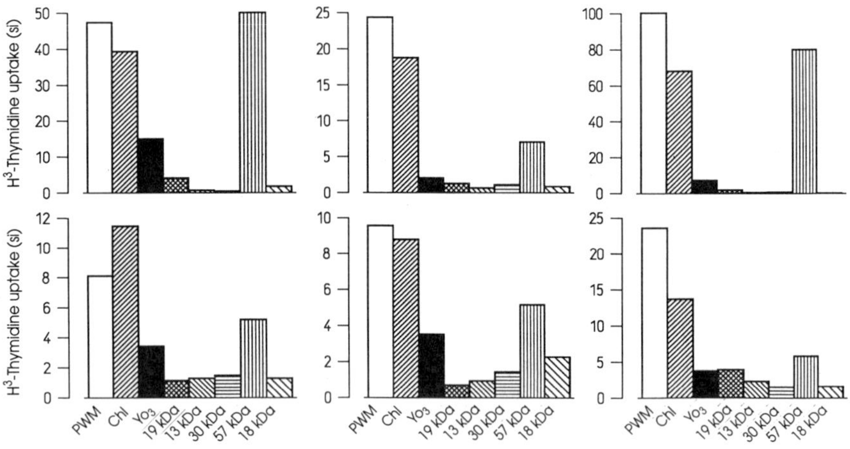

Fig. 36.2 Proliferative response of synovial fluid mononuclear cells of *Chlamydia* induced ReA to chlamydial or yersinial conserved proteins. Synovial fluid mononuclear cells of six patients with *Chlamydia*-induced ReA were stimulated for proliferative response with recombinant forms of chlamydial conserved proteins: the 57 kDa heat shock protein and the 18 kDa histone-like protein, and yersinial conserved proteins: the β-urease subunit (19 kDa), the L23 ribosomal protein (13 kDa) and the L2 ribosomal protein (30 kDa). Proliferative response was considered positive when stimulation index (SI) was >5.

Yersinia-specific CTL lines from HLA-B27$^+$ ReA patients recognize peptides derived from 13 kDa (L23) and 60 kDa proteins with B27 binding motif

Two HLA-B27$^+$ *Yersinia*-specific CTL lines were selected for further investigation of *Yersinia*-derived HLA-B27 restricted epitopes. The list of nonapeptides used in this study is shown in Table 36.1. EBV cell lines matched for the HLA-B27 molecule, but mismatched for all other HLA class I molecules, were pulsed with relevant peptides at the concentration of 50 μM, incubated overnight and used as targets. The concentration of peptides during cytotoxic assay was 10 μM.

Although the 19 kDa protein is relevant for CD4$^+$ T-cell response, nonapeptides derived from this protein did not induce a cytotoxic response, whereas HLA-B27-matched Epstein–Barr virus cells prepulsed with pooled 13 kDa peptides were specifically lysed by both lines (Fig. 36.5). As shown in the same figure, both lines also recognized pooled peptides of 60 kDa. Figure 36.5b shows that a strong binder derived from the 60 kDa. figure 36.5b shows that a strong binder derived from the 60 kDa protein (60 kDa 284–292) induces specific ^{51}Cr release, whereas its homologue, *Chlamydia* 57 kDa

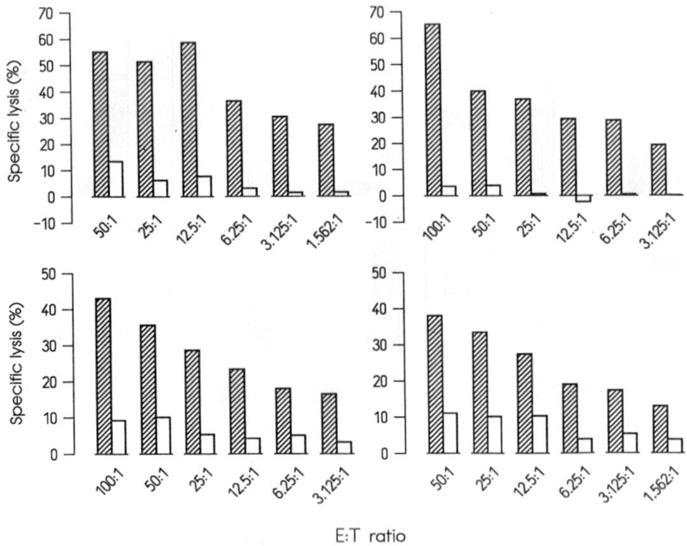

Fig. 36.3 Lysis of *Yersinia* infected target cells by *Yersinia* CTL lines. *Yersinia* CTL lines, derived from 4 HLA-B27 + *Yersinia*-induced ReA patients, were stimulated for 3 weeks with macrophages infected with live *Yersinia* and tested in ^{51}Cr release assay either with macrophages infected with *Yersinia* (shaded bars) or macrophages alone (white bars). Spontaneous release of ^{51}Cr was less than 20%.

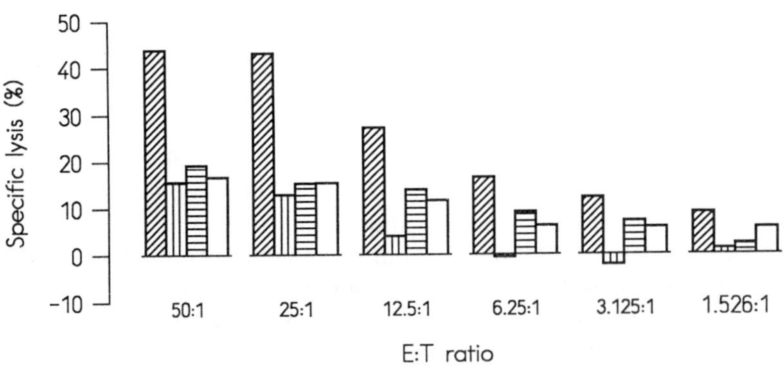

Fig. 36.4 MHC class I restricted lysis of target cells by a *Yersinia* specific line. A *Yersinia* specific CTL line derived from the synovial fluid of an HLA-B27 negative ReA patient was tested for a specific cytotoxic response either with macrophages infected with *Yersinia* (diagonal shading), macrophages pre-incubated with heat-inactivated *Yersinia* (vertical shading) or in the presence of anti-class I Ab (horizontal shading). White bars are results for Mϕ alone.

Table 36.1 *Yersinia*- and *Chlamydia*-derived peptides, and their binding affinity to HLA-B27. The single letter amino acid code is used. The binding affinity of all peptides was determined in an in vitro assembly, except for the 18 kDa (Chl.HC1) protein where HLA-B27 binding motif was used as the only criterion. The strong binders are in italics. The non-binders are not shown.

Chl. HC1 33–41	Q	R	V	R	T	E	S	I	K
Chl. HC1 80–88	V	R	A	T	K	T	V	A	K
Chl. HC1 93–101	K	R	T	C	A	T	K	A	K
Y.e. L23 11–19	L	R	A	P	H	V	S	E	K
Y.e. L23 67–75	K	R	H	G	Q	R	V	G	R
Y.e. L23 75–83	R	R	S	D	W	K	K	A	Y
Y.e. U-β 60–68	V	R	N	T	G	D	R	P	I
Y.e. U-β 93–101	K	R	L	N	I	S	S	T	T
Y.e. U-β 103–111	I	R	F	E	P	G	D	E	T
Y.e. U-β 153–161	*R*	*R*	*A*	*A*	*E*	*R*	*G*	*F*	*K*
Chl. groEL 12–20	A	R	K	K	I	Q	K	G	V
Chl. groEL 117–125	K	R	G	I	D	K	A	A	K
Chl. groEL 284–292	*R*	*R*	*K*	*A*	*M*	*F*	*E*	*D*	*I*
Chl. groEL 379–387	I	R	V	G	A	A	T	E	I
Y.e. GroEL 12–20	A	R	I	K	M	L	R	G	V
Y.e. GroEL 57–65	A	R	E	I	E	L	E	D	K
Y.e. groEL 117–125	K	R	G	I	D	K	A	V	I
Y.e. groEL 284–292	*R*	*R*	*K*	*A*	*M*	*L*	*Q*	*D*	*I*
Y.e. groEL 344–352	K	R	V	V	I	N	K	D	T
Y.e. groEL 349–357	I	R	Q	Q	I	E	E	A	T
Y.e. groEL 446–454	L	R	A	M	E	S	P	L	R

284–292 peptide, does not. This might be due to differences in residues 6 and 7 (Table 36.1) which are important for TcR recognition.

DISCUSSION

In ReA, Reiter's syndome and ankylosing spondylitis, the mechanisms whereby the MHC class I antigen HLA-B27 confers disease susceptibility have remained unknown. One hypothesis is that binding of bacteria-derived and/or autologous 'arthritogenic peptides' to the HLA-B27 molecule could induce CD8 CTLs as a crucial event in the initiation of ReA and the other spondyloarthropathies (14). Information acquired to date indicates that synovial response of T cells to bacterial antigens has, with few exceptions (9), been confined to CD4$^+$ cells in ReA (3). Since antigens of intracellular pathogens (e.g. viruses, but also bacteria associated with ReA) may have preferential access to class I MHC antigen for presentation to T cells (15), and since the triggering bacteria, in most cases of ReA, can be identified

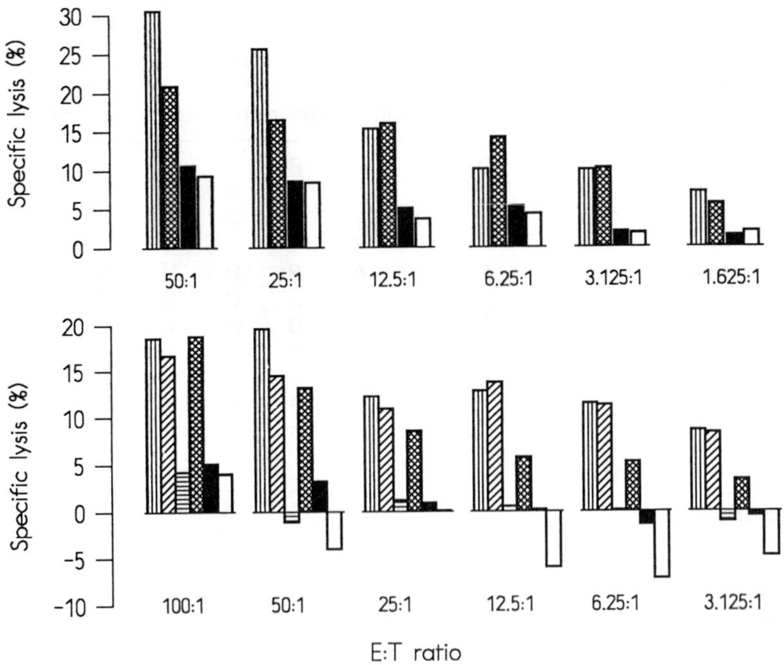

Fig. 36.5 HLA-B27 restricted lysis of target cells incubated with *Yersinia*- or *Chlamydia*-derived peptides. An EBV cell line matched for HLA-B27, but mismatched for all other MHC class I molecules was preincubated with pools of HLA-B27-restricted peptides derived either from *Yersinia* GroEL (60 kDa heat shock protein) (vertical shading), GroEL strong binder (diagonal shading), 13 kDa protein (cross-hatching), 19 kDa protein (black); or *Chlamydia*-derived 57 kDa strong binder (horizontal shading). Concentration of each peptide during the standard ^{51}Cr release assay was 10 μM. EBV cells without peptides were used as the negative control (white bars).

by means of an antigen-specific proliferative response, both CD4$^+$ and CD8$^+$ synovial fluid T cells might play a role in the pathogenesis of ReA. For us, the crucial question was whether synovial-fluid-derived T cells would recognize conserved bacterial proteins and peptides. Several immunodominant proteins of *Chlamydia* and *Yersinia* seem to be highly conserved, not only between different bacterial species but also between procaryotes and eucaryotes. The L23 ribosomal protein has 32% identity and an overall homology of 56% between *Yersinia* and humans (5). The 57 kDa heat shock protein of *Chlamydia* and 60 kDa heat shock protein of *Yersinia* have set up to 50% of homology with human proteins. furthermore, there are animal models describing the *Chlamydia* 57 kDa heat shock protein in DTH (16) and the 19 kDa protein of *Yersinia* inducing arthritis in rats after intra-articular injection (17). We found that the 57 kDa protein and 19 kDa protein can induce a proliferative response in *Chlamydia* or *Yersinia*-induced ReA, respectively. The 19 kDa is, except in *Klebsiella*, not found in other ReA-associated bacteria, and therefore may not be a shared antigen.

However, Hermann and colleagues (12) described a clone which recognizes 19 kDa-derived HLA-B27 peptides in one patient with early ReA. CTL lines from HLA-B27 patients recognizing Mϕ infected with live *Yersinia*, but not EBV pulsed with 19 kDa-derived peptides, suggest that these might not get access to the pathway I of antigen presentation. The L23 ribosomal protein elicited a proliferative response in 10 ReA patients. Furthermore, an HLA-B27 matched EBV cell line pulsed with L23-derived peptides was lysed by two *Yersinia*-specific CTL lines. Although the distribution of CD4 and CD8-epitopes on one protein is not clear, these data suggest that the L23 ribosomal protein may be relevant both on the level of CD4$^+$ and CD8$^+$ T-cell immune response. The proliferative response to the 60 kDa heat shock protein of *Yersinia* was not determined, although its homologue, 57 kDa of *Chlamydia*, induced a strong proliferative response in patients with *Chlamydia*-induced ReA. The 60 kDa derived pool of peptides and the strong binder (284–292) elicit a cytotoxic response in the *Yersinia* CTL line. However, when an HLA-B27-matched EBV cell line was pulsed with 57 kDa-derived strong binder, no cytotoxic response was observed. The 50 kDa strong binder and 57 kDa strong binder differ only in residues 6 and 7 which are responsible for binding to TCR (18). Work is now in progress to generate *Chlamydia*-specific CTL lines. This will allow us to see whether homologous epitopes are recognized by different bacteria CTLs. The 'arthritogenic-peptide' theory suggests that such a peptide, or its mimic, is found in a joint-specific protein. At present, there are no data on homology between bacterial and joint-specific protein. Furthermore, it is still not clear whether ReA arthritis is due to the persistent bacterial infection in the joint (19,20) or some process which leads to autoimmunity (21).

CONCLUSION

This study shows that conserved proteins seem to be relevant both for CD4 and for CD8 T-cell responses in the pathogenesis of ReA.

Two main antigens recognized by CD4$^+$ T cells in *Yersinia*-induced ReA patients are the L23 ribosomal protein (13 kDa) and the 19 kDa subunit of urease. In *Chlamydia*-induced ReA patients only 57 kDa heat shock protein was able to induce a proliferative response, suggesting that a cross-reactivity between different bacterial strains at the level of CD4 T-cell recognition is not likely.

Yersinia-specific CTL lines generated from synovial fluid of ReA showed specific cytotoxic response to L23 and 60 kDa nonapeptides using EBV transformed lines matched for HLA-B27 but mismatched for all other class I molecules as targets, indicating that these responses are HLA-B27 restricted.

The ongoing investigations with *Chlamydia* and *Chlamydia*-specific CTL lines will hopefully tell us if these CD8 epitopes are shared between different bacteria involved in ReA.

REFERENCES

1. Keat, A. 1983. Reiter's syndrome and reactive arthritis in perspective. *N. Engl. J. Med.* **309**:1606–15.
2. Brewerton, D. A., F. D. Hart, M. Caffrey *et al.* 1973. Ankylosing spondylitis and HLA-B27. *Lancet* **1**:904–7.
3. Gaston, J. S. H., P. F. Life, K. Granfors *et al.* 1989. Synovial T lymphocyte recognition of organisms that trigger reactive arthritis. *Clin. Exp. Immunol.* **76**:348–53.
4. Sieper, J., G. Kingsley, A. Palacios-Boix *et al.* 1991. Synovial T lymphocyte-specific immune response to *Chlamydia trachomatis* in Reiter's disease. *Arthritis Rheum.* **34**:588–98.
5. Mertz, A., A. Daser, M. Skurnik *et al.* 1994. The evolutionary conserved ribosomal protein L23 and the cationic urease β-subunit of *Yersinia enterocolitica* 0:3 belong to immunodominant antigens in *Yersinia* triggered reactive arthritis: implication for autoimmunity. *Mol. Med.* **1**:44–5.
6. Deane, K., R. Jeacock, A. Hassell *et al.* 1994. Identification of two target antigens recognized by synovial fluid T cells in *Chlamydia*-induced reactive arthritis (abstract). *Arthritis Rheum.* **37** (suppl. 9): S364.
7. Pfeifer, J. D., M. J. Wick, R. L. Roberts *et al.* 1993. Phagocytic processing of bacterial antigens for class I MHC presentation to T cells. *Nature* **361**:359–62.
8. Pope, M., I. Kotlarski and K. Doherty. 1994. Induction of Lyt-2+ cytotoxic T lymphocytes following primary and secondary *Salmonella* infection. *Immunology* **81**:177–82.
9. Hermann, E., D. T. Y. Yu, K.-H. Meyer zum Büschenfeld and B. Fleischer. 1993. HLA-B27-restricted CD8 T cells derived from synovial fluids of patients with reactive arthritis and ankylosing spondilitis. *Lancet* **342**:646–50.
10. Beatty, P. R. and R. S. Stephens. 1994. CD8+ T lymphocyte-mediated lysis of *Chlamydia* infected L cells using an endogenous antigen pathway. *J. Immunol.* **153**:4588–95.
11. Starnbach, M. N., M. Bevan and M. Lampe. 1994. Protective cytotoxic T lymphocytes are induced during murin infection with *Chlamydia trachomatis. J. Immunol.* **153**:5183–9.
12. Ackermann, B., D. T. Y. Yu, G. Kuipers *et al.* 1995. A *Yersinia* urease-β-subunit derived peptide is recognized by HLA-B27 restricted cytotoxic T cells in *Yersinia*-induced reactive arthritis (abstract). *Arthritis Rheum.* **38**: (suppl. 9): S201.
13. Bowness, P. 1995. The link between CD8+ cells and HLA-B27: arthritogenic peptide or a failure to respond? *Third International Workshop on Reactive Arthritis. Abstract Book.*
14. Benjamin, R. J. and P. Parham. 1990. Guilt by association: HLA-B27 and ankylosing spondilitis. *Immunol. Today* **11**: 137–42.

15. Morrison, L. A., A. E. Lukacher, V. L. Braciale *et al.* 1986. Differences in antigen presentation to MHC class I- and class II-restricted influenza virus specific cytolytic T lymphocyte clone. *J. Exp. Med.* **163**:903–8.
16. Morrison, R., K. Lyng and H. Caldwell. 1989. *Chlamydia* disease pathogenesis. Ocular hypersensitivity elicited by genus-specific 57kD protein. *J. Exp. Med.* **169**:663–75.
17. Mertz, A., S. R. Batsford, E. Curschellas *et al.* 1991. Cationic *Yersinia* antigen-induced chronic allergic arthritis in rats: a model for reactive arthritis in humans. *J. Clin. Invest.* **87**: 632–42.
18. Guo, H. C., D. R. Madden, M. L. Silver *et al.* 1993. Comparation of the P2 specificity pocked in three human histocompatibility antigens: HLA-A*6801, HLA-A*0201, and HLA-B*2705. *Proc. Natl. Acad. Sci.* USA **90**:8053–7.
19. Taylor-Robinson, D., C. B. Gilroy, B. J. Thomas and A. C. S. Keat. 1992. Detection of *Chlamydia trachomatis* DNA in joints of reactive arthritis patients by polymerase chain reaction. *Lancet* **340**:81–2.
20. Nikkari, S., R. Merilahti-Palo, R. Saario *et al.* 1992. *Yersinia* triggered reactive arthritis: use of polymerase chain reaction and immunocytochemical staining in the detection of bacterial components from synovial fluid. *Arthritis Rheum.* **35**:682–7.
21. Sieper, J. and J. Braun, 1995. Pathogenesis of spondyloarthropathies. Persistent bacterial infection, autoimmunity, or both?*Arthritis Rheum.* **38**:1547–54.

37

Production and Characterization of Monoclonal Antibodies to Antigens of *Borrelia burgdorferi* Strain Košutnjak-K1

Edita Grego, Miodrag Čolić, Vilma Jovičić and Branislav Lako

Lyme borreliosis is an infectious disease with worldwide distribution, caused by the tick-borne spirochete *Borrelia burgdorferi* (1,2). The disease may involve many organs, most commonly the skin, joints, heart and nervous system (3).

Borrelia burgdorferi has to date been isolated from humans, small mammals, birds and arthropods in North America and Europe (3). Although these spirochete isolates have shown considerable homogeneity in their PAGE protein profiles (4), there also were indications of significant genotypic and phenotypic heterogeneity among strains associated with Lyme borreliosis from different origins (3). These findings may explain differences in the clinical symptoms of Lyme disease and *B. burgdorferi* infections in different regions and countries (3). It was shown that *B. burgdorferi* sensu lato responsible for Lyme disease is a complex of three genospecies, *B. burgdorferi* sensu stricto, *B. garinii* and *B. afzelii* (5). Thus, *B. burgdorferi* sensu stricto, the prevailing species in the USA, is commonly associated with rheumatological manifestations of Lyme disease (6). On the other hand, the most common Eurasian species of Lyme disease borreliae, *B. garinii* and *B. afzelii*, are mainly associated with neurological and dermatological manifestations, respectively (3). Polymorphism of borrelial antigens may also influence the serodiagnosis of Lyme disease (7).

An epidemiological study in Yugoslavia showed that rate of ticks which are infected with *B. burgdorferi* is about 30%, and the number of patients

Immunoregulation in Health and Disease
ISBN 0-12-459460-3

with Lyme disease is found to be similar to the number of patients in other countries (8). The first isolation of *B. burgdorferi* in Yugoslavia was from the spleen of *Apodemus flavicollis* from Košutnjak-K1 (9).

The aims of the study described here were basically to characterize this isolate electrophoretically and identify it to a genospecies level. In addition, we wanted to produce monoclonal antibodies (mAb) to antigens of this strain and compare their reactivity with the antigens of referent strains of *B. burgdorferi* B31 in an effort to develop a better diagnostic method for Lyme borreliosis and contribute to the understanding of the epidemiology and pathogenesis of this disease in our country.

MATERIALS AND METHODS

Spirochete strains

The type strain of *B. burgdorferi* B31 (ATCC 35210) isolated from *I. dammini* (10) and the strain K1 were used in antigen preparation. The spirochetes were grown in BSK II medium (10).

Monoclonal antibody production

BALB/c mice, female, 6 week olds, were immunized intraperitoneally with 10 mg *B. burgdorferi* strain K1 in 0.5 ml PBS/$MgCl_2$. The immunization procedure was repeated twice at 10-day intervals. Fusion was performed 3 days after the last challenge with P3X-63-Ag8.653 myeloma cells using polyethylene glycol 1500 (Serva, Heidelberg, FRG) suspended in RPMI 1640 medium (Serva) with 10% fetal calf serum (FCS) hybridoma grade (Serva). The cells were plated out into 96-well plates (Flow Laboratories). Peritoneal macrophages were used as feeder cells. Hybridomas were selected for in hypoxantine–aminopterin–thymidine (HAT) medium (Serva), according to Kohler and Milstein (11). Supernatants of growing hybridomas were screened by indirect immunofluorescent assay (IFA).

IFA

The isolate was grown in BSK II medium to the early stationary phase, washed three times in PBS/$MgCl_2$ and adjusted to a density to produce smears of about 100 separate borreliae per microscopic field of $\times 400$. The slides were air dried, fixed in cold acetone, and incubated with undiluted supernatants. After that, sheep anti-mouse Igs (INEP, Zemun, Yugoslavia), was added to the slides of a 1:25 dilution in PBS. The slides were examined in epifluorescence light on a Leitz Ortolux microscope with a $\times 40$ objective.

Sodium dodecyl sulfate-polyacrylamide gel electrophoresis (SDS–PAGE)

Electrophoresis in 12.5% polyacrylamide gels, 1.5 mm thick, was performed according to the method of Laemmli (12). Electrophoretic separation of *B. burgdorferi* strains B31 and K1 was done in an LKB-vertical system for electrophoresis, at 15°C, at 40 mA constant current. Electrophoresis buffer pH 8.3, was used as electrolyte. Gels were stained with Coomassie brilliant blue R-250 (Bio-Rad). Molecular weight standards were obtained from Pharmacia (Sweden).

Western blotting (immunoblot) analysis

After electrophoresis, proteins were transferred to polyvinylidene difluoride (PVDF) membranes by semi-dry graphite blotting (LKB) for 1.5 h at 170 mA constant current. The membranes were then saturated with 1% bovine serum albumin (Serva) for 30 min at room temperature and incubated overnight at 4°C with undiluted supernatants and serum of immunized mice at 1:120 dilution. After three washes, membrane were incubated for 2 h at room temperature with peroxidase conjugated goat anti-mouse IgG (Nordic) at 1:1000 dilution. The protein bands were visualized by addition of 3,3′ diaminobenzidine – DAB (Serva), 6 mg/ml, and 0.01% hydrogen peroxide.

RESULTS AND DISCUSSION

For examination of antigenic characteristic of *B. burgdorferi* strain K1 we analysed whole-cell lysates of this strain by SDS–PAGE and compared with the results obtained by using the referent B31 strain (Fig. 37.1). In general, the SDS–PAGE protein profiles of K1 and B31 were similar, but few exceptions among outer surface proteins (Osp) were detected.

The first difference was observed in range of 30–35 kDa low-molecular-mass major proteins, OspA and OspB. B31 has the OspA band of 31 kDa and the OspB band of 34 kDa (Fig. 37.1B), characteristically for *B. burgdorferi* sensu stricto group, to which this strain belongs (4). K1 has the OspA and OspB bands of 32 and 35 kDa, respectively. We also noticed that OspA and OspB in K1 are less abundant than these proteins in B31 strain (Fig. 37.1A).

The second difference is linked to a major band in K1 with an estimated molecular mass of 22–23 kDa, OspC, which is absent in B31, as expected (13).

On the basis of results obtained for the K1 strain concerning the expression of OspA (32 kDa), OspB (35 kDa) and OspC (23 kDa) proteins, we can

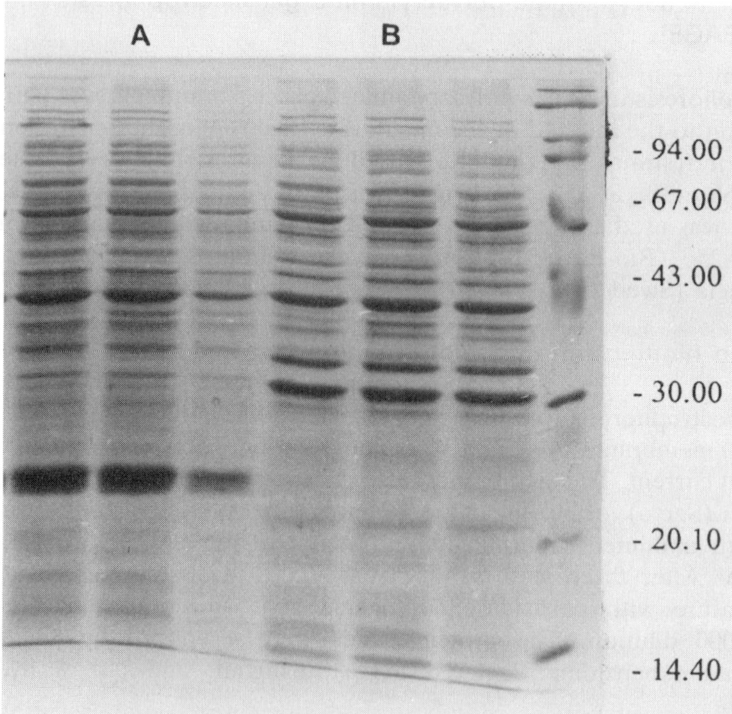

Fig. 37.1 The SDS–PAGE profiles of K1 and B31 strains of *B. burgdorferi*. Coomasie blue-stained SDS–12% PAGE of the whole cell of *B. burgdorferi* K1 (A) and B31 (B). Sizes of molecular mass standards (in kDa) are shown on the right.

conclude that this strain belongs to group VS461 or *B. afzelii* (14). It is known that *B. afzelii* has strong expression of OspC and this is associated with weaker bands of OspA and OspB. The reverse relationship between OspA/OspB and OspC has already been described (14). Large genotypic and phenotypic heterogeneity have been noticed among different strains of *B. burgdorferi*. Furthermore, it has been shown that the prevalence of *B. burgdorferi* with variable Osps, the rate of osp mutations within ticks, the number of different *B. burgdorferi* isolates and their relative concentrations in individual ticks, and the infectivity and pathogenicity of different isolates, represent variables that may influence on reliable clinical diagnosis and successful therapy (15). Most of these variables can be monitored by specific mAbs (16). So far several mAbs to particular antigens of *B. burgdorferi* have been produced (17–24). Owing to their high sensitivity and predetermined specificity they are very useful for detection of the microorganisms or their shed or degraded antigenic components in tissues and in fluids (16).

In an effort to collect more information about antigenic characteristics of our isolate we have developed mAbs directed against the K1 strain. From a fusion eight mAbs have been raised and characterized by indirect immunofluorescence and western blot using K1 and the referent strain, B31. The results are presented in Fig. 37.2.

Western blot analysis shows that six mAbs (E5E4, E5C3, E1E2, E1E12, E5A5, E4G3) recognize the antigenic determinants in a K1 protein with an apparent molecular weight of 35 kDa OspB (Fig. 37.2a). The first five mAbs do not recognize this B31 protein. Only MAb E4G3 binds to the antigenic determinant of OspB which is common for both strains (Fig. 37.2b).

The OspB lipoprotein of *B. burgdorferi* is a major component of the borrelial protein profile and has been shown to be highly immunogenic in experimentally immunized and infected mammals. This antigen, together with OspA, plays an important role in the adhesion and invasion process (17). However, the OspB loci of different strains show considerable heterology at the nucleic acid sequence level. The heterogeneity is also confirmed by several mAbs which detect different epitopes of OspB (17–19).

Shoberg *et al.* (20) demonstrated a highly conserved domain of OspB in a region of the lipoprotein which has been proposed to function in virulence, suggesting that this domain may play an important functional role in some aspect of the bacterium's existence. The mAb E4G3, which recognizes a common epitope for K1 and B31 strains, may recognize this epitope.

We also developed an mAb against p93 (E4G2), and this antigen was detected by immunoblot analysis in K1 and B31 strains of *B. burgdorferi* (Fig. 37.2c) and MAb E5H3 which specifically recognizes the protein OspC with 23 kDa molecular mass only in immunoblot analysis using proteins of K1 (Fig. 37.2d). This is in agreement with the fact that B31 is phenotypically OspC negative (13).

p93 antigen is located on the protoplasmatic cylinder of the organism (21). Two previously described mAbs, D4 (22) and 181.1 (21) also recognized this protein. The cellular function and possible pathogenic implications of p93 have not been finally clarified, but it is frequently recognized both in the early and late clinical stages of Lyme borreliosis (15).

OspC is immunodominant protein of the early humoral immune response in humans (23). First studies using a recombinant OspC protein for serodiagnosis have been carried out and showed that OspC is a specific and sensitive marker for the early stage of Lyme borreliosis (13). Furthermore, in a gerbil model of Lyme disease, active immunization with OspC protected rodents from infection, particularly against challenge with European *B. burgdorferi* strains that express little or no OspA (24).

A great OspC variability (23,25) may suggest that the OspC protein plays an important role in evasion of the immune system of the vertebrate reservoir host. On the other side, the high degree of conservation of OspC sequences within the isolates (even in strains isolated from different geographic regions)

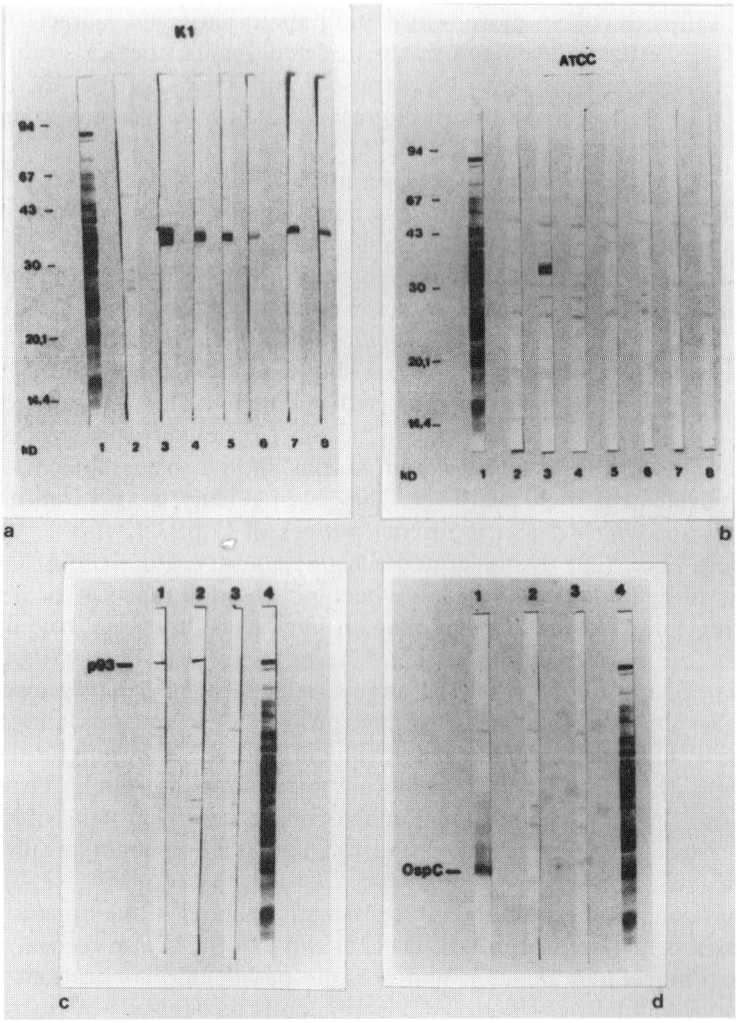

Fig. 37.2 Immunoblot reactions of K1 and B31 strains by mAbs. (a) Immunoblot reactions of K1 isolate by mAbs directed against the OspB protein (lanes 3–8). The first lane shows immunoblot reaction with serum of immunized mice at 1:120 dilution as positive control, and, as negative control, lane 2 was incubated with RPMI + 10% FCS. (b) Immunoblot reactions of B31 (ATCC 35210) strain by mAbs directed against the OspB proteins (lanes 3–8) and lane 1 is positive, and lane 2 is negative control. (c) Immunoblot reactions of K1 (lane 1) and B31 (lane 2) isolates by mAb directed against P93 compared with negative (lane 3) and positive (lane 4) control. (d) Immunoblot reactions of K1 (lane 1) and B31 (lane 2) isolates by mAb directed against OspC antigen compared with negative (lane 3) and positive (lane 4) control.

suggests that immune selection of OspC might be occurring in the vertebrate host (25).

It has been shown that the 41 kDa flagellar protein, OspC and p93 are antigens which first induce antibody responses in Lyme borreliosis (15). Consequently, these antigens are of primary interest for serological diagnosis and vaccine development. This would be especially useful in Europe where patient isolates occasionally lack OspA but where a strong immunological response is usually mounted against OspC (23).

One of the major problems associated with the effective laboratory diagnosis of Lyme disease is the lack of a good marker antigen for Lyme disease spirochaetes that is highly conserved, yet restricted to these species. In addition, this disease is followed by a species-specific immune response. Thus, the reliability of a serological investigation of Lyme disease increases when one measures antibody titres against the Osps of Lyme disease *Borrelia* species occurring in a particular geographic region (23). Therefore, a panel of mAbs which we developed could be very useful for resolving most of these problems.

CONCLUSION

According to the protein profile of *B. burgdorferi*, strain Košutnjak-K1, it was concluded that it belongs to *B. afzelii* group of *B. burgdorferi* sensu lato. The antigenic characteristics of this strain were determined by a panel of eight newly developed mAbs using K1 as immunogen. Five mAbs were specific for the outer surface protein OspB of K1, and one was specific for OspB of K1 and the reference strain, B31, which belongs to *B. burgdorferi* sensu stricto. One mAb was reactive with p93 protein, present on both strains. The last mAb recognized OspC antigen only in K1 strain.

REFERENCES

1. Burgdorfer, W., A. G. Barbour, S. F. Hayes *et al.* 1982. Lyme disease – a tick borne spirochetosis? *Science* **216**:1317–19.
2. Sehmid, G. P. 1985. The global distribution of Lyme disease. *Rev. Infect. Dis.* **7**:41–50.
3. Steere, A. C. 1989. Lyme disease. *N. Engl. J. Med.* **321**:586–96.
4. Baranton, B., D. Postic, I. Saint Girous *et al.* 1992. Delineation of *Borrelia burgdorferi* sensu stricto, *B. garinii* sp.nov. and group VS461 associated with Lyme borreliosis. *Int. J. Syst. Bacteriol.* **42**:378–83.
5. Jaenson, T. G. T. 1991. The epidemiology of Lyme borreliosis. *Parasitol. Today* **7**:39–45.
6. Assonss, M. V., D. Postic, G. Pauel *et al.* 1993. Western blot analysis of sera from Lyme borreliosis patients according to the genomic species of 8the *Borelia* strains used as antigens. *Eur. J. Clin. Microbiol. Infect. Dis.* **12**:261–8.

7. Dressler, F., R. Ackermann and A. C. Steere. 1994. Antibody responses to the three genomic groups of *Borrelia burgdorferi* in European Lyme borreliosis. *J. Infect. Dis.* **169**:313–18.
8. Đorđević, D., R. Dmitrović, V. Đerković. 1993. Problem i značaj lajmske bolesti u humanoj medicini. *Glas SANU* **43**:3–8.
9. Stajković, N., M. Obradović, B. Lako *et al.* 1993. Prva izolacija *Borrelia burgdorferi* iz *Apodemus flavicolis* u Jugoslaviji. *Glas SANU* **43**:99–106.
10. Barbour, A. G. 1984. Isolation and cultivation of Lyme disease spirochetes. *Yale J. Biol. Med.* **57**:521–5.
11. Kohler, G. and C. Milstein. 1975. Continuous cultures of fused cells secreting antibody of predefined specificity. *Nature* **227**:680–5.
12. Laemmli, U. K. 1970. Cleavage of structural proteins during assembly of the head of bacteriophage T4. *Nature (London)* **227**:680–5.
13. Padula, S. J., F. Dias, A. Sampiri *et al.* 1994. Use of recombinant OspC from *Borrelia burgdorferi* for serodiagnosis of early Lyme disease. *J. Clin. Microbiol.* **32**:1733–8.
14. Wilske, B., V. Preac–Mursic, G. Schierz *et al.* 1988. Antigenic variability of *Borrelia burgdorferi. Ann. NY Acad. Sci.* **539**:124–43.
15. Bunikis, J., B. Olsen, G. Westman and S. Bergstrom. 1995. Variable serum immunoglobulin responses against different *Borrelia burgdorferi* sensu lato species in a population at risk for and patients with Lyme disease. *J. Clin. Microbiol.* **33**:1473–8.
16. Aguila, H. L., R. R. Pollack, G. Spira and M. D. Scharff. 1986. The production of more useful monoclonal antibodies. *Immunol. Today* **7**: 380–3.
17. Barbour, A. G. and M. E. Schrumpf. 1986. Polymorphism of major surface proteins of *Borrelia burgdorferi. Zentralbl Bacteriol. Hyg. A.* **263**:83–91.
18. Schiable, U. E., R. Walich, S. E. Moter *et al.* 1990. Characterization of *Borrelia burgdorferi* associated antigens by monoclonal antibodies. *Immunobiology* **181**:357–66.
19. Stanek, G., B. Jurkowitch, C. Kochl *et al.* 1990. Reactivity of European and American isolates of *Borrelia burgdorferi* with different monoclonal antibodies by means on microimmunoblot technique. *Zbl.Bact.* **272**:426–36.
20. Shoberg, R. J., M. Jonsson, A. Šadziene *et al.* 1994. Identification of highly cross-reactive outer surface protein B epitope among diverse geographic isolates of *Borrelia burgdorferi* spp. causing Lyme disease. *J. Clin. Microbiol.* **32**:489–500.
21. Luft, B. J., S. Mudri, W. Jiang *et al.* 1992. The 93-kilodalton protein of *Borrelia burgdorferi*: an immunodominant protoplasmatic cylinder antigen. *Infect. Immun.* **60**:4309–21.
22. Volkman, D. J., B. J. Luft, P. D. Gorevic *et al.* 1991. Characterization of an immunoreactive 93 kDa core protein of *Borrelia burgdorferi* with a human IgG monoclonal antibody. *J. Immunol.* **146**:3177–82.
23. Wilske, B., S. Jauris, R. Lobentanzer, I. Pradel *et al.* 1995. Phenotypic analysis of outer surface protein C (OspC) of *Borrelia burgdorferi* sensu lato by monoclonal antibodies: relationship to genospecies and OspA serotype. *J. Clin. Microbiol.* **33**:103–9.
24. Preac-Mursic, V., B. Wilske, E. Patsorius *et al.* 1992. Active immunization with pC protein of *Borrelia burgdorferi* protects gerbils against *B. burgdorferi* infection. *Infection* **20**:342–8.
25. Wilske, B., V. Preac–Mursic, S. Jauris *et al.* 1993. Immunological and molecular polymorphism of OspC, an immunodominant major outer surface protein of *Borrelia burgdorferi. Infect. Immun.* **61**:2182–91.

38

Direct Anticryptococcal Activity of Rat T Cells

Valentina Arsić, Sanja Mitrović, Aleksandar Džamić, Ivana Kranjčić-Zec, Danica Milobratović and Marija Mostarica Stojković

T-cell mediated immunity plays a major role in the protection against infection with encapsulated fungus *Cryptococcus neoformans*. However, the mechanisms by which T lymphocytes facilitate elimination of the yeast cells have not been completely understood. It is generally thought that T lymphocytes reactive with *C. neoformans* indirectly function by production of cytokines which recruit and activate non-specific effector cells such as monocyte/macrophages, neutrophils and NK cells (1,2) or might lyse *C. neoformans*-laden unactivated phagocytes after recognizing the peptides derived from fungal proteins bound to major histocompatibility complex (MHC) molecules expressed on the infected cell, similar to the function of cytotoxic T cells during infections with other intracellular pathogens (3,4). Recently, a novel mechanism has been discovered by which freshly isolated human and mouse T lymphocytes from uninfected individuals can inhibit the growth of *C. neoformans* (5–7), an opportunistic yeast-like fungus with the tendency to infect patients with impaired T-cell functions.

In this report we extend these observations to rats. We compared anticryptococal activity of mononuclear cells derived from different peripheral lymphoid tissues of normal rats. We further determined the phenotype of effector cells and demonstrated that immunization with cryptococcal antigen enhanced the ability of rat T lymphocytes to exert cryptococcal growth inhibition capacity.

MATERIALS AND METHODS

Animals

Dark August (DA) rats 12–16 weeks old, sex matched in each experiment, were obtained from the animal colony maintained at the Institute for Biological Research, University of Belgrade, Yugoslavia.

Immunoregulation in Health and Disease
ISBN 0-12-459460-3

C. neoformans

The encapsulated strain of *C. neoformans* used in this study was isolated from cerebrospinal fluid of a patient with AIDS who had developed cerebral cryptococcosis. Yeast cells were kept frozen at −70°C. Before being used in the growth inhibition assay, cells were thawed, plated on fresh Sabouraud agar slants for one day and then cultivated in RPMI 1640 medium supplemented with 10% fetal calf serum (FCS, ICN Flow) for next 24 h, washed and after counting in a haemocytometer adjusted to the desired concentration. Heat-killed *C. neoformans* cells used for immunization were prepared by incubating a suspension of cryptorocci in PBS for 1 h at 80°C. Soluble culture filtrate antigen was produced as previously described (8).

Preparation of effector cell populations

Mononuclear cells from peripheral blood (PB), lymph nodes (LN) and spleen of DA rats were obtained after centrifugation on density gradient. Non-adherent cells were prepared by filtration over the nylon wool column (9). Negative selection of cells by panning out either $CD4^+$ or $CD8^+$ subpopulation of T lymphocytes on the basis of cell surface markers was done by the indirect panning method (10). The efficacy of depletion was confirmed by flow cytometry.

Immunization with *C. neoformans*

Rats were immunized with heat-killed *C. neoformans* organisms by intradermal injection of 0.1 ml of suspension containing 2×10^7 cells into each hind footpad. Five days later the rats were boosted by injection 0.5 ml suspension containing 1×10^8 yeast cells intraperitoneally. Control rats were injected with an equal volume of PBS by the same routes. Eight days after the first injection rats were sacrificed and their spleens removed for the analysis of specific proliferative response and anticryptococcal activity.

C. neoformans growth inhibition assay

Antifungal activity was determined as described (5). Briefly, effector cells were cultivated at different effector/target ratios ranging from 400 : 1 to 25 : 1 with 5×10^3 cryptococcal target cells in a total volume of 0.2 ml RPMI 1640 medium in quadruplicate wells of a flat-bottom 96-well microtitre plate (Linbro, Flow Lab). Control wells contained only 5×10^3 cryptococcal target cells in medium. After 24 h incubation at 37°C in 5% carbon dioxide test samples and control samples were resuspended in 0.1% Triton X-100 (US Biochemical Corporation) in water to lyse the effector cells, the treatment previously shown to have no effects on the viability of cryptococci. The content of each well was serially diluted in sterile PBS and plated in duplicate on Sabouraud agar slants. After 3 days of incubation at 26°C, colony-forming units (CFU) were counted and the percentage of cryptococcal growth inhibition was determined according to the following formula:

$$\frac{\%\ cryptoccal}{growth\ inhibition} = \frac{mean\ control\ CFU - mean\ experimental\ CFU}{mean\ control\ CFU} \times 100$$

Proliferation assay

Mononuclear spleen cells (4×10^5) from *C. neoformans*-immunized and PBS-injected rats were cultivated in triplicates in 0.2 ml RPMI 1640 medium supplemented with 5% FBS in flat-bottom 96-well microtitre plates alone or in the presence of 1% soluble culture filtrate antigen. After 72 h incubation at 37°C in 5% carbon dioxide in humidified atmosphere cell cultures were pulsed with 37 kBq/well of methyl-^{3}H-thymidine (^{3}H-TdR, specific activity 185 GBq/mmol, Amersham) and were harvested 18 h later on to glass fibre filters.

RESULTS AND DISCUSSION

Initial experiments were performed to establish whether mononuclear cells derived from lymphoid tissues of normal, non-immunized and non-infected rats exerted the anticryptococcal activity in the microassay similar to that described with human and mouse lymphocytes. Our results have shown that rat mononuclear cells exerted a fungistatic effect in all tested effector : target ratios, but the optimal effect was obtained at 100 : 1 ratio (data not shown) and all further experiments were done using this ratio. Significant inhibition of in vitro growth of yeast cells was observed after cocultivation with mononuclear cells as well as with non-adherent populations highly enriched in T lymphocytes derived from all tested rat lymphoid tissues (Fig. 38.1). As antifungal activity of non-adherent lymphoid cells was even enhanced in comparison with non-separated population of the respective tissue, it was obvious that cells other than T lymphocytes were not required for this interaction to occur. The results showing that as cell populations were enriched for T lymphocytes the anticryptococcal activity of the effector cell population concomitantly increased (Fig. 38.1) are in accordance with data obtained with murine lymphocytes (7). As shown in Fig. 38.1, rat peripheral blood mononuclear cells, both unseparated and non-adherent, exerted maximal fungistatic activity while lymph node cells were the least effective. Bearing in mind that rodent natural killer cells (NK) have the ability to interact directly with cryptococcal cells and kill them (11) and that order of

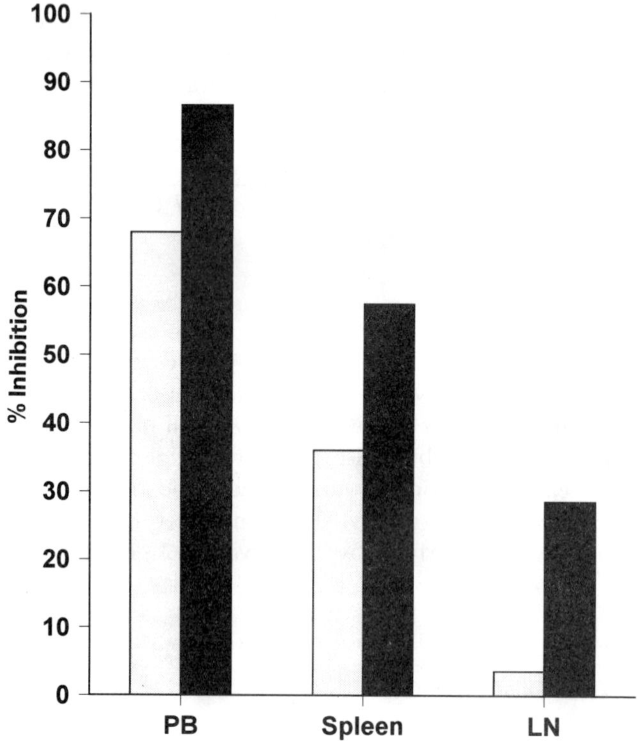

Fig. 38.1 Growth inhibition of *C. neoformans* mediated by unseparated (light bars) and non-adherent (black bars) mononuclear cell populations of rat peripheral lymphoid tissues. Effector cells (5×10^5/well) were incubated with *C. neoformans* (5×10^3/well). After 24 h the number of live yeast cells was determined by counting CFU following dilution and spread plates. Data are representative of three experiments performed in quadruplicate.

frequency of NK cells in rat lymphoid organs (PBL > spleen > lymph node, 12) correlated to the magnitude of anticryptococcal activities of the respective tissues demonstrated in these experiments, it was reasonable to assume that the observed fungistatic effect could be ascribed to NK cells and not to T lymphocytes. We therefore analysed the membrane phenotype of the effector cells and demonstrated that more than 95% are T lymphocytes (data not shown). Further, we separated non-adherent mononuclear spleen cells into $CD4^+$ and $CD8^+$ population by an indirect panning technique and compared the anticryptococcal activity of the effector cell populations before and after applying the separation procedure (Fig. 38.2). Over 90% of the cells expressed the cell surface antigen selected for (data not shown). The $CD8^+$ population had slightly a higher effect in growth inhibition than the $CD4^+$ cells, but these latter cells were almost as effective as unseparated non-

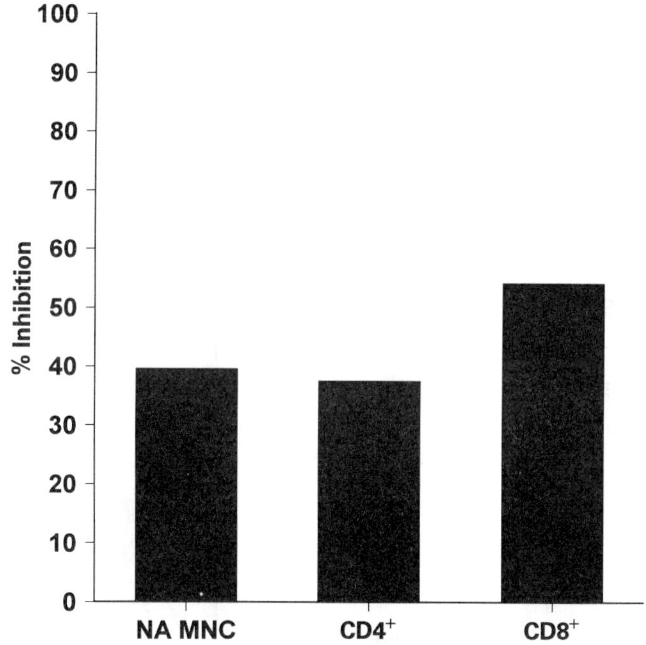

Fig. 38.2 Both $CD4^+$ and $CD8^+$ cell populations are responsible for the antifungal activity of rat spleen non-adherent mononuclear cells. Nylon-wool non-adherent mononuclear spleen cells were separated into $CD4^+$ and $CD8^+$ population by indirect panning method. Unseparated and negatively selected cells (5×10^5/well) were incubated with *C. neoformans* (5×10^3/well). After 24 h the number of live yeast cells was determined by counting CFU following dilution and spread plates. Results shown are from a representative experiment. Two other experiments yielded similar results.

adherent spleen mononuclear cells. This result strongly points to the fact that T lymphocytes are responsible for the observed fungistatic effects. It also demonstrates that both $CD4^+$ and $CD8^+$ cells can inhibit in vitro growth of *C. neoformans*, as has been shown for human T lymphocytes (13). It was shown that both T-cell subpopulations are required in vivo for resistance against *C. neoformans*, as indicated by the fact that elimination of either $CD4^+$ or $CD8^+$ cells impaired the ability to clear the yeast from the infected host (14, 15). The stronger inhibitory effect of the $CD8^+$ population observed in this study could be explained by the concomitant antifungal activity of NK cells (11), which are $CD8^+$ in rats (16).

To determine whether previous in vivo exposure to *C. neoformans* enhanced the ability of T lymphocytes to display direct anticryptococcal activity we compared non-adherent mononuclear spleen populations from *C. neoformans*-immunized rats with a similar T-cell-enriched population of

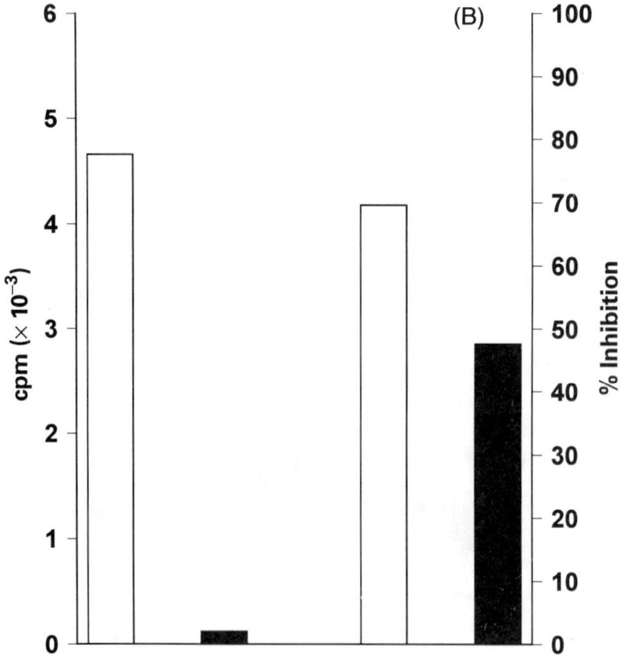

Fig. 38.3 Lymphocytes activated in vivo with specific antigen are more efficacious in *C. neoformans* growth inhibition. A. Mononuclear spleen cells (4×10^5) obtained from rats immunized as described in Materials and Methods (white bars) or from control rats (black bars) were cultivated in the presence of soluble crytococcal antigen (1%) for 4 days and pulsed with ^{3}H-TdR for the last 18 h. Results are expressed as mean cpm of the triplicate cultures. SD did not exceed 10% of the mean. B. The same cell populations were depleted of adherent cells and incubated (5×10^5/well) with *C. neoformans* (5×10^3/well). After 24 h the number of live yeast cells was determined by counting CFU following dilution and spread plates.

saline-treated control rats for the ability to mediate growth inhibition of cryptococcal cells. The efficacy of the immunization was demonstrated by assessing proliferative response of spleen mononuclear cells obtained from *C. neoformans*-injected and control rats after in vitro stimulation with specific cryptococcal antigen. Results (Fig. 38.3A) showing that only cells derived from immunized rats proliferated in the presence of cryptococcal antigen indicate that *C. neoformans*-injected rats developed specific anticryptococcal response. The anticryptococcal activity of T lymphocytes obtained from immunized rats was significantly greater than that mediated by lymphocytes from control rats (Fig. 38.3B). These data are in accordance with the results obtained in a murine model showing that immunization with intact *C. neoformans* induced, in lymph nodes and spleens, T lymphocytes which have enhanced abilities to bind and inhibit *C. neoformans* cell growth compared to control T lymphocytes (7,17).

CONCLUSION

The data presented here provide evidence that freshly isolated rat peripheral T lymphocytes act directly on *C. neoformans* to inhibit or kill it. Fractionation of lymphocytes into CD4^{+} and CD8^{+} revealed that both cell populations exerted anticryptococcal effect, although the in vitro growth inhibition mediated by the CD8^{+} fraction was more efficient. Rats given heat-killed *C. neoformans* developed sensitized splenic T lymphocytes with augmented ability to inhibit the in vitro growth of *C. neoformans.* There is ample evidence that human and murine T lymphocytes inhibit *C. neoformans* growth in vitro. To our knowledge the data presented here are the first demonstration that rat T lymphocytes also can directly inhibit the growth of a fungal target. Therefore, these results suggest that direct antifungal activity is a general property of T lymphocytes irrespective of species they are derived from, but it remains to elucidate the extent of its contribution to the host defense against infectious agents.

REFERENCES

1. Huffnagle, G. B., M. F. Lipscomb, J. A. Lovchick *et al.* 1994. The role of CD4+ and CD8+ T cells in protective inflammatory response to a pulmonary cryptococcal infection. *J. Leukocyte Biol.* **55**:34–42.
2. Kawakami, K., S. Kohno, J. Kadota *et al.* 1995. T. cell-dependent activation of macrophages and enhancement of their phagocytic activity in the lungs of mice inoculated with heat-killed *Cryptococcus neoformans:* Involvement of IFN-gamma and its protective effect against cryptococcal infection. *Microb. Immunol.* **39**:135–43.
3. Kaufmann, S. H. E., E. Hug and G. DeLibero. 1986. *Listeria monocytogenes* restrictive T lymphocyte clones with cytolytic activity against infected target cells. *J. Exp. Med.* **164**:363–8.
4. Silva, C. L., M. F. Silva, R. C. L. R. Pietro and D. B. Lowrie. 1994. Protection against tuberculosis by passive transfer with T-cell clones recognising mycobacterial heat-shock protein 65. *Immunology* **83**:341–6.
5. Murphy, J. W., M. R. Hidore, and S. C. Wong. 1993. Direct interaction of human lymphocytes with the yeast-like organism, *Cryptococcus neoformans. J. Clin. Invest.* **91**:1553–66.
6. Levitz, S. M., M. P. Dupon, and E. H. Smail. 1994. Direct activity of human T lymphocytes and natural killer cells against *Cryptococcus neoformans. Infect. Immun.* **62**:194–202.
7. Muth, S. and J. W. Murphy. 1995. Direct anticryptococcal activity of lymphocytes from *Cryptococcus neoformans*-immunized mice. *Infect. Immun.* **63**:1637–44.
8. Buchanan, K. L. and J. W. Murphy. 1993. Characterization of cellular infiltrates and cytokine production during the expression phase of the anticrytococcal delayed-type hypersensitivity response. *Infect. Immun.* **61**:2854–65.

9. Julius, M. H., E. Simpson and L. A. Herzenberg. 1973. A rapid method for the isolation of functional thymus-derived murine lymphocytes. *Eur. J. Immunol.* **3**:645–9.
10. Wysocki, L. J. and V. L. Sato. 1978. 'Panning' for lymphocytes: a method for cell selection. *Proc. Natl. Acad. Sci. USA* **75**:2844–8.
11. Hidore, M. R., N. Nabavi, F. Sonleitner and J. W. Murphy. 1991. Murine natural killer cells are fungicidal to *Cryptococcus neoformans*. *Infect. Immun.* **5**:1747–54.
12. Reynolds, C. W., T. Timonen and R. B. Herberman. 1981. Natural killer (NK) cell activity in the rat. I. Isolation and characterization of the effector cells. *J. Immunol.* **127**:282–7.
13. Levitz, S. M. and M. P. Dupont. 1993. Phenotypic and functional characterization of human lymphocytes activated by interleukin-2 to directly inhibit growth of *Cryptococcus neoformans* in vitro. *J. Clin. Invest.* **91**:1490–8.
14. Hill, J. C. and A. G. Harmsen. 1991. Intrapulmonary growth and dissemination of an avirulent strain of *Cryptococcus neoformans* in mice depleted of CD4+ or CD8+ T cells. *J. Exp. Med.* **173**:755–8.
15. Huffnagle, G. B., J. L. Yates and M. F. Lipscomb. 1991. Immunity to a pulmonary *Cryptococcus neoformans* infection requires both CD4+ and CD8+ T cells. *J. Exp. Med.* **173**:793–800.
16. Reynolds, C. W., S. O. Sharrow, J. R. Ortaldo and R. B. Herberman. 1981. Natural killer (NK) cell activity in the rat II. Analysis of surface antigens on LGL by flow cytometry. *J. Immunol.* **127**:2204–8.
17. Muth, S. and J. W. Murphy. 1995. Effects of immunization with *Cryptococcus neoformans* cells or cryptococcal culture filtrate antigen on direct anticryptococcal activities on murine T lymphocytes. *Infect. Immun.* **63**:1645–51.

39

Pro-IL-1β Processing is an Essential Step in the Autocrine Regulation of Acute Myeloid Leukaemic Cell Growth

Stanislava Stošić-Grujičić, Nadežda Basara
and Charles A. Dinarello

The abnormal growth and maturation arrest of leukaemia progenitors in patients with acute myeloid leukaemia (AML) include the production of various cytokines and growth factors, some of which may be produced by neoplastic cells themselves (1,2). Increasing evidence indicates a central pathophysiologic role for IL-1β, which includes induction of other growth factors and up-regulation or down-regulation of receptors (1,3). Thus, one of the possible ways to inhibit the abnormal growth in AML could be the blockade of IL-1. To prove a role for IL-1, a variety of modalities has been used to block the production and/or activity of the cytokine. These include agents which inhibit IL-1 transcription and synthesis, the processing of pro-IL-1β into its mature forms, the secretion of IL-1β, the activity of IL-1 using neutralizing antibodies or soluble (extracellular) IL-1 receptors, the ability of IL-1 to bind to its receptors using receptor blockade, the availability of surface receptors using agents which down-modulate receptor expression, or agents which affect IL-1 mediated signal transduction (4). By using some of these strategies, classical extracellular regulation of the AML blast cell growth including autocrine and paracrine loops mediated by IL-1 has been well documented (5). However, there is evidence that intracellular autocrine loops involving GM-CSF may also be operative in some cases of AML cells (2). Here we have studied whether intracellular autocrine loops involving the IL-1 system are operative in autonomous growth of AML cells. We therefore analysed the effect of antisense oligonucleotide to the IL-1β converting enzyme (ICE), a specific cysteine protease which mediates processing of endogenously produced non-functional pro-IL-1β into its mature form (6),

Immunoregulation in Health and Disease
ISBN 0-12-459460-3

and we compared it with the effects obtained by IL-1 receptor antagonist (IL-1RA), an agent which blocks the binding of IL-1 to its receptors (3).

MATERIALS AND METHODS

Leukaemia cells of 19 randomly selected AML patients were obtained at diagnosis from bone marrow (BM) and peripheral blood (PB) samples. Informed consent was obtained from the patients and the study was approved by an Institutional Human Research Committee. The diagnoses were established according to the FAB criteria (7). Low-density leukaemia cells were prepared using Ficoll-Hypaque density gradient. Cells were grown continuously in the presence of recombinant human IL-1RA (Upjohn, Kalamazoo), or phosphorothioate-derived 16-mer antisense oligonucleotide for human IL-1β converting enzyme CCT-TGT-CGG-CCA-TGG-C (2032-2, Genta, San Diego, CA, USA). A control oligonucleotide was CTG-AAG-GGC-TTC-TTC-C (2042-2, Genta). The effects of the agents on AML cell growth were assessed by using two complementary systems: colony formation (CFU-AML) and AML cell proliferation.

CFU-AML assay was performed according to Marie *et al.* (8). Briefly, 2×10^4 T-cell depleted (by sheep red blood cell rosseting) leukaemia blast cells were plated in 96-well microplates in Iscove's modification of Dulbecco's medium (IMDM, Gibco) with 0.8% methycellulose, 20% fetal calf serum (FCS, Flow Laboratories, Irvine, Scotland) and 10% phytohaemagglutinin stimulated leukocyte conditioned medium (PHA-LCM) and incubated at 37°C in a humidified atmosphere with 5% carbon dioxide. Colony numbers (aggregates of greater than 20 cells) were scored after 7 days of incubation. Results were expressed as the mean obtained from 6 replicate cultures, with the SEM less than 10%. The percent inhibition of CFU-AML by IL-1RA, or antisense oligonucleotide was calculated by comparison with growth of control cells in medium only.

Proliferation assay was performed in the liquid system in 96-well microplates containing 5×10^4 BM-derived cells/well, or 1×10^5 PB-derived cells/well in RPMI 1640 medium with 10% FCS. Spontaneous proliferation in triplicate cultures was determined by the incorporation of ^{3}H-thymidine (6.7 Ci/mmol, 1 μCi/well, ICN Radiochemicals, Irvine) added for the final 18 h of the 66 h incubations. Results were expressed as mean cpm with the SEM less than 10%, or as a percentage inhibition of ^{3}H-thymidine incorporation, calculated in relation to individual control proliferation where the agent was omitted, i.e. without IL-1RA, or antisense oligonucleotide.

Statistical significances were evaluated by the Student's *t* test. $p < 0.05$ was considered significant.

RESULTS AND DISCUSSION

We have shown previously that freshly obtained AML cells show some degree of autonomous growth in culture, whereas blood leukocytes from healthy donors do not unless stimulated (5,9). Table 39.1 summarizes the clinical and the growth characteristics of the AML samples studied. As shown, both BM-derived and PB-derived AML cells displayed autonomous growth. Spontaneous cell proliferation varied, as well as CFU-AML colony formation, and did not correlate with the type of AML according to FAB criteria.

To assess the effect of antisense ICE oligonucleotide on autonomous growth of AML blast cells, a dose–response experiment was performed using AML cell samples from a few randomly selected AML patients (i.e. patients No. 2, 3, 4, 9, 10, 11 and 16 from Table 39.1). As assessed by ^{3}H-thymidine incorporation, increasing concentrations of the antisense oligonucleotide in the range from 10 to 75 μM in a dose-dependent way inhibited spontaneous proliferation, while the same concentrations of control oligonucleotide had no effect on cell growth (data not shown). Therefore, 50 μM of oligonucleotides were used for further experiments. Similarly, a dose-dependent inhibition of growth was obtained in a pilot study with recombinant IL-1RA when applied in concentrations between 0.8 and 50 μg/ml (9), and 10 μg/ml was therefore used for comparative analysis.

Figure 39.1 compares the effects of the interruption of intracellular IL-1 loops by antisense ICE oligonucleotide and interruption of extracellular loops by IL-1RA on AML cell proliferation. Inhibition of DNA synthesis was seen with the antisense oligonucleotide in all of the samples tested. The degree of inhibition of BM-derived and PB-derived samples varied from 20 to 97% and from 4 to 97%, respectively. On the other hand, IL-1RA inhibited both BM-derived and PB-derived cell proliferation only in 8 of 18 AML cases. The mean inhibitory effect on AML cell proliferation obtained by antisense oligomer was significantly higher in comparison to IL-1RA induced inhibition (Fig. 39.1).

The comparison of the effects of antisense oligomer and IL-1RA at a progenitor cell level is presented in Fig. 39.2. The growth of leukaemia blast progenitors was significantly affected in a majority of cases, both with antisense ICE oligonucleotide and IL-1RA. The degree of inhibition of CFU-AML is much higher in the presence of antisense ICE oligonucleotide in comparison to the treatment with IL-1RA.

As previously shown (1,5,9), we confirmed by using IL-1RA that blocking the interaction between IL-1 and leukaemia cells through prevention of IL-1 binding to receptors results in growth arrest of malignant AML cells. Further studies using antisense strategy for interruption of pro-IL-1β processing by targeting ICE revealed the role of an intracellular autocrine loop involving IL-1 in the control of the autonomous growth of AML cells. As suggested recently, the effect of inhibiting ICE may not be entirely straightforward (10),

Table 39.1. Clinical and growth characteristics of AML samples

Patient no.	Age/Sex	Diagnosis (FAB)	BM blasts (%)	PB blasts (%)	Hb (g/dL)	Plt ($\times 10^9$/l)	WBC ($\times 10^9$/l)	CFU-AML BM	CFU-AML PB	^{3}H-TdR uptake BM	^{3}H-TdR uptake PB
1	41/M	M0	60	80	10.0	40	240.0	23.8	47.5	26 693	38 228
2	52/F	M1	92	n.d.	12.0	80	1.5	53.0	n.d.	692	8489
3	77/F	M1	95	43	3.4	94	2.3	14.3	n.d.	705	1485
4	58/F	M2	60	33	7.9	24	30.0	123.8	2.5	4147	2295
5	44/M	M2	55	1	8.6	14	2.0	n.d.	n.d.	190	108
6	63/M	M2	77	17	5.8	14	17.0	11.3	10.2	4979	9893
7	31/M	M3	95	85	9.4	21	13.0	42.0	37.0	78	89
8	56/F	M3	90	37	8.1	15	2.0	51.0	48.0	85	103
9	64/M	M4	75	47	8.4	65	29.3	8.0	9.3	1546	444
10	62/F	M4eo	40	18	11.5	23	95.0	n.d.	114.0	n.d.	35 738
11	60/M	M4	50	20	6.8	20	16.0	16.7	0	6973	12 674
12	59/M	M4	59	37	9.3	32	31.0	13.0	0	1252	1223
13	41/M	M4	67	69	11.6	17	90.0	192.0	388.0	571	1039
14	66/F	M4	74	22	12.1	186	122.0	20.7	65.9	4909	6649
15	58/M	M4	42	56	8.8	14	17.0	5.1	7.6	4655	16 278
16	24/M	M5	90	11	7.2	68	23.0	29.2	90.7	2671	4203
17	16/M	M5	85	88	9.9	18	74.0	3.0	20.0	2316	6371
18	33/F	M5a	95	94	13.8	30	32.0	68.6	21.0	392	541
19	66/M	M5a	83	8	7.8	35	33.0	52.4	25.3	3358	10 178

FAB, French–American–British criteria for diagnosis of AML; BM, bone marrow; PB, peripheral blood; Hb, haemoglobin; Plt, platelets; WBC, white blood cells.

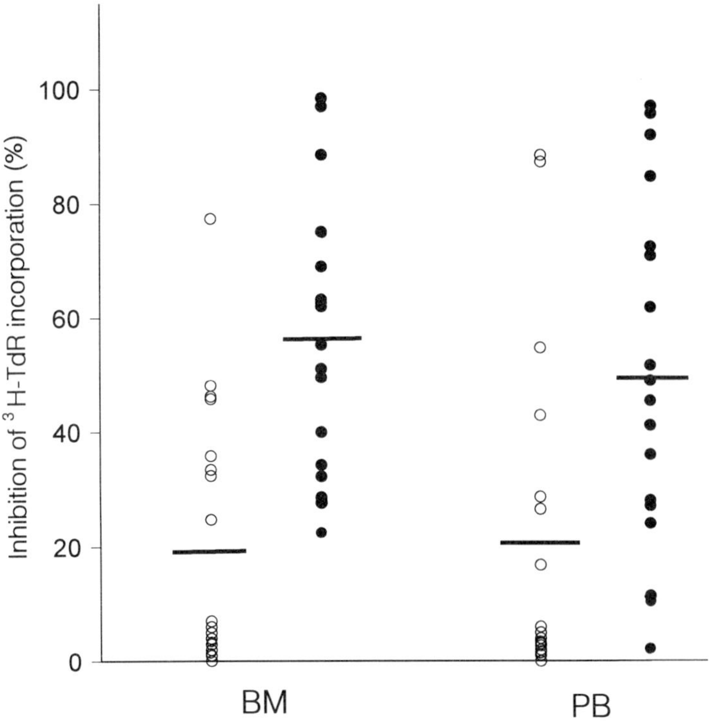

Fig. 39.1 The effect of IL-1RA and antisense oligonucleotide to ICE on spontaneous bone marrow (BM) and peripheral blood (PB) AML cell proliferation. Results obtained from patients 1–19 are depicted. The data are presented as the percent of the inhibition of mean ^{3}H-TdR incorporation obtained from each patient in the presence of IL-1RA (○), or antisense ICE oligonucleotide (●) as compared to control culture. Significantly higher inhibition ($p < 0.05$) was produced by antisense ICE oligonucleotide compared with IL-1RA (horizontal bar indicates the mean inhibition value of each group).

since it is possible that this treatment reduces apoptosis, as the ICE gene belongs to the family of 'cell-death' genes (11). If inhibition of ICE reduces natural apoptotic mechanisms, there would be an increase in the proliferation or viability of cells that would otherwise undergo apoptosis. However, we have shown that in vitro treatment of AML cells with antisense ICE oligonucleotide did not increase, but rather reduced AML cell proliferation. In addition, the treatment did not change leukaemia blasts viability, as judged by trypan blue exclusion and flow cytometric analysis of propidium-iodine stained cells (data not presented). Thus, it seems likely that specific inhibition of ICE by antisense oligomer is not associated with defects in apoptosis, but with inhibition of processing and release of mature IL-1β. In

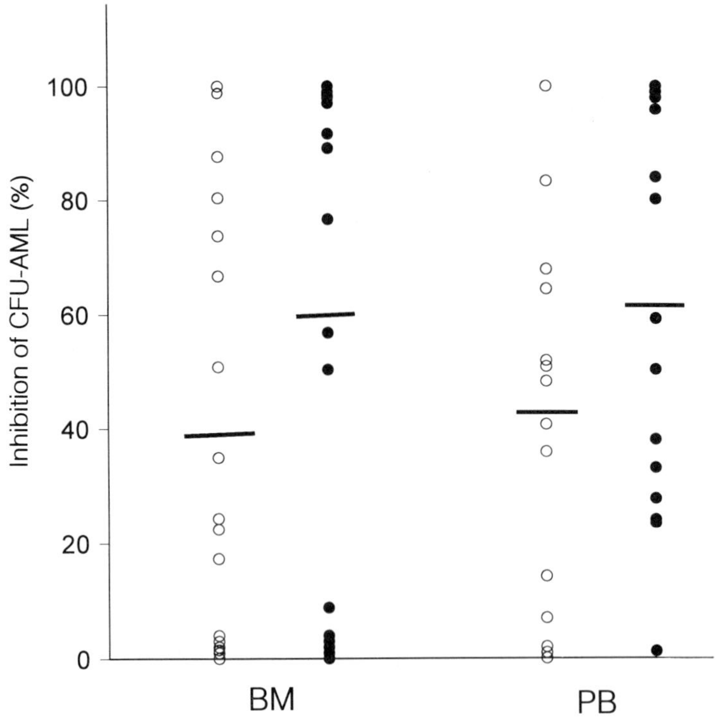

Fig. 39.2 The effect of IL-1RA and antisense oligonucleotide to ICE on bone marrow (BM) and peripheral blood (PB) CFU-AML colony formation. Results obtained from patients 1–19 are depicted. The data are presented as the percent of inhibition of mean colony numbers obtained from each patient in the presence of IL-1RA (○), or antisense ICE oligonucleotide (●) as compared to control culture. Significantly higher inhibition ($p < 0.05$) was produced by antisense ICE oligonucleotide compared with IL-1RA (horizontal bar indicates the mean inhibition value of each group).

support of this, it was recently shown that ICE blockade by the other ICE-specific inhibitors suppresses the proliferation of malignant cells from patients with AML (10, 12). Although the physiological function of mammalian ICE homologues is unknown, overexpression of the ICE gene is observed in a number of leukaemias (6) suggesting a role for ICE in driving the leukaemia process. Therefore, our data might suggest improvement in therapeutic potential by targeting ICE genes responsible for disease.

CONCLUSIONS

In the present study, it was shown that autonomous growth of AML cells is inhibited by antisense oligonucleotide to IL-1β converting enzyme and by

IL-1RA. IL-1 blockade affects not only AML cell proliferation, but AML cell progenitors as well. Since the inhibitory effect of antisense ICE oligonucleotide was more efficient when compared to the effect of IL-1RA, our results suggest that pro-IL-1β processing is an essential step in the regulation of AML cell growth.

ACKNOWLEDGEMENT

We acknowledge the financial support of the Scientific Fund of Serbia. We also thank Dr. Nada Kraguljac and Dr. Dijana Šefer for expert technical assistance.

REFERENCES

1. Kurzrock, R., M. Wetzler, Z. Estrov and M. Talpaz. 1995. Interleukin-1 and its inhibitors: A biologic and therapeutic model for the role of growth regulatory factors in leukemias. *Cytokines Mol. Therapy* **1**:177–84.
2. Rogers, S. Y., D. Bradbury, R. Kozlowski and N. H. Russell. 1994. Evidence for internal autocrine regulation of growth in acute myeloblastic leukemia cells. *Exp. Hematol.* **22**:593–8.
3. Dinarello, C. A. 1991. Interleukin-1 and interleukin-1 antagonism. *Blood* **77**:1627–52.
4. Dinarello, C. A. 1994. Interleukin-1 in disease. *Keio J. Med.* **43**:131–6.
5. Rambaldi, A., M. Torcia, S. Bettoni *et al.* 1991. Modulation of cell proliferation and cytokine production in acute myeloblastic leukemia by interleukin-1 receptor antagonist and lack of its expression by leukemic cells. *Blood* **78**:3248–53.
6. Cerretti, D. P., C. J. Kozlosky, B. Mosley *et al.* 1992. Molecular cloning of the interleukin-1β converting enzyme. *Science* **256**:97–100.
7. Bennet, J. M., D. Catovsky, M. T. H. Daniel *et al.* 1985. Proposed revised criteria for the classification of the acute leukemias. French-American-British (FAB) co-operative group. *Ann. Int. Med.* **103**:620–5.
8. Marie, J. P., C. A. Izaguirre, C. I. Civin *et al.* 1981. Granulopoietic differentiation in AML blasts in culture. *Blood* **58**:670–4.
9. Stošić-Grujičić, S., N. Basara, P. Milenković, and C. A. Dinarello. 1995. Modulation of acute myeloblastic leukemia (AML) cell proliferation and blast colony formation by antisense oligomer for IL-1 beta converting enzyme (ICE) and IL-1 receptor antagonist (IL-1Ra). *J. Chemotherapy* **7**: 67–70.
10. Dinarello, C. A. and N. H. Margolis. 1995. Cytokine-processing enzymes. *Curr. Biol.* **5**: 587–90.
11. Kumar, S., M. Kinoshita, M. Noda, N. G. Copeland and N. A. Jenkins. 1994. Induction of apoptosis by the mouse Nedd2 gene, which encodes a protein similar to the product of the Caenorhabditis elegans cell death gene ced-3 and the mammalian IL-1 beta-converting enzyme. *Genes Dev.* **8**:1613–26.
12. Estrov, Z., R. A. Black, R. Kurzrock *et al.* 1994. IL-1β converting enzyme (ICE) inhibitor suppresses AML blast proliferation. *Blood* **84**:380.

40

Modulation of Acute Myeloid Leukaemic Cell Growth by Human Macrophage Inflammatory Protein-1α

Nadežda Basara, Stanislava Stošić-Grujičić, Dijana Šefer, Zoran Ivanović, Nina Radošević, Darinka Bošković and Pavle Milenković

Acute myeloid leukaemia (AML) is a clonal neoplastic disorder characterized by the proliferation and accumulation in the bone marrow and peripheral blood of abnormal leukaemia blast cells (1). The mechanisms involved in regulation of AML cell proliferation are not fully understood (2). It has been shown that AML progenitor cells are responsive to stimulatory molecules that regulate normal haemopoietic stem cell proliferation (3). On the other hand, the regulatory role of inhibitors of stem cell proliferation on AML progenitors and AML cell proliferation has not yet been established (4,5).

Recently, a stem cell proliferation inhibitor has been characterized (6) and found to be identical to macrophage inflammatory protein-1α (MIP-1α). MIP-1α, an 8 kDa glycoprotein, inhibited proliferation of immature haemopoietic progenitors in normal bone marrow both in vitro and in vivo (7,8). The inhibition of normal bone marrow progenitors might therefore be used for protection of these cells from the cytotoxic drugs effective on leukaemia cells. However, more recently it has been shown that MIP-1α also inhibits early and mature AML progenitors and prevents AML progenitors from entering the proliferative phase of the cell cycle, thus indicating possible clinical benefits in AML therapy (9).

The aim of our study was to investigate the effect of the peptide LD78, the human homologue of murine MIP-1α, which shows 747 amino acid sequence homology with MIP-1α (10), on bone marrow AML progenitor cells, as measured by in vitro CFU-AML growth. In addition, proliferative status of the bone marrow in the presence of LD78 was evaluated.

Immunoregulation in Health and Disease
ISBN 0-12-459460-3

Table 40.1 Clinical characteristics of AML patients at diagnosis

Patient no.	Age/sex	FAB	Hb (g/dl)	WBC ($\times 10^9$/l)	Plt ($\times 10^9$/l)	BM (blasts) %
1	55/M	M1	8.7	68	6.0	90
2	52/M	M2	8.6	115	10	56
3	53/F	M2	11.9	60	23	70
4	44/M	M2	8.6	2.0	14	55
5	61/M	M2	9.2	14	4	70
6	69/F	M2	8.6	7.2	112	37
7	58/M	M2	11.0	26	22	72
8	69/F	M2	9.0	27	45	76
9	19/F	M3	11.5	2	73	70
10	27/F	M3	10.3	16	7	90
11	18/F	M3	7.4	1.7	14	95
12	31/F	M3	9.4	13	21	99
13	29/F	M3	8.7	17	12	95
14	34/F	M4	7.2	45	19	40
15	70/F	M4	10.0	50	10	80
16	35/M	M4	8.0	65	27	90
17	58/F	M4	9.0	56	54	78
18	59/M	M4	9.3	31	32	35
19	38/F	M4	8.5	25	47	67
20	28/M	M4	11.6	92	4.0	40
21	60/F	M5b	10.0	20	68	80
22	53/M	M5	8.0	65	27	85
23	16/M	M5	9.9	5.2	188	71

FAB, French–American–British criteria for diagnosis of AML (13); Hb, haemoglobin; WBC, white blood cells; Plt, platelets; BM, bone marrow; PB, peripheral blood.

MATERIAL AND METHODS

Patients

Bone marrow and peripheral blood samples from 23 adult, previously untreated, AML patients (Table 40.1) were studied. In all cases, informed consent was obtained from the patients. The study was approved by an Institutional Human Research Committee. The diagnosis and classification were established according to the FAB criteria (11). There were one M1, seven M2, five M3, seven M4 and three M5. Median age was 52 years (range from 16 to 70 years) and sex distribution was 10 males and 13 females (1 : 1.3 ratio).

The bone marrow (BM) cells were aspirated from the sternum; mononuclear cells were separated by density gradient (Lymphoprep, density

1.077 g/cm^3, Nyegaard, Oslo, Norway) washed and resuspended in Iscove's modification of Dulbecco's medium (IMDM, Gibco).

LD78

We have used recombinant human MIP-1α (R&D Systems, Minneapolis, MN, USA), sometimes referred to as LD78 as described by Obary *et al.* (10). Due to the high structural homology between the two genes encoding MIP-1α and LD78, the two terms are used interchangeably, as suggested recently by Lord (12).

CFU-AML assay

The technique of blast colony formation was used as previously described by Marie *et al.* (13). Briefly, 2×10^4 T-cell depleted BM cells in 0.1 ml of IMDM were plated in a culture mixture of methylcellulose (0.8%), 20% fetal calf serum (FCS, Gibco) and 10% phytohaemagglutinin-leukocyte conditioned medium in 96-multiwell culture plates, 0.3 ml per well (Becton-Dickinson). Aggregates of more than 20 cells were counted as CFU-AML colonies at day 7. The percentage of inhibition of CFU-AML growth in the presence of increasing concentrations (50–400 ng/ml of culture) of LD78, was calculated by comparison of the growth of colonies in the experimental to the growth of these colonies in control plates without LD78.

Proliferation assay

For the liquid proliferation system (spontaneous proliferation), cells were plated for 66 h in RPMI 1640-10% FCS in 96-well microplates at 5×10^4 BM cells/well, in the continuous presence of increasing concentrations of LD78 or in the absence of LD78. Spontaneous proliferation was determined by incorporation of ^{3}H-TdR added 18 h before harvesting as already described (14). Results were expressed as the mean cpm obtained in triplicate cultures or as percentage of inhibition of control ^{3}H-TdR incorporation, obtained in the absence of LD78.

RESULTS

It was apparent that AML cells of 4 out of 20 patients studied (20%) did not form bone marrow CFU-AML colonies, so the effect of LD78 in those cases could not be evaluated. Inhibition of bone marrow CFU-AML growth with LD78 was obtained in 14/16 samples which formed colonies (Table 40.2).

Table 40.2 Effect of LD78 on CFU-AML colony formation and AML cell proliferation

Patient no.	CFU-AML BM			AML cell proliferation BM		
FAB	Control	+LD78	% inhibition	Spontaneous	+LD78	% inhibition
1 (M1)	0	0	/	122 ± 21[b]	233 ± 37	0
2 (M2)	46.4 ± 11.8[a]	0	100	639 ± 27	456 ± 19	28.6
3 (M2)	0	0	/	3304 ± 136	2373 ± 116	28.2
4 (M2)	nd	/	/	190 ± 12	185 ± 26	0
5 (M2)	37.4 ± 2.7	11.6 ± 1.2	69.0	nd	/	/
6 (M2)	9.2 ± 0.8	0.7 ± 0.2	92.4	nd	/	/
7 (M2)	21.8 ± 2.4	1.0 ± 0.3	95.4	nd	/	/
8 (M2)	10.2 ± 0.9	2.0 ± 0.3	80.4	nd	/	/
9 (M3)	nd	/	/	102 ± 8	69 ± 5	32.3
10 (M3)	84.3 ± 4.9	36.0 ± 2.1	57.3	174 ± 18	194 ± 35	0
11 (M3)	0	0	/	158 ± 35	173 ± 10	0
12 (M3)	42.0 ± 4.9	29.0 ± 3.3	31.0	78 ± 5	67 ± 7	14.1
13 (M3)	32.1 ± 2.9	0	100	nd	/	/
14 (M4)	24.8 ± 1.7	9.2 ± 0.5	62.9	9559 ± 593	7616 ± 490	20.3
15 (M4)	0	0	/	605 ± 103	584 ± 51	3.5
16 (M4)	29.6 ± 2.3	0.5 ± 0.2	98.3	198 ± 10	119 ± 23	39.9
17 (M4)	34.8 ± 1.8	20.0 ± 1.3	42.5	2666 ± 69	1865 ± 74	30.0
18 (M4)	13.0 ± 0.5	12.4 ± 1.6	0	1252 ± 156	1342 ± 172	0
19 (M4)	19.0 ± 1.2	0	100	nd	/	/
20 (M4)	50.4 ± 3.6	17.8 ± 1.2	64.7	nd	/	/
21 (M5b)	18.6 ± 1.1	17.3 ± 0.6	7.0	715 ± 32	635 ± 15	11.2
22 (M5)	113.7 ± 4.3	111.8 ± 0.8	1.7	6839 ± 207	3646 ± 97	46.7
23 (M5)	nd	/	/	272 ± 12	256 ± 20	5.9

[a]Results are expressed as the number of CFU-AML per 2×10^4/BM cells (mean $\pm$ SEM of 6 microwells).
[b]Results are expressed as cpm of ^{3}H-TdR incorporation/5×10^4 BM cells (mean $\pm$ SEM of triplicate cultures).
nd – not done; (/) – % inhibition could not be estimated since CFU-AML were not detected in control cultures.

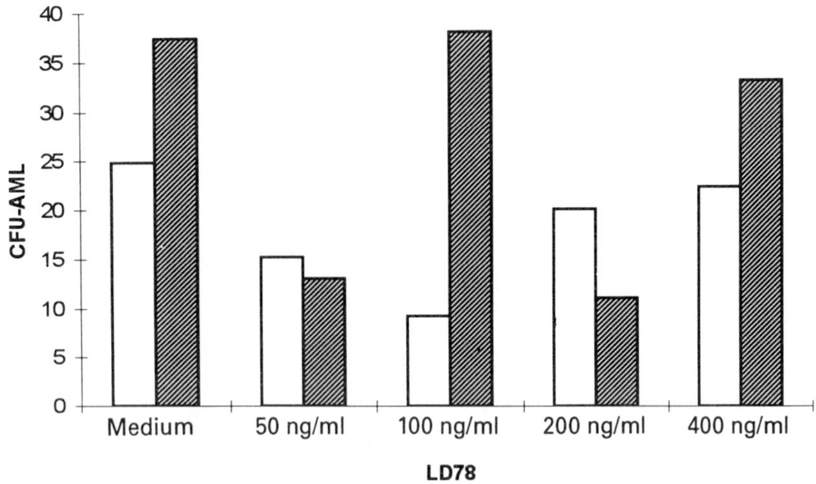

Fig. 40.1 Typical dose-dependent effect of LD78 on bone marrow CFU-AML colony formation in two AML patients (no. 14, white bars and no. 5, shaded bars). Results are expressed as mean colony number per 2×10^4/cells, obtained from each sample in the presence of increasing concentrations of LD78.

The overall frequency of bone marrow CFU-AML varied from 9 to 114 colonies per 2×10^4 cells plated. However, the concentration of LD78 inducing maximal inhibition of bone marrow CFU-AML growth varied. The maximal inhibition was most often obtained with 100 ng/ml and 200 ng/ml, but in the bone marrow of patient no. 17 the inhibition was significant even at the smallest concentration of LD78 (25 ng/ml) (data not shown) used. The average maximal percent of inhibition of BM CFU-AML was 62.7 ± 9.1 ($x \pm$ SEM, for this and following results) when compared to the control cultures. The typical dose response inhibition of CFU-AML growth with LD78 peaked at 100 or 200 ng/ml, with less inhibitory effect at higher doses in most of the samples studied (Fig. 40.1).

To further clarify the role of LD78 in AML cell growth, bone marrow, AML cells from 16 patients were cultured in a liquid proliferation assay system with or without increasing concentrations of LD78. Bone marrow AML cell spontaneous ^{3}H-thymidine uptake varied from 78 to 9559 cpm and was significantly inhibited in 9/16 samples (over 10% in comparison to medium control) when LD78 was added (Table 40.2). The average maximal percent of inhibition of BM AML cell proliferation was 16.3 ± 4.0 when compared to medium control. Dose-dependent inhibition with LD78 was bell shaped, peaked at 100–200 ng/ml with less inhibitory effect at higher doses (Fig. 40.2). In summary, the inhibitory effect of LD78 was significantly ($p < 0.001$) more pronounced on BM AML progenitors (62.7 ± 9.1) when compared to more mature leukaemic cells (16.3 ± 4.0).

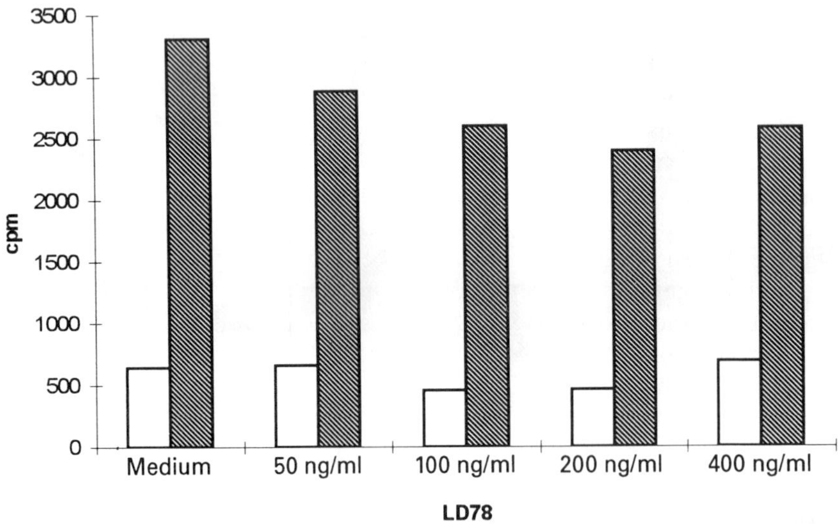

Fig. 40.2 Typical dose-dependent effect of LD78 on bone marrow leukaemia cell proliferation in two AML patients (no. 2, white bars and no. 3, shaded bars). Results are expressed as mean ^{3}H-TdR incorporation obtained from each sample in the presence of increasing concentrations of LD78.

DISCUSSION

The results presented demonstrate the inhibitory effect of LD78 on AML cell growth of bone-marrow-derived progenitors, probably mediated by an effect on AML cell proliferation. This suggests that the normal inhibitory control mechanisms mediated by LD78 are still intact in AML progenitor cells. The observed inhibitory effect of LD78 in CFU-AML growth was not related to the type of AML as evaluated by FAB criteria for classification of AML. Furthermore, in the same FAB group of patients the inhibitory effect was not present in all cases tested.

An inhibitory effect of rhMIP-1α on AML progenitors was recently also described (9) using other culture techniques. The difference of the degree of inhibition in the results obtained by Ferrajoli *et al.* (9) who found less pronounced inhibition of AML progenitors in the presence of MIP-1α and our study could be ascribed to the different molecules used for the study (rhMIP-1α vs LD78), higher concentrations of MIP-1α in their study (up to 1600 μg/ml) compared to our study (up to 400 ng/ml) and the different culture techniques.

Proliferation of haemopoietic progenitors is influenced by a balance of stimulatory and inhibitory effects of defined haemopoietic growth factors and cytokines (8). The overall effects of these molecules on the growth of haemopoietic progenitors are the consequence of combined effects on cell growth. MIP-1α was recently described as a proliferation inhibitor (6) which is shown to act at the level of CFU-S and CFU-A of the murine stem cell compartment in vitro and in vivo (8,15,16). In addition MIP-1α is able to protect the multipotent progenitor CFU-S population from the effect of S-phase specific agents like hydroxyurea (8) and cytosine arabinoside. Broxmeyer *et al.* (7,17) demonstrated the activity of MIP-1α on normal human progenitors in vitro indicating that MIP-1α is inactive on more mature lineage restricted progenitor cells. Furthermore, MIP-1α seems to be a bidirectional regulator of haemopoietic progenitor growth whose effect is dependent on other growth factors present in the culture and the maturation stage of progenitors (18). This may in part explain the heterogeneity of the effect of LD78 on CFU-AML growth observed here and the difference in degree of inhibition on spontaneous AML cell proliferation and CFU-AML growth originating from the same patient. The mechanism of the effect of LD78 on normal progenitor cells as well as on leukaemic cells is not clear. It has been shown recently (19) that the effect of MIP-1α is direct on singly plated CD34$^+$ cells from human bone marrow and that it is not mediated via contaminating accessory cells. The effect of MIP-1α on the proliferation of T-lymphocytes seems to be mediated in part by the inhibition of IL-2 production (20). Thus, elucidation of the precise mechanism of action of MIP-1α will require further studies.

The inhibitory effect of LD78 observed in our study on AML leukaemic progenitors and cell proliferation is unlike the effects seen with chronic myeloid leukaemic progenitors. Eaves *et al.* (21) have recently shown that the response of normal primitive haemopoietic cells and primitive chronic myeloid leukaemic cells is different. The cycling of normal bone marrow haemopoietic cells may be inhibited by the action of MIP-1α, while primitive chronic myeloid leukaemic cells show unresponsiveness to MIP-1α.

The question of the mechanisms of the overgrowth of AML cells to normal marrow cells in vivo is not yet solved. One explanation is that AML cells have become unresponsive to inhibitors of normal haematopoiesis thus gaining a growth advantage. The effect of inhibitory factors in leukaemic cells has been investigated only to a limited degree (9,21,22). This study has shown that LD78 is more active on AML progenitors than on AML cell proliferation, suggesting that the limited activities of LD78 on more mature leukaemic cells are present in AML, contrary to their effects in CML.

CONCLUSIONS

In the present study, we have shown that LD78 is more active on AML progenitors than on AML cell proliferation. Inhibition of the AML cells although less than that of the progenitors, indicates that more limited activity of LD78 on more mature leukaemic cells is present in AML.

ACKNOWLEDGEMENT

We acknowledge Žana Janković for excellent technical assistance. This work is partly supported by the Scientific Fund of Serbia.

REFERENCES

1. Miller, K. B. 1995. Clinical manifestations of acute myeloid leukaemia. In: *Hematology, basic principles and practice* (R. Hoffman, E. J. Benz Jr., S. J. Shattil, B. Furie, H. J. Cohen and L. E. Silberstein, eds.), Churchill Livingstone, Edinburgh, 993–1014.
2. McCulloch, E. A. 1986. Regulatory mechanism affecting the blast stem cells of acute myeloblastic leukemia. *J. Cell. Physiol.* **4** (suppl):27–33.
3. Löwenberg, B. and I. Touw. 1993. Hematopoietic growth factors and their receptors in acute leukemia. *Blood* **81**:281–92.
4. Tessier, N. and T. Hoang. 1988. Transforming growth factor beta inhibits the proliferation of the blast cells of acute myeloblastic leukemia. *Blood* **72**:159–64.
5. Nara, N., S. Tohda, K. Nagata and Y. Yamashita. 1989. Inhibition of the in vitro growth of blast progenitors from acute myeloblastic leukemia patients by transforming growth factor beta. *Leukemia* **3**:572–7.
6. Graham, G. J., E. G. Wright, R. Hewick *et al.* 1990. Identification and characterization of an inhibitor of haemopoietic stem cell proliferation. *Nature* **6265**:442–4.
7. Broxmeyer, H. E., B. Sherry, L. Lu *et al.* 1990. Enhancing and suppressing effects of recombinant murine macrophage inflammatory proteins on colony formation in vitro by bone marrow myeloid progenitor cells. *Blood* **76**:1110–16.
8. Lord, B. I., T. M. Dexter, J. M. Clements *et al.* 1992. Macrophage-inflammatory protein protects multipotent hematopoietic cells from the cytotoxic effects of hydroxyurea in vivo. *Blood* **79**:2605–9.
9. Ferrajoli, A., M. Talpaz, T. F. Zipf *et al.* 1994. Inhibition of acute myelogenous leukemia progenitor proliferation by macrophage inflammatory protein 1-alpha. *Leukemia* **8**:798–805.
10. Obary, K., M. Fukida, S. Maeda and K. Shimada. 1986. A cDNA clone used to study mRNA inducible in human tonsillar lymphocytes by a tumour promoter. *J. Biochem.* **99**:885–94.
11. Benett, J. M., D. Catovsky, M. T. H. Daniel. 1985. Proposed revised criteria for the classification of the acute leukemias. French–American–British (FAB) Cooperative group. *Ann. Int. Med.* **103**:620–5.
12. Lord, B. I. 1995. MIP-1α: biological and clinical perspectives. *FORUM* **5**:125–41.
13. Marie, J. P., R. Zittoun, D. Thevenin *et al.* 1983. In vitro culture of clonogenic leukemic cells in acute myeloid leukemia; growth pattern and drug sensitivity. *Br. J. Haematol.* **55**:427–32.
14. Stošić-Grujičić, S., N. Basara, P. Milenković and C. A. Dinarello. 1995. Modulation of acute myeloblastic leukemia (AML) cell proliferation and blast colony formation by antisense oligomer for IL-1 beta converting enzyme (ICE) and IL-1 receptor antagonist (IL-1ra). *J. Chemotherapy* **7**:67–70.
15. Quesniaux, V. F. J., G. J. Graham, I. Pragnell *et al.* 1993. Use of 5-fluorouracil

to analyse the effect of macrophage inflammatory protein-1α on long-term reconstituting stem cells in vivo. *Blood* **81**:1497–504.

16. Cooper, S., C. Mantel and H. E. Broxmeyer. 1994. Myelosuppressive effects in vivo with very low dosages of monomeric recombinant murine macrophage inflammatory protein-1α. *Exp. Hematol.* **22**:186–93.
17. Broxmeyer, H. E., B. Sherry, S. Cooper, L. Lu *et al.* 1993. Comparative analysis of the human macrophage inflammatory protein family of cytokines (chemokines) on proliferation of human myeloid progenitor cells. *J. Immunol.* **150**:3448–58.
18. Keller, J. R., S. H. Barteimez, E. Sitnicka *et al.* 1994. Distinct and overlapping direct effects of macrophage inflammatory protein-1α and transforming growth factor β on hematopoietic progenitor/stem cell growth. *Blood* **84**:2175–81.
19. Lu, L., M. Xiao, S. Grisby, W. X. Wang *et al.* 1993. Comparative effects of suppressive cytokines on isolated single CD34^{+++} stem/progenitor cells from human bone marrow and umbilical cord blood plated with and without serum. *Exp. Hematol.* **21**:1442–6.
20. Zhou, Z., Y. J. Kim, K. Pollok *et al.* 1993. Macrophage inflammatory protein-1α rapidly modulates its receptors and inhibits the anti-CD3 mAb mediated proliferation of T-lymphocytes. *J. Immunol.* **151**:4333–41.
21. Eaves, C. J., J. D. Cashman, S. D. Wolpe and A. C. Eaves. 1993. Unresponsiveness of primitive chronic myeloid leukemia cells to macrophage inflammatory protein 1α, an inhibitor of primitive normal hematopoietic cells. *Proc. Natl. Acad. Sci. USA* **90**:120 15–19.
22. Holyoake, T. L., M. G. Freshney, A. M. Sproul *et al.* 1993. Contrasting effects of rhMIP-1α and TGF-β_1 on chronic myeloid leukemia in vitro. *Stem Cells* **11** (suppl. 3):122–8.

41

Interference at the Respiratory Burst Level Between the Signals Delivered *in vitro* in Human Peripheral Neutrophils via fMLP, Complement and Fc Receptors

Marinela Bostan, Alexandra Livescu, Monica Neagu, Gina Manda, Maria Chirilã, Elena Mazîlu, Alexandru Constantin Bancu and Laurentiu Mircea Popescu

The polymorphonuclear granulocytes (PMNs) represent one of the first non-specific lines of defence against pathogens. Gradients of chemotactic factors such as *N*-formylated peptides (1) and chemokines (2) recruit the circulating PMNs from the blood vessels into the surrounding tissue (3). At the inflammatory site, PMNs non-specifically destroy the pathogens by oxygen-dependent and -independent mechanisms. Phagocytosis and degranulation, triggered by Fcγ and complement receptors, are generally accompanied by a sustained oxidative activity that generates reactive oxygen species (ROS) such as superoxide anion, hydrogen peroxide, singlet oxygen and hydroxyl radical (4). Cellular enzymatic systems such as NADPH-oxidase (5), myeloperoxidase (MPO) (6,7) and superoxide dismutase are mainly involved in ROS generation. ROS are partly released in the extracellular space by degranulation and exert an oxidative stress both on pathogens and bystander cells. Certain specific regulatory mechanisms protect the normal cells against the damaging effects of ROS (6).

The aim of the present report is to establish the influence of the

Immunoregulation in Health and Disease
ISBN 0–12–459460–3

chemotactic signals on the phagocytosis-associated respiratory burst of PMNs. The functional interference of the signals simultaneously delivered in vitro by the chemotactic synthetic peptide fMet-Leu-Phe (fMLP) and zymosan particles not opsonized (Z), or opsonized with heat-inactivated normal serum (ZO), was investigated. Our results indicate the existence of a functional interference between chemotactic peptides receptors and the complement or Fc receptors at the level of the PMN respiratory burst.

MATERIALS AND METHODS

Reagents

Luminol (Sigma) dissolved in a minimal amount of DMSO was diluted with Hank's balanced salt solution supplemented with 0.1% glucose and 20 mM HEPES (HBSS). Cytochrome c (Sigma) was dissolved in HBSS. Sepcel was produced in our laboratory.

Stimuli and modulatory agents

Zymosan particles were obtained in our laboratory according to the method described by Lachman (8). Zymosan particles were opsonized with heat-inactivated human normal serum. Cytochalasin B and f-Met-Leu-Phe (Sigma) were dissolved in a minimal amount of DMSO and diluted before use in HBSS. The final DMSO concentration did not exceed 0.1%.

Cells

Fresh blood was collected by venepuncture from healthy volunteers (Haemathology Centre, Bucharest). Polymorphonuclear granulocytes were isolated by density gradient centrifugation on Sepcel (9) and red blood cells lysed with 0.83% ammonium chloride 0.084% sodium hydrogen carbonate (10). Isolated PMNs were resuspended in HBSS. Cellular viability, estimated by eosin exclusion test, exceeded 96%.

Cytochrome c reduction test

The test was performed according to the method of Olinescu (11). Briefly, test samples containing 0.98 mg/ml cytochrome c, 1×10^6 cells/ml, in the presence or absence of various combinations of stimulatory/modulatory agents, adjusted to 1 ml with HBSS, were incubated 30 min at 37°C. The control sample contained 0.98 mg cytochrome c/ml. the reaction was stopped on ice and supernatants were collected. the optical densities of the test samples supernatants were measured by differential spectrophotometry at 535 nm and 550 nm using as reference the control sample. The superoxide anion release was estimated as difference of optical densities [(OD550−OD535) × 1000].

Luminol amplified chemiluminescence

Evaluation of MPO-mediated ROS production was performed according to the method described by Allen (4). Test samples containing 1 μM luminol, 1×10^6 cells/ml, in the presence or absence of various stimulatory/modulatory agent combinations, adjusted to 500 μl with HBSS, were incubated for 30 min at 37°C. The control sample contained 1 μM luminol. The chemiluminescence was continuously measured using an LKB-Wallac Chemiluminometer. Chemiluminescence data, expressed as electric pulses/time (mV/min), were analysed as maximum intensity of chemiluminescence [CI_{max}].

Statistics

Experimental results were expressed as mean value ± standard deviation (SD) for five experiments performed with cells isolated from different human normal subjects.

RESULTS AND DISCUSSION

The effect of (10^{-8}, 10^{-7}, 10^{-6})M fMLP on the respiratory burst developed by PMNs stimulated with 2 mg/ml non-opsonized (Z) or opsonized (ZO) zymosan particles was investigated in comparison with the cellular response of PMNs independently activated with the same stimuli. The cellular responses were measured in the presence and absence of 4 μg/ml cytochalasin B (CB), an agent that favours exocytosis by hindering actin polymerization (12).

Both the ranges of fMLP concentrations known to induce selectively chemotaxy and respiratory burst (13) were studied. Zymosan particles, *Saccharomyces cerevisiae* wall structures recognized by CR3, trigger cellular adhesion, endocytosis and respiratory burst of phagocytes (14), apparently activating only the NADPH-oxidase, without further inducing MPO-mediated generation of ROS (15). Zymosan opsonized with heat-inactivated normal serum (ZO) interacts with neutrophils mainly via Fc receptors and induces phagocytosis, degranulation and oxidative response, activating the MPO system. As fMLP induces superoxide generation but fails to trigger associated exocytosis, we also investigated the oxidative response of PMNs in the presence of cytochalasin B (CB). This experimental model mimics some conditions characteristic for the cells heading towards the inflammatory site. During this movement PMNs are simultaneously activated by cytotoxicity-inducing stimuli and by ascending chemotactic factor concentrations.

The effect of fMLP on the respiratory burst of PMN in vitro stimulated with Z

Superoxide anion release

The experimental results (Fig. 41.1a) indicate that the signals delivered by fMLP and Z are not just additive, suggesting the existence of a functional interference dependent on the relative concentrations of the stimuli. Thus, PMNs costimulated with Z and $(10^{-7}, 10^{-6})$M fMLP develop cellular responses similar to those induced by fMLP alone. PMNs costimulated with Z and 10^{-6}M fMLP release superoxide anion, similarly to those independently activated by Z. In the presence of 4 μg/ml CB, the release of superoxide anion by PMNs, independently or concomitantly stimulated with Z and fMLP, is amplified (Fig. 44.1b). The signals delivered to PMNs by the stimuli are not additive. Thus, the cellular response induced by fMLP is dominant at high doses (10^{-6}M) of chemoattractant, whereas those triggered by Z govern the oxidative activity in the presence of lower concentrations of $(10^{-8}, 10^{-7})$M fMLP.

MPO-mediated ROS generation

The experimental data (Fig. 41.2a) indicate that, unlike fMLP, Z does not deliver activating signals to the MPO system and abolishes the stimulatory effects exerted by fMLP in the case of costimulated cells. Cytoskeleton disturbances induced by 4 μg/ml CB affect neither the response induced by Z nor the functional cooperation between the stimuli (Fig. 41.2b).

The effect of fMLP on the respiratory burst of PMNs in vitro stimulated with ZO

Superoxide anion release

The results presented in Fig. 41.3a indicate that, the signals delivered at the level of superoxide anion release by fMLP and ZO are not just additional, suggesting the existence of a functional interference. Thus, fMLP amplifies the superoxide anion release induced by ZO for all the chemotactic peptide concentrations investigated.

In the presence of 4 μg/ml CB superoxide anion release is significantly potentiated when the stimuli were either independently or concomitantly applied (Fig. 41.3b), indicating that actin polymerization hinders the radical exocytosis. At high non-chemotactic doses of fMLP (10^{-6}M), the signals

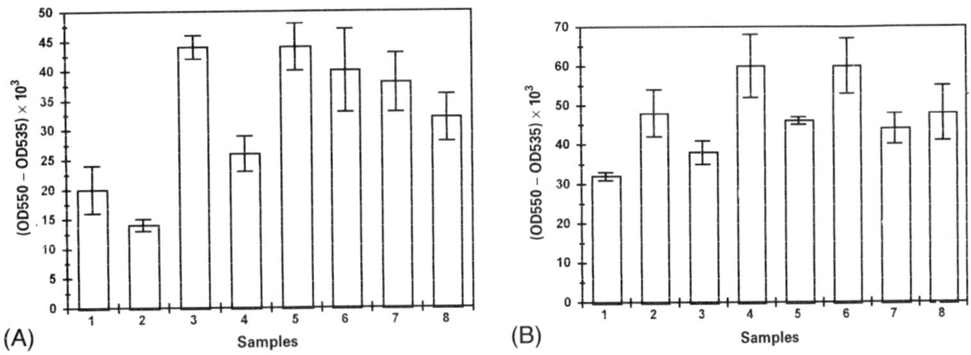

Fig. 41.1 The superoxide anion release by PMNs in vitro costimulated with fMLP and 2 mg/ml Z, in the absence (A) and presence (B) of 4 μg/ml cytochalasin B. 1, non-stimulated cells; 2, Z; 3, 0.01 μM fMLP; 4, Z + 0.01 μM fMLP; 5, 0.1 μM fMLP; 6, Z + 0.1 μM fMLP; 7, 1 μM fMLP; 8, Z + 1 μM fMLP.

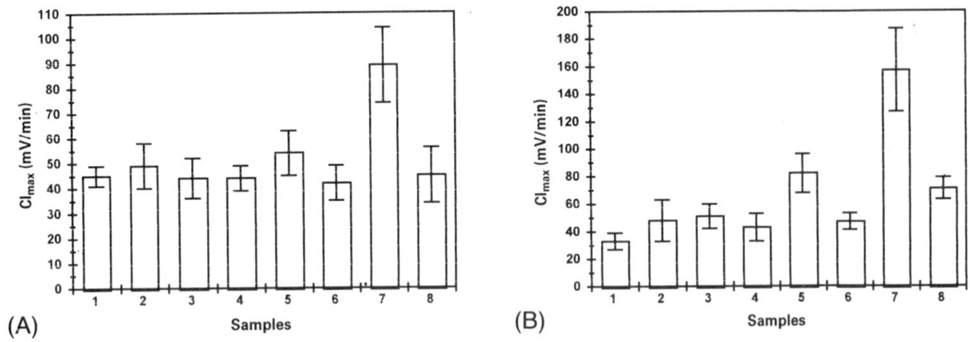

Fig. 41.2 The MPO-mediated ROS generation by PMNs in vitro costimulated with fMLP and 2 mg/ml Z, in the absence (A) and presence (B) of 4 μg/ml cytochalasin B. 1, non-stimulated cells; 2, Z; 3, 0.01 μM fMLP; 4, Z + 0.01 μM fMLP; 5, 0.1 μM fMLP; 6, Z + 0.1 μM fMLP; 7, 1 μM fMLP; 8, Z + 1 μM fMLP.

delivered by FcγR and fMLP-R tend to become additive, suggesting that microfilament relaxation seems to abolish the functional interference of the mentioned receptors. At lower, potentially chemotactic concentrations of fMLP (10^{-8}M, 10^{-7}M), PMNs develop non-additional cellular responses, similar to those induced by ZO when applied independently, indicating that CB exerts no major effect on the receptor functional interference.

MPO-mediated ROS generation

The experimental results (Fig. 41.4a) indicate that, in the absence of CB, ZO abolishes the stimulatory signals delivered by fMLP for all the

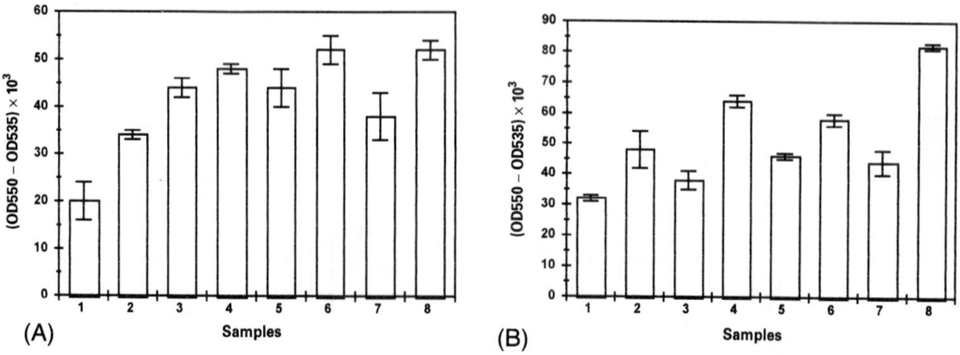

Fig. 41.3 The superoxide anion release by PMNs in vitro costimulated with fMLP and 2 mg/ml ZO, in the absence (A) and presence (B) of 4 μg/ml cytochalasin B. 1, non-stimulated cells; 2, ZO; 3, 0.01 μM fMLP; 4, ZO + 0.01 μM fMLP; 5, 01 μM fMLP; 6, ZO + 0.1 μM fMLP; 7, 1 μM fMLP; 8, ZO + 1 μM fMLP.

investigated chemoattractant concentrations, suggesting the existence of a negative interference between the receptors.

According to the data presented in Fig. 41.4b, the cellular responses induced by FcγR and fMLP-R in the presence of 4 μg/ml CB are additive for all the chemoattractant concentrations investigated. These results suggest that actin filament relaxation favours the MPO-mediated ROS generation and, hence, that the functional interference of the receptors seems to be dependent on microfilament integrity.

CONCLUSION

Our experimental results suggest that neutrophils simultaneously challenged via fMLP receptors and CR3 develop only a weak respiratory burst, especially at high doses of *N*-formylated peptides, apparently a characteristic of the inflammatory site. This mechanism could be effective in protecting the bystander cells against the non-discriminating cytotoxic action of the oxidative stress. A different interference pattern was observed when FcγR and *N*-formylated chemotactic peptide receptors are costimulated. The chemotactic peptide sustains the respiratory burst, mainly its early phase. Our experimental results with cytochalasin B-treated cells indicate that the receptors' functional cooperation is generally independent on actin filament integrity. We noticed an exception: the MPO-mediated ROS generation by PMNs costimulated via FcγR and *N*-formylated chemotactic peptides receptors.

The chemotactic factors exert a modulatory action on the microbicidal oxygen-dependent functions of PMNs. As our results suggest, the respiratory

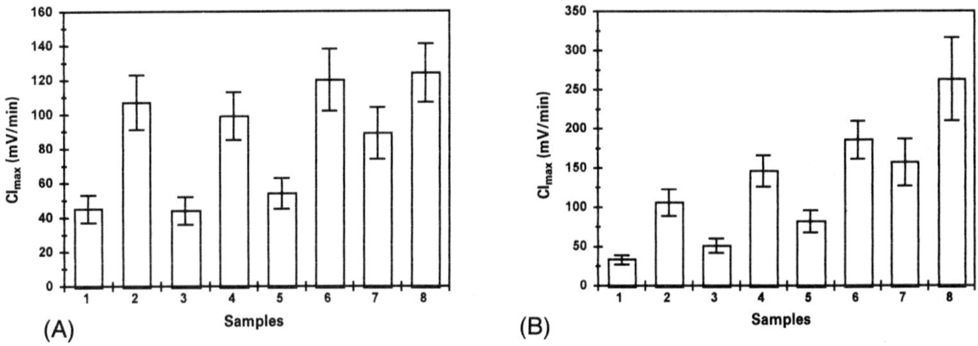

Fig. 41.4 The MPO-mediated ROS generation by PMNs in vitro costimulated with fMLP and 2 mg/ml ZO, in the absence (A) and presence (B) of 4 μg/ml cytochalasin B. 1, non-stimulated cells; 2, ZO; 3, 0.01 μM fMLP; 4, ZO + 0.01 μM fMLP; 5, 0.1 μM fMLP; 6, ZO + 0.1 μM fMLP; 7, 1 μM fMLP; 8, ZO + 1 μM fMLP.

burst elicited in the neutrophil subjected to low (chemotactic) concentration of fMLP is mainly represented by ROS elicited by phagocytosis-inducing stimuli, while inside the inflammatory site, a high (non-chemotactic) concentration sustains the oxidative response elicited by IgG opsonized particles.

REFERENCES

1. Oppenheim, J. J., C. O. C. Zachariae, M. Mukaida and K. Matsushima. 1991. Properties of the novel proinflamatory supergene 'intecrine' cytokine family. *Annu. Rev. Immunol.* **9**:617–48.
2. McDonald, P. P., M. Pouliot, P. Borgeat and S. R. McCall. 1993. Induction by chemokines of lipid mediator synthesis in granulocyte-macrophage colony stimulating factor-treated human neutrophils. *J. Immunol.* **151**:6109–399.
3. Downey, G. P. 1994. Mechanisms of leukocyte motility and chemotaxis. *Curr. Opin. Immunol.* **6**:113–24.
4. Allen, R. C. 1986. Phagocytic leukocyte oxygenation activities and chemiluminescence: a kinetic approach. *Meth. Enzymol.* **133**:449–509.
5. Bastian, N. R. and J. B.-Jr. Hibbs, 1994. Assembly and regulation of NADPH-oxidase and nitric oxide synthase. *Curr. Opin. Immunol.* **6**:131–9.
6. Basaga, H. S. 1990. Biochemical aspects of free radicals. *Biochem. Cell. Biol.* **68**:989–98.
7. Tobler, A. and H. P. Koeffler. 1991. Myeloperoxidase: localization, structure and function. In: *Blood Cell Biochemistry* (J. R. Harris, ed.) Plenum, New York, pp. 255–88.
8. Lachman, P. J., M. J. Hobart and W. P. Aston, 1973. Complement technology. In: *Handbook of Experimental Immunology* (D. M. Weir, ed.) Blackwell Scientific Publications, Oxford, chapter 5:p. 8.
9. Boyum, A. 1968. Isolation of mononuclear cells and granulocytes from human blood. *Scand. J. Clin. Lab. Invest.* **21**:77–89.

10. Edwards, W. S. 1987. Luminol- and lucigenin-dependent chemiluminescence of neutrophils: role of degranulation. *J. Clin. Lab. Immunol.* **22**:35–9.
11. Olinescu, A., G. Manda, M. Neagu *et al.* 1993. Action of some proteic and carbohydrate components of *Symphytum officinale* upon normal and neoplastic cells. *Rom. Arch. Microbiol. Immunol.* **52**:73–80.
12. Hoffstein, S. C. and H. M. Korchak. 1983. Early consequences of neutrophil activation and their association with degranulation. In: *Phagocytosis – Past and Future* (M. L. Karnovsky and L. Bolis, eds.) Academic Press, London, p. 47.
13. Walker, B. A. M., B. E. Hagenlocker, E. B. Stubbs Jr. *et al.* 1991. Signal transducing events and FcgR engagement in human neutrophils stimulated with immune complexes. *J. Immunol.* **146**:735–41.
14. Fallmann, M., R. Andersson and T. Andersson, 1993. Signaling properties of CR3 (CD11b/CD18) and CR1 (CD35) in relation to phagocytosis of complement-opsonized particles. *J. Immunol.* **151**:330–8.
15. Manda, G., M. Neagu, A. Livescu *et al.* 1996. Functional interference of CR3 and *N*-formylated peptide receptors in the respiratory burst of human normal polymorphonuclear granulocytes stimulated with zymosan and fMet-Leu-Phe. *Rev. Roum. Biochim.* **33** (in press).

42

HLA DQA1/DQB1 Heterogeneity in DRB1*11/12 Haplotypes in a Greek Population

Katerina Tarassi, Chryssa Papasteriades, Helen Pappas, Kjersti S. Rønningen and William Ollier

The major histocompatibility complex (MHC) is the most polymorphic genetic system in humans and as such is a valuable tool for population studies (1). HLA-DR, -DQ and -DP antigens are transmembrane glycoprotein heterodimers (α,β chain) (2) encoded by genes (DRA, DRB, DQA, DQB, DPA, DPB) located in the MHC class II region (3). Recently molecular techniques have revealed high polymorphism, particularly in the HLA-DRB1, -DQA1 and -DQB1 genes. Allele frequency and haplotype combinations of these genes have been found to differ between various ethnic groups studied (4).

Although HLA antigen and haplotype frequencies in Greeks show much similarity to those reported for other European caucasoids (5), certain differences have been found to characterize this population (6,7). HLA-DR5, and in particular DR11, is one of the most frequent -DR antigens, serologically defined, in the Greek population (5,8).

The aim of the present work was to further determine the subtypes of HLA-DR5 by molecular techniques and to define DRB1/DQA1/DQB1 haplotypes in DR5-positive subjects.

MATERIAL AND METHODS

We studied 87 randomly selected healthy, unrelated individuals of Greek origin, 53 males and 34 females.

HLA class II typing was performed

- by classical serological technique (two-step microlymphocytotoxicity) using well-characterized sera (9) and B lymphocytes separated by immunomagnetic beads (10)

Immunoregulation in Health and Disease
ISBN 0-12-459460-3

- by PCR-SSO molecular technique (11) using 32 probes for DRB1, 10 probes for DQA1 and 15 probes for DQB1 alleles.

RESULTS AND DISCUSSION

HLA-DR5 defined by molecular techniques presented with a gene frequency of 28.7% in our population. DRB1*11 prevailed (26.9%), whereas DRB1*12 was much less common (1.8%). These results were in full agreement with those obtained by serology. Comparing these findings with those presented in the data book of the 11th International Histocompatibility Workshop and Conference (12), it appears that Greeks are characterized by a high frequency of HLA-DR5. As found in this set of Greek controls, a higher frequency of -DR11 than of -DR12 was found in all caucasoids and negroids studied, while -DR12 was more frequent in most orientals.

Among the four DRB1*11 subtypes we could identify, DRB1*1104 was the most frequent (15.6%), followed by DRB1*1101 (8.4%), DRB1*1102 (2.3%) and DRB1*1103 (0.6%). Two subtypes of DR12 were found in our population, DRB1*1201 (1.2%) and DRB1*1202 (0.6%) (Table 42.1).

With regard to the DRB1*11 subtypes, it is of interest that while DRB1*1101 is the most common allele in almost all populations (caucasoids, negroids and orientals) studied, DRB1*1104 is the most frequent one among Spaniards (4%), Indians (4.6%) and Greeks (15.6%). DRB1*1102, with a frequency of 2.3% in our population, is almost absent among other caucasoids and orientals but characterizes negroid populations, especially Senegalese (6.6%). DRB1*1103 was found with the lowest frequency among Greeks and is also very rare in other populations. Concerning DRB1*12, DRB1*1201 is the most common allele in caucasoids and negroids and in the majority of oriental populations DRB1*1202 appears with the highest frequency.

Several haplotype combinations between DRB1*11/12 and DQA1/DQB1 were observed, DRB1*11/DQA1*0501/DQB1*0301 being the most frequent one (22.6%). In addition to this association, usually seen in all other

Table 42.1 Frequency (%) of DRB1*11/12 subtypes

DRB1*	Phenotype frequency (%)	Gene frequency (%)
1101	16.1	8.4
1102	4.6	2.3
1103	1.1	0.6
1104	28.7	15.6
1201	2.9	1.2
1202	1.1	0.6

Table 42.2 DQA1/DQB1 heterogeneity in DRB1*11/12 haplotypes

Haplotype			HF%
DRB1*11-	DQA1*0501	- DQB1*0301	22.6
DRB1*1101-	DQA1*0501	- DQB1*0301	5.8
DRB1*1102-	DQA1*0501	- DQB1*0301	2.3
DRB1*1104-	DQA1*0501	- DQB1*0301	12.8
DRB1*12-	DQA1*0501	- DQB1*0301	1.2
DRB1*11-	DQA1*0101	- DQB1*0501	0.005
DRB1*11-	DQA1*0101	- DQB1*0502	0.005
DRB1*1101-	DQA1*0501	- DQB1*0201	0.005
DRB1*1104-	DQA1*0501	- DQB1*0201	0.005
DRB1*1103-	DQA1*0101	- DQB1*0503	0.005

populations studied (12), certain unexpected allele combinations were also noticed (Table 42.2). So, it is obvious that a reasonable heterogeneity in DRB1*11 haplotypes was seen in our population.

In conclusion, it seems that the Greek population differs from other European populations, with respect to HLA-DR11, DRB1*11 subtype frequency and the unusual DRB1*11/DQ associations found. These data can be used for anthropological studies, in order to estimate population relationships. They may also be of importance in the practical applications of histocompatibility, as in the study of disease associations and bone marrow transplantation.

REFERENCES

1. Mattiuz, P. L., D. Inde, A. Piazza *et al.* 1970. New approaches to the population genetic and segregation analysis of the HLA system. In: *Histocompatibility Testing 1970* (P. I. Terasaki, ed.) Munksgaard, Copenhagen, pp. 193–205.
2. Strominger, J. L. 1987. Structure of class I and class II HLA antigens. *Br. Med. Bull.* **43**:81–93.
3. Bodmer, W. F., E. D. Albert, J. G. Bodmer *et al.* 1988. Nomenclature for factors of the HLA system, 1987. *Immunobiology* **177**:465–76.
5. Pachoula-Papasteriadis, C., W. Ollier, S. Cutbush *et al.* 1989. HLA antigen and haplotype frequencies in Greeks. *Tissue Antigens* **33**:488–90.
6. Awad, J., W. Ollier, S. Cutbush *et al.* 1990. Heterogeneity of HLA-DR4 in Greeks including a unique DR4-DQW2 association. *Tissue Antigens* **35**:40–1.
7. Cuccia, M., P. Astolfi, E. Gyodi *et al.* 1992. HLA in five populations of southern Europe. In: *HLA 1991. Proceedings of the Eleventh International Histocompatibility Workshop and Conference* (K. Tsuji, M. Aizawa, T. Sasazuki (eds.) Oxford University Press, Oxford, Vol. 1, pp. 655–6.
8. Tarassi, K., N. Bikas, A. Tsirogianni *et al.* 1994. HLA antigens and auto-antibodies in women with gestational diabetes melitus. *Abstract Book of 9th International Congress of Immunology, San Francisco*, p. 114.

9. Terasaki, P. I. and J. D. McClelland. 1964. Microdroplet assay of human serum cytotoxins. *Nature* **204**:998–1000.
10. Ebrinchmann, J., F. Vartdal, G. Gaudernack *et al*. 1988. Direct immunomagnetic quantification of lymphocyte subsets in blood. *Clin. Exp. Immunol.* **71**:182–6.
11. Wordworth, B. P., C. E. M. Alsopp, P. Young and J. I. Bell. 1990. HLA-DR typing using DNA amplifications by the polymerase chain reaction and sequential hybridization to sequence-specific oligonucleotide probes. *Immunogenetics* **32**:413–18.
12. The Data Book. 1991. *11th International Histocompatibility Workshop and Conference, Yokohama, Japan*, p. 1166.

43

Experimental Trauma and the Complement System

Bojana Rodić, Čedomir Radojičić and Vojislav D. Miletić

It is well known that the complement system is an important immediate host defence mechanism in trauma and that it undergoes significant changes in the post-traumatic period (1,2). Complement activation is usually beneficial to the host, but if such activation is profound and persistent, a depletion of essential complement components and its functional activities can be observed. Burn injury, for example, activates and depletes the complement system; the resultant hypocomplementemia can influence the processes of opsonization, chemotaxis and bacteriolysis. Also, active complement cleavage products, which are generated during the activation process, may contribute to vascular injury, shock lung, and phagocytic cell dysfunction, and can induce immunosuppression and protein catabolism (1,3).

Investigations performed so far mostly refer to the influence of thermal injury on the haemolytic complement activity (1,2). There is scant information on other models of experimental trauma (such as radiation, chemical, mechanical) and no information at all on complement capability to control formation and elimination of precipitating immunocomplexes after trauma, a function of outstanding biological importance. Solubilization of preformed immunoprecipitates, complex-release activity (CRA) (4), and complement mediated inhibition of immune precipitation (CMI) (5), are the expression of this function. The central event in both reactions is the incorporation of C3b fragments into immunocomplexes (IC). In case of CRA, the C3b fragments (generated preferentially during the alternative pathway of complement activation) affect the Fc–Fc interactions in the immunoprecipitates, causing their degradation. In case of CMI, the C3b fragments (generated preferentially during the classical pathway of complement activation) hinder the Fc–Fc interactions in the early phase of antigen-antibody reaction, disabling immunoprecipitation. CRA and CMI are not only expressed in case of certain antigen–antibody reactions, but represent general biological phenomena. Both processes will result in

Immunoregulation in Health and Disease
ISBN 0–12–459460–3

generation of IC with incorporated C3b fragments, which react with CR1 (specific receptor for C3b) on erythrocytes, become transported to the liver, hereby being eliminated from the circulation.

Only few data exist concerning radiation trauma. After radiation trauma (single doses, 4 Gy), certain alterations of haemolytic complement activity in the classical activation pathway and appearance of circulating immunocomplexes and specific autoantibodies can be observed (6). Bearing in mind the substantial differences between the classical and alternative pathway, based on immune mechanisms which activate the classical pathway, and non-immune mechanisms which activate the alternative pathway, we compared changes caused by radiation and thermal trauma within the complement system of experimental animals. Our previous results demonstrated deficiency in complement alternative pathway caused by experimental burns (7). As an indicator of the functionality of the complement system, the activity of the complement alternative pathway (CAHU) and complement mediated inhibition of immune precipitation (CMI) were measured. The results were compared within types and doses of trauma and time of sampling (1 h, 3 h, 24 h, 7 d, 14 d, 30 d after trauma).

MATERIALS AND METHODS

BALB/c strain mice (males, 20–24 weeks of age) were used for this investigation. In case of radiation trauma, the animals were irradiated by X-rays on a linear accelerator with doses of 1, 3, and 5 Gy. Blood samples were taken from the retro-orbital plexus before trauma (0 time), 1 h, 3 h, 24 h, 7 d, 14 d and 30 d after trauma (10 animals each). Sera were stored at −80°C until analysis.

In case of thermal injury, BALB/c male mice (20–24 weeks of age) were submitted to Arturson's thermal injury (8) for 3 s (sublethal trauma). Blood samples were taken before trauma (0 time), 1 h, 3 h, 24 h, 7 d, 14 d, and 30 d after trauma (10 animals each). Sera were stored at −80°C until analysis.

Complement haemolytical activity by alternative pathway of activation (CAHU) was determined using the laser-nephelometry method, in which non-sensitized rabbit erythrocytes, suspended in GVB–Mg^{++}-EGTA buffer, were used (9). CAHU was expressed in haemolytic units (HU/ml). Due to low haemolytic activity in the majority of the samples, the results were scored in the following way: CAHU activity $<$ 0.06 HU/ml = 1; 0.06–0.10 = 2; 0.11–0.15 = 3; 0.16–0.20 = 4; 0.21–0.25 = 5 and $>$ 0.26 = 6.

To perform complement mediated inhibition of immune precipitation (CMI), isolated bovine serum albumin (BSA) and rabbit anti-bovine albumin (anti-BSA) were used (10). Immune precipitates were formed at equivalence. Registration of precipitation kinetics was performed for 20 min by measuring laser light scattering, using a Behring laser nephelometer (helium–neon,

4 mV, 632 nm), with automatic recorder (PYE Unicam AR 55). The percentage of precipitation was calculated planimetrically.

Student's *t* test was applied for statistical analysis of the results obtained.

RESULTS AND DISCUSSION

In this work, the effects of experimental radiation and thermal trauma on the complement system of experimental animals were studied.

The influence of thermal and radiation trauma on murine complement alternative pathway activity is presented in Table 43.1.

Experimental thermal injury has shown specific influence on alternative pathway activity. Immediately after trauma (up to 3 h) the alternative pathway expresses a sudden, statistically significant increase of activity, followed by a significant, but transitory, activity decrease (after 24 h). This is in agreement with our previously published results (7). Another report, suggesting preferential activation through the alternative pathway after burn injury, published by Gelfand *et al.* (11), has shown that

- massive activation of the complement system occurred in the initial 2 h after injury
- the alternative pathway was the primary pathway of activation
- the terminal complement components were not depleted to the same degree.

Similar results were obtained in case of radiation trauma. After experimental radiation trauma (doses: 5 Gy), a sudden statistically significant ($p < 0.001$) increase of CAHU activity was noted during the first 3 h. Twenty-four hours after irradiation, a significant decrease of activity, compared to

Table 43.1 Influence of radiation exposure and thermal injury on CAHU

Time of sampling	Radiation exposure			Thermal injury
	1 Gy	3 Gy	5 Gy	
0 time	1.30 ± 0.48	1.30 ± 0.48	1.30 ± 0.48	1.30 ± 0.48
1 h	1.20 ± 0.42	2.80 ± 1.03	2.91 ± 0.71	3.26 ± 1.23
3 h	1.27 ± 0.42	3.86 ± 0.70	5.43 ± 1.42	5.93 ± 0.48
24 h	1.40 ± 0.52	2.30 ± 0.48	3.00 ± 0.60	3.85 ± 1.03
7 d	1.54 ± 0.53	2.87 ± 1.45	2.91 ± 0.88	3.92 ± 0.78
14 d	1.30 ± 0.76	1.92 ± 0.72	2.60 ± 1.90	2.91 ± 1.01
30 d	1.41 ± 0.81	1.63 ± 0.91	1.95 ± 0.97	2.04 ± 0.81

the previous value ($p < 0.01$), was observed, but this value still exceeded the initial one. In the following (7 d, 14 d, 30 d), a decrease of activity (without approaching initial values), was observed. The 3 Gy dose causes similar, although less pronounced, effects. The 1 Gy dose does not lead to significant changes in the CAHU activity.

No reliable data are available on the mechanism of these changes and their biological significance. Most complement proteins are acute-phase proteins, whose plasma concentration increases following tissue injury and inflammation (12). Their distinguished feature is that synthesis of most of them is regulated by IL-1-type cytokines, IL-6-type cytokines and mostly by IFNγ (which is not generally considered as a major inducer of acute-phase proteins), not only in the liver but also in extrahepatic sites, where they are produced by macrophages, fibroblasts and epithelial and endothelial cells. As their concentration is increased due to enhanced synthesis, it is reasonable to expect their functionality to be increased, but functionality decrease which occurs after 24 h and fast recovery is a phenomenon based on unrevealed biological mechanisms. A possible explanation for changes in complement alternative pathway activity can be the presence of inhibitors which are generated after trauma. Although 'anti-complement' activity was not shown in our previous work (7), the possibility of existence of inhibitors, not detectable by known anti-complementary assays, cannot be excluded.

Although in case of complement haemolytic activity the complement system acts as an acute phase reactant, a completely different pattern is observed for complement-mediated inhibition of immune precipitation (Table 43.2).

Investigations on CMI have shown that changes occur in the first hour after trauma (first CMI-value decrease), and this trend is continued until the day 30 in case of radiation trauma, while in case of thermal trauma, a trend towards recovery is observed after 14 days. If we compare the time of CMI deficiency appearance, it is worth noting that CMI deficiency precedes AP

Table 43.2 Influence of radiation exposure and thermal injury on CMI

Time of sampling	Radiation exposure			Thermal injury
	1 Gy	3 Gy	5 Gy	
0 time	88.41 ± 3.36	88.41 ± 3.36	88.41 ± 3.36	88.41 ± 3.36
1 h	89.70 ± 4.20	74.72 ± 5.45	71.75 ± 6.98	80.21 ± 4.20
3 h	84.21 ± 6.36	70.63 ± 5.88	63.74 ± 5.34	70.24 ± 5.83
24 h	85.31 ± 2.82	57.49 ± 5.83	36.81 ± 3.58	48.39 ± 4.42
7 d	83.65 ± 6.88	59.32 ± 3.47	33.72 ± 4.28	52.58 ± 5.31
14 d	80.65 ± 5.37	54.28 ± 4.30	30.65 ± 6.63	63.72 ± 5.28
30 d	72.03 ± 8.33	47.58 ± 6.61	21.14 ± 4.24	65.32 ± 5.37

deficiency and that it may serve as a significant parameter of changes within the complement system. In this work, for the first time, a new deficiency in the complement functionality after experimental trauma is presented. The host's inability to correctly handle and control the behaviour of immunocomplexes formed in traumatized animals might be critical for the early recovery period after trauma. These changes in complement functionality, especially in the case of radiation trauma, may be related to complications developed as late manifestations of radiation exposure. Our present knowledge on the mechanisms of complement-dependent processes of IC elimination is insufficient for complete elucidation of the observed phenomena. Further investigations using genetical and artificial manipulation of complement activity in experimental animals should lead to more complete explanation.

CONCLUSIONS

In this work, the effects of experimental thermal and radiation trauma on the complement system of experimental animals were studied. As an indicator of the functionality of the complement system, CAHU and CMI were measured. It was shown that both types of trauma activate complement to a major degree. In case of CAHU, the lowest activity was detected 24 h after trauma, being preceded by significant rise, suggesting typical acute phase reaction. Statistically significant decrease of CMI occurs after 24 h continuing after 14 and 30 days in case of radiation trauma; slight recovery of CMI was observed after 14 days in case of thermal trauma. It is worth noticing that CMI values are more sensitive indicators of changes within the complement system after experimental trauma than CAHU values. Our findings suggest that experimental trauma probably releases inhibitory substances for complement activity in the regulation of the immunoprecipitation process. Further investigations, using genetical and artificial manipulation of complement activity in experimental animals, should confirm this assumption.

REFERENCES

1. Yamada, Y. and J. A. Gelfand. 1986. Role of complement following thermal injury. In: *Advances in Host Defense Mechanisms*, Vol. 6 (Gallin and Fauci, eds.) Raven Press, New York.
2. Gallinaro, R., W. G. Cheadle, K. Applegate and H. C. Polk 1992. The role of the complement system in trauma and infection. *Surg. Gynecol. Obstet.* **174**:435–40.
3. Gelfand, J. A. 1984. How do complement components and fragments affect cellular immunological function? *J. Trauma* **24**(9), S118–24.

4. Czop, J. and V. Nussenzweig. 1976. Studies on the mechanism of solubilization of immune aggregates by complement. *Exp. J. Med.* **143**:615–22.
5. Shifferly, J. A., P. Woo and D. K. Peters. 1982. Complement-mediated inhibition of immune precipitation. *Clin. Exp. Immunol.* **47**:555–62.
6. Balsalobre, A. 1991. Circulating immunocomplexes, autoantibodies and complement after ionizing radiation exposure. *Rev. Esp. Fisiol.* **47**(3):147–50.
7. Miletić, V., G. Lukić, Č. Radojičić *et al.* 1983. Activity of murine complement alternative pathway after thermal injury. *Period. Biol.* **85**:163–4.
8. Arturson, G. 1964. The infliction and healing of large standard burns. *Acta Pathol. Microbiol. Scand.* **61**:353–7.
9. Miletić, V. D., Č. Radojičić and A. Dujić. 1982. A laser nephelometric method for measuring alternative pathway complement activity of human and murine serum. *Immunol. Lett.* **5**:49–53.
10. Miletić, D. and B. Rodić. 1984. Study of complement effects on kinetics of immune precipitation. *Complement* **1**:194–200.
11. Gelfand, J. A., M. B. Donelan and A. Hawiger. 1982. Alternative pathway activation increases mortality in a model of burn injury in mice. *J. Clin Invest.* **70**:1170–6.
12. Colten, H. R. 1993. The acute phase complement proteins. In: *Acute Phase Proteins* (A. Mackiewicz, I. Kushner, H. Baumann, eds.) CRC, Boca Raton, FL, pp. 207–21.

44

Investigation of Some Factors That May Modulate the Activity of NK Cells

Gordana Konjević and Ivan Spužić

Natural killer (NK) cells, as a part of native immunity, participate in the first line of defence against malignant processes (1,2). Data indicate a deterioration in their cytotoxic potential depending on the extent of the disease and the fact that numerous factors in their environment may modulate their activity (3,4). In this study NK cytotoxic activity was investigated primarily in terms of its modulation by external factors, cytokines and their receptors.

MATERIALS AND METHODS

Investigations were performed on 50 healthy controls and on 71 patients in different clinical stages of breast cancer.

In vitro 18 h cultures of PBL were performed in culture medium RPMI 1640 (CM) (Gibco, England) supplemented with 10% v/v FCS (Gibco, England), healthy control sera (HS), sera of patients with breast cancer in clinical stages I–III (CaSa), sera of patients with breast cancer in clinical stage IV (CaSm), these pooled sera (CaSp) and dialyzed sera depleted of molecules below 10 000 Da (CaSd). Treatments of PBL were also done with rh IL-2 (Amersham, England) 100 U/ml of CM. CaSp was treated with anti-TNFα mAb (Endogen, USA) 20, 40 μl/ml, concentration 0.1 mg protein/ml, for 2 h at 37°C. Mouse anti-human mAb for TNFα receptor I (p60) and Rc II (p80), 0.1 mg protein/ml (Genzyme, USA) were used for neutralization in concentration of 20 μl/ml of PBL suspension 2×10^6/ml.

Evaluation of NK cell activity was performed by the standard ^{51}Cr release cytotoxicity assay (5). 100 μl of PBL, as effector cells (E) at concentration of 4.0×10^6/ml of culture medium and two 1 : 1 dilutions (2.0×10^6/ml and

Immunoregulation in Health and Disease
ISBN 0-12-459460-3

1.0×10^6/ml) were mixed with 100 μl of the tumour cell line K 562, as target cells (T), at concentration of 0.05×10^6/ml, prelabelled with radioactive ^{51}Cr (Na_2CrO_4, As = 3.7 MBq, Amersham, England), resulting in three effector-to-target (E : T) cell ratios of 80 : 1, 40 : 1 and 20 : 1. Each E : T ratio was done in triplicate.

The assay was done in 96-hole round-bottom microwell plates (Flow, USA) which were incubated for 4 h at 37°C in a humidified atmosphere containing 5% carbon dioxide. After that the plates were centrifuged for 5 min at 200 *g* and 100 μl of supernatants from each well was used on a gamma counter (Berthold, Germany) for determination of the amount of released ^{51}Cr from lysed K 562 tumour cells in counts per minute (cpm). The NK cell cytotoxic activity was calculated using the following formula:

$$\frac{cpm\ in\ experimental\ release - cpm\ in\ spontaneous\ release}{cpm\ in\ maximal\ release - cpm\ in\ spontaneous\ release} \times 100$$

Maximal release was obtained by incubation of target K 562 tumour cells in the presence of 5% Tryton, and spontaneous release was obtained by incubation of tumour cells in culture medium alone.

Data analysis was done by a Wilcoxon test of equivalent pairs.

RESULTS AND DISCUSSION

An evaluation of NK cell activity has shown that it is, compared to healthy control subjects, significantly reduced in breast cancer patients, especially in advanced clinical stages of disease (6,7). It was therefore interesting to see whether this phenomenon is due to the cells themselves, or whether it is caused by the factors which are present in their environment. In this sense, the sera of patients with different clinical stages of breast cancer were used for the investigation of their effect on NK cell activity of patients and controls, and it was shown (Fig. 44.1) that the sera of patients in early clinical stages (CaSa) had an enhancing effect on NK cell activity compared to control normal sera ($p < 0.01$). This could be due to the presence of protective stimulative factors in the sera of patients with localized malignancy reported also by Adrianov *et al.* (8). However, sera of patients in advanced stages (CaSm) had an inhibitory effect ($p < 0.05$) on NK cytotoxic activity of both controls and patients (Fig. 44.1). These phenomena were found by other investigators (9), who state that they are cancer-related, as they disappear after surgical removal of the tumours (10). Considering the consequences of the inhibitory effect of these sera, we proceeded to further analyse this effect.

Dialysis of CaSp by which molecules of low molecular mass were removed (CaSd) gave even greater and time-dependent inhibition of NK cell activity

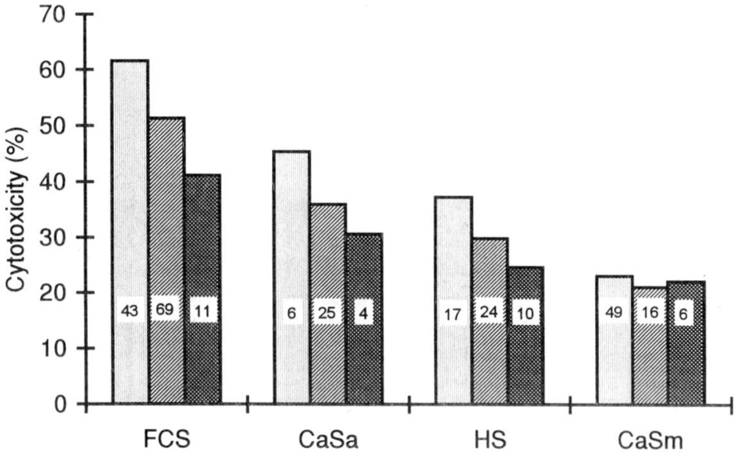

Fig. 44.1 The effect of different sera on NK cell cytotoxicity of breast cancer patients and controls. PBL of healthy controls (light bars) and two groups of breast cancer patients in different clinical stages, in concentration 2.0×10^6/ml, were pretreated for 18 h in CM RPMI 1640 supplemented with 10% v/v inactivated FCS, CaSa, HS and CaSm. The cells were then collected and used for the evaluation of NK cell cytotoxicity. Results are expressed as mean values at E:T ratio 80:1 and the numbers in columns indicate the number of people investigated. Diagonal shading, clinical stage I–III; cross-hatching, clinical stage IV.

of controls (Fig. 44.2). This indicates that the effect was not due to prostaglandins or other molecules of low molecular mass, but rather to the remaining molecules of higher molecular mass, i.e. TNFα (11), which are now more concentrated. In support of this are the findings by Guidi *et al.* (12), who showed that the inhibitory effect of sera of breast cancer patients with metastasis was in the fraction of 25–125 kDa.

Considering that CaSp exhibited such an inhibitory effect on NK cell activity, further study was designed to show whether these sera interfere with the activity of IL-2. In this sense, simultaneous treatment with CaSp, CaSd and IL-2 showed interference with IL-2 stimulation, but this was of a reversible nature, as washing out of the applied sera after 4 h and then the addition of IL-2 led to almost optimal stimulation (Fig. 44.3). A possible cause of this may be due to factors that bind the present IL-2 or IL-2 receptors on NK cells (13). However, evaluation of these sera for their content of soluble IL-2 Rs showed that they were increased only in a few cases (14).

In order to see whether the effect of CaSm is dependent on TNFα, as this cytokine is often increased in the sera of patients with malignancies (15), the sera were treated with mAb for this cytokine. However, only insignificant

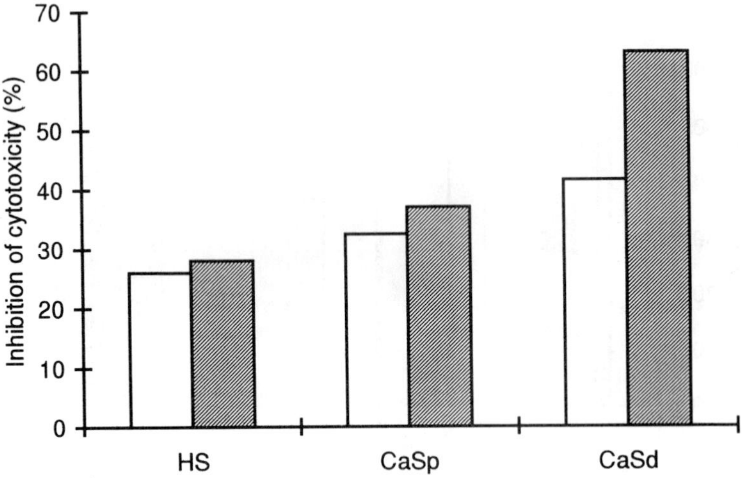

Fig. 44.2 Time-dependence of inhibitory effect of different sera on NK cell activity. Healthy control PBL (total number of 8.0×10^6) were pretreated with 10% HS, CaSp and CaSd for 4 h (white bars) and 18 h (dark bars) after which the cells were collected, washed and adjusted to concentration of 4.0×10^6/ml for determination of NK cytotoxicity. Results are expressed as percentage inhibition of NK cell activity compared to control sera at E : T ratio 80 : 1.

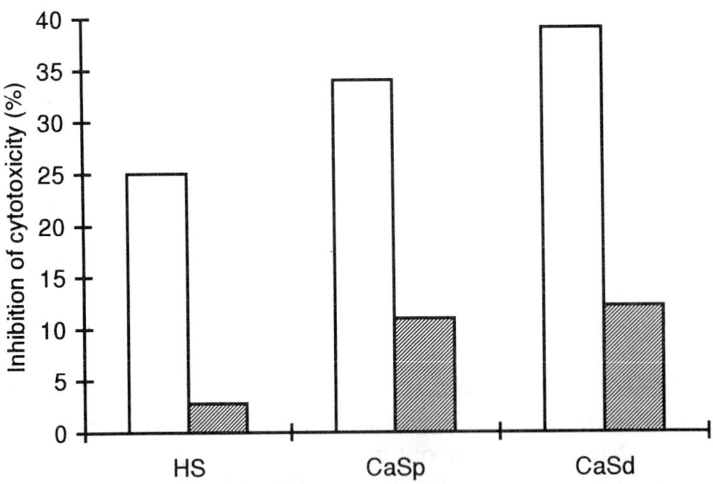

Fig. 44.3 The effect of the presence of different sera on IL-2 stimulation of NK cell activity. The total number of 8.0×10^6 PBL of healthy controls was treated simultaneously for 18 h in CM with 10% v/v of different sera and rh IL-2, 100 U/ml (light bars), and also, first, for 4 h with each serum after which the cells were washed and further treated up to 18 h with the given concentration of IL-2 alone (dark bars). Results are expressed as percentage inhibition of NK cell activity compared to control sera at E : T ratio 80 : 1.

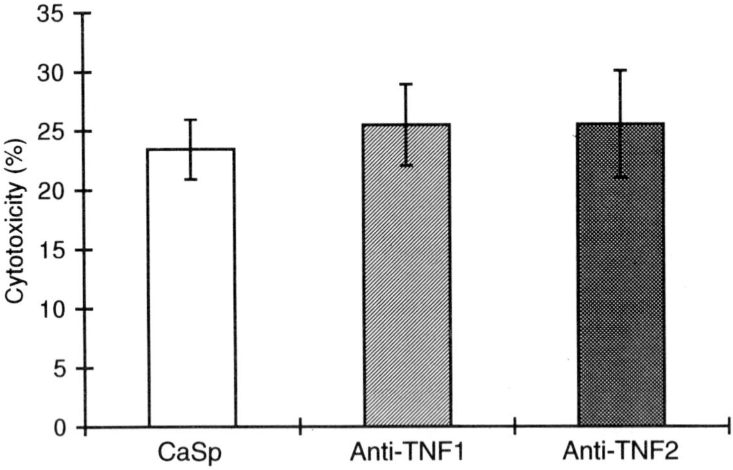

Fig. 44.4 The effect of anti-TNFα mAb on breast cancer patients' sera-induced inhibition of NK cell cytotoxicity. CaSp was pretreated for 2 h at 37°C with anti-TNFα mAb in concentration 20 μl/ml (anti TNF1) and 40 μl/ml (anti TNF2) and subsequently used as 10% v/v supplementation of CM for an 18 h treatment of PBL. Results of the effect of untreated (CaSp) and treated (TNF1, TNF2) sera on NK cytotoxicity are expressed at E : T ratio 80 : 1 as $\bar{x} \pm$ SE.

Table 44.1 The effect of blocking TNF Rs I and II during IL-2 induced stimulation of NK cell cytotoxicity

	IL-2	IL-2 + mAb TNF Rc I	IL-2 + mAb TNF Rc II	IL-2 + mAb TNF Rc I,II
NK cell cytotoxicity (%)	47.09	39.75 (84.41%)[a]	35.63 (75.66%)	29.19 (61.99%)

[a]Percent of NK cytotoxicity obtained by treatment with IL-2 alone (100 U/ml).

change in the effect on NK cell activity was obtained by neutralizing TNFα (Fig. 44.4), suggesting that TNFα did not participate in the inhibitory effect of investigated sera.

IL-2 stimulation induces TNFα production by NK cells (16), T helper cells and, indirectly, by macrophages, as well as the expression of TNFα receptors on NK cells, which, otherwise, in resting state do not express the two types of TNF receptors (17). Blocking of TNFα Rc I and II, separately or together, by mAbs during IL-2 treatment gave a decrease of NK activity compared to the effect of IL-2 alone (Table 44.1), confirming the findings of Zambello *et al.* (18) of a potentiating role of TNFα in NK cell activation by IL-2.

CONCLUSION

Considering that numerous factors may influence the natural activity of NK cells, both of healthy controls and of people with malignancies, the effect of some of these factors was investigated. It has been shown that IL-2, TNFα and the sera of patients with localized breast cancer potentiate their cytotoxicity to a different degree, while sera of patients in advanced clinical stages of breast cancer, after dialysis and blocking mAbs for TNF Rcs, decrease NK cell cytotoxicity.

REFERENCES

1. Herberman, R. B. and J. R. Ortaldo. 1981. Natural killer cells and their role in defences against disease. *Science* **214**:24–31.
2. Barlozzari, T., J. Leonhardt, R. H. Wiltrout *et al.* 1985. Direct evidence for the role of LGL in the inhibition of experimental tumor metastases. *J. Immunol.* **134**:2783–9.
3. Robertson, M. J. and J. Ritz. 1990. Biology and clinical relevance of human natural killer cells. *Blood* **76**:2421–38.
4. Brenner, B. G., S. Benarrosh and R. G. Margolese. 1986. Peripheral blood NK cell activity in human breast cancer patients and its modulation by T-cell growth factor and autologous plasma. *Cancer* **58**:895–902.
5. Ortaldo, J., R. Winker, C. Morgen *et al.* 1987. Analysis of rat NKCF produced by rat NK cell lines and the production of a murine monoclonal antibody. *J. Immunol.* **139**:3159–62.
6. White, D., D. B. Jones, T. Cooke and N. Kirkham. 1982. Natural killer (NK) activity in peripheral blood lymphocytes of patients with benign and malignant breast disease. *Br. J. Cancer* **46**:617–20.
7. Konjević, G. and I. Spužić. 1993. Stage dependence of NK cell activity and its modulation by interleukin-2 in patients with breast cancer. *Neoplasma* **40**:81–5.
8. Adrianov, I. G. and T. N. Katashova. 1989. The effect of autoplasma of patients with breast cancer on the functional activity of natural killer cells and adhering mononuclear cells in peripheral blood in vitro. *Exp. Oncol.* **11**: 64–6.
9. Kumazawa, H., M. Minamino, N. Yukawa and M. Hess. 1995. Suppression of natural killer cell activity by serum derived from head and neck cancer patients. *Cancer Detection and Prevention* **19**: 494–502.
10. Pislarisu, M., A. Opriou, D. Taranu *et al.* 1988. Modulation of natural killer cell activity by serum from cancer patients: Preliminary results of a study of patients with colorectal adenocarcinoma or other types of cancer. *Cancer Res.* **48**: 2596–603.
11. Mannel, D. N., A. Kist, A. D. Ho *et al.* 1989. Tumor necrosis factor production and natural killer cell activity in peripheral blood during treatment with recombinant tumor necrosis factor. *B. J. Cancer* **60**: 585–8.
12. Guidi, L., S. Specter, C. Bartolini *et al.* 1990. Inhibitory activity on IL-2 production and response of serum from cancer patients. EOS-J. *Immunol. Immunopharmacol.* **X**: 22–7.
13. Yokose, N., K. Ogata, T. Ito *et al.* 1994. Elevated plasma soluble interleukin 2 receptor level correlates with defective natural killer and $CD8^+$ T-cell in myelodysplastic syndromes. *Leukemia Res.* **18**: 777–82.

14. Konjević, G. and I. Spužić. 1995. Suppressive interaction of breast cancer patients' sera on interleukin-2 induced stimulation of natural killer cells. *J. Exp. Clin. Cancer Res.* **14**: 31–7.
15. Teppo, A. M. and C. P. Maury. 1987. Radioimmunoassay of tumor necrosis factor in serum. *Clin. Chem.* **33**: 2024–7.
16. Aramburu, J., M. A. Balboa, A. Rodriguez *et al.* 1993. Stimulation of IL-2-activated natural killer cells through the Kp43 surface antigen up-regulates TNFα production involving the LFA-1 integrin. *J. Immunol.* **151**: 3420–9.
17. Tartaglia, L. A., R. F. Weber, I. S. Figari *et al.* 1991. The two different receptors for tumor necrosis factor mediate distinct cellular responses. *Proc. Natl. Acad. Sci. USA* **88**: 9292–6.
18. Zambello, R., L. Trentin, P. Bulian *et al.* 1992. Role of tumor necrosis factor-alpha and its specific 55-kD and 75-kD receptors in patients with lymphoproliferative disease of granular lymphocytes. *Blood* **80**: 2030–7.

Index